POSTANESTHETIC CARE

POSTANESTHETIC CARE

Elizabeth A. M. Frost, MD
Professor
Department of Anesthesiology
Albert Einstein College of Medicine
Montefiore Medical Center
Bronx, New York

Paul L. Goldiner, MD, DDS
Professor and Chairman
Department of Anesthesiology
Albert Einstein College of Medicine
Montefiore Medical Center
Bronx, New York

With a Foreword by
Christopher Bryan-Brown, MD
Professor
Department of Anesthesiology
Albert Einstein College of Medicine
Vice Chairman for Clinical Affairs
Department of Anesthesiology
Montefiore Medical Center
Bronx, New York

APPLETON & LANGE
Norwalk, Connecticut/San Mateo, California

Notice: Our knowledge in clinical sciences is constantly changing. As new information becomes available, changes in treatment and in the use of drugs become necessary. The author and the publisher of this volume have taken care to make certain that the doses of drugs and schedules of treatment are correct and compatible with the standards generally accepted at the time of publication. The reader is advised to consult carefully the instruction and information material included in the package insert of each drug or therapeutic agent before administration. This advice is especially important when using new or infrequently used drugs.

Copyright © 1990 by Appleton & Lange
A Publishing Division of Prentice Hall

90 91 92 93 94 / 10 9 8 7 6 5 4 3 2 1

Prentice Hall International (UK) Limited, *London*
Prentice Hall of Australia Pty. Limited, *Sydney*
Prentice Hall Canada, Inc., *Toronto*
Prentice Hall Hispanoamericana, S.A., *Mexico*
Prentice Hall of India Private Limited, *New Delhi*
Prentice Hall of Japan, Inc., *Tokyo*
Simon & Schuster Asia Pte. Ltd., *Singapore*
Editora Prentice Hall do Brasil Ltda., *Rio de Janeiro*
Prentice Hall, *Englewood Cliffs, New Jersey*

Library of Congress Cataloging-in-Publication Data

Postanesthetic care / [edited by] Elizabeth A. M. Frost, Paul L.
  Goldiner.
      p.   cm.
    ISBN 0-8385-7895-0
    1. Postoperative care. 2. Surgical intensive care. I. Frost,
  Elizabeth A. M. II. Goldiner, Paul L.
  RD51.P655 1990
  617'.919—dc20   90-107
                                                      CIP

Acquisitions Editor: R. Craig Percy
Production Editor: Jeff vonLiebermann
Designer: Janice Barsevich

PRINTED IN THE UNITED STATES OF AMERICA

Contributors

David Amar, MD
Assistant Professor
Department of Anesthesiology
Albert Einstein College of Medicine
Montefiore Medical Center
Bronx, New York

Jeffrey Askanazi, MD
Associate Professor
Division of Critical Care Medicine
Department of Anesthesiology
Albert Einstein College of Medicine
Director, Nutrition Support Service
Division of Critical Care Medicine
Montefiore Medical Center
Bronx, New York

Steven A. Blau, MD
Associate Professor
Department of Surgery
Albert Einstein College of Medicine
Director, Burn Center
Jacobi Hospital
Bronx Municipal Hospital Center
Bronx, New York

Svetlana Bonner, MD
Fellow in Neuroanesthesia
Department of Anesthesiology
Albert Einstein College of Medicine
Montefiore Medical Center
Bronx, New York

Mathelyn Claudio, RN, BSN
Clinical Associate
Division of Pain Management
Department of Anesthesiology
Montefiore Medical Center
Bronx, New York

Thomas J. DeKornfeld, MD
Professor Emeritus
Department of Anesthesiology
University of Michigan Medical School
Ann Arbor, Michigan

Nashaat Eissa, MD
Fellow in Critical Care Medicine
Albert Einstein College of Medicine
Bronx, New York

Joanne L. Floyd, MD
Assistant Professor
Division of Critical Care Medicine
Departments of Anesthesiology and
    Internal Medicine
Albert Einstein College of Medicine
Bronx, New York

Elizabeth A. M. Frost, MD
Professor
Department of Anesthesiology
Albert Einstein College of Medicine
Montefiore Medical Center
Bronx, New York

Paul L. Goldiner, MD, DDS
Professor and Chairman
Department of Anesthesiology
Albert Einstein College of Medicine
Montefiore Medical Center
Bronx, New York

Sheldon Goldofsky, MD
Assistant Professor
Department of Anesthesiology
Albert Einstein College of Medicine
Bronx, New York

Gary Hartstein, MD
Instructor
Department of Anesthesiology
Albert Einstein College of Medicine
Bronx, New York

Ingrid B. Hollinger, MD
Associate Professor of Anesthesiology
Assistant Professor of Pediatrics
Albert Einstein College of Medicine
Clinical Director
Department of Anesthesiology
Montefiore Medical Center
Bronx, New York

Griselda A. Jones, MD
Fellow
Department of Anesthesiology
Albert Einstein College of Medicine
Montefiore Medical Center
Bronx, New York

Ronald Kaplan, MD
Associate Professor
Department of Anesthesiology
Albert Einstein College of Medicine
Director, Division of Pain Management
Department of Anesthesiology
Montefiore Medical Center
Bronx, New York

Olli Kirvelä, MD, PhD
Visiting Research Fellow
Division of Critical Care Medicine
Department of Anesthesiology
Albert Einstein College of Medicine
Bronx, New York
Senior Staff Attending
Department of Anesthesiology
Turku University Central Hospital
Turku, Finland

Claudia Komer, MD
Instructor
Department of Anesthesiology
Albert Einstein College of Medicine
Montefiore Medical Center
Bronx, New York

Vladimir Kvetan, MD
Associate Professor
Division of Critical Care Medicine
Department of Anesthesiology
Albert Einstein College of Medicine
Director
Division of Critical Care Medicine
Departments of Anesthesiology and Medicine
Montefiore Medical Center
Bronx, New York

Soomyung Lee, MD
Assistant Professor
Department of Anesthesiology
Albert Einstein College of Medicine
Montefiore Medical Center
Bronx, New York

Rhoda D. Levine, MD
Associate Professor of Anesthesiology
Albert Einstein College of Medicine
Bronx, New York

Ross A. Malley, MD
Staff Anesthesiologist
Department of Anesthesia
Naval Hospital
Portsmouth, Virginia

Gertie F. Marx, MD
Professor
Department of Anesthesiology
Albert Einstein School of Medicine
Bronx, New York

Hideo Nagashima, MD
Professor
Director, Anesthesiology Research
Department of Anesthesiology
Albert Einstein College of Medicine
Montefiore Medical Center
Bronx, New York

Gene Pesola, MD
Research Fellow
Memorial Sloan-Kettering Cancer Center
New York, New York

Werner K. Pfisterer, MD, MS, EdDoct
Assistant Professor
Director, Medical Education
Department of Anesthesiology
Albert Einstein College of Medicine
Bronx, New York

Steven S. Schwalbe, MD
Assistant Professor
Department of Anesthesiology
Albert Einstein College of Medicine
Director, Obstetric Anesthesia
Jacobi Hospital
Bronx Municipal Hospital Center
Bronx, New York

Michael D. Umanoff, MD
Assistant Professor
Department of Anesthesiology
Seton Hall University School of Graduate
  Medical Education
South Orange, New Jersey
Attending Anesthesiologist
Department of Anesthesiology
St. Joseph's Hospital and Medical Center
Paterson, New Jersey

Patricia S. Underwood, MD
Associate Professor
Department of Anesthesiology
Albert Einstein College of Medicine
Vice-Chairman, Academic Affairs
Department of Anesthesiology
Montefiore Medical Center
Bronx, New York

Contents

Foreword

Within a few years of the first public demonstration of the use of ether to perform surgical procedures (October 16, 1846), it was realized that the consequences of anesthesia could be both dire and manifest *after* the operation. The very origin of the recovery room was a phenomenon of the Victorian era, when at times anesthesia was an ordeal as formidable as the surgery itself. Special areas were set aside near the operating rooms where there was a concentration of personnel versed in the management of the postanesthetic patient. The patient was watched (an effective and well-established form of monitoring!), revived and fortified with brandy, the more painful sensations dulled with morphine, and the patient's vomit cleaned up before transfer to the ward. As both surgery and anesthesia improved, the need for recovery areas became less apparent, and a good idea was temporarily lost.

With the advent of thoracic, intracranial, and cardiac surgery, the need for a recovery area became obvious again, but now for surgical reasons rather than anesthesia-related ones. There were strongholds against this wave of reform. Particularly in the larger cities of the United States, hospital administrators did not wish to provide recovery room management, and tried to maintain that a private duty nurse could provide the necessary care (at the patient's expense!). When insurance companies began to pick up the costs, the recovery room became well established.

Most of the life-support techniques and monitoring we use today were developed so that surgeons could perform more invasive and radical surgery. Mechanical ventilation through a cuffed endotracheal tube made open-chest surgery possible and overcame the pneumothorax problem. As long ago as the 1920s, a device to provide artificial respiration in the postoperative patient with severe atelectasis or pneumonia (a very frequent cause of mortality before the antibiotic era) was very seriously suggested, and even occasionally used. From the knowledge and skills acquired in the care of the patient during surgery, anesthesiologists were able to introduce ventilator therapy not only during the postoperative period, but also to the patient with causes of respiratory failure other than an operation.

The basis of critical care monitoring is intraoperative monitoring. It resulted from a need to find out both how the patient was faring and how he or she was responding to the ever-increasing number of drugs and manipulations available in the operating room. It is not surprising that the continuum of the nonoperative management of patient care should extend into the recovery room (now more correctly called the postanesthetic care unit, or PACU), and often even beyond to the intensive care unit (ICU) and pain service.

A large part of postanesthetic care has become very much critical care, and for the more compromised patient, the two are the same. The everyday issues of the ill surgical patient are the same in the PACU and the ICU. It may not sit well with the health authorities and those who provide the reimbursment, but a PACU in any facility dealing with the sick has to be able to provide critical care. One of the political reasons that there is some difficulty about accepting this within organized nursing is that there are now several special-interest groups—representing critical care, postanesthetic, and neurosurgical practitioners—all taking considerable amounts of responsibility for the patient after surgery. Fortunately *collaborative practice* is the watchword of the day, and all these groups are eager to learn and work with physicians on *supplying the force* (sic Nightingale) needed to restore the critically ill to health. An anesthesiology-generated text on the management of the patient following anesthesia and surgery can provide valuable information that will help strengthen a care plan with well-prioritized medical as well as nursing actions. This is one of the major goals of this book.

There is a venerable adage that *patients do not come into hospital for anesthesia*. It has become a maxim among some members of the legal profession that *an anesthetic death is an avoidable death*. With the staggering awards won by plaintiffs (and their attorneys) over the past two decades, there is increasing public apprehension. This has resulted in both an external introduction of somewhat confusing regulations, mandating certain actions and monitoring apparatus (some of which is unstandardized); and a very rigorous self-imposed set of guidelines for improving patient safety. The result has been a reduction of *near misses*; a reduction of mortality and morbidity from preventable causes; and decreased legal liability. Patient safety concerns have moved into the PACU, because it is realized that anesthesia care is not completed, nor responsibility ended until the patient has at least concluded the postanesthesia phase of his or her management.

Patients are coming to surgery in an unhealthier status than would have been considered compatible with survival only a few years ago. Emergency procedures are being performed successfully on patients with recent myocardial infarcts, severe respiratory failure, and those who have had no food by mouth for months. Exsanguination is being effectively managed, and total by pass of the heart and lungs has become so commonplace that it is hardly given a second thought. During surgery and into the postoperative period drugs are used to control the blood pressure and cardiac output and to treat cardiac arrhythmias. The period of arousal from anesthesia is a treacherous time for the unskilled and inexperienced because the variations in sympathetic tone give rise to tremendous alterations in cardiac function and peripheral vascular resistance. The risk of myocardial infarction is greatly increased at this point by potentially avoidable hypertension and tachycardia. Assessment of the patient's volume status can also be very confusing, because peripheral blood pressures can be normal and ventricular filling pressures high in the face of severe hypovolemia. The organ function deficits, delayed awakening from anesthesia, confusional states, oliguria, cardiac arrhythmias, pulmonary arteriovenous admixture, and so on, need to be sorted out both in terms of pathophysiology and pharmacodynamics. These frequently have to be recognized against a background of preexisting disease, endocrine disorder, sepsis, and the extremes of life. Often the picture can be further confused by physical pain and distress. A systematically planned approach with protocols designed to meet the contingencies used by people who understand them is the patient's best defense.

Postanesthetic care must have plans and procedures for the effective investigation and management of the patient who does not wake up as expected after general anesthesia; is unable to ventilate adequately; appears to have residual curarization, excessive narcotic administration, or inadequate fluid resuscitation or pulmonary function; or is uncontrollably restless.

The exciting field of critical care obstetrics (with its aggressive management of the patient with eclampsia or pregnancy-associated hypertension) has resulted in a gratifying decrease in fetal mortality, infant morbidity, and improved maternal well-being, and it is an area that is now involving anesthetic practice. The obstetric unit is an area where postanesthetic care has increased in need even for the normal patient. One of the results of the expanding use of cesarean section for delivery has been an increase in maternal mortality and morbidity from anesthesia-related incidents. There is an appreciable incidence of aspiration of gastric contents in the postoperative period, when patients may become renarcotized or have residual weakness from muscle relaxant or spinal anesthesia. Understanding the problems and the development of proper recovery facilities can go far to minimize the risk to the patient and from the often very costly medicolegal retribution for neglect.

Much time and effort has been spent in getting patients in a reasonable state out of the operating room. As the skill and expertise of those caring for patients in the OR increases, so too will the management of the patient in the postanesthetic phase become ever more complex and time consuming. The ramifications of postanesthetic care run through the whole field of surgical and anesthesia practice, and may run far beyond the immediate operative period. Success is based on sound preparation and grounding in the material presented in the subsequent chapters. Success is providing the postanesthetic care that will see the patient on the road to recovery following surgery.

Christopher Bryan-Brown
Bronx, New York

Introduction

Involvement of anesthesiologists outside the operating room in direct patient care has expanded greatly in recent times. As more and complicated procedures under many different circumstances are undertaken, the anesthesiologist's knowledge, skill, adaptability, and ability to predict outcome are tested repeatedly.

In the early days of anesthesia, intraoperative morbidity and mortality were frequent occurrences. As a second-year medical student, Harvey Cushing substituted for Dr. Frank Lynam, anesthetist at the Massachusetts General Hospital. Dr. Lynam had warned Cushing that the first case, a woman with a strangulated hernia, might not survive. From his own experience and that of others, Lynam taught that such patients usually died shortly after induction. True to expectations, Cushing's patient survived only a few minutes after Cushing began to administer ether. In this textbook *Chloroform and other Anesthetics*, written in 1848, John Snow devotes 150 pages to describing the complications associated with chloroform inhalation.

Modern technology and increased safety of anesthetic agents have reduced the risks of adverse outcomes such that an "anesthetic death" is fortunately a rarity. The emphasis now is on further improving operative outcome and has shifted to the postanesthetic care period. After hours of intense monitoring and minute-by-minute adjustment of physiologic parameters, the patient is returned to an area where surveillance and physician availability may be reduced.

As the importance of postanesthetic care has been increasingly realized, at both national and state levels associations have formed dedicated to defining standards for appropriate care (see Appendix A). Anesthesiologists have frequently held key positions in preparing these standards. Appropriately, the anesthesiologist has, in most instances, been recognized as the physician ultimately responsible for postanesthetic care units (PACUs).

We hope this text will provide a ready, comprehensive reference for all aspects of postanesthetic care. The management of more routine cases is considered as well as that of patients often transferred directly to other intensive care areas (cardiac and neurosurgical patients) or patients treated in separate hospital areas (obstetric suites). We here tried to include a general broad base of information while emphasizing the involvement by other specialists such as internists, risk management groups, respiratory therapists, and, of course, the nursing staff.

The book is intended primarily for anesthesiologists, surgeons, and internists. We realize that nationally there are great differences in patient requirements, staffing, and physical structures of postanesthetic care areas. Contributions to this text are based on the experiences of physicians working in both academic and private practice settings and in large university and small community hospitals. We trust that given this wide area, readers will find some common ground that can be applied in their setting.

We express our gratitude to our contributors for their diligence in preparing their manuscripts; and to the secretarial staff of the Albert Einstein College of Medicine/Montefiore Medical Center, especially Ms. Leida Colon and Ms. Belinda Fortsch, for their patience.

Elizabeth A. M. Frost
Paul L. Goldiner
Bronx, New York

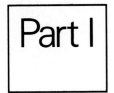

Part I General Considerations

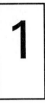

1 | Admission and Discharge Criteria

Svetlana Bonner

One late October morning in 1846, a messenger brought a short letter from Dr William Morton to the house of Dr Horace Wells. The message read: ''Dear Sir, I write to inform you that I have discovered a preparation, by inhaling which a person is thrown into sound sleep. The time required to produce sleep is only a few moments, and the time in which persons remain asleep can be regulated at pleasure. While in this state, the severest surgical or dental operations may be performed, the patient not experiencing the slightest pain.''[1] The compound was ether and its administration ushered in the era of surgical anesthesia.

The development of this new field opened up possibilities of surgical procedures thus far unheard of. It took, however, close to one hundred years for the medical community to realize that patients who have undergone the ''severest'' surgical procedures under anesthetics, required intensive monitoring well after the completion of both surgery and anesthesia. In 1863, Florence Nightingale wrote on the use of special areas put aside in country hospitals for the recovery of patients from the immediate effects of surgery.[2] But it is Dandy and Firor who deserve the credit for the first recovery room—the neurosurgical three-bed unit that they opened at Johns Hopkins Hospital in 1923.[3] The annual report of the section on anesthesia of the Mayo Clinic in 1943 mentioned a postanesthesia observation room caring for 2000 patients.[4] After two immediate postoperative deaths, one in a neurosurgical patient during transport, and the other in an inadequately monitored patient after a hysterectomy, an area adjacent to the operating rooms was designated as the recovery room at the Hospital of the University of Pennsylvania in 1946. Today hospitals frequently have not one, but several recovery rooms (eg, a separate obstetrical or ambulatory unit) in addition to specialized intensive care units which frequently provide postanesthesia care for patients recovering from cardiothoracic or neurosurgical procedures. The currently recognized importance of the recovery room was summarized in a supreme court decision in 1969:

The function of this room is to provide highly specialized care, frequent and careful observation of patients who are under the influence of anesthesia. They remain in this room until they have regained consciousness and their bodies return to their normal functions. The nurses in this room are there for the purpose of promptly recognizing any respiratory problem, cardiovascular problem, or hemorrhaging. The patient is more prone to crises after the operation than while in the operating room where the respiration is being controlled. This is the most important room in a hospital and one in which the patient requires the greatest attention because it is fraught with the greatest potential dangers to the patient. As the dangers or risks are ever-present there should be no relaxing of vigilance.[5]

No emphasis is strong enough to bring forth the importance of recovery room observation, for it is the immediate next step after the operating room, where the patient's every heartbeat and every breath, whether it be taken by the patient or given to the patient, has been carefully monitored by the anesthesiologist.

All patients after general or regional anesthesia should be nursed in a specially designated recovery area.[6] Patients who receive local anesthesia with intravenous sedation sufficient to alter their level of consciousness should also recover in the postanesthetic care unit (PACU). Occasionally exceptions can be made to these rules, and patients may be transferred directly from the operating room to the ward if

1. Local anesthesia only was used and the patient's condition is stable.
2. The patient is an infection risk and no isolation area is available.
3. There is an intensive care unit specially designed for particular care.
4. By agreement with the surgeon and anesthesiologist, the patient wishes to make arrangements for special care on the wards.[7]

If the reason for the patient's transfer to the ward is infection or personal wishes, nursing care should be arranged for the first two to four hours of postanesthesia time that is comparable to PACU standards.[8]

The PACU and operating room should be in close proximity. The maximum safe limit of transfer time is five minutes.[8] It is unwise to include a trip in an elevator as part of the transfer, because emergencies cannot be adequately treated and elevator equipment malfunction is always a possibility. Two individuals must accompany the patient during transfer, one of whom must be part of the anesthesia care team. Availability of adequate monitoring, oxygen, and all resuscitative measures is recommended during transport, including continuous ECG and pulse oximetry. Recent reports indicate that clinically significant desaturation frequently occurs during the immediate postanesthesia time period.[9,10] On arrival to the PACU three basic steps are essential:

1. Provision of oxygen.
2. Measurement and recording of vital signs by the nurse and communication of these data to the anesthesiologist (in most hospitals this step also involves establishment of electrocardiographic monitoring).
3. A report given by the anesthesiologist to the PACU nurse including the following:
   - Brief personal history, patient's name, age, sex, comprehension limits (eg, native language), etc.
   - Diagnosis, surgical procedure, surgeon of record.
   - Anesthetic course, anesthetic technique, anesthesiologist of record, complications, anticipated need for pain medications, estimated time of reversal of regional block, agents (if appropriate), intraoperative fluid balance.
   - Pretransfer laboratory data (eg, Hct, K^+).
   - Time when medications were administered that are to be continued postoperatively (eg, antibiotics, steroids).
   - Brief medical history, allergies, chronic conditions, previous illnesses, and maintenance medications.
   - Anticipated problems.
   - Postanesthetic orders (eg, O_2 administration, endotracheal tube care, vital sign "alarms" requiring the presence of an anesthesiologist, such as systolic blood pressures over 160 or under 100, heart rates above 110 or below 60, etc.

On accepting the patient, the PACU nurse can complete a short form (Fig. 1–1) which is frequently incorporated into the recovery room flowchart. The same chart usually includes a table for the Aldrete score,[11] a postanesthetic evaluation scale based on the Apgar score (Table 1–1). The range is 10 for complete recovery to 0 for comatose patients. The score should be recorded on admission and at 15- to 30-minute intervals to document improvement or deterioration. The Aldrete score is a convenient PACU aid but has obvious limitations, because patients with cardiac dysrhythmias, oliguria, or severe nausea and vomit-

RECOVERY ROOM ADMISSION

Vital Signs: temperature _____   BP _____   PR _____   RR _____

Anesthesia: regional _____   general _____   other _____

Regional: level of analgesia _____

General: unresponsive _____   drowsy _____   awake _____

airway oral _____   nasal _____   none _____

endotracheal tube _____   tracheostomy _____

Figure 1–1. Short form which the recovery room nurse may complete to record patient data at time of admission. BP = blood pressure; PR = pulse rate; RR = respiratory rate.

TABLE 1–1. ALDRETE'S POSTANESTHESIA RECOVERY SCORE

Activity
Voluntary movement of all limbs to command	2
Voluntary movement of 2 extremities to command	1
Unable to move	0

Respiration
Breathe deeply and cough	2
Dyspnea, hypoventilation	1
Apneic	0

Circulation
Blood pressure equals 20% of preanesthetic level	2
Blood pressure equals 20–50% of preanesthetic level	1
Blood pressure equals 50% of preanesthetic level	0

Consciousness
Fully awake	2
Arousable	1
Unresponsive	0

Color
Pink	2
Pale, blotchy	1
Cyanotic	0

Patients should score at least 7 prior to discharge from the PACU.

ing can all score the highest 10 but may not be recovered from anesthetic effects. This point once again underscores the importance of vigilance on the part of the PACU team (nurses, anesthesiologists, and surgeons) in providing adequate care. The original authors reported in their study that patients who scored 7 or below consistently required further intensive care observation (in a PACU or other intensive care unit). The Carignan's postanesthetic score (Table 1–2) is rarely applicable in the PACU setting, because assessments are made on the second, fifth, and fifteenth day following surgery.[12] Routine postoperative monitoring in the recovery room includes pattern and rate of respirations, cardiac rate and rhythm, blood pressure, and temperature monitoring, as well as careful assessment of fluid intake and output. Pulse oximetry is used increasingly as a simple, noninvasive mean to evaluate oxygen saturation and volume status. In addition, systems with preexisting disease or those whose function might have been jeopardized as a result of the surgical procedure must be under constant observation.

RESPIRATORY SYSTEM

On admission to the recovery area, the patient's respiratory rate is measured, and again at 15-minute intervals (Table 1–3). Patients recovering after general anesthesia with potent inhalation agents are likely to manifest respiratory rates in the normal to high range (16 to 30/min) while those whose maintenance was primarily with opioids will breathe at 10 to 16/min. Regular respiratory pattern is to be expected, while phasic variations (eg, Cheyne-Stokes), use of accessory muscles, snoring, or wheezing indicate problems of excessive anesthetic effect, respiratory obstruction, or neurologic complications. Auscultation is irreplaceable in assessing adequacy of respiration. Measurements of tidal volume (TV) and vital capacity (VC) can be easily performed with bedside spirometric equipment. It is important to realize that unlike tidal volume, the VC maneuver is effort-dependent and therefore requires an awake, cooperative patient. Estimation of ventilatory reserve may be necessary in circumstances in which a VC measurement is not obtainable. A reasonable substitute measurement is that of negative inspiratory pressure (NIP).[13] In normal healthy individuals the NIP exceeds −80 cm of water

TABLE 1–2. CARIGNAN'S POSTANESTHETIC SCORING SYSTEM[a]

	0	1	2	3	4
Circ	BP stable, pulse always under 100	BP change less than 30%, pulse 100–120	Vasopressors or Digitalis	BP under 100 in spite of treatment	Decompensated
Resp	Rate under 15 breath-holding more than 25 sec	Rate 15–20, productive cough	Rate over 20 rales or temp up to 100°F	Temp over 100°F, partial atelectasis	Major
CNS	Amnesic satisfied	Confused or recalls induction	Dissatisfied with anesthesia for any reason	Extrapyramidal signs	Major neurologic complications
GI	Nothing	No more than 3 episodes of nausea	Nausea, vomited once only	Vomiting	Ileus
Renal	Voids over 800 cc	Over 800 cc per catheter	Voids 500–800 cc	500–800 cc per catheter	Under 500 cc

[a]Even though the creators of this system do not group total scores, it is obvious that the lower the score, the better the patient's condition.

TABLE 1-3. COMMON PARAMETERS USED TO ASSESS RESPIRATORY FUNCTION IN THE PACU

Parameters	Normal Values
Auscultation	Clear, bilaterally equal
Respiratory rate	10–30/min
Respiratory pattern	Regular
Tidal volume	At least 7–9 mL/kg
Vital capacity	At least 15 mL/kg
Negative inspiratory pressure	At least −20 cm H_2O within 20 sec
Arterial pCO_2	30–50 mm Hg
Arterial pO_2	At least 60 mm Hg on room air

within 10 seconds. Clinical experience has shown that an individual who can generate a NIP of −20 cm H_2O within 20 seconds can be assumed to have a VC of 15 mL/kg or greater, which is the minimum VC requirement to maintain adequate ventilation over a prolonged period of time.[14] Blood gas analyses reflect the status of cardiopulmonary homeostasis and are therefore most useful in assessment of the critically ill or pulmonary-depressed patient. Alveolar ventilation is directly reflected in the partial pressure of carbon dioxide ($PaCO_2$) in the arterial blood. The dissolved oxygen gas tension (PaO_2) is closely related to the oxygen content of arterial blood. (See Table 1–3 for respiratory parameter guidelines.) Pulse oximeters are the new standard monitors in the operating rooms and should be available for PACU use.

CARDIOVASCULAR SYSTEM

Blood pressure, heart rate, and auscultation of heart sounds are routinely monitored in the PACU. Continuous electrocardiographic monitoring complete with a printer to provide a permanent record is standard. An acceptable heart rate and rhythm are essential for proper cardiovascular functioning. A rate that is too rapid will decrease diastolic filling of the ventricles and allow less time for effective coronary perfusion, thus simultaneously diminishing cardiac output and increasing myocardial oxygen demands. Heart rates below 50 beats/min are usually detrimental except in healthy athletic young adults (see Table 1–4 for causes of heart rate alterations). Cardiac monitors in the PACU aid in the diagnosis of myocardial ischemia, but a formal 12-lead electrocardiogram is required to confirm the diagnosis. Blood pressure is measured as an indicator of blood flow and tissue perfusion. If central venous or pulmonary artery pressure monitors have been placed, more accurate assessment of hemodynamic status can be made (Table 1–5).

FLUID AND ELECTROLYTE BALANCE

Close monitoring of fluid balance and electrolyte levels are as important in the PACU as they are intraoperatively. On one hand, the task of balancing fluid status might seem easier in a stable awakening patient. However, equilibrating volumes and changing catecholamine levels when the stimulation of skin closure and endotracheal intubation is removed, can make appropriate fluid management a most challenging task. Routine postoperative intravenous fluid orders may not be adequate to maintain a homogeneous state and close cooperation of PACU physicians and nurses is essential. Most electrolyte measurements are performed in the appropriate labs in a separate area in the hospital. We, however, found the immediate availability of Na^+, K^+, Ca^{2+} (Nova 6 Electrolyte Analyzer, Nova Biomedical, Waltham, MA), glucose (Accu-chek II, Boehringer Manheim, Indianapolis, IN), and hematocrit (Microhemocrit Centrifuge and Microcapillary Reader, Damon-IEC Division, Needham Heights, MA) determinations useful both for the operating room and the PACU. Urine output is a guide to the adequacy of renal perfusion, and as such reflects the general hemodynamic status.

TABLE 1-4. COMMON CAUSES OF ALTERATIONS IN HEART RATE

Tachycardia	Bradycardia
Pain	Previous condition
Volume overload	Beta blockade
Hypovolemia	Narcotic overdose
Drug effect	Heart block
Hyperthermia	Excess vagal tone
Alteration of cerebral blood flow	Severe hypoxia
Hypoxia	Hypothermia
Hypercarbia	Brain stem injury

TABLE 1-5. VALUES USED TO ASSESS CARDIOVASCULAR FUNCTION

Parameters	Normal Values
Heart rate	50–100/min
Blood pressure	90/50–160/100 mm Hg
Central venous pressure	2–8 mm Hg
Pulmonary artery pressure	20/8–30/12 mm Hg
Pulmonary capillary wedge pressure	8–12 mm Hg
Cardiac output (70-kg patient)	5L/min
Cardiac index	2.5–3.5 L/min/m²

However, the lack of urine output may reflect primary kidney malfunction and not perfusion deficits.

temperature better than all of the above methods, but some aural probes may injure the ear canal.

NEUROLOGIC FUNCTION

The sensorium serves as a reflector of perfusion and oxygenation. Several scoring systems pertaining to different clinical situations have been developed, such as the Aldrete, Apgar, Carignan, and Glasgow coma scales. In addition, portable electroencephalographic monitors are now available that have an option of presenting electrophysiologic brain activity in the form of spectral arrays that can be easily interpreted at the bedside. Caution should be exercised in using these monitors, for they are not yet confirmed diagnostic tools, but rather indicate trends. Pupillary reflexes should be monitored for all patients, and recorded on the PACU charts at 15- or 30-minute intervals.

TEMPERATURE

Intraoperatively, temperature is altered by administration of cold fluids and gases, exposure of both the interior and the exterior of the body to the cool environment, vasodilatation, and depression of the thermoregulatory center by anesthetic agents.[7,15] Moderate hypothermia can be protective by decreasing oxygen consumption. In the recovery period rebound shivering can increase oxygen demand by 400%,[16] which can be catastrophic for critically ill patients with coronary or cerebrovascular diseases.[17]

Although shivering is best prevented, it is not always possible to control all the contributing factors. Certain drugs such as methylphenidate[18] (Ritalin) and opiates[19] have been used with partial success, and injection of amino acid taurine has been effective in monkeys.[20] A recent report describes successful application of radiant heat for rapid control of shivering.[21]

Skin temperature measurements can be useful in very small infants, or adults after minor operations where precision is not required. Oral recordings are inaccurate and can be somewhat hazardous in patients who are not fully awake but possess a full set of healthy teeth. Esophageal temperature recordings (from the lower third of the esophagus) are best indicators of core temperature but are not feasible if the patient is awake.[22] The rectal temperature, therefore, becomes the most common measurement, though it changes slowly compared to the core temperature. Tympanic membrane temperature may follow brain

DISCHARGE PLANNING

Should any deviations from the expected recovery course occur, it is the responsibility of the PACU nurse to notify the anesthesiologist or the surgeon, who can then evaluate the problem and correct it (Chapter 9). Even in cases of uncomplicated recovery, a physician must assess the patient prior to discharge from the PACU (Joint Commission on Accreditation of Hospitals Guidelines):

> A mechanism for the release of patients from any postanesthesia care unit: The basis for the decision to discharge a patient from any postanesthesia care unit shall be made only by a physician or, in the case of a patient without medical problems admitted by the qualified oral surgeon, by that oral surgeon, and not by nursing service personnel. However, the actual release of a postanesthesia patient by a physician or, when appropriate, by a qualified oral surgeon, and documentation thereof does not necessarily require the presence or signature of a specified physician or qualified oral surgeon at the time of release. When discharge criteria are used, they shall be comprehensive, approved by the medical staff to assure the same standard of care for all patients, and rigidly enforced. When the responsible physician or qualified oral surgeon has not issued a written order or authenticated a verbal release, the name of the physician or qualified oral surgeon responsible for the patient's release shall be recorded in the medical record.[23]

It is routine practice in most institutions that patients spend at least an hour in the PACU. During the discharge evaluation at the completion of the recovery room stay, the physician (usually an anesthesiologist) has to determine whether the patient is ready to leave the environment of intensive care monitoring. Several major issues must therefore be considered:

- Level of consciousness. The patient must be oriented enough to summon help when necessary. Reflexes must be intact. The patient must be able to cough to clear secretions, and to protect the airway should vomiting occur.
- Hemodynamic status. Heart rate and blood pressure should stabilize at a level comparable though not necessarily identical to the preanesthetic parameters (see Aldrete's score, Table 1–1). The PACU nurses should note if the

patient voided postoperatively, and communicate the information to the care team.

- Motor/sensory function (important following regional anesthesia. The patient must recover enough motor strength to change position in bed, and sufficient sensory function to prevent possible injury.
- Waiting periods. These commonly include
  1. A minimum 30-minute observation period following intravenous narcotic administration (peak effect at 10 to 20 minutes), or naloxone
  2. A one-hour observation period following intramuscular administration of narcotics, antiemetics, or antibiotics.
  3. A one-hour observation period following extubation.
  4. A 30-minute observation period following discontinuation of oxygen therapy.
  5. Other medication-related waiting periods as determined by the anesthesiology department.[24]
- Surgical procedure effects. Dressings should be dry. All tubes, drains, and catheters should be patent and working properly. No new deficits should be present (eg, neurologic, vascular) and those that were corrected during the operation should remain corrected.

The anesthesiologist in the PACU writes a short note in addition to the discharge orders (Fig. 1–2). It should be obvious that numerous considerations will change discharge planning depending on the character of the procedure and general condition of the patient.

The above guidelines need not be met under some circumstances:

1. Patient is being transferred to another intensive care area. These patients need not be awake or extubated, and their hemodynamic status frequently depends on intravenous administration of vasoactive antidysrhythmic or inotropic drugs. The condition, however, should be optimized at a level appropriate for transfer. Thus infusions should be titrated to desired effects, monitors should be available for transfer, and any special requirements should be met, such as positive end-expiratory pressure (PEEP) valves for ventilating devices used during transfer if necessary, portable suction devices, and so on. Usually such patients require at least one physician present for the transport.

2. Ambulatory patients. Stringent criteria must be met.[24] The patient must be able to tolerate oral fluids and walk without assistance. Most units require that patients void urine prior to discharge home. It is also a universal requirement that a responsible adult accompany the patient. These patients also receive explicit written instructions (Fig. 1–3).

Staff in each PACU develop admission and discharge criteria that meet the needs, standards, and specific requirements of the operating rooms and PACU. These should incorporate the JCAH, the American Society of Anesthesiologists, and the American Society of Postanesthesia Nursing guidelines. Yet however detailed the rules, and however many possibilities and instances they might cover, no rule, regulation, or criterion replaces good clinical judgment based on vigilance.

RECOVERY ROOM DISCHARGE

Vital signs stable _____ _____
Patient awake (obeys commands) _____ _____
Laryngeal reflexes present _____ _____
Regional block: Sensation _____ _____
                 Motion _____ _____
To room _____   To ICU _____   To home _____

Figure 1–2. A stamp such as this one may conveniently be put in the patient's chart. The anesthesiologist should also add a note in the record.

SAME DAY CARE CENTER

Post Procedure Instructions
(Circle Appropriate)

1. A responsible adult must accompany you home at discharge and be with you for 24 hour period.

2. Diet: Begin with liquids or light foods and progress slowly to your regular diet.

3. No alcoholic beverage (beer, wine, liquor) for 24 hours.

4. Do not drive, or operate any machinery or power-tools for 24 hours after procedure.

5. Do not make important legal or personal decisions for 24 hours after procedure.

6. If you have received general anesthesia, you may experience a sore throat for the first 24 hours. This is harmless and will disappear.

7. Analgesics or other medication may be ordered by your physician if he/she feels that it is necessary

      <u>Medication</u>   <u>Route & Dosage</u>

    _____   _____

    _____   _____

8. Resume your normal activities one day following procedure unless otherwise indicated.

    A. Activity restrictions: _____

9. If any unusual bleeding; respiratory problems or acute pain occurs after discharge from the hospital, notify your physician immediately, or proceed to the Emergency Room of the nearest hospital.

       Physician's Name & Phone #: _____ _____
       MMC Emergency Room #   _____

10. Follow up appointment made: _____

11. Other instruction (Specialized treatment, equipment, etc.)

    _____

    _____

12. The nursing staff of the Same Day Care Center will telephone you the day after surgery. This is a routine call to find out how you are doing.

Figure 1–3. Outpatient postanesthesia teaching information (Montefiore Hospital, New York).

REFERENCES

1. Morton WTG: *Remarks on the proper mode of administering sulfuric ether by inhalation.* Boston, Dutton & Wentworth, 1947.
2. Nightingale F: *Notes on Hospitals.* London, Longman, Roberts-Green, 1863, p. 89.
3. Harvey AM: Neurosurgical genius—Walter Edward Dandy. *Johns Hopkins Med J* 1974; 135:358.
4. Dripps RD, Eckenhoff JE, Van Dam LO: The immediate postoperative period: Recovery and intensive care, in: *Introduction to Anesthesia: The Principles of Safe Practice,* ed 7. Philadelphia, Saunders, 1988, pp 430–440.
5. Fischer TL: Responsibility for care in recovery rooms. *Can Med Ass J* 1970; 102:78.
6. Practice advisory for recovery room. Anesthesia practice advisory, no. 2. *ASA Newsletter,* May 1978.
7. Frost EAM: Admitting assessment and monitoring, in Frost EAM (ed): *Recovery Room Practice.* Boston, Blackwell, 1985, pp. 3–11.
8. Brody DC, Shapiro AG, Caine MM: Criteria for Patient Care. In: Israel JS, DeKornfeld TJ (eds): *Recovery Room Care* ed 2. Chicago, Year Book, 1987, pp 85–105.
9. Buschman A, Morris R, Warren D, et al: Pulse oximetry and the incidence of hypoxemia during recovery from anesthesia. *Anesthesiology* 1987; 67(3A):A481.
10. Bissonette B, Scott A: Oral presentation, 44th meeting of the Canadian Anaesthetists' Society, Calgary, Alberta, 1987.
11. Aldrete JA, Kronlik D: A postanesthetic recovery score. *Anesth Analg* 1970; 49:924–933.
12. Carignan G, Keeri-Szanto M, Lavellee J-P: Postanesthetic scoring system. *Anesthesiology* 1964; 25:396–397.
13. Bendixen HH, Bunker JP: Measurement of inspiratory force in anesthetized dogs. *Anesthesiology* 1962; 23:315.
14. Shapiro BA, Harrison RA, Kacmarek RM, Cane RD: Assessment of cardiopulmonary reserves. In: *Clinical Application of Respiratory Care,* ed 3. Chicago, Year Book, 1985, p 343.

15. Hammel HT: Anesthetics and body temperature regulation. *Anesthesiology* 1988; 68:833–835.

16. Bay J, Nunn JF, Prys-Roberts C: Factors influencing arterial PO_2 during recovery from anaesthesia. *Br J Anaesth* 1968; 40:398–406.

17. Cullen DJ: Recovery room care of the surgical patient. *ASA Refresher Courses* 1980; 8:13–28.

18. Brichard G, Johnstone M: The effect of methyl-phenidate (Ritalin) on post-halothane muscular spasticity. *Br J Anaesth* 1970; 42:718–721.

19. Pauca AL, Savage RT, Simpson S, Roy RC: Effect of pethidine, fentanyl and morphine on post-operative shivering in man. *Acta Anesthesiol Scand* 1984; 28:138–143.

20. Murphy MT, Lipton JM, Loughran P, Giesecke AH: Postanesthetic shivering in primates: Inhibition by peripheral heating and by taurine. *Anesthesiology* 1985; 63, 161–165.

21. Sharkey A, Lipton JM, Murphy MT, Giesecke AM: Inhibition of postanesthetic shivering with radiant heat. *Anesthesiology*, 1987; 66:249–252.

22. Rupp SM, Severinghaus JW: Hypothermia. In: Miller RD (ed): *Anesthesia*, ed 2. New York, Churchill Livingston, 1986, pp 1995–2022.

23. Joint Commission on Accreditation of Hospitals (JCAH): Anesthesia services: Standard IV, p 5. In: *Accreditation Manual for Hospitals*, 1984.

24. Hartwell PW: Discharge criteria in recovery room care, in Frost EAM (ed): *International Anesthesiology Clinics*. Boston, Little, Brown, 1983, pp 107–114.

2 Delayed Return to Consciousness

Ross A. Malley

The problem of delayed emergence confronts the anesthesiologist frequently in the postanesthetic care unit (PACU). It represents a challenge to rapidly and accurately diagnose and treat the etiology, which may be minor or life threatening. This is similar to the diagnostic problem facing a physician in the emergency room when presented with a comatose patient. Indeed, the same principles of management can be used. The fact that the patient has recently undergone a surgical and anesthetic procedure will certainly change the focus of the physician but also provides current information about the patient. This is a luxury rarely available to an emergency room physician.

Delayed emergence is an emergency until proven otherwise and, similar to treating victims of cardiac arrest or trauma, diagnostic and therapeutic maneuvers are performed almost concurrently. An understanding of the mechanism of consciousness and the problems affecting it in the perioperative period is critical for timely and appropriate therapy of the patient.

CENTRAL NERVOUS SYSTEM FUNCTION AND CONSCIOUSNESS

The central nervous system is a complex organ, both in terms of structure and function. This complexity has been achieved at the cost of significant limitations. The brain has limited energy and substrate stores and high oxygen requirements, which make it dependent upon an uninterrupted supply for normal function.[1] The brain is also a "fastidious" organ that "operates" within a relatively narrow physiologic milieu. Whether a disease process or anesthetic effect perturbs this system, the effect is the same: functional derangement. Structures that must function normally for consciousness include the reticular activating system (RAS) in the brainstem and the cerebral cortexes.[2] Interruption, either structurally or functionally, of their normal activity will decrease consciousness.

DIFFERENTIAL DIAGNOSIS

A review of the causes of altered consciousness as presented by Plum and Posner reveals a long and detailed list of the structural, metabolic, and psychiatric processes found as the cause of the patient's "coma."[3] For the anesthesiologist, this list may be organized into several broad categories that will provide a more useful framework for evaluating the patient in the recovery room. As presented in Table 2–1, these are categorized as (1) neurologic injury (the hardware is broken); (2) metabolic abnormalities (other organ systems are not functioning and the environment is hostile); and (3) drug effects. In the PACU setting, the third category will be the most common cause encountered.

TABLE 2–1. DIFFERENTIAL DIAGNOSIS OF DELAYED EMERGENCE

Neurologic Injury

Ischemia
Mass lesions
Seizure disorders

Metabolic Abnormalities

Hypoglycemia
Diabetic ketoacidosis
Nonketotic hyperosmolar hyperglycemic coma
Hepatic dysfunction
Electrolyte disturbances
Renal dysfunction
Thyroid dysfunction
Adrenocortical dysfunction
Cardiorespiratory failure
Hypothermia
Malignant hyperthermia

Drug Effects

Inhalational anesthetics
Opioids
Barbiturates
Benzodiazepines
Ketamine
Anticholinergics
Muscle relaxants

CEREBRAL DYSFUNCTION

A patient may fail to regain consciousness in an appropriate manner due to structural injury to the brain itself. Two broad categories of problems can occur—ischemia or mass lesions. A third subcategory of patients are those with seizure disorders who will be unresponsive in the ictal and postictal period.

Ischemia

The brain will not function unless it is supplied with an uninterrupted supply of oxygen and energy substrates. If the supply is interrupted either globally or regionally, unconsciousness may occur.

Prolonged hypotension may produce irreversible neurologic damage even in patients with normal cerebral vasculature. Normal cerebral blood flow averages 50 mL/100 g/min divided to 80 mL for gray matter, 20 mL for white matter. Critical flow levels for normothermic patients are approximately 15 mL/min when the EEG becomes flat and under 10 mL/min when irreversible damage occurs.[4]

Cerebral perfusion pressure is equal to the mean arterial pressure (MAP) minus the intracranial pressure (ICP). The brain is able to maintain perfusion constant over a range of approximately 50 to 150 mm Hg MAP by autoregulation. Cerebral blood flow becomes pressure-dependent above and below these levels. The curve is shifted to the right in hypertensive patients.[5]

In patients with preexisting cerebrovascular disease, tolerance of hypotensive events is even less as the perfusion beyond stenotic areas may already be tenuous. In this group, the need to maintain blood pressure is critical and rapid restoration to or above preanesthetic levels is indicated. Therapy includes the use of volume, inotropes, and vasopressors as appropriate to restore circulating blood volume and cardiac output.

Pulmonary problems also produce ischemic events if there is failure of gas exchange. Exposure to hypoxic gas mixtures, pulmonary emboli, pulmonary edema, losses of airway, and aspiration are some causes of reduced arterial oxygen content that lead to ischemic events in the perioperative period.

Embolization

Intravascular particles may be produced and travel into the cerebral circulation to obstruct large or small arteries. Atherosclerosis is a common disease in the American population and the cerebral circulation is commonly involved. The carotid artery is a common site of plaque formation and fragments of cholesterol and thrombus can embolize to the brain.[6] This may occur spontaneously or during carotid endarterec-

tomy when residual fragments of the resected atheroma are present when the carotid clamp is released.

The heart is also a prime source of embolic phenomena. Plaques from diseased valves are seen in subacute bacterial endocarditis. Thrombus formation in the atria (chronic atrial fibrillation) and ventricles (following infarctions) predisposes to embolic events.

Venous thrombosis could lead to cerebral embolization in the presence of a patent foramen ovale, especially if right-sided heart pressures are elevated such as seen following pulmonary embolization.

Gas bubbles also produce an embolization syndrome. Situations where this may occur include cardiac surgery where the heart chambers are entered. Air may also be injected into the arterial circulation from the use of arterial lines. Bubbles can be "flushed" retrograde up the artery to the central circulation and into the brain. "Paradoxical" air emboli also may occur in the patient with a patent foramen ovale.[7] The use of nitrous oxide in these situations may potentiate the problem be diffusion into the bubble and expansion of its size.

Thrombosis

Cerebral thrombotic events disrupt normal perfusion of cerebral structures and reduce the level of consciousness. An increased risk of thrombosis is associated with certain disease states such as brain tumors. Coagulopathies may occur in patients with sickle cell disease or its variants (sickle thalassemia, for example), disseminated intravascular coagulation (DIC), thrombocytosis, polycythemia, or in women taking oral contraceptives.

Thrombosis can occur in patients with intrinsic vascular diseases. Examples include vasculitides (temporal arteritis, collagen vascular diseases, hypersensitivity reactions to drugs, Kawasaki's disease) and dissection of the aorta.

Mass Lesions

Intracerebral masses will produce a decrease in the function of the brain. These masses include tumors, hemorrhage, and gas.

Tumors will decrease the level of consciousness due to their infiltration into or pressure upon brain structures. Clearly tumors do not grow sufficiently to produce a marked change in the level of consciousness of the patient during the perioperative period. Increases in the degree of edema surrounding the tumor from vigorous hydration, cauterization of vessels, or bleeding into the tumor are more common mechanisms.

Intracranial hemorrhages produces mass lesions. Bleeding may be intraparenchymal, epidural, or subdural.[8] The bleeding may result from rupture of preexisting cerebral aneurysms, trauma, or bleeding diathesis. Cerebral aneurysms are at risk of rupture in the setting of rapidly increasing blood pressure that will stress the defective wall beyond its burst strength. This may occur during the induction period with laryngoscopy.[9] Such increases may be blunted with incremental doses of narcotics, barbiturates, lidocaine, or deepening of inhalational anesthesia prior to manipulating the trachea.

Patients who have sustained trauma may present with intracerebral hemorrhage. Of special mention are those who have sustained an epidural hematoma due to arterial disruption. The initial loss of consciousness following the trauma may have resolved and the patient may have a "lucid interval" where he or she is responsive.[10] This is replaced by progressive decreased level of consciousness as the arterial bleed continues and the expanding hematoma compresses vital structures and causes edema. If the patient was anesthetized during the lucid period, delayed return of consciousness may present, until the swelling subsides, despite release of the hematoma.

Gas can also act as a mass lesion intracranially, as after craniotomy, especially in the sitting position.[11] Cerebrospinal fluid is lost and brain volume is reduced by diuresis during the operative period. When the calvarium is closed, air fills the remaining voids. Postoperatively, swelling of the brain tissue, increase in body temperature, and reaccumulation of cerebrospinal fluid may occur more rapidly when the insoluble nitrogen is reabsorbed, leading to elevated intracranial pressure. The same problem can occur in closed-head procedures such as following air contrast encephalography or transphenoidal hypophysectomy where air is injected into the subarachnoid space. If nitrous oxide is used to anesthetize a patient during or soon after these procedures, the nitrous oxide can diffuse into the existing bubbles and produce a tension pneumocephalus.[12]

Seizure Disorders

Patients with preexisting seizure disorders may have decreased levels of consciousness due to the disease itself or the sedating effects of the drug used to treat it. Anesthetic agents have been associated with the induction of seizures. Of the intravenous induction agents, methohexital and ketamine have been implicated. Enflurane, in high concentrations and during profound hypocarbic conditions, produces "spike and wave" activity on the electroencephalogram.[13] If the patient is manifesting evidence of ongoing seizure activity, termination of the event with barbiturate, benzodiazepines, or phenytoin is required. Protection of the airway and maintenance of hemodynamic stability is also crucial. Termination of the

"seizure activity" with muscle relaxants is ineffective in reducing the high metabolic rate of the brain, although these drugs can reduce lactic acidosis by preventing muscle action.

METABOLIC ABNORMALITIES

Hypoglycemia

Glucose is the critical energy substrate for the brain. There is approximately 2 grams of glucose and glycogen stored in the adult brain, which serves to support survival of tissue but is insufficient for normal function. Generally, at a blood glucose level of 30 mg/dL, confusion will occur, and at less than 15 mg/dL the patient will be comatose. Individuals at risk for this process include those receiving exogenous insulin, oral hypoglycemics, those with severe hepatic dysfunction, and patients with hypopituitarism, hypothyroidism, and endogenous overproduction of insulin from insulinomas. The primary goal is prevention of the hypoglycemic state.[14] Currently, the availability of test strip glucose determination and glucometry allow for frequent real-time determination of the patient's glucose level and should serve to limit the incidence of significant hypoglycemia in the postoperative period. This test also enables the anesthesiologist to monitor the patient in the PACU. If necessary, rapid replacement with injectable 50% dextrose in water is indicated followed by maintenance infusions containing glucose.

Diabetic Ketoacidosis

On the other end of the spectrum are patients with diabetic ketoacidosis (DKA). This process occurs when there is insufficient circulating insulin to meet the metabolic demands of the patient. The phenomena may occur in diabetic patients when "stressed" by a surgical procedure or infection. In its full-blown manifestation, diabetic coma is characterized by hyperglycemia, ketonemia, metabolic acidosis, and osmotic diuresis produced by the high levels of osmotically active metabolites.[15] These metabolic changes result in a decreased level of consciousness (serum glucose greater than 800 to 1000 mg/dL). Associated abnormalities include a loss of total body potassium and hypophosphatemia. The loss of potassium may not be apparent when serum levels are measured, due to the shift of potassium from intracellular stores that occurs as hydrogen ions move intracellularly and metabolic acidosis develops. Hypokalemia may be a complication of rapid correction of acidosis if supplemental potassium is not provided. Treatment involves replenishment of intravascular volume and restoration of circulating insulin to halt further ketogenesis and allow for the cellular utilization of the high circulating glucose. Electrolyte levels must be monitored and appropriate correction made to prevent unacceptable shifts as noted previously.

Nonketotic Hyperosmolar Hyperglycemic Coma

This process may complicate the anesthetic recovery in patients with overt diabetes, normal patients under stressful conditions, or elderly, debilitated patients who have been unable to drink or have received insufficient intravenous fluid replacement. Differing from DKA in that there is no ketosis, this process shares the characteristics of hyperglycemia (glucose levels under 800 mg/dL), hyperosmolality, and electrolyte and fluid disequilibrium. The severe osmolality increase causes intracerebral dehydration and brain dysfunction. The lack of ketosis is produced by the level of circulating insulin, which is sufficient to suppress fat metabolism but unable to control the blood glucose levels. The associated osmotic diuresis results in hypovolemia with hemoconcentration, hypotension, and potentially, poor peripheral perfusion.[16]

The syndrome has been seen in patients receiving parenteral hyperalimentation, presumably because hypertonic infusions have been given during a stressful event.

The principles of treatment are similar to those for DKA except that these patients are very sensitive to small doses of insulin. Administration of insulin to promote the intracellular transport of the circulating glucose is necessary. Hypovolemia must be corrected carefully with intravenous electrolyte solutions; special attention must be paid to monitoring serum potassium levels. Too vigorous rehydration is dangerous since diffuse cerebral edema can result as water moves intracerebrally in response to the preexisting cellular hyperosmolality.

Hepatic Dysfunction

Hepatic dysfunction is a potential cause of delayed emergence for a number of reasons. The liver is responsible for multiple functions that maintain the normal homeostasis of the patient including glucose and protein metabolism and degradation and clearance of toxic metabolites and drugs.[17] As the major site of protein synthesis, dysfunction can decrease albumin levels and thus allow increased circulating free drug levels. The liver is responsible for the clearance of nitrogen from protein as urea and dysfunction can result in elevated levels of ammonia.

Dysfunction can be seen in patients with a history of prolonged hypotension or hypoxia since the liver is sensitive to decreased oxygen supply due to its high metabolic rate. Decreased perfusion may be seen in patients with cardiac dysfunction and congestive failure. Therapy for the cardiac disease may worsen hepatic function if high-dose sympathomimetics and vasopressors are used that decrease hepatic and splanchnic perfusion. Infectious etiologies such as viral hepatitides (hepatitis A, B, non-A non-B, Epstein-Barr virus, and cytomegalovirus) can damage the liver. Hepatic dysfunction can be caused by anesthetic agents either directly (halothane hepatitis rarely) or indirectly by hypoperfusion. Extrahepatic problems such as cholelithiasis or bile-duct obstruction due to pancreatic tumor can also produce dysfunction.

Electrolyte Disturbances

Hyponatremia, hypocalcemia, and hypermagnesemia are three electrolyte disturbances commonly implicated as causes of depressed level of consciousness.

Hyponatremia. Hyponatremia or water intoxication is encountered relatively frequently in the recovery period. The two common etiologies include the syndrome of inappropriate antidiuretic hormone release (SIADH) and free water absorption during transurethral resection of the prostate (TURP). The stress of a surgical procedure along with the effects of positive pressure ventilation, pulmonary carcinomas, and diseases of the pituitary system are all associated with SIADH.[18] Free water absorption occurs during TURP when the irrigating solution used (glycine in water, for example) is forced into open venous channels during the course of the prostatic resection, a process that can occur very rapidly.[19]

The signs and symptoms of hyponatremia vary directly with the speed of development. At sodium levels of approximately 120 mEq/L, somnolence and confusion are likely. When levels reach 110 mEq/L, seizures and coma occur. Below 110 mEq/L cardiovascular instability and dysrhythmias occur. Other associated findings include pulmonary dysfunction, congestive failure, and jugular venous distension due to volume overload. The emergency treatment of significant symptoms (seizures, coma, and dysrhythmias) includes the use of hypertonic saline, so-called ''hot salt.'' This must be infused carefully with appropriate monitoring to avoid iatrogenically increasing volume overload or producing neurologic injury.[20] In an emergent situation, gradual replacement with normal saline with concurrent diuresis using furosemide is acceptable to correct the hyponatremia.

Hypocalcemia. Hypocalcemia occurs when serum levels (total serum calcium) drop below 4.5 mEq/L. Of equal importance is the concentration of ionized calcium (normal range is 2 to 2.5 mEq/L). Individuals with low serum albumin from chronic disease, hepatic failure, or massive volume replacement may demonstrate low total calcium but normal ionized calcium.[21]

Etiologies include acute pancreatitis, hypoparathyroidism following parathyroid or thyroidectomy, and patients with end-stage renal disease. Acute decreases in ionized calcium are associated with respiratory alkalosis (overvigorous hyperventilation) or metabolic alkalosis (bicarbonate injection). Rapid infusion of blood products containing citrate can cause chelation of available calcium, but this requires rapid (> 0.5 to 1 mL/kg/min) infusion.[22]

The signs and symptoms of hypocalcemia include confusion, seizures, and coma. Associated findings include cardiac dysfunction with hypotension, decreased contractility, and variable Q-T prolongation.[23] Diffuse muscle spasm (tetanus) may occur including laryngeal muscle spasm.

Therapy for true serum hypocalcemia is calcium replacement with calcium chloride (3 to 6 mg/kg over 10 to 15 min) or calcium gluconate. Hyperventilation causing low ionized calcium, should be corrected first.

Hypermagnesemia. Hypermagnesemia occurs when plasma concentrations exceed 2.5 mEq/L. Patients with preeclampsia/eclampsia treated with exogenous magnesium and individuals with end-stage renal disease are most susceptible. The therapeutic range of magnesium treatment of the preeclamptic patient is 4 to 6 mEq/L, which produces the desired suppression of CNS irritability. Plasma levels in excess of this level produce suppression of deep tendon reflexes, sedation, and coma.[24] Peripheral muscle weakness with respiratory insufficiency is associated with levels in the 10 to 15 mEq/L range. Cardiovascular collapse occurs at higher levels.

Treatment of hypermagnesemia includes discontinuation of exogenous sources, support of ventilation and cardiac function, and counteraction of the effects of the existing magnesium load with intravenous calcium.

Renal Dysfunction

Adequate kidney function is critical for maintaining water and electrolyte homeostasis. It is also involved in the metabolism and excretion of endogenous wastes and exogenously administered medications. In the presence of long-standing renal failure, multiple complications can occur, which may affect CNS function. Accelerated hypertension can be seen with cerebrovascular accidents and cardiovascular dysfunction. Volume overload and congestive failure may occur. Electrolyte abnormalities such as hyperkalemia, hypermagnesemia, and hypocalcemia can

occur. Platelet dysfunction predisposes to bleeding diathesis, which can affect the CNS. Acid–base disturbances resulting from the inability to excrete fixed acid metabolites and uric acid also have the potential of depressing consciousness.[25]

Thyroid Dysfunction

Thyroid disorders prolong recovery of consciousness. Both decreased function of the thyroid (hypothyroidism) and over activity (hyperthyroidism/thyroid storm) are responsible.

Hypothyroidism. This process is caused by disease processes that affect different levels of the pituitary–thyroid axis and are classified as either primary or secondary hypothyroidism (Table 2–2). Overall, individuals demonstrate a decreased metabolic function as a result of the reduction in circulating thyroid hormones. Clinically this is manifested by decreased cardiac output, bradycardia, and exquisite sensitivity to depressive medications.[26] In its full-blown manifestation (myxedema coma) hypothyroidism can produce congestive heart failure, respiratory insufficiency, hypothermia, and coma.[27] There may also be associated adrenal insufficiency.

Therapy for these patients includes exogenously administered thyroid hormone along with general supportive care.

Hyperthyroidism. Hyperthyroidism as an etiology of decreased consciousness is most likely to occur when frank thyrotoxicosis or ''thyroid storm'' occurs. This condition is precipitated by excessive release of thyroid hormone from the thyroid gland potentiated by its ability to store large quantities of preformed hormone, unlike other endocrine glands. Release can be precipitated by stress (surgery, infections). Central nervous system manifestations include tachycardia, hypertension, or hypotension with congestive failure

---

TABLE 2–2. CLASSIFICATION OF HYPOTHYROIDISM

Primary—Inhibition occurs in thyroid gland

Hashimoto's thyroiditis
Radioactive iodine
Surgical resection
Thyroid-inhibiting drugs
    Excessive iodine
    Propylthiouracil
    Methimazole
    Lithium carbonate

Secondary—Dysfunction occurs outside of gland

Hypothalamic dysfunction
    Loss of thyrotropin-releasing hormone (TRH)
Pituitary dysfunction
    Loss of thyrotropin-stimulating hormone (TSH)

and shock. The associated hyperthermia and dehydration worsen hemodynamic instability.

Treatment of thyrotoxicosis is based upon reducing further release of the hormone and blocking its peripheral effects while supporting the cardiorespiratory system and correction of metabolic problems. Pharmacologic therapy includes intravenous sodium iodide to acutely suppress hormone release, beta blockers to control tachycardia (these drugs should be used with caution in patients with congestive heart failure or bronchospastic disease), and supplemental corticosteroids to supplement the patient during this hypermetabolic state.[28] Hyperthermia is controlled with infusion of cold electrolyte solutions and surface cooling. The differential diagnosis is between thyroid storm or a malignant hyperthermia episode.[29]

Malignant Hyperthermia

Malignant hyperthermia (MH) is characterized by uncontrolled intracellular calcium fluxes in muscle with activation of the excitation–contraction coupling mechanism. The syndrome occurs in genetically susceptible individuals when exposed to potent inhalational agents or succinylcholine or any anesthetic technique. Once triggered, the patient will present with evidence of accelerated metabolism that is nonspecific except for the production of muscle spasm. Symptoms include hyperthermia, spasm of muscles including the masseters (trismus), hypoxia, and hypercarbia due to hypermetabolism and metabolic acidosis. Cardiac dysrhythmias may occur and serum potassium is elevated. Rhabdomyolysis can occur and result in acute tubular necrosis (ATN). The respiratory and metabolic acidosis and hyperthermia are chiefly responsible for the CNS symptoms. The appearance of these symptoms may occur for the first time in the postoperative period in a fulminant manner or they may evolve slowly.[30] Among the differential diagnoses are malignant neurolept syndrome (MNS), which is associated with administration of neuroleptic analgesics. A common pathway of hypermetabolism may exist between MH and MNS.[31]

Treatment of the MH process is based upon terminating the use of triggering agents and the use of dantrolene sodium to disrupt the abnormal calcium fluxes and reduce the metabolic activation. Successful use of this drug requires a high degree of suspicion to treat the process early before significant hemodynamic and metabolic instability occur. Additional support includes intubation and hyperventilation with oxygen to correct hypoxia and hypercarbia. External cooling is indicated along with infusion of cold electrolyte solutions or gastric lavage. A brisk diuresis with osmotic diuretics should be initiated to reduce the risk of ATN. The use of these supportive measures will not be sufficient to treat this disease without the use of dantrolene, which has reduced the morbidity and mortality of this disease (2 to 5 mg/kg—7 to 10 vials). A protocol for the treatment of MH as advocated by the Malignant Hyperthermia Association of the United States is outlined in Table 2–3.

Adrenocortical Dysfunction

Patients with depressed function of the adrenal cortex are at risk for delayed return of consciousness following trauma or surgical stress. Dysfunction may be due to destruction of the adrenal glands, deficient production of adrenocorticotropic hormone (ACTH) by the anterior pituitary, or suppression of the gland by exogenous corticosteroids. Whatever the cause, the adrenals are unable to respond to the stress by releasing additional cortisol.[32]

In the PACU, the patient may manifest circulatory collapse. Serum electrolytes reveal hyponatremia and hyperkalemia. Serum glucose is low. Hematocrit may be elevated due to hypovolemia but this finding can be masked by surgical losses and intraoperative crystalloid replacement. The diagnosis can be established

---

TABLE 2–3. MALIGNANT HYPERTHERMIA PROTOCOL

1. Have a high index of suspicion!

2. Stop all triggering agents and ventilate with 100% oxygen. Change tubing/CO_2 canisters or entire machine if potent agents have been used.

3. Call for assistance! Mixing dantrolene, monitoring the patient, drawing laboratory studies, etc, is very difficult to do alone!

4. Stop or expeditiously complete the surgery.

5. Administer 2–3mg/kg of dantrolene intravenously. This is the specific therapy for this pathologic process! Repeat as necessary to control the hypermetabolic state. (100mg/kg or more)

6. Start cooling the patient with cold intravenous fluids, gastric lavage, or bladder irrigation.

7. Continue routine monitoring with BP, ECG, temperature, pulse oximetry and capnography. Addition of arterial and central venous lines is useful.

8. Monitor urine output with a Foley catheter and maintain urine output at 1–2mL/kg with appropriate fluids and furosemide if necessary. Myoglobin-induced renal failure can occur in this setting.

9. Monitor arterial and mixed venous blood gasses and treat metabolic acidosis with hyperventilation and sodium bicarbonate as indicated.

10. Monitor serum electrolytes, especially potassium, along with CPK, LDH, and myoglobin to assess muscle damage. Treat hyperkalemia with insulin/glucose infusions.

11. Monitor CBC, clotting factors, and fibrin split products to assess for disseminated intravascular coagulation.

12. Transfer to ICU for monitoring. Dantrolene, 1–2mg/kg Q 4–6hrs IV, should be given following initial stabilization for 24–48 hrs.

13. Cardiac dysrhythmias may be treated with procainamide IV if unresponsive to correction of electrolytes and pH.

14. Continued vigilance for recurrence of malignant hyperthermia in the postoperative/ICU phases of treatment is vital!

by measuring urinary or plasma corticosteroid levels although it may be difficult to obtain the results of these tests quickly.

Emergency resuscitation of the patient is accomplished with replacement of volume and correction of electrolyte imbalances and hypoglycemia with appropriate intravenous solutions. Steroid replacement is provided with intravenous hydrocortisone 100 mg, followed by 50 mg every 6 hours.[33]

Respiratory Problems

Respiratory problems are relatively common in the PACU and can delay awakening because of hypoxemia or hypercarbia. Additionally, the effects of the inhalation anesthetics are prolonged as excretion is delayed.

The etiologies of pulmonary dysfunction seen in the PACU are diverse (Table 2–4). They include processes intrinsic to the lung and upper airway, cardiac dysfunction, neuromuscular diseases affecting the muscles of respiration, and depression of central nervous system control of respiration. Regardless of the etiology, prompt identification of these patients is imperative to restore appropriate gas exchange.[34]

Hypoxemia is associated with conditions producing areas of atelectasis and intrapulmonary right-to-left shunting. Preexisting pneumonia, perioperative aspiration, inspissation of secretions, bronchospasm, pulmonary emboli, and pulmonary edema all pro-

TABLE 2–4. DIFFERENTIAL DIAGNOSIS OF PULMONARY DYSFUNCTION

Airway Obstruction
Pharyngeal obstruction from tongue
Laryngospasm
Endotracheal tube problems
    Kinking, secretions
    Mainstem intubation
Foreign bodies

Intrinsic Lung Disease
Chronic obstructive pulmonary disease
Bronchospastic disease
Atelectasis
Pulmonary edema
Pneumo/hemothorax

Cardiovascular Problems
Myocardial failure
Pulmonary embolization
Hypovolemia

Respiratory ''Pump'' Failure
Preexisting neuromuscular disease
Residual neuromuscular blockade
Unstable chest wall (flail chest)
Splinting

Central Respiratory ''Drive'' Dysfunction
Drug-induced depression
Loss of hypercarbic drive in patients with COPD

duce arterial hypoxemia. The availability of pulse oximetry or blood gas analyses aids in identification of hypoxemia. Treatment with supplemental oxygen, mechanical ventilation, positive end-expiratory pressure (PEEP), diuretics, and bronchodilators is directed to maximize arterial oxygenation and minimize the potential toxic effects of prolonged oxygen administration.[35]

Hypercarbia occurs when alveolar ventilation is insufficient to excrete the carbon dioxide produced by the body. In the postoperative period, this may occur because of preexisting chronic obstructive pulmonary disease (COPD), respiratory muscle dysfunction, elevated CO_2 production, or suppression of central respiratory drive. If the patient is intubated, capnography can provide continuous on-line monitoring of exhaled CO_2 levels. Blood gas analyses also reveal elevated CO_2 levels. Therapy includes mechanical ventilation, judicious analgesia, optimizing volume status, bronchodilators, suctioning, antibiotics, and warming or cooling as needed.

Cardiovascular Instability

Impaired cardiovascular function depresses the CNS by decreasing brain perfusion, leading to decreased delivery of oxygen and energy substrates. Hypotension is an important manifestation of this instability and may be due to hypovolemia, myocardial dysfunction, or decreased peripheral vascular resistance.

Hypovolemia may be caused by inadequate volume resuscitation during surgery to replace losses from bleeding, ''third spacing,'' evaporative losses from exposed bowel, and excessive diuresis. Even if the patient was normovolemic during the course of the surgery, these losses will continue in the recovery period and fluid replacement must be continued.

Myocardial dysfunction is common in the postoperative period due to intrinsic depression of myocardial contractility or rhythm disturbances. Contractility may be decreased due to preexisting cardiac disease, perioperative ischemia/infarction, profound hypothermia, or residual anesthetic effect. Electrolyte imbalances (hyper- or hypokalemia), acidosis, hypoxia, hypercarbia, and sympathetic and parasympathetic stimulation may induce tachycardia, nodal rhythms, and ventricular premature beats. These increase myocardial oxygen consumption, disrupt sequential contraction of the atria and ventricles, and predispose to malignant ventricular rhythm disturbances.[36]

Changes in the tone of the peripheral vasculature affect blood pressure. Systemic vascular resistance is decreased by residual sympathetic block from regional anesthetics, septic shock, rewarming, and premature discontinuation of vasopressor drugs.

Yet another etiology of hypotension occurring in

the PACU is monitor failure. Precipituous treatment of ''hypotension'' in the awake mentating patient should be preceded by exclusion of automatic blood pressure cuff error and assurance that direct arterial measurements are indeed correct and the transducer has not been closed to the cannula and opened to atmospheric pressure for calibration purposes.

The patient with hypotension must be aggressively evaluated to determine the etiology. Frequent measurements of blood pressure, heart rate and rhythm, quality of pulse, or other evidence of peripheral hypoperfusion and determination of the perioperative fluid balance and continued losses must be made. If a question as to adequate central filling pressure or myocardial performance exists, the use of central venous pressure or pulmonary artery catherization should be considered. Based upon the etiology determined, appropriate therapy with fluids, inotropes, vasopressors, dilators, or other therapy is indicated.

Hypertension can alter the level of consciousness. Acute and severe elevations in blood pressure can overwhelm cerebral vascular autoregulation, leading to hypertensive encephalopathy and cerebral vascular accidents. The heart may fail because of increased afterload. Causes of postoperative hypertension include preoperative cardiovascular disease, pain, excessive fluid replacement, or rebound phenomena from withdrawal of antihypertensive drug therapy.[37] Treatment based on the precipitating event is required to reduce the risk of cerebral or myocardial damage.

Hypothermia

Hypothermia progressively decreases consciousness. Sedation, in the absence of other drug or disease effects, occurs at approximately 33°C with progression to coma at lower levels. Surgical patients are at risk for hypothermia due to exposure in cold operating rooms, open abdomen and chest procedures, infusion of ambient temperature intravenous fluids, washing with cold disinfecting solutions, or deliberate cooling for cardiovascular or cerebral procedures. Transurethral resection of the prostate or urethroscopic bladder procedures with the use of large volumes of irrigating solution are also associated with cooling. Children are at increased risk due to their large surface-to-weight ratios. Anesthesia compounds these problems. Regional techniques profoundly effect sympathetic tone causing vasodilatation and extremity heat loss. The use of high flows of dry anesthetic gases promotes respiratory water loss with concomitant heat loss. Despite using heated fluids, warming blankets, heated humidifiers, wrapping extremities, and covering exposed viscera, many patients are hypothermic on admission to the PACU.

Besides the direct depression of CNS function, hypothermia has other effects that promote delay of emergence. The metabolism and excretion of anesthetic gases, opioids, sedatives, and muscle relaxants are delayed. Myocardial function may be decreased or increased depending upon the activity of the sympathetic nervous system. Dysrhythmias are seen with profound hypothermia (under about 30°C).[38]

The treatment of hypothermia is based upon gradual rewarming using surface warming and warmed intravenous solutions. If hypothermia is minimal, covering with blankets and allowing the patient to passively warm is sufficient. Vital signs should be monitored for hypotension due to peripheral dilation with rewarming. Dysrhythmias may be caused by passive movement of limbs, forcing cold blood into the central compartment. Shivering can be hazardous in the cold patient as it will increase oxygen consumption and elevate CO_2 production. Shivering may be suppressed by phenothiazines, meperidine, or muscle relaxants and assisted ventilation.[39]

ANESTHETIC DRUGS

Drug effects are the most common cause of delayed or prolonged emergence in the post-operative period. Factors responsible include relative or absolute overdosage, individual patient variation, and drug interactions.

The approach to identifying a drug-induced problem requires reviewing the chart and obtaining a good history, including the preanesthetic assessment, inpatient drug administration record, and anesthetic record. For this database, the provider should be guided in a rapid and organized identification of the drug(s) responsible and institute appropriate support or treatment.

Inhalational Anesthetics

Inhalational anesthetics will depress the level of consciousness at relatively low concentrations. Except for nitrous oxide, the remaining hydrocarbon anesthetics are varyingly soluble in the lipid phase and significant amounts may accumulate in the body fat mass during prolonged surgical procedures. These agents are also eliminated primarily by the lungs with minimal metabolism. However, these agents have a depressant effect upon cardiopulmonary function that serves to limit the delivery to and ventilation of the alveoli for elimination. At the conclusion of the anesthetic, when the patient is transported to the PACU and the level of stimulation decreases, there is the potential for these agents to leave the fat tissue, raise the blood and brain levels, and reduce the rate of elimination and delay emergence.

Multiple patient factors have been identified that reduce the minimum alveolar concentration (MAC) and place the patient at risk for delayed emergence even with subanesthetic levels of agent. Hypothermia will reduce MAC requirements in animal models and man.[40] Age is an important factor as MAC decreases with advancing age. Pregnancy also reduces MAC.[41]

Several medications interact with residual potent inhalation agents and reduce the level of consciousness. Narcotics, benzodiazepines, barbiturates, and other induction agents are immediately obvious. Not to be neglected are antisialogues, psychotropic drugs, alcohol (acutely ingested), or use of other "street drugs." Antihypertensives such as alpha-methyldopa, which reduce the central nervous system concentration of neurotransmitters, have also been implicated in a dose-dependent decrease of MAC.[42]

Once a residual potent inhalational agent has been identified as the etiology of the delayed emergence, the primary treatment is support of ventilation and circulation, protection of the patient's airway, and careful observation. If the patient is intubated, objective evidence of the excretion of the anesthetic may be obtained if infrared or mass spectrometry equipment is available in the PACU.

Narcotics

Narcotic compounds are used extensively not only to provide analgesia as part of a "balanced" anesthetic technique but as complete anesthetic agents. Whether used as a bolus or infused by a pump, these agents are ubiquitous in today's anesthetic practice. Also, recurrent respiratory depression after apparent recovery from the administration of fentanyl have been reported.[43] Secondary rises in plasma fentanyl concentrations may or may not be causative.[44,45] Alfentanil, an opioid analgesic with a short terminal elimination half-time, has been associated with recurrent apnea in the PACU.[46] Signs and symptoms of continued narcotic activity besides somnolence include a slow respiratory pattern due to direct depression of brain stem centers. Minute ventilation may be preserved by increased tidal volumes. Examination of the pupils reveals miosis. Responsiveness to elevated $PaCO_2$ is depressed and respiration does not increase.

Metabolism of narcotics occurs primarily in the liver and kidneys. Decreased functioning of these organ systems is associated with increased elimination half-times, leading to prolonged somnolence in the recovery period.[47] Sensitivity to opiates remains stable with aging until about age 60, when it increases. Patients with reduced metabolic rates due to hypothermia or hypothyroidism are also at risk of narcotic overdose.

Multiple drug interactions are associated with narcotic utilization. Most significant combinations resulting in prolonged emergence are due to psychotropic agents (Table 2–5). Monoamine oxidase inhibitors are responsible for significant and potentially lethal interactions, especially with meperidine. This interaction is associated with respiratory depression, hypotension, and hyperpyrexia.[48] These agents also may be responsible for the metabolism of both narcotics and barbiturates.[49] The other agents listed generally intensify the sedative properties of the narcotics, an action that is used to limit the amount of opioid used.

Treatment of a suspected narcotic overdose is specific and supportive. The patient's airway and ventilation must be protected. The sedative or respiratory–depressive effects of narcotics can be terminated by the use of antagonists (naloxone). Care must be used in reversing the narcotic depression, however, as analgesia is also diminished, sympathetic activation occurs, and the occurrence of hypertension, tachycardia, acute pulmonary edema, and cardiac dysrhythmias has been described.[50] Titration of small doses (25 to 50 micrograms) slowly is the key if reversal is desired. An alternative specific reversal agent is nalbuphine, a mixed agonist–antagonist, which can reverse the respiratory depression while maintaining an acceptable level of analgesia.

TABLE 2–5. COMMON PSYCHOTROPIC AGENTS

Monoamine Oxidase Inhibitors

Tranylcypromine
Isocarboxizide
Phenelzine
Deprenyl

Tricyclic Antidepressants

Imipramine
Doxepin
Desipramine
Amitriptyline
Nortriptyline
Protriptyline

Phenothiazines

Chlorpromazine
Perphenazine
Trifluoperazine
Thioridazine
Fluphenazine

Thioxanthenes

Thiotixene
Chlorprothixene

Butyrophenones

Droperidol
Haloperidol

Lithium Carbonate

Benzodiazepines

This class of agents is extensively used in anesthesia for anxiolytic, amnestic, and sedative properties. The most commonly used drugs are diazepam, lorazepam, and midazolam. The drugs are dependent upon oxidative metabolism in the liver and are highly (> 96%) protein bound. They also demonstrate high lipid solubility, which terminates their action by redistribution to inactive binding sites in the fat. Accumulation of the drug from repeated doses may occur. Sedation in the postoperative period along with small but variable degrees of respiratory depression is not uncommon.

Patients at risk for prolonged or exaggerated effects of the benzodiazepines include the elderly and those with significant hepatic dysfunction. The elimination half-life for diazepam is prolonged from approximately 30 hours in the young adult to greater than 90 hours in the elderly.[51] Patients with cirrhosis demonstrate increased sensitivity to these agents presumably due to both decreased metabolism and decreased protein-binding sites with increased "free" drug.

Multiple drug interactions are possible with the benzodiazepines. The sedative properties of opioids, barbiturates, ketamine, acute alcohol ingestion, and potent inhalational agents are all augmented.[52] A significant interaction with the H_2 blocker cimetidine has been described, leading to prolonged sedation and elimination half-life of both diazepam and its active metabolites.[53]

Treatment is primarily supportive. A specific antagonist, flumazenil, is not yet available in the United States although it has been shown to be effective in European studies in reversing benzodiazepine-induced anesthesia at a dose of 6 mg/kg.[54]

Barbiturates, especially the thiobarbiturates thiopental and thiamylal, are extensively used as induction agents. These medications are highly protein bound but lipid soluble and thus rapidly cross the blood–brain barrier to suppress neural transmission in the CNS. A rapid redistribution into nonneural tissues terminates their activity while final elimination of the drug is dependent upon hepatic metabolism.

Prolonged activity of these agents is produced if repeated doses are utilized. Accumulation in the fat tissues and slow release maintains levels in the circulation. Obese patients have prolonged elimination half-lives and may be at risk for postoperative sedation.[55] Hepatic dysfunction predisposes to prolonged effects and patients with renal disease may have more "free" drug available due to competition for protein binding sites by metabolic waste products.[56] Barbiturates are ionized compounds and pH changes will modify the amount of lipid-soluble drug present.

An example is the effect of acidosis on deepening the level of thiopental sedation.s[57]

The treatment for relative or absolute overdosage is supportive.

Ketamine

Ketamine is a phencyclidine compound that produces "dissociative anesthesia." Its activity is terminated by redistribution with final elimination following hepatic degradation.

Emergence delirium appears in approximately 10 to 30% of patients. White and associates reported an increased incidence in patients older than 16 years; women; patients receiving more than 2 mg/kg; and those with preexisting personality disorders.[58] A proposed mechanism is continued dissociation and abnormal processing of visual, auditory, and position information. This problem may occur more frequently if droperidol, which can cause dysphoric reactions alone, is used with ketamine.[59]

Treatment is primarily supportive. If the cardiorespiratory systems are stable the delirium can be blunted with small doses of narcotics or benzodiazepines with careful monitoring.

Anticholinergics

The tertiary amines, atropine and scopolamine, are lipid soluble and readily cross the blood–brain barrier. Glycopyrrolate, another commonly used anticholinergic, is a quaternary amine compound and is excluded from the CNS.

The tertiary amines are responsible for CNS effects ranging from sedation to the more intense central anticholinergic syndrome, which is characterized by restlessness, somnolence, unresponsiveness, and hallucinations. Scopolamine is much more potent in this regard but the effect may be seen with atropine especially if used as part of reversal of neuromuscular blockade.[60] The central anticholinergic syndrome can be treated with the use of physostigmine.[61] Dosages in the range of 20 to 40 micrograms/kg will increase the availability of acetylcholine in the CNS and reverse the symptoms of this process. Physostigmine, a tertiary amine, is able to cross the blood–brain barrier and act centrally.

Scopolamine enhances the sedative effects of opioids, benzodiazepines, and barbiturates.

Muscle Relaxants

Multiple criteria are used to determine level of consciousness including respiratory pattern and movement. Residual effects of muscle relaxants may "mask" the central wakefulness of a patient in the PACU. The availability of peripheral nerve stimulators allows for rapid and objective assessment of the presence or absence of residual neuromuscular blockade.

Depolarizing Muscle Relaxants. Succinylcholine is the most commonly used depolarizing muscle relaxant in the United States. Its characteristics of rapid onset and rapid degradation and termination of action when used in appropriate doses make it a very useful agent. Several conditions may prolong the duration of paralysis. Phase II block occurs when the muscle membrane is exposed to large or repeated doses of depolarizing agents, which desensitize the receptors to further stimulation and disrupt the normal transmembrane fluxes of sodium, potassium, and calcium. Generally, the dosage range necessary to produce a Phase II block is about 2 to 4 mg/kg, but this is variable. The response to peripheral muscle stimulation is similar to that produced by nondepolarizing agents: (1) decreased twitch to single stimulus; (2) fade to continuous stimuli; (3) posttetanic potentiation; and (4) antagonism of block by anticholinesterase agents.[62] Of note is that this antagonism seems to occur during a "window" in the development of the block and may not be seen at other times.

A qualitative defect in plasma cholinesterase may cause prolonged blockade. Approximately one in 3200 patients are homozygous for atypical plasma cholinesterase, have a low dibucaine number when tested, and will demonstrate a prolonged blockade to succinylcholine.[63] The incidence of patients heterozygous for atypical plasma cholinesterase is approximately one in 480 patients, and they demonstrate a mild to moderate prolongation of the blockade. This prolonged effect is due to the continued presence of active drug at the muscle membrane. Patients may also present with low levels of normal cholinesterase, which usually occurs with severe hepatic dysfunction. Serum cholinergic activity is also decreased during the puerperium and the effects of succinylcholine is prolonged.[64]

Finally, the patient may have a normal quantity and quality of plasma cholinesterase but this is inhibited by drugs or chemicals. Patients with glaucoma or myasthenia gravis may be treated with anticholinesterase drugs (neostigmine or echothiophate). Individuals who are exposed to organophosphate inhibitors used as insecticides are also at risk of prolonged neuromuscular blockade.[65]

Whatever the mechanism of prolongation, the treatment of these patients entails the maintenance of respiration and airway control. This, and watchful waiting for the spontaneous recovery, is all that is required.

TABLE 2–6. NONDEPOLARIZING MUSCLE RELAXANTS

Long-Acting
D-Tubocurarine
Pancuronium
Gallamine
Metocurine

Intermediate-Acting
Vecuronium
Atracurium

Nondepolarizing Muscle Relaxants. Nondepolarizing agents may be classified into two broad categories—long-acting and intermediate–acting drugs (Table 2–6). The liver and kidney are responsible for the majority of metabolism and excretion of these drugs with the exception of atracurium, which is metabolized by plasma esterases and Hofmann degradation.[66]

Prolongation of action of these agents can occur by multiple mechanisms. Hepatic and renal disease have a marked effect upon the termination of activity of these drugs, affecting principally the long-acting agents, while atracurium and vecuronium are less affected.[67] Hypothermia will slow metabolism even in normal patients. The use of combinations of nondepolarizers is associated with duration of action beyond that of the individual compounds. This is presumed to be due to a combined pre- and postsynaptic action.[68]

Drug interactions are significant factors. Antibiotics, especially the aminoglycosides, can potentiate the activity of muscle relaxants.[69] Elevated serum magnesium (as seen in patients treated for pregnancy-induced hypertension) increases the sensitivity to blockade. Residual potent inhalational agents produce a dose-dependent increase in the degree of blockade,[70] as does the presence of adrenergic blocking agents.

Once the presence of continued blockade is confirmed, reversal, with anticholinesterase/anticholinergic agent combinations (neostigmine–glycopyrrolate, for example), can be accomplished. Alternatively, support of ventilation and airway can be provided and neuromuscular transmission allowed to recover spontaneously.

Miscellaneous Drugs

If drug-induced depression is suspected after the common anesthetic agents have been excluded, a thorough review of the patient's drug history is indicated. Discussion with family members, emergency response personnel, or any other source of information concerning the patient's prehospital history is indicated. A high index of suspicion is needed especially if illicit drug use is suspected. Toxicology screens of blood and urine may be indicated although access to results may be delayed.

Agents not considered "sedating" may produce these effects in certain populations. The example of the reaction of the elderly patient to elevated blood levels of cimetidine is instructive, as this is an agent that can produce profound confusion in this population.[71]

CLINICAL APPLICATION

The individual who displays delayed return of consciousness postoperatively should be treated as critically unstable until proven otherwise! A systematic approach is indicated.

Similar to any patient found unresponsive, the basic "ABCs" of airway, breathing, and circulation will identify immediately life-threatening problems that may be the cause or a side effect of the underlying process. When the patient has been stabilized, attention can be turned to further diagnostic and therapeutic measures based upon the information generated from patient records, monitoring, and laboratory investigation.

Communication among anesthesiologist, PACU staff, surgeon, and other consultants is imperative in ensuring appropriate care for the patient with delayed emergence.

REFERENCES

1. Raichle ME: The pathophysiology of brain ischemia. *Ann Neurol* 1983;13:2–10.
2. Adams RD, Victor M: *Principles of Neurology*, ed 3. New York, McGraw-Hill, 1985, pp 255–256.
3. Plum F, Posner JB: *The Diagnosis of Stupor and Coma*, ed 3. Philadelphia, Davis, 1980, p 2.
4. Lassen NA, Christensen MS: Physiology of cerebral blood flow. *Br J Anaesth* 1976;48:719–734.
5. Shapiro HM: Anesthesia effects upon cerebral blood flow, cerebral metabolism, electroencephalogram, and evoked potentials, in Miller RD (ed): *Anesthesia*, ed 2. New York, Churchill Livingstone, 1986, pp 1249–1288.
6. Sundt TM, Meyer FB, Anderson RE: Patterns of cerebral atherosclerosis and pathophysiology of ischemia, in Sundt TM (ed): *Occlusive Cerebrovascular Disease: Diagnosis and Surgical Management*. Philadelphia, Saunders, 1987, pp 11–18.
7. Perkins-Pearson NAK, Marshall WK, Bedford RF: Atrial pressures in the seated position: Implications for paradoxical air embolism. *Anesthesiology* 1982;57:493–497.
8. Kistler JP, Ropper AH, Martin JB: Cerebrovascular disease, in Braunwald EB, Isselbacher KJ, Petersdorf RG,

et al (eds): *Harrison's Principles of Internal Medicine*. New York, McGraw-Hill, 1987, pp 1931–1959.
9. Hamill JF, Bedford RF, Weaver DC, Colohan AR: Lidocaine before endotracheal intubation: Intravenous or laryngotracheal? *Anesthesiology* 1981;55:578–581.
10. Baker EP, Wepsic JG: Neurosurgical emergencies, in Wilkins EW (ed): *MGH Textbook of Emergency Medicine*. Baltimore, Williams & Wilkins, 1983, pp 600–602.
11. Kitahata LM, Katz JD: Tension pneumocephalus after posterior fossa craniotomy, a complication of the sitting position. *Anesthesiology* 1976;44:448–450.
12. Artru AA: Nitrous oxide plays a direct role in the development of tension pneumocephalus intraoperatively. *Anesthesiology* 1982;57:59–61.
13. Leibowitz MH, Blitt CB, Dillion JB: Enflurane-induced central nervous system excitation and its relation to carbon dioxide tension. *Anesth Analg* 1972;51:355–363.
14. Walts FL, Miller J, Davidson MB, Brown J: Perioperative management of diabetes mellitus. *Anesthesiology* 1981;55:104–109.
15. Kreisberg RA: Diabetic ketoacidosis: New concepts and trends in pathogenesis and treatment. *Ann Intern Med* 1978;88:681–695.
16. Arieff AI, Carroll HJ: Nonketotic hyperosmolar coma with hyperglycemia. *Medicine* 1972;51:73–94.
17. Mazoit J-X, Sandouk P, Zetlaoui P, Scherrmann J-M: Pharmacokinetics of unchanged morphine in normal and cirrhotic subjects. *Anesth Analg* 1987;66:293–298.
18. Chung H-M, Kluge R, Schrier RW, Anderson RJ: Postoperative hyponatremia: A prospective study. *Arch Intern Med* 1986;146:333–336.
19. Hurlbert BJ, Wingard DW: Water intoxication after 15 minutes of transurethral prostatic resection. *Anesthesiology* 1979;50:355–356.
20. Sterns RH, Riggs JE, Schochet SS: Osmotic demyelination syndrome following correction of hyponatremia. *N Engl J Med* 1986;314:1535–1542.
21. Stoelting RK: *Pharmacology and Physiology in Anesthetic Practice*. Philadelphia, Lippincott, 1987, p 536.
22. Delinger JK, Nahrwold ML, Gibbs PS, Lecky JH: Hypocalcemia during rapid blood transfusion in anaesthetized man. *Br J Anaesth* 1976;48:995–1000.
23. Delinger JK, Nahrwold ML: Cardiac failure associated with hypocalcemia. *Anesth Analg* 1976;55:34–36.
24. Elliott J: Magnesium sulfate as a tocolytic agent. *Am J Obstet Gynecol* 1983;147:277–285.
25. Muller MG: Anesthesia for the patient with renal dysfunction. *Int Anesth Clin* 1984;22:169–187.
26. Levelle JP, Jopling MW, Sklar OS: Perioperative hypothyroidism: An unusual postanesthetic diagnosis. *Anesthesiology* 1985;63:195–197.
27. Blum J: Myxedema coma. *Am J Med Sci* 1972;264:432–443.
28. Stehling LC: Anesthetic management of the patient with hyperthyroidism. *Anesthesiology* 1974;41:585–595.
29. Peters KR, Nance P, Wingard DW: Malignant hyperthyroidism or malignant hyperthermia? *Anesth Analg* 1981;60:613–615.
30. Gronert GA: Malignant hyperthermia. *Anesthesiology* 1980;53:395–423.

31. Guze BH, Baxter LR: Neuroleptic malignant syndrome. *N Engl J Med* 1985;313:163–166.

32. Weatherill D, Spence AA: Anaesthesia and disorders of the adrenal cortex. *Br J Anaesth* 1984;56:741–747.

33. Liddle GW: Addison's disease, in Wyngaarden JB, Smith LH (eds): *Cecil Textbook of Medicine*, ed 16. Philadelphia, Saunders, 1982, p 1229.

34. Catley DM: Postoperative analgesia and respiratory control. *Int Anesth Clin* 1984;22:4:95–111.

35. Davis WB, Rennard SI, Bitterman PB, Crystal RG: Pulmonary oxygen toxicity: Early reversible changes in human alveolar structures induced by hyperoxia. *N Engl J Med* 1983;309:878–883.

36. Mecca RS: Postanesthetic recovery, in Barash PG, Cullen BF, Stoelting RK (eds): *Clinical Anesthesia*. Philadelphia, Lippincott, 1989, pp 1399–1406.

37. Brodsky JB, Bravo JJ: Acute postoperative withdrawal syndrome. *Anesthesiology* 1976;44:519–520.

38. Wong KC: Physiology and pharmacology of hypothermia. *West J Med* 1983;138:227–232.

39. Rodriquez JL, Weissman C, Damask MC, et al: Physiologic requirements during rewarming: Suppression of the shivering response. *Crit Care Med* 1983;11:490–497.

40. Vitez TS, White PF, Eger EI II: Effects of hypothermia on halothane MAC and isoflurane MAC in the rat. *Anesthesiology* 1974;40:80–86.

41. Palahniuk RJ, Shnider SM, Eger EI: Pregnancy decreases the requirement of inhaled anesthetic agents. *Anesthesiology* 1974;41:82–83.

42. Miller RD, Way WL, Eger EI II: The effect of alphamethyldopa, reserpine, quanethidine, and iproniazid on minimum alveolar anesthetic requirement (MAC). *Anesthesiology* 1969;29:1153–1158.

43. Becke LD, Paulson BA, Miller RD, et al: Biphasic respiratory depression of fentanyl-droperidol: a fenterylalene used to supplement nitrous oxide anesthesia. *Anesthesiology* 1976;44:291–296.

44. Jaffe RS, Moldenhauer CC, Hug CC, et al: Nalbuphine antagonism of fentanyl induced ventilatory depression: A randomized trial. *Anesthesiology* 1988;68:254–260.

45. McQuay HJ, Moore RA, Paterson GMG, et al: Plasma fentanyl concentrations and clinical observations during and after operation. *Br J Anesth* 1979;51:543–550.

46. Jaffe RS, Coalson D: Recurrent respiratory depression after alfentanil administration. *Anesthesiology* 1989;70:151–153.

47. Don HF, Dieppa RD, Taylor P: Narcotic analgesics in anuric patients. *Anesthesiology* 1975;42:745–747.

48. Brown TCK, Cass NM: Beware—The use of MDA inhibitors is increasing again. *Anaesth Intensive Care* 1979;7:65–68.

49. Eade NR, Renton KW: The effect of phenelzine and tranylcypromine in the degradation of meperidine. *J Pharmacol Exp Ther* 1970;173:31–36.

50. Flacke JW, Flacke WE, Williams GD: Acute pulmonary edema following naloxone reversal of high dose morphine anesthesia. *Anesthesiology* 1977;47:376–378.

51. Klotz U, Avant GR, Hoyumda A, et al: The effect of age and liver disease on the disposition and elimination of diazepam in adult man. *J Clin Invest* 1975;55:347–359.

52. Gyermek L: Clinical effects of diazepam prior to and during general anesthesia. *Curr Ther Res* 1975;17:175–188.

53. Greenblatt DJ, Abernathy DR, Morse DS, et al: Clinical importance of the interaction of diazepam and cimetidine. *N Engl J Med* 1984;310:1639–1643.

54. Duvaldstin P, Lebrault C, Guirimand F, et al: Efficacy of flumazenil reversal after midazolam induced anesthesia. *Anesthesiology* 1988;69 3A 560.

55. Jung D, Mayersohn DR, Perrier D, et al: Thiopental disposition in lean and obese patients underoing surgery. *Anesthesiology* 1982;56:269–274.

56. Ghoneim MM, Pandya H: Plasma protein binding of thiopental in patients with impaired renal or hepatic function. *Anesthesiology* 1975;42:545–549.

57. Stoelting RK: *Pharmacology and Physiology in Anesthetic Practice*. Philadelphia, Lippincott, 1987, p 106.

58. White PF, Way WL, Trevor AJ: Ketamine—Its pharmacology and therapeutic uses. *Anesthesiology* 1982;56:119–136.

59. Erbguth PH, Reiman B, Klein RL: The influence of chlorpromazine, diazepam and droperidol on emergence from ketamine. *Anesth Analg* 1972;51:693–700.

60. Baraka A, Yared J-P, Karam A-M, Winnie A: Glycopyrrolate-neostigmine and atropine-neostigmine mixtures affect postanesthetic arousal times differently. *Anesth Analg* 1980;59:431–434.

61. Duvoisin RC, Katz RL: Reversal of central anticholinergic syndrome in man by physostigmine. *JAMA* 1968–206:1963–1965.

62. Standaert FG: Basic physiology and pharmacology of the neuromuscular junction, in Miller RD (ed): *Anesthesia*, ed 2. New York: Churchill Livingstone, 1986, p 855.

63. Kalow W, Genest K: A method for the detection of atypical forms of human serum cholinesterase. Determination of dibucaine numbers. *Can J Biochem* 1957;35:339–353.

64. Shnider SM: Serum cholinesterase activity during pregnancy, labor and the puerperium. *Anesthesiology* 1965;26:335–341.

65. Milby TH: Prevention and management of organophosphate poisoning. *JAMA* 1971;216:2131–2133.

66. Fisher DM, Canfell PC, Fahey MR, et al: Elimination of atracurium in humans: Contribution of Hofmann elimination and ester hydrolysis verses organ-based elimination. *Anesthesiology* 1986;65:6–12.

67. Duvaldestin P, Agoston S, Henzel E: Pancuronium pharmacokinetics in patients with liver cirrhosis. *Br J Anesth* 1978;50:1131–1136.

68. Taylor P: Are neuromuscular blocking agents more efficacious in pairs? *Anesthesiology* 1985;63:1–3.

69. Sokoll MD, Gergis SD: Antibiotics and neuromuscular function. *Anesthesiology* 1981;55:148–159.

70. Waud BE: Decrease in dose requirements of d-tubocurarine by volatile anesthetics. *Anesthesiology* 1979;51:298–302.

71. Schentag JJ, Cerra FB, Calleri G, et al: Pharmacokinetic and clinical studies in patients with cimetidine associated mental confusion. *Lancet* 1979;1:177–178.

3 | Postoperative Drug Interactions

Hideo Nagashima

A study by Smith and associates showed an exponential increase in incidence of adverse drug interactions in relation to the number of drugs given.[1] Patients coming to the postanesthetic care unit (PACU) have been subjected to an enthusiastic drug administration and treatment by the anesthesiologist during surgery together with other drugs given before surgery or administered for the control of chronic ailments. Furthermore, these patients probably will receive more medications in the PACU, such as analgesics for pain control, antibiotics for prophylactic infection control, drugs that attenuate noxious hyper- or hypoactive autonomic nervous system symptoms, (alpha, beta blockers or stimulants, Ca^{2+} channel blockers, etc), or antiemetics.

A survey of drug therapy given to 100 patients, ranging in age from 7 months to 96 years old, consecutively admitted to our PACU revealed that an average of 4, 7.6, and 4.5 different drugs have been given to these patients before, during, and after surgery, respectively (Table 3-1). An overall average of 16 different drugs was given perioperatively. Although there were few adverse drug reactions encountered in the patients surveyed, a higher incidence of drug interactions may be anticipated among surgical patients, particularly after complicated surgical procedures and anesthetic treatments. Knowledge of drug actions and interactions and understanding of pathophysiologic conditions of patients for drug therapy lead to proper institution of treatment.

In this chapter, basic information on drug actions and interactions commonly encountered during perioperative periods is briefly presented since there are many informative articles on this subject available.[2-4]

Possible or anticipated adverse drug interactions and the undesirable responses will be discussed and illustrated with case presentations.

GENERAL PRINCIPLES OF DRUG INTERACTIONS

Responses after combined use of two or more drugs administered concomitantly or sequentially are either enhancement or diminution of the individual effects. These responses could be beneficial or hazardous to patients. Drug interactions are mostly based on physical, chemical, pharmacokinetic, and pharmacologic reactions.

Physical and chemical interactions are well exemplified by the mechanism of action of protamine sulfate for reversal of the anticoagulant activity of heparin, which is based on acid–base reaction. The diminished effects of muscle relaxants (pancuronium bromide, succinylcholine chloride, vecuronium bromide, atracurium besylate) mixed with thiopental sodium, causing precipitation, are also results of acid–base reaction.

Pharmacokinetic interactions may be the results of altered absorption, distribution, metabolism, or elimination. Drug distribution depends on apparent kinetics as well as kinetic volume of distribution, plasma protein binding of drugs, and degree of biologic membrane permeability. Alteration of these factors governing drug distribution results in unexpected responses to the drug given. For example, protein binding of neostigmine may be 95%.[5] Since the free fraction of the drug is capable of reaching its site of action, an increased effect of neostigmine, which may be undesirable, such as strong muscarinic action, may result if it is displaced from plasma protein by other drugs with high protein binding like diazepam. Another example is patients with liver disease in whom verapamil disposition is markedly prolonged.[6] The combined use of propranolol and verapamil for the treatment of supraventricular tachycardia must be carefully administered. An enhanced effect of verapamil may be seen and severe bradycardia, which may lead to disastrous outcome,

TABLE 3-1. SURVEY OF DRUG THERAPY GIVEN TO 100 PATIENTS

Periods	Number of Drugs Received (Mean ± SEM)
Preoperative	4.0 ± 0.3
Intraoperative	7.6 ± 0.3
Postoperative	4.5 ± 0.4
Perioperative	16.0 ± 0.8

may develop. Sudden withdrawal of phenobarbital used as an anticonvulsant in patients with a convulsive disorder may cause an increase of anticoagulant activity of bishydroxycoumarin (Dicumarol), since phenobarbital induces enzymes that increase the rate of metabolic biotransformation of Dicumarol.

An example of pharmacologic interactions is the interaction of succinylcholine or decamethonium with cholinergic receptors, resembling the effect of the physiologic transmitter. Competitive inhibition of d-tubocurarine to prevent the adsorption of acetylcholine to the cholinergic receptors is another example of pharmacologic interactions. Interaction at the site of action is demonstrated by potentiation of the neuromuscular blocking effect of certain antibiotics (such as kanamycin sulfate, polymyxin B sulfate) by calcium channel blockers (such as verapamil).[7] Verapamil causes reduction of the available intercellular calcium iron, which is responsible for the release of acetylcholine.

POSSIBLE OR ANTICIPATED ADVERSE DRUG INTERACTION AND THE UNDESIRABLE RESPONSES

In our small survey (100 patients), various surgical procedures such as pediatric, general orthopedic, gynecologic, cardiac, neurosurgical, and peripherovascular surgeries are included. Depending on pathologic conditions, surgical procedures, and age, perioperative medications, including anesthetics, differ from one to the other. Several cases are presented.

Case 1. A 2-year-old girl, weighing 9.6 kg, diagnosed to have tetralogy of Fallot with pulmonary atresia, was admitted for surgical repair. The patient had had an uneventful right Blalock-Taussig shunt performed at the age of 4 months. Cardiac catherterization under basal narcosis, consisting of meperidine 2 mg/kg and phenergan 1 mg/kg intramuscularly (IM), demonstrated a considerable right-left shunt with unsaturation of the left-sided blood (O_2 percent saturation: right atrium = 57, right ventricle = 63; left ventricle = 79; aorta = 75). Prior to the surgery she was cyanotic but not on any medication. On the day of surgery the patient was premedicated with pentobarbital 30 mg IM and atropine 0.1 mg two hours preoperatively. Anesthesia was induced with 100% O_2 containing 0.5 to 1.0% halothane and increments of fentanyl. A nasotracheal intubation with #4.0 Portex tube was facilitated by intravenous administration of 1.0 mg pancuronium. Anesthesia was maintained solely with increments of fentanyl, and muscular relaxation (monitored by arrest of diaphragmatic movement) was achieved with pancuronium. Before com-

mencement of bypass the patient received 30 mg of heparin. Arterial blood gas analyses revealed pH 7.39, P_{CO_2} 33.0 mm Hg, P_{O_2} 60.1 mm Hg. During extracorporeal circulation moderate hypothermia (24°C) was used and the perfusion pressure was kept at around 30 mm Hg with incremental use (7 times) of 20 μg neosynephrine. Surgical repair was uneventful after 2 hours and 20 minutes perfusion. Weaning from extracorporeal circulation was uneventful. Total protamine given was 40 mg. After the surgical repair arterial blood gas analyses was pH 7.37, P_{CO_2} 40.5 mm Hg, P_{O_2} 279.2 mm Hg, and O_2 saturation 99.7%.

After seven hours of surgery and anesthesia the patient was responsive and transferred to the PACU, her ventilation supported. Other drugs given during the procedure were oxicillin as a prophylactic antibiotic and dopamine drip (8 to 25 μg/kg/min) near the end of surgery to support cardiac performance. In the PACU the infusion of dopamine was discontinued and dobutamine 10 μg/kg/min was started. Vital signs at that time were BP 80/50, HR 160/min, CVP 14, LA 15 mm Hg, pH 7.34, P_{CO_2} 45.5 mm Hg, P_{O_2} 136.5 mm Hg, HCO_3 24.0. Her condition remained satisfactory for the next two hours and then she was transferred to the pediatric ICU. In the late evening of the same day (six hours later), an excess salivation was noted, requiring suctioning. During suctioning, the patient became agitated and extubated herself. The patient was ventilated via mask immediately. An anesthesiologist was called and succinylcholine 10 mg was given through the central cannula. An attempt to intubate was unsuccessful. A second dose of succinylcholine 10 mg was given. Immediately thereafter, severe bradycardia ensued and cardiac arrest followed. Cardiopulmonary resuscitation consisting of open chest massage, administration of atropine, epinephrine $NaHCO_3$, $CaCl_2$, was unsuccessful. The patient expired after an hour of resuscitation attempt.

It has been reported that sinus bradycardia after a second dose of succinylcholine develops among infants and children with higher incidence than in adults, due to stimulation of muscarinic receptors in sinus nodes.[8] It is suggested that succinylmonocholine and choline, metabolites of succinylcholine after hydrolysis, may sensitize the myocordium. In this case, the interaction of a mother compound and its metabolite was probably responsible for the arrest. The intravenous use of anticholinergics, such as atropine and glycopyrbolate, prior to the administration of succinylcholine (especially if two doses are given) prevents this complication.

Case 2. A 4-year-old, 15.0-kg, boy with bronchopulmonary dysplasia resulting from prolonged mechanical ventilation after meconium aspiration at birth, was admitted for bronchoscopy, laryngoscopy, and possible decannulation of the tracheostomy tube. The boy had a history of chronic asthma. His daily maintenance medications included theophylline (Theo-Dur) orally (PO) 100 mg tid, prednisone 15 mg PO daily, and use of albuterol (Ventolin) inhalation aerosol. On the day of surgery pentobarbital 30 mg and atropine 0.2 mg were given IM as premedication an hour prior to scheduled surgery. Anesthesia was induced with N_2O and O_2 containing halothane via a tracheostomy tube. After the patient was well anesthetized, the tracheostomy tube was replaced with #3.5 endotracheal tube orally. The remaining anesthetic procedure was uneventful and revision of the tracheal stoma was successfully performed. At the end of the procedure a prophylactic antibiotic cefazolin (Kefzol) 250 mg was given intravenously. The patient was alert and breathing spontaneously on transfer to the PACU. Upon arrival, his breath sounds were good with a few scattered rhonchi. Lips and nail beds were pink and he was lying on his left side. Vital signs were satisfactory. About 15 minutes after arrival in the PACU the patient became agitated and started to cry. A nurse noted that his face was swelling and his eyes were puffy. Subcutaneous emphysema of his chest and shoulders became more obvious. Diphenhydramine 25 mg and epinephrine 0.1 mg were given intravenously. His respiration became labored and O_2 saturation began to fall. After sedation with morphine sulfate and diazepam, an orotracheal intubation was accomplished and assisted ventilation established. After a stormy three days in the pediatric ICU, the patient was successfully weaned off from the ventilator. There were no apparent consequences from this incidence.

The case presented is not clearly due to drug interaction but rather to an anaphylactoid reaction to cefazolin. Detailed investigation of this boy revealed that he once developed a rash after the use of penicillin. Because of the similarity in chemical structure of penicillin and cephalosporin (cefazoline is a first-generation cephalosporin), patients who are allergic to penicillin may manifest cross-reactivity to cephalosporins (as many as 20% of patients who are allergic to penicillin).[9] Particularly the patient who exhibited recent allergic reaction to penicillin should probably not receive cephalosporins.

Case 3. An 80-year-old female, weighing approximately 50 kg, was scheduled for left hemiarthroplasty for intratrochanteric fracture. The patient was hospitalized ten days prior to the proposed surgery after a fall that caused the fracture. Because of complex medical conditions, she required extensive preoperative medical assessment, including admission to the medical intensive care unit where a pulmonary artery catheter was inserted for optimal fluid therapy, treatment of atrial fibrillation (AF) (ventricular rate of 170/min), and control of urinary tract infection (fever 102°F at admission).

After intense medical treatment, consisting of combinations of digoxin, propranolol, and procainamide, her medical condition improved (BP 130/70, HR 100/min, RR 24). Fever, however, persisted (at around 101 to 102°F) and pulmonary infection developed. Fixation of her fractured hip and institution of early mobilization was proposed. Cardiac parameters were within acceptable values. Anesthesia was commenced with a sleeping dose of thiamylal (100 mg total), fentanyl, and isoflurane with oxygen. An orotracheal intubation was facilitated with vecuronium 8 mg. Soon after the induction of anesthesia, hypertension and tachycardia developed, and additional digoxin and a nitroglycerine drip were given with satisfactory results. Arterial blood gas analyses (ABG) and hemodynamics of the patient were monitored throughout surgery. Surgery was completed after four hours.

Upon arrival in the PACU, the patient's vital signs were stable, she was alert and agitated by the orotracheal tube in situ which was removed. Soon after, her O_2 saturation began to fall and ABG indicated inadequate ventilation.

Reinsertion of the orotracheal tube was performed and mechanical ventilation initiated. Her cardiac function, however, began to deteriorate and vigorous treatment, including dobutamine (10 μg/kg/min) and dopamine (2 μg/kg/min) together with digoxin was started.

Her condition improved gradually and she was weaned over five days. A survey of medication given to this patient during the postoperative period revealed that dobatamine, dopamine, digoxin, procainamide, nitropaste, pilocarpine, ranitidine (Zantac), metamucil, metronidazole (Flagyl), gentamycin, heparin, vistaril, morphine, and lorazepan (Ativan), were administered.

In spite of numerous medications given to this patient perioperatively, no adverse drug interactions were observed. Undesirable drug interactions could, however, be anticipated in this case. For instance, hypokalemia resulting from rapid fluid replacement for the treatment of dehydration may precipitate digitalis toxicity. The use of quinine also increases digoxin toxicity probably due to (1) reduction of renal clearance of the drug; and (2) displacement of digoxin from tissue binding sites, which subsequently increases the plasma level of the drug.

Since phenothiazines and antipsychotic drugs have dopanergic receptor blocking action, the effect of dopamine may be reduced in the presence of these drugs. Although ranitidine, a histamine H_2 blocker, has fewer side effects and interactions with other drugs, some of the significant drug interactions must be considered. Decrease in clearance of warfarin[10] and phenytoin[11] by H_2 blockers leads to increase in prothrombin time and toxic effects of phenytoin,[11] respectively. Other drugs that interact with H_2 blockers include benzodiazepines[12] (prolongs their effects) and propranolol (increases the incidence of bradycardia).[13]

Lorazepam possesses an anticonvulsant effect. A shorter-acting benzodiazepine is, however, preferred over lorazepam for the treatment of local-anesthetic-induced convulsions.[14]

Case 4. A 70-year-old-male, weighing 134 pounds, who presented with an ischemic right foot for 8 months, was admitted for reconstructive vascular procedure of the foot. The patient's past medical history included right bundle branch block, myocardial infarction (1969, 1984) and coronary arteriosclerosis. Daily maintenance medications were furosemide 40 mg PO bid, digoxin 0.25 mg PO od, nitroglycerine 6.5 mg PO qid, captopril 6.25 mg PO qid, and acetaminaphen with codeine (Tylenol #3) one to two tablets PO q four to six hours. An hour prior to the surgery, the patient received diphenhydramine 25 mg and morphine sulfate 5.0 mg IM as premedication. During eight and a half hours of surgical and anesthetic intervention, the patient received nitrous oxide, isoflurane, thiamylal, vecuronium, fentanyl, diazepam, lidocaine, pancuronium, nitroglycerin infusion, heparin, cefazolin, diphenhydramine, and protamine. Surgery and anesthesia were uneventful. In the PACU, together with daily maintenance medications for his cardiac condition, meperidine, phenergan, and oxycodone hydrochloride (Percocet) were given for pain relief. Later pain medication was changed to morphine, given intravenously through a patient-controlled analgesia device. Dipyridamole (Persantine), insulin, aspirin, and KCl solution were also prescribed. The patient was discharged home a week after the procedure.

Although no adverse drug interactions were observed in this patient after receiving 26 different medications during his hospitalization, several drugs are to be considered for possible undesirable drug effects. A concomitant use of furosemide, a potent diuretic, with digoxin must be carefully regulated. Hypokalemia resulting from diuresis may potentiate the action of digitalis[15] and lead to cardiac dysrhythmias. Overdose or prolonged use of nitroglycerin infusion may cause methemoglobinemia and more than 7 μg/kg/min infusion may be dangerous.[16] Although captopril, an angiotensin-converting enzyme inhibitor, has very few side effects, the use of this drug in patients with renal dysfunction may cause a high incidence of neutropenia. A concommitant use of capto-

pril with a recently instituted diuretic therapeutic agent may result in augmentation of the hypotensive effect of captopril. A potentiating effect of captopril by other vasodilating agents is quite common.

Case 5. A 64-year-old male with arteriosclerotic heart disease and severe postinfarction angina requiring an intraaortic balloon pump assist was scheduled for quadruple coronary artery vein bypass graft on an emergency basis. The patient complained of right upper quadrant pain with fever of 101°F, suspicious of mild acute cholecystitis. Medications included diazepam 5.0 mg PO PRN, which was changed to lorazepam 2 mg for sedation, acetaminophen for pain and fever, cefaxitin 2 g every eight hours, regular insulin coverage for IV infusion of 5% dextrose in water, chlorpropamide (Diabinese) 250 mg od, isosorbide dinitrate (Isordil) 30 mg tid, propranolol 30 mg PO tid, diltiazem (Cardizam) 60 mg tid, and furosemide 80 mg PO qid. Anesthesia was induced with 50 mg of ketamine IV, increments of sufentanil, midazolam, vecuronium for intubation, and pancuronium for maintenance of muscular relaxation, and occasional use of neosynephrine 0.1 mg to maintain adequate blood pressure and perfusion pressure during extracorporeal circulation. After two and a half hours of bypass, epinephrine, dobutamine, and dopamine drips were required for support of cardiac function for approximately one hour. These infusions were later replaced with nitroglycerin. In addition to the nine medications given intraoperatively, cefazolin, heparin, and protamine were administered. The patient's condition was unstable in the PACU, requiring mechanical and pharmacologic support for adequate cardiac performance. After five days of intensive care, the patient expired. The total number of drugs given to this patient perioperatively was 29.

We believe there were no adverse drug interactions responsible for the unfortunate outcome. Several drugs that this patient had taken, however, have possible important drug interactions worthy of discussion. The hypoglycemic action of chlorpropamide may be potentiated by nonsteroidal antiinflammatory agents that are highly protein bound. In patients receiving salicylates, sulfonamides, chloramphenicol, coumarins, and monoamine oxidase inhibitors, a hypoglycemic response should be anticipated. The concommitant use of beta-adrenergic blockers (propranolol in this patient) or digitalis with calcium-channel blockers (diltiazem in this patient) is quite effective in prolonging the AV node refractory period, thus slowing the heart rate. Caution must be taken not to cause an undesirable additive effect from combinations. The use of ketamine for the induction of anesthesia to this patient was appropriate because anesthetic doses of ketamine stimulate the cardiovascular system.[17] In large doses, however, ketamine depresses myocardial function.[18] One must remember that ketamine, like cocaine, enhances the dysrhythmogenicity of epinephrine.[19]

Case 6. A 62-year-old female, with a history of hypertension for many years, underwent left pterional craniotomy for clipping of a left posterior communicating artery aneurysm. The patient had had angina for two years. Her daily medications included nifedipine (Procardia) 10 mg tid, digoxin 0.25 mg od, aspirin 325 mg od, and nitroglycerin sublingually for anginal pain. Aspirin was, however, discontinued four days prior to the surgery. On the morning of surgery, in addition to the nifedipine, nitroglycerin, and digoxin, metoprolol (Lopressor) 100 mg, dexamethasone (Decadron) 10 mg, diazepam 10 mg, ranitidine 150 mg, and oxacillin were given. Anesthesia was induced with sufentanil and a sleeping dose of thiamylal. An orotracheal intubation was facilitated by the use of pancuronium. Lidocaine 75 mg was given intravenously to alleviate sympathetic response during intubation. Anesthesia was maintained with oxygen with air containing isoflurane. To control hypertension during the course of the procedure, 5 mg increments of labetalol were given intravenously. Other medications given were mannitol, KCl, and a mixture of glycopyrrolate and pyridostigmine for reversal of neuromuscular blockade. Naloxone was also given to antogonize the effect of sufentanil. Anesthesia was uneventful.

In the PACU, she was appropriately responsive, vital signs stable. Approximately two hours later, she became hypotensive, BP 80/50, and the level of consciousness decreased. The trachea was reintubated and an infusion of neosynephrine started. Four hours later, the blood pressure stable, she was again extubated.

Labetalol is a blocker of both peripheral alpha- and beta-receptors. Because of minimal effect on heart rate and cardiac output, labetalol has more desirable and predictable effects on a decrease in both blood pressure and vascular resistance.[20] The bioavailability of labetalol is greatly affected by the concommitant use of cimetidine and subsequently the hypotensive effect of labetalol is enhanced. The use of labetalol during halothane anesthesia requires special attention because the hypotensive effect of both agents are synergistic. The anticonvulsant phenytoin is used to reduce the epileptic incidence after craniotomy. Although this patient had not received phenytoin, pharmacokinetics of dexamethasone is affected by phenytoin and plasma clearance of the steroid is markedly shortened.[21] Naloxone was administered to reverse the effect of sufentanyl at the end of surgery. Naloxone is effective in antagonizing narcotic-

induced central nervous system and respiratory depressions. The use of naloxone, however, causes nausea and vomiting. Although it was been reported that a large dose of naloxone (4 and 8 mg) given intravenously to a normal (unanesthetized or unpremedicated) subject did not cause central nervous system excitation or cardiovascular stimulation,[22] possible stimulating effects on this system would be expected.[23] Serious consequences after the use of naloxone include acute pulmonary edema.[24]

Case 7. A 19-year-old white female had reflex sympathetic dystrophy for two years, manifested after a ball hit the right medial aspect of her ankle while she was playing softball. She developed chronic severe pain, was admitted for 22 days, and was treated with epidural bupivacaine. Subsequently, she became symptom-free until she reinjured her ankle. She developed severe pain. Epidural bupivacaine treatment did not alleviate the pain this time. She was referred for quanethidine Bier block. Her medications consisted of meperidine (Demerol) 100 mg PO q three hours, nortriptyline (Pamelor) 50 mg PO, and baclofan 20 mg PO bid. The patient complained that while she was receiving the pain treatment she felt dizzy and became unconscious (seizures?). Electroencephalograms were taken and repeatedly showed ''epileptiform'' activity. The patient was given phenytoin (Dilantin) 300 mg medication once a day at bedtime. She became tremulous and had intermittent gastrointestinal distress. She was referred for quanethidine Bier block. Her last meperidine dose was at 6:30 AM. While the tourniquet was applied on her thigh prior to intravenous guanethidine instillation she complained of discomfort followed by oposthitonic activity, hyperextension of her body, and tonic activity with hyperventilation. Diazepam 20 mg followed by 375 mg of thiopental were given intravenously to control seizures. To rule out meperidine withdrawal, fentanyl (total of 100 μg in increments) was given intravenously. Soon after this, the patient became quiet, and shortly thereafter regained orientation and stable vital signs.

The patient was admitted to the intensive care unit (ICU). She continued to receive daily maintenance doses of meperidine, phenytoin, and Lioneral. Diazepam, hydrotizine, and lorazepam were added to the above medications. In the late evening of the same day in the ICU the patient manifested similar seizure activity, which was controlled with lorazepam 2 mg and phenytoin 250 mg IV. The following day at around noon, she had another episode of seizures. Phenytoin 10 mg/kg was given to control the seizures. Neurologic consultations were made and a diagnosis of pseudoseizures caused by emotional problems or other causes was made. Meperidine was discontinued and was replaced with oxycodone tablets q four hours in lieu of the neurotoxic of meperidine. The patient continued to have brief periods of seizures but the intensity and duration lessened. Two days after the discontinuation of meperidine no seizures were observed. The patient stated pain on her foot became considerably less and she was able to move it freely. After three days of hospitalization (two days after discontinuation of meperidine) the patient was discharged home with oxycodone tablets PRN.

In terms of drug interactions, phenytoin possesses two important pharmacologic properties: (1) it enhances drug metabolizing enzymes although it is a weak hepatic microsomal enzyme inducer; and (2) it binds strongly (about 90%) to plasma protein, mainly albumin. The former probably shortens the action of a compound by rapid metabolism on one hand, but increases plasma concentration of metabolites of the compound on the other. The latter increases the active free fraction of other drugs by occupying plasma protein and subsequently enhances the pharmacologic effect of the other drugs. In this case, it appears that the institution of phenytoin for her mild seizure manifestation a week prior to the guanethidine treatment accelerated meperidine metabolism and subsequently increased plasma concentration of one of the metabolites of meperidine, normeperidine. Normeperidine is a proconvulsant.[25,26] A significant correlation between plasma concentration of normeperidine level and manifestations of central nervous system irritability has been reported.[27] A mean plasma normeperidine level of 530 mg/mL causes apprehension, tremors occur at 643 mg/mL, and clonic movement and seizures occur at 1286 mg/mL. A long plasma half-life of normeperidine (14 to 20 hours), in contrast to that of meperidine (3 to 4 hours), increases the undesirable effects. Although there was no determination of plasma level of normeperidine in this case, from the point of view of her clinical course, it is apparent that her abnormal neurologic manifestations were caused by normeperidine, a resultant product of phenytoin–meperidine interaction.[28]

SUMMARY

Because of the many reports on drug actions and interactions available, an outline of some principles and mechanisms of drug actions and interactions has been briefly presented here. With case presentations, drug actions and interactions commonly encountered perioperatively were discussed. As stated before, fortunately there are not many adverse drug reactions seen perioperatively. Close communication of pre- and intraoperative drug surveillance, correct diagnosis, knowledge of pharmacology of drugs and void of iatrogenesis are important. All members of the medical team should avoid addition of another drug to a patient's regimen unless its therapeutic effect is clearly indicated. Anticipation of possible adverse drug responses can alleviate undesirable consequences or quickly institute appropriate treatment.

REFERENCES

1. Smith JW, Seidl LG, Cluff LE: Studies on the epidemiology of adverse drug reactions. V clinical factors susceptibility. *Ann Intern Med* 65:629, 1966.
2. Nagashima H: Drug interactions in the recovery room, in Andrews IC, Frost EA (eds): *The Recovery Room*. Boston, Little, Brown, 1983, pp 93–105.
3. Hansten PD: *Drug Interactions*. Philadelphia, Lea & Febiger, 1971.
4. Griffin JP, D'Arcy PF: *A Manual of Adverse Drug Interactions*. Bristol, England, Wright, 1975.
5. Ty Smith N, Corbascio AN: *Drug Interactions in Anesthesia*. Philadelphia, Lea & Febiger, 1986.
6. Foldes FF, Forbat AF: Fundamental considerations of drug interactions. *Excerpt Medica*, series no. 347, Sept 1974.
7. Woodcock BG, Rietbrock I, Wohringer HF, Reitbrock N: Verapamil disposition in liver disease and intensive-care patients: Kinetics, clearance and apparent blood flow relationships. *Clin Pharmacol Ther* 1981;29:27–34.
8. Bikhazi GB, Flores C, Foldes FF: The neuromuscular (NM) effect of verapamil–antibiotic combinations. *Pharmacologist* 1984;26:127.
9. Craythorne NWB, Turndorf H, Dripps RD: Changes in pulse rate and rhythm associated with the use of succinylcholine in anesthetized children. *Anesthesiology* 1960;21:465–470.
10. Sande MA, Mandell GL: Antimicrobial Agents, in Gilman AG, Goodman LS, Rall TW, Murad F (eds): *Goodman and Gilman's the Pharmacological Basis of Therapeutics*. New York, Macmillan, 1980, pp 1066–1094.
11. Silver BA, Bell WR: Cimetidine potentiation of the hypoprothrombinemic effect of warfarin. *Ann Intern Med* 1979;90:348–349.
12. Hetzel DJ, Bochner F, Hallpike JF, Shearman DJC: Cimetidine interaction with phenytoin. *Br Med J* 1981;282:1512.
13. Koltz U, Reimann I: Delayed clearance of diazepam due to cimetidine. *N Engl J Med* 1980;302:1012–1014.
14. Feely J, Wilkinson GR, Wood AJJ: Reduction of liver blood flow and propranalol metabolism by cimetidine. *N Engl J Med* 1981;304:692–695.
15. Feinstein MB, Lenard W, Mathias J: The antagonism of local anesthetic induced convulsions by the benzodiazepine derivative diazepam. *Arch Int Pharmacodyn Ther*, 1970;187:144.
16. Merin RG, Bastron RD: Diuretics, in Smith N, Carbascio AN (eds): *Drug Interactions in Anesthesia*. Philadelphia, Lea & Febiger, 1986, pp 145–162.
17. Gibson GR, Hunter JR, Raabe DS Jr, et al: Methemo-

globinemia produced by high-dose intravenous nitro-glycerin. *Ann Intern Med* 1982;96:615–616.

18. Traber DL, Wilson RD: Involvement of the sympathetic nervous system in the pressor response to Ketamine. *Anesth Analg* 1969;48:248–252.

19. Dowdy EG, Kaya K: Studies of the mechanism of cardiovascular response to CI-581. *Anesthesiology* 1968;29:931–943.

20. Koehntop DE, Liao J-C, Van Bergen FH: Effects of pharmacologic alterations of adrenergic mechanisms by cocaine, tropolone, aminophylline and ketamine on epinephrine induced arrhythmias during halothane–nitrous oxide anesthesia. *Anesthesiology* 1977;46:83–93.

21. Wallin JD, O'Neill WM: Labetalol. Current research and therapeutic status. *Arch Intern Med* 1983;143:485–490.

22. Chalk JB, Ridgeway K, Brophy T, et al: Phenytoin impairs the bioavailability of dexamethasone in neurological and neurosurgical patients. *J Neurol Neurosurg Psych* 1984;47:1087–1090.

23. Duncalf D, Nagashima H, Duncalf RM: Naloxone fails to antagonize thiopental anesthesia. *Anesth Analg* 1978;57:558–562.

24. Tanaka GY; Hypertensive reaction to naloxone. *JAMA*, 1974;228:25.

25. Flacke JW, Flacke WE, Williams GD: Acute pulmonary edema following naloxone reversal of high-dose morphine anesthesia. *Anesthesiology* 1977;47:376–378.

26. Shochet RB, Murray GB: Neuropsychiatric toxicity of meperidine. *J Intensive Care Med* 1988;3:246.

27. Tang R, Shimomura SK, Rotblatt M: Meperidine-induced seizures in sickle cell patients. *Hospital Formulary* 1980 (October): 764.

28. Kaiko R, Foley K, Heidrich G, et al: Normeperidine plasma levels and central nervous system irritability in cancer patients. *Fed Proc* 1978;37:568.

29. Szeto HH, Inturrisi CE, House R, et al: Accumulation of normeperidine in patients with renal failure or cancer. *Ann Intern Med* 1977;86:738.

4 Infection Control and Infectious Diseases

Gary Hartstein

Infection control assumes crucial importance in the postanesthetic period. A considerable number of patients undergo surgery with infections, either as the indication for operation or as a coexisting process. Furthermore, the susceptibility to infection is increased in surgical patients, because of breaks in the integrity of skin or mucosal barriers, the presence of invasive devices (intravascular cannulae, urinary catheters, drains, and so on), and the possible effects of anesthesia on immune function.[1] In this chapter the principles of infection control, the precautions currently applied to protect patients and personnel from infection, and the care of the patient with sepsis are reviewed.

GENERAL PRINCIPLES

The process of infection is multifactorial, involving source factors, transmission from the source to the host, and host factors. Infection, defined as "invasion and multiplication of microorganisms in body tissues, resulting in local cellular injury,"[2] must be distinguished from colonization, wherein organisms multiply but do not invade or cause tissue damage or a clinical response. All humans are colonized, with the habitual organisms present at a given site defined as the normal flora for that site. Risk factors, generically, are those that increase the virulence of the normal flora, decrease resistance to invasion, or increase chances or efficiency of transmission. Many elements increasing the risk of infection are present in postoperative patients, including advanced age, poor general condition, concomitant medical therapy, and the presence of invasive devices (Table 4–1).[3] Nosocomial infections are of particular concern because of their impact on morbidity and mortality, their economic impact, and because these are the infections likely to be seen in or transmitted to the postanesthetic patient.[4,5]

The sources of infections, especially nosocomial infections, include humans, with special emphasis on health care personnel. Visitors can also harbor infectious organisms, but are rarely allowed into postanesthetic areas. Other patients can also serve as sources

of infection. When human beings are the sources, the organisms are often *Staphylococcus aureus* and group A streptococci. More exotic bacteria, such as Acinetobacter, are common when factors such as dermatitis are present in the host.[6]

Inanimate sources also threaten patients. Because of high-efficiency filtration, the air is rarely a source. Water, however, can carry *Pseudomonas* or *Legionella* organisms.[3] Respiratory therapy equipment, especially that containing liquid reservoirs, has been well described as a source, as have arterial line flush solution containers and stopcocks.[7,8] Much of this equipment is relatively hard to disassemble, clean, and sterilize, or is intolerant of sterilization techniques. Of potential importance to the postanesthetic patient is the occasional contamination of handwashing and skin-preparation solutions, usually with gram-negative rods.[9] Air-fluidized (Clinitron) beds can also be contaminated, and they present significant difficulties in cleaning and disinfecting.[10]

Host factors are vitally important in influencing susceptibility to infection, and many of these factors are present in the postanesthetic period. Host susceptibility can be considered as a continuum from immunity or resistance, through a colonized or carrier state, and on to clinical infection. Passage from one state to another can be modified by concurrent diseases, such as diabetes, cancer (especially leukemias and lymphomas), and uremia.[11] These diseases are common in surgical patients. The host's state of nutrition is likely related to his or her ability to resist infection. The prevalence of malnutrition is surprisingly high in hospitalized patients.[12] It is known that protein/calorie malnutrition in children increases

TABLE 4–1. FACTORS INCREASING INFECTION POSTOPERATIVELY[a]

Prolonged surgery
Advanced age
Poor general condition
Malnutrition
Invasive monitors
Other medical diseases

[a]Several factors combine to increase the incidence of infection in the postoperative period.

their susceptibility to infection, that poor preoperative nutritional status increases the risk of perioperative pneumonia, and that successful nutritional support decreases postoperative infectious complications.[3,13,14] The presence of invasive devices is common in the postoperative period. These devices provide a pathway to what are usually sterile body areas (bladder, intravascular space, intracranial space, and so on), bypassing natural defense mechanisms.[3]

Medical treatments can also have varied and dramatic effects on susceptibility to infection. Cancer chemotherapeutic drugs have profound effects on cells mediating immune function, both qualitatively and quantitatively. These drugs can also cause alterations in the integrity of mucosal barriers. Antibiotic therapy, by changing the normal flora, can decrease resistance to multiplication and invasion by pathogenic organisms. The use of H_2 blockers reduces the gastric pH and diminishes the barrier function of the stomach's acidity.[3,11]

Infections are transmitted from source to host by four major routes. The most frequent and most important in the postanesthetic period is through contact. This can be either direct contact between host and source, or indirect via an intermediate object or person. Droplets of infected fluids can remain airborne for approximately 3 feet, and can therefore serve as a contact medium. A second route of transmission is vehicle-borne. In the postanesthetic period this usually implies infection via contaminated blood products, drugs or drug diluents, or intravenous fluids. Airborne transmission of infection is usually via droplet nuclei, the residual particles left after evaporation of droplets. These nuclei are light enough to be held in suspension by normal indoor air currents, and as such can carry infectious particles long distances. For completeness, vector-borne (by insects or animals) transmission must be mentioned. These are rarely if ever involved in nosocomial, perianesthetic infections.[11]

The above information allows us to understand the pathogenesis of nosocomial infections. These infections depend on exposure of a susceptible host to a source via a route of transmission. Colonization occurs (the host can also be the source if an alteration of the endogenous flora gives rise to a virulent strain). Then multiplication occurs. The speed with which a patient becomes colonized depends on the above-mentioned host factors, the site in question, the presence of foreign bodies, and the virulence of the organism. For example, in the presence of a tracheostomy tube, the upper respiratory tract is colonized within 48 hours.[15] Once colonization is established, clinical response (infection) occurs when a threshold level of multiplication and invasion have occurred. Once established, the patient often remains colonized by these frequently multiply resistant organisms for years, with obvious implications for subsequent hospitalizations.[16]

Intervention to prevent infection can occur at several stages in the postanesthetic period. The step most vulnerable is the process of transmission, to prevent or forestall colonization. It has been documented that patients who become colonized with new organisms while in the hospital are more likely to develop infections.[17] Most host factors are fixed and cannot be altered, with the exception perhaps of early and vigorous nutritional support.

The thrust, then, of infection control in the postanesthetic period involves the application of precautions designed to interrupt the transmission of organisms.

INFECTION CONTROL

Design Factors

Infection control begins with the physical design of the postanesthetic care unit (PACU). Interpatient spread of infection is reduced with single-patient cubicles; this is clearly not practical for the PACU, but if significant numbers of patients requiring strict or respiratory isolation (discussed later) are to be cared for, isolation rooms with nonrecirculated air at negative pressure should be provided.[15]

Sinks (for handwashing) should be placed near entrances and exits, and adequate floor space must be allocated to allow personnel and equipment access to patients, and to discourage contact with adjacent patients without handwashing. Ideally, 7 feet should be allowed between beds, and 120 square feet of floor space per patient should be provided.[18]

Traffic control is important when caring for infected patients. PACUs should be situated at the end of corridors, and infected patients within the PACU should be placed in cul-de-sacs, to minimize through traffic.

Clean disposal facilities must be separate from contaminated facilities, and sinks for handwashing should not be used for equipment.[3]

Handwashing

The most important infection control measure is without question the rigorous application of handwashing.[19] This is defined as a "vigorous rubbing together of all surfaces of lathered hands followed by rinsing under a stream of water".[19] The importance of handwashing is great enough to warrant more detailed study, especially because this act forms the basis of all subsequent precautions.

The bacterial population on the hands can be divided into resident bacteria, which can be repeatedly cultured from the hands because they survive and multiply in the superficial layers of the skin, and transient flora. The latter organisms have limited survival potential on the hands, and are rarely recultured. Resident bacteria are generally not highly virulent, with a few exceptions. After surgery or other procedures causing or allowing deep penetration of these organisms, or in the presence of immune compromise or a foreign body, or with overt skin infections, these organisms can be significantly more virulent than is usually the case. The transient flora on the hands of health care personnel often derive from the bacteria of colonized or infected patients, and are often at the origin of nosocomial infections. These distinctions are important, because they influence the ease of killing of the organisms.

Normal soaps or detergents will usually eliminate most transient flora, while antimicrobial products are necessary to kill or inhibit the resident flora. Soaps and detergents serve to suspend the organisms, and allow them to be rinsed off (mechanical removal). Antimicrobials either kill or inhibit the growth of microorganisms (chemical removal).[19]

The indications for handwashing should be specified. Hands should be washed:

- Before all invasive procedures.
- Before caring for infection-prone patients (those who are immune-compromised, and newborns).
- After any situation when microbial contamination of the hands is likely, especially after mucous membrane, blood, or body fluid contact, or contact with secretions or excretions.
- After contact with inanimate surfaces or objects likely to be contaminated with virulent or epidemiologically significant organisms.
- After caring for patients who are either infected or likely to be colonized with significant (eg, multiply resistant) organisms.
- Between all contacts in high-risk units (the PACU should be considered as such).[19]

The above indications apply even if gloves are used. Antimicrobial products should be used for handwashing before caring for newborns, in high-risk units, and before caring for severely immune-compromised patients. Plain soaps are acceptable for other situations. Bar soaps should be stored on racks that allow drying, and the dispensers of liquid soaps should be cleaned and filled with fresh product when empty. Because of the risk of contamination with gram-negative organisms, half-filled containers should not be refilled.[19]

Poor compliance by medical staff with handwashing has been well documented.[20] Some possible reasons are a perceived lack of time, inadequate prioritization of the procedure, the imposed inconvenience due to poor location of sinks, cutaneous reactions to what are often unpleasant solutions, or a lack of "example setting" by medical and nursing leadership.[3]

Universal Precautions

The next level of infection control is called universal precautions. This is a relatively new concept that has grown out of a recognition of the weaknesses of previously used procedures for applying precautions. The isolation of body substances of patients with bloodborne infections has the obvious rationale of preventing health care workers from exposure to bloodborne pathogens. Previously, patients who carried or were suspected of carrying a diagnosis of an infectious disease requiring body substance isolation had an order written and a "flag" placed on their chart signaling the need to apply "blood and body fluid precautions."[21] Thus, the application of precautions is dependent on suspicion or diagnosis. Unfortunately, clinical or laboratory diagnosis of diseases caused by bloodborne pathogens (HIV, hepatitis B, non-A non-B hepatitis, and so on) often lacks sensitivity, with consequent risk of undiagnosed patients failing to have precautions applied. For this reason, in 1987 the Centers for Disease Control (CDC) recommended the universal application of body fluid precautions.[22] These precautions are designed to eliminate contact with blood, body fluids containing visible blood, and those known to contain infectious titers of bloodborne organisms. These include all tissues, semen, vaginal secretions, and cerebrospinal, synovial, peritoneal, pleural, pericardial, and amniotic fluids.[21] The precautions do not apply to feces, nasal secretions, sputum, sweat, tears, urine, or vomitus, unless visibly bloody, because these fluids are either free of bloodborne pathogens, or have such small quantities as to pose no risk for these infections. Vaccination against hepatitis B virus (HBV) is considered to be an important adjunct to these precautions.[21] Furthermore, these universal precautions in no way reduce the need for specific, disease-related precautions (eg, enteric precautions for infectious diarrhea).

Universal precautions, as prescribed by the CDC, are detailed in Table 4–2.[22] A few facts about these precautions will help to clarify several common questions.

The selection of gloves has been an issue in many hospital areas, including PACUs. No difference in the barrier effectiveness of intact vinyl versus intact latex gloves has been reported. It is clear that sterile gloves (usually latex) should be used for contact with sterile body areas. When sterile gloves are not required—as, for example, for mucous membrane contact and other diagnostic or therapeutic patient contacts—nonsterile examination gloves are acceptable. Gloves should be

TABLE 4-2. UNIVERSAL PRECAUTIONS

1. Barriers should be used by health-care workers (HCW) when contact with blood or applicable body fluids is anticipated. These include gloves for contact with blood, fluids, mucous membranes, non-intact skin, contaminated surfaces, for venipuncture or vascular access. Gloves must be changed after contact. Masks and protective eyewear (or faceshields) should be used if droplets will be created. Gowns or aprons should be worn if splashes are anticipated.

2. Hands and involved skin should be immediately and thoroughly washed after removal of gloves and if contaminated.

3. Special care with sharps is required. Recapping, bending, or removal from syringes should be discouraged. Disposal in puncture resistant containers should be used. In-line stopcocks may help avoid recapping.

4. In areas where the need for resuscitation is predictable, mouthpieces, resuscitation devices, or ventilation devices should be available to decrease the need for mouth to mouth breathing.

5. HCW with weeping dermatitis or exudate skin lesions should be temporarily relieved of direct patient or equipment care responsibilities.

6. Because pregnant HCW place a fetus at risk, they should be especially familiar with and careful about using these precautions.

From Centers for Disease Control. Recommendation for prevention of HIV transmission in health care settings. MMWR (suppl) 1987;6:15–1.

changed between patient contacts, and should not be reused. As mentioned in Table 4–2, hands should be washed after removing gloves.[21]

Specific Situations

Universal precautions are applied to all patients. Some specific precautions are relevant to the care of the postanesthetic patient. Categories of precautions have been applied to certain diseases.

The first category is called *strict* isolation (Table 4–3). Diseases requiring strict isolation are transmitted by both direct contact and the airborne route, and these precautions are designed to interrupt this transmission.

These patients require private rooms with handwashing facilities. The door should be kept closed, and gowns, masks, and gloves must be donned by all persons before entering the room, and discarded before leaving it. Hands must be washed before

TABLE 4-3. DISEASES REQUIRING STRICT ISOLATION

Pharyngeal diphtheria
Viral hemorrhagic fevers, including Lassa fever and Marburg
   virus disease
Measles
Pneumonic plague
Varicella
Disseminated zoster

entering and after leaving the patient. All room contents are considered contaminated, and require decontamination prior to leaving the room. Health care workers caring for patients with diphtheria, rubella, or varicella must be immune to these diseases. A sphygmomanometer and stethoscope should be dedicated to the patient; sterilization is necessary only if contaminated with infectious fluids. Dressings and tissues must be double bagged, and placed in containers labeled as contaminated waste. Urine and feces should be flushed into the unit's isolation hopper without exposing others. Rectal thermometers should be washed with soap, and kept in 70 to 90% ethyl or isopropyl alcohol with 0.2% iodine. Oral thermometers should be washed with soap, wiped with an alcohol swab, and stored dry. These should be discarded when the patient is discharged. Linen should be double bagged, with a water-soluble inner bag. Aerosol formation should be avoided by avoiding vigorous shaking. Pillows and mattresses should be covered with impervious plastic, which should be wiped with a germicide or removed and laundered at the time of terminal sterilization.

Small parts of equipment used in patient care should be double bagged, labeled "contaminated," and sent to central supply for decontamination. Larger parts should be wiped with a germicide and sent for decontamination. Terminal cleaning should be by personnel wearing the same protective clothing as when the patient was in the room. If adequate ventilation is present, an airing out period is not necessary. If an air conditioner is present, the filter should be disposed of in contaminated trash. Mop heads should be soaked in a germicide and decontaminated. Walls, blinds, and curtains need be washed only if visibly contaminated.

Contact isolation is required for organisms spread by direct contact that are highly transmissible, epidemiologically significant, or both (Table 4–4). Single rooms with sinks are necessary. If there is a likelihood of soilage, gowns should be worn, while masks are only necessary for rubella, and staphylococcal or group A streptococcal pneumonias. Gloves must be worn for direct contact with the infected area. Gloves should be changed after removing soiled dressings prior to applying new dressings. Hands should be washed before entering and on leaving the room, before and after wound care, and when changing the site of care. The dressings should be handled with sterile instruments, placed into zip-locked plastic bags, and discarded with contaminated waste. Thermometers are treated as for strict isolation. Clean dressings and a clean towel should be placed on the wound just prior to transport.

Interruption of droplet transmission is the object of *respiratory* precautions. These patients should be

TABLE 4-4. DISEASES REQUIRING CONTACT ISOLATION

Cutaneous diphtheria

Group A streptococcal endometritis

Severe primary disseminated herpes simplex

Localized herpes zoster

Impetigo

Staphylococcus aureus or group A streptococcal pneumonias

Rabies

Rubella

Scabies

Scalded skin syndrome

Vaccinia

Infection or colonization with multiply resistant bacteria
    Gram-negative rods sensitive to one or no antibiotics
    Methicillin-resistant *Staph aureus*
    Penicillin-resistant *Strep pneumoniae*
    Ampicillin- and chloramphenicol-resistant *Haemophilus influenzae*
    Others judged clinically or epidemiologically significant by the infection-control team

TABLE 4-6. DISEASES REQUIRING ENTERIC PRECAUTIONS

Amebic dysentery

Cholera

Suspected acute infectious diarrhea

Echovirus disease

Chlostridium difficile or *Staphylococcus aureus enterocolitis*

Enterovirus disease

Gastroenteritis
    Campylobacter
    Cryptosporidium
    E coli
    Dientamoeba fragilis
    Giardia lamblia
    Salmonella sp
    Shigella sp
    Vibrio parahaemolyticus
    Viral (including norwalk agent and rotavirus)
    Yersinia enterocolitis
    Presumed infectious
    Type A hepatitis

Herpangina

Pleurodynia

Poliomyelitis

Typhoid fever

---

cared for in private rooms with sinks and closed doors. Masks are absolutely necessary, as is handwashing on entering and leaving. Anything contaminated with sputum should be wiped with a germicide. The patient should be transported while wearing a disposable mask. Respiratory equipment should be double bagged, labeled with specific instructions as to what organisms(s) are involved and what precautions are necessary, and sent for decontamination and sterilization. Disposable equipment should be used when possible. Filters should be placed between breathing circuits and ventilators (Table 4-5).

Diseases transmitted by the fecal-oral route are subject to *enteric* precautions (Table 4-6). Private rooms are only necessary for patients with poor personal hygiene. Gowns are needed only for direct

TABLE 4-5. DISEASES REQUIRING RESPIRATORY ISOLATION

H influenza epiglottitis

Meningitis
    H influenza (known or suspected)[a]
    Meningococcal (known or suspected)[a]

Meningococcal pneumonia[a]

Meningococcemia[a]

Mumps

Pertussis

Tuberculosis with positive sputum smear, or chest x-ray strongly suggestive of active tuberculosis, or patients with the diagnosis "rule-out TB." Laryngeal TB is included.[b]

[a]Precautions necessary for 24 hours following institution of effective antimicrobial treatment.

[b]Duration of isolation for TB can be guided by clinical response and reduction in numbers of organisms on sputum smear. Usually this occurs 2 to 3 weeks after therapy is started. The pulmonary or infectious disease services should be consulted prior to discontinuing precautions.

care, or if there will be contact with excretions. Hands should be washed on entering and leaving the room. Masks are not necessary; gloves are needed for contact with the patient or with potentially contaminated objects.

The precautions and procedures regarding placement and maintenance of intravascular devices at the Bronx Municipal Hospital Center are outlined in Table 4-7.

SEPSIS

Presentation

Patients with sepsis present among the most difficult and challenging problems in the postanesthetic period. Multiple hemodynamic, metabolic, and respiratory abnormalities occur, and mortality is high. A systematic approach to these patients requires an understanding of the pathophysiology of the syndrome; such an approach helps to make caring for these desperately ill patients less intimidating and contributes to decreased morbidity and mortality.

Definition

Dorland's Medical Dictionary defines sepsis as "the presence in the blood or other tissues of pathogenic microorganisms or their toxins; the condition associated with such presence."[23] For our purpose, sepsis will be defined as a characteristic systemic manifestation of infection, whether or not bacteria are present

TABLE 4–7. STANDARDS AND PRECAUTIONS FOR VASCULAR ACCESS DEVICES

Type of Intravascular Device	Site Change	Tubing Change	Dressing Change	Comments
Routine peripheral IV (plastic or steel cannula)	72 h	72 h (after blood, blood products, lipid, and triple mix TPN)	Daily if site not changed in 72 h	1. Site preparation: 2% tincture of iodine, allowing 30 sec for drying. Wipe off with alcohol before insertion. 2. Gloves worn during insertion.
Heparin locks	72 h	Same	Same	Same
Peripheral central line	72 h (except brachial Broviac cannulas)	Same	Same (Brachial Broviac, 72 hr)	1. Mask, gown, and sterile gloves worn during insertion. 2. Mask and sterile gloves during dressing change.
Central line: multilumen, single lumen (subclavian or jugular site)	If needed longer than 14 days consider long-term cannulas	Same	72 h gauze dressings, 4 days transparent	May change *once* over a guidewire if in less than 3 days.
Long-term central line: Hickman, Broviac Porta-cath	Varies	Same	Daily if site not changed in 72 h	1. Insertion to be done in OR or designated treatment room. 2. Mask and sterile gloves during dressing change.
TPN lines	See type of intravascular device column	Same	See type of intravascular device column	1. Lipid or triple mix lines must be changed every 24 h.
Arterial and Swan-Ganz	4 days	48 h	48 h	1. Flush solution and tubing to be changed every 48 h. 2. Transducer and other accessories discontinued in 4 days with site change.

in the blood (bacteremia). The syndrome usually, but not always, consists of hypotension, with a normal or elevated cardiac output, and a low systemic vascular resistance. Septic shock implies organ hypoperfusion—that is, central nervous system dysfunction, pulmonary failure, renal insufficiency, and most significantly, progressive lactic acidosis.

Precipitating Factors
The sepsis syndrome is occurring more commonly because of several recent trends in medical practice, including more frequent use of invasive monitors and catheters, aggressive cytotoxic and immunosuppressive therapies, frequent use of corticosteroids, and the emergence of multiply resistant strains of microorganisms. Furthermore, the patient population is aging, and increased survival of patients with diseases such as diabetes and cancer has dramatically increased the size of the population at risk.

Gram-negative bacteremia is one of the most common events leading to the sepsis syndrome.[24] Approximately 70,000 to 300,000 cases of gram-negative bacteremia occur each year.[25] Of these, 40 to 50% develop shock, which is fatal in 40 to 90%.[25] If sepsis due to gram-positive organisms, viruses, and fungi is included, up to 100,000 deaths from this syndrome occur annually in the United States.[25] From 1965 through 1974, 7 to 12 gram-negative bacteremic events per 1000 hospital admissions were estimated to have occurred.[25] This represents an approximately 25-fold increase in incidence over two decades.[24] These statistics translate to very frequent postanesthetic contact with these patients.

Certain factors are known to increase the risk of bacteremia, sepsis, and resultant death. Patient characteristics associated with high risk of bacteremia include advanced age, the presence of severe debilitating illnesses, and burns. Iatrogenic factors include instrumentation of the genitourinary, respiratory, or gastrointestinal tracts; intraarterial or intravenous cannulation; mechanical ventilation; surgical or gastrointestinal endoscopic procedures; septic abortion or premature rupture of membranes; use of steroids, cytotoxic, and antimetabolite drugs; and failure to drain purulent collections. Mortality from bacteremia is increased in the presence of cirrhosis, a hematologic cancer, or surgery associated with steroid use, cancer, or diabetes. Failure to mount a febrile response to bacteremia is also associated with high mortality as is hypotension.[26] Gram-negative bacteremia carries a mortality of 7 to 10% if shock is not present; if the patient is in shock, the mortality increases to 47%.[27] For gram-positive bacteremia, the corresponding figures are 8 and 33%.[27] In normotensive patients, polymicrobial bacteremia is associated with a higher mortality than is bacteremia, where only one organism is isolated. If shock is present, the mortality is similar, suggesting that once the full-blown syndrome of septic shock develops the shock state itself is the major determinant of outcome, not the source of the bacterial insult.[27]

Diagnosis

Although the majority of patients with sepsis in the postanesthetic period will already carry the diagnosis, due to the high morbidity and mortality of the sepsis syndrome, the clinical index of suspicion must remain high, especially in unstable patients at high risk. Clinical findings can be divided into those caused by the infection itself and those related to the sepsis syndrome (that is, the systemic response to the infection).

Usually patients present with fever, often with rigors if bacteremia is present. The patient may have signs or symptoms relating to the source of the infection (such as purulent sputum with rales, abdominal signs, or urinary symptoms). Some or all of these may be masked by the residual effects of anesthesia.

The following signs can all be associated with the sepsis syndrome, whether as isolated findings, or in groups. The earliest sign of sepsis is frequently tachypnea with respiratory alkalosis. Altered mental status is often noted, especially in the elderly in whom agitation or sudden onset or worsening of dementia may be seen. The appearance of seizures may also herald the sepsis syndrome, while oliguria, thrombocytopenia, hypothermia, and leukocytosis (or a decreased white blood cell count) may be noted. Hypotension is often a late sign, and may be associated with acidosis and shock. The need for a high clinical index of suspicion is apparent when one considers the subtlety of the above signs, especially if only one is present.[24,28]

The rapid determination of the source of the in-

fection, and the prompt institution of appropriate definitive therapy (defined as therapy directed at eradicating the infection as contrasted with supportive therapy) is of primary importance in treating sepsis.[29] Studies have documented that prompt institution of appropriate antibiotic therapy significantly reduces mortality from gram-negative bacteremia, whether or not shock is present.[26] When the diagnosis of sepsis is made or suspected, all invasive catheters should be changed, appropriate cultures should be obtained, and all suspected fluids should be stained and examined microscopically. Since certain groups of bacteria are often found in association with particular sites of infection, a knowledge of these relations is useful in initiating empiric antibiotic therapy (Table 4-8). Once cultures are obtained, empiric antibiotic therapy should be instituted, taking into consideration the patient's status, the likely organisms, and the local epidemiology, including antibiotic sensitivities of endemic hospital species.

Intraabdominal sources present a special problem; they should be suspected in all surgical or trauma patients who have sustained even minimal violation of intestinal integrity. Diagnosis can be difficult. Ultrasound followed by PIPIDA scintigraphy will usually correctly diagnose acute acalculous cholecystitis, a not infrequent cause of sepsis in the critically ill patient.[30] CT scan of the abdomen will demonstrate 80 to 90% of intraabdominal abscesses.[30]

TABLE 4-8. ORGANISMS COMMONLY ASSOCIATED WITH INFECTION OF VARIOUS ORGAN SYSTEMS

Origin	Organism
Respiratory	Pseudomonas
	E. coli
	Klebsiella
	Enterobacter
	Acinetobacter
	Serratia
Vascular	Pseudomonas
	Serratia
	Enterobacter
Urinary	E. coli
	Klebsiella
	Enterobacter
	Proteus
	Serratia
Gastrointestinal	E. coli
	Klebsiella
	Enterobacter
	Serratia
	Bacteroides
	Salmonella
Biliary	E. coli
	Klebsiella
	Enterobacter
	Serratia

Repeat laparotomy should be considered in the high-risk patient (such as those with trauma or previous surgery) if multiple organ failure develops without an apparent etiology. Percutaneous CT or ultrasound-guided catheter drainage of single abdominal abscesses is useful, if the access tract does not cross bowel.[31]

Pathophysiology

Not all bacteremic events lead to sepsis, and conversely, not all sepsis is associated with bacteremia. The crucial event leading to sepsis is elaboration by the infecting organism of mediators, which in turn produce the clinical, biochemical, and pathophysiologic manifestations of sepsis. The nature and identity of these mediators is the subject of intensive and ongoing research, controversy, and interest. The literature of mediator involvement in sepsis is extensive and often confusing.[32] The lipopolysaccharide component of the gram-negative bacterial cell wall (endotoxin), when injected into animals, reproduces several of the manifestations of sepsis. It is likely that endotoxin (in gram-negative infections), or some other structural bacterial component (in other bacterial infections), is involved in the release or activation of mediators in the organism.[33] These include the protein cascades (the complement, kinin, and coagulation systems), wherein inactive precursors are proteolytically activated.

Activation of complement possibly via the alternate pathway appears to occur early in septic shock, although this has been questioned.[34,35] In a murine model of sepsis, a strain deficient in the C5 component of complement survived longer, and had reduced alveolar–arterial oxygen gradients, and higher arterial O_2 tensions than C5-sufficient twins.[36] Activated C3 and C5 (C3a and C5a) are potent chemotactic substances for white blood cells, act to aggregate granulocytes, and dramatically increase vascular permeability, causing diffuse capillary leak. C3a and C5a are called anaphylotoxins because of the similarity of their effects to some of those of histamine. Complement-induced granulocyte activation and aggregation probably underly several clinical consequences of sepsis, such as the adult respiratory distress syndrome (ARDS).[37]

Products of arachidonic acid metabolism (the prostanoids) include prostaglandins, prostacyclin, thromboxane, and the leukotrienes, and are also likely involved in the pathogenesis of sepsis.[38]

The cardiovascular response to sepsis seems to include a reversible decrease in myocardial performance, as indicated by a marked fall in ejection fraction. The serum from septic patients with low ejection fractions contains a peptide that produces myocardial depression in an in-vitro preparation.[39]

Clinical Aspects

The hemodynamic, pulmonary, and metabolic effects of sepsis are complicated and varied.

The classic description of human septic shock defines two phases, a phase of "warm" shock, with peripheral vasodilation, high cardiac output, and hypotension, followed by the preterminal phase of "cold" shock, characterized by cold, clammy skin, low cardiac output, and hypotension. This classic description, however, does not describe the clinical picture seen in most cases of human septic shock. It is based on a frequently used model of sepsis, the canine endotoxin model, wherein dogs are injected with a lethal bolus of endotoxin. This model rapidly produces a low cardiac output state with massive bloody diarrhea (which is rarely if ever seen in human sepsis). Most human deaths from septic shock are from either refractory hypotension, with normal to high cardiac output maintained until death, or from multiple organ failure. Few humans die with a low cardiac output state.[33,40] Cardiac output is a rather poor indicator of global myocardial performance, since the intact organism is capable of altering rate, contractility, and loading conditions to maintain output in the face of compromised pump function. Results of nuclear ejection fraction (EF) studies on patients in septic shock indicate that one half of the patients studied had EFs below 0.4, suggesting relatively severe depression of ventricular function. However, 76% of the survivors, but none of the nonsurvivors, had depressed EFs. Importantly, in those with depressed EFs, stroke volume was maintained by an increase in both end-diastolic and end-systolic volumes. EFs in survivors gradually returned to normal by ten days after the onset of shock.[41] These findings were confirmed in a canine model that accurately simulates the hemodynamic findings in human sepsis.[42] This study showed reversible systolic dysfunction, with ventricular dilation and maintenance of stroke volume in response to volume infusion. Inadequate myocardial perfusion or global ischemia was excluded as a cause of this reversible ventricular dysfunction.[43] Septic shock can also give rise to segmental ventricular dysfunction, with ECG and echocardiographic findings similar to myocardial infarction.[44]

The sepsis syndrome is one of the major causes of ARDS. The mediators mentioned above are all capable of inducing damage to the alveolar–capillary membrane, the most likely site of the initial injury of ARDS.

Septic patients are in a hypermetabolic, hypercatabolic state. Large amounts of endogenous protein are broken down, a process that is not inhibited by glucose administration. Relative insulin resistance is seen, and elevated rates of lipolysis are noted. This metabolic situation can be reproduced by infusion of epinephrine, norepinephrine, cortisol, and glucagon in amounts similar to those present in septic patients (Shamoon H, personal communication).

Supportive Treatment

The initial treatment consists of establishing the diagnosis of sepsis, obtaining appropriate culture materials, and treating the infection (with antibiotics and drainage if necessary). Removal of any necrotic tissue is also necessary.

At our institution, a hypotensive, septic patient receives a fluid challenge with 500 to 1000 mL of crystalloid. If this does not restore blood pressure to normal (at least 90 mm Hg systolic), invasive hemodynamic monitoring is initiated, with placement of arterial and pulmonary artery catheters. Fluid resuscitation is carried out until a pulmonary artery wedge pressure of 12 to 18 mm Hg is reached. The rationale for this is threefold. First, these patients are often dehydrated, as fever and tachypnea have usually increased insensible losses, while decreased oral intake is often associated with the initiating illness. Second, the diffuse capillary leak seen in sepsis necessitates large volumes of fluid to establish normal intravascular volume. Third, in sepsis total body oxygen consumption becomes dependent on oxygen delivery over a wide range.[45,46] Thus, as long as calculated O_2 delivery (equal to the product of cardiac output times the arterial O_2 content) to the periphery increases, oxygen uptake rises, presumably reflecting improvement in the metabolic status of the tissues.

If restoration of adequate intravascular volume does not restore blood pressure to at least 90 mm Hg systolic, vasopressor therapy is indicated. No controlled studies exist to determine the pressor of choice in sepsis. At our institution, if cardiac output is deemed to be "adequate" (admittedly a difficult assessment in sepsis!), a norepinephrine infusion is titrated to maintain a systolic blood pressure of 90 mm Hg. Concomitantly, a low-dose dopamine infusion (0.5 to 2.5 μg/kg/min) is initiated to preserve renal perfusion. If cardiac output is low (that is, a mixed cardiogenic/septic situation), an acceptable blood pressure is established as above, at which point dobutamine is titrated to effect on cardiac output.

All patients in shock in our ICU are sustained with mechanical ventilation to decrease the work of breathing. Standard goals are achievement of an arterial oxygen saturation of 90% or higher at an F_IO_2 of no higher than 0.5; positive end-expiratory pressure (PEEP) is used as necessary to achieve this value with careful attention to PEEP effect on cardiac output and O_2 delivery.

Nutritional support is initiated as soon as feasible after the septic insult, to minimize the adverse effects of excessive endogenous protein catabolism. The enteral route, while desirable, is often not possible in this group of critically ill patients. Nutritional goals, roughly speaking, are to provide 35 to 40 nonprotein kcal/kg/day, and 1.5 to 2 g protein/kg/day. The calories are divided between carbohydrate and fat with two constraints: (1) no more than 60% of total calories are given as lipid; and (2) the rate of administration of carbohydrate should not exceed 5 to 6 mg/kg/min.

Despite several anecdotal reports of favorable blood pressure responses to naloxone administration, and extensive literature reports of its use in various animal models of sepsis, we do not use this drug in septic patients. No controlled studies exist to document improved hemodynamics or, more importantly, outcome, after naloxone administration.

Although the literature is replete with articles studying the effects of high-dose corticosteroids given before, during, and after sepsis, an article in 1984 reports the outcome of a randomized prospective trial of methylprednisolone versus dexamethasone versus placebo. The groups treated with steroids had higher percentages of patients with reversal of shock within 24 hours; overall mortality, however, was not different among the groups. It is speculated that early in septic shock (within the first four hours), in certain subgroups of patients (as yet undefined), corticosteroids may be useful.[47]

Two randomized, prospective, double-blind, placebo-controlled studies reported in 1987 also failed to show any benefit from steroid administration.[48,49] More deaths due to secondary infections were noted in the steroid-treated group.[48]

REFERENCES

1. Hansbrough JF, Zapata-Sirvent RL, Battle EJ, et al: Alterations in splenic lymphocyte subpopulations and increased mortality from sepsis following anesthesia in mice. *Anesthesiology* 1985;63:267–273.
2. Taylor EJ: *Dorland's Illustrated Medical Dictionary*, ed 27. Philadelphia, Saunders, 1988, p 834.
3. Massanari RM, Hierholzer WJ: The intensive care unit, in Bennett JV, Brachman PS (eds): *Hospital Infections*, ed 2. Toronto, Little, Brown, 1986.
4. Haley RW: *Managing Hospital Infection Control for Cost-Effectiveness: A Strategy for Reducing Infectious Complications*. Chicago, American Hospital Publishing, 1986.
5. Donowitz LG, Wenzel RP, Hoyt JW: High risk of hospital acquired infection in the ICU patient. *Crit Care Med* 1982;10:355–357.
6. Buxton AE, Anderson RL, Werdegar D, Atlas E: Nosocomial respiratory tract infection and colonization with Acinetobacter calcoaceticus: Epidemiologic characteristics. *Am J Med* 1978;65:507–513.
7. Craven DE, Connolly MG, Lichtenberg DA, et al: Contamination of mechanical ventilators with tubing

changes every 24 or 48 hours. *N Engl J Med* 1982;306:1505–1509.

8. Shimozaki T, Deane RS, Mazuzan JE, et al: Bacterial contamination of arterial lines. *JAMA* 1983;249:223–225.

9. Morse LJ, Schonbeck LE: Hand lotions: A potential nosocomial hazard. *N Engl J Med* 1968;278:376–378.

10. Scheidt A, Drusin LM: Bacteriologic contamination in an air-fluidized bed. *J Trauma* 1983;23:241–242.

11. Garner J, Simmons BP: Rationale and responsibilities for isolation precautions, *CDC Guide for Infection Precautions in Hospitals*. Washington, DC, USDOHHS, CDC, 1983, pp 7–8.

12. Bistran RB, Blackburn GL, Vitale J, et al: Prevalence of malnutrition in general medical patients. *JAMA* 1976;235:1567–1570.

13. Garibaldi RA, Britt MR, Coleman ML, et al: Risk factors for postoperative pneumonia. *Am J Med* 1981;70(3):677–80.

14. Starker PM, LaSala PA, Askanazi J, et al: The influence of preoperative total parenteral nutrition upon morbidity and mortality. *Surg Gynecol Obstet* 1986;162:569–574.

15. Northey D, Adess ML, Hartsuch JM: Microbial surveillance in a surgical intensive care unit. *Surg Gynecol Obstet* 1974;139:321–325.

16. Goldman DA: Bacterial colonization and infection in the neonate. *Am J Med* 1981;70:279–287.

17. Burke JF, Quinby WC, Bondoc CC, et al: The contribution of a bacteriologically isolated environment to the prevention of infection in seriously burned patients. *Ann Surg* 1977;186:377–385.

18. U.S. Department of Health and Human Services, PHS, Health Resource Administration: *Minimum Requirements of Construction and Equipment for Hospitals and Medical Facilities*. Washington, DC: U.S. Government Printing Office, DHEW(HRA) publ no 79-14500,1978.

19. Garner JS, Favero MS: *Guidelines for Handwashing and Hospital Environmental Control, 1985*. U.S. Department of Health and Human Services, Public Health Service, Centers for Disease Control, HHS publ no 99-1117,1985.

20. Albert RK, Condie F: Handwashing patterns in medical intensive care units. *N Engl J Med* 1981;304:1465–1466.

21. Centers for Disease Control: Update: Universal precautions for prevention of transmission of human immunodeficiency virus, hepatitis B virus, and other blood-borne pathogens in health care settings. *MMWR* 1988;37:377–387.

22. Centers for Disease Control: Recommendations for prevention of HIV transmission in health care settings. *MMWR(suppl)* 1987;36:15–185.

23. DeGroot-Kosolcharoen J, Jones JM: Permeability of latex and vinyl gloves to water and blood. *Am J of Infection Control* 1989;17:196–201.

24. Greenman RL: Gram-negative bacteremia, in Gardner LB (ed): *Acute Internal Medicine*. New York, Medical Examination Publishing, 1986, pp 393–399.

25. McCabe WR: Gram-negative bacteremia. *Adv Intern Med* 1974;19:135–158.

26. Kreger BE, Craven DE, McCabe WR: Gram-negative bacteremia IV. Re-evaluation of clinical features and treatment in 612 patients. *Am J Med* 1980;68:344–355.

27. Jacoby I: Septic shock, in Rippe JM, Irwin RS, Alpert JS, Dalen JE (eds): *Intensive Care Medicine*. Boston, Little, Brown, 1985, pp 666–675.

28. MacLean LD: Shock: Causes and management of circulatory collapse, in Sabiston DC (ed): *Davis-Christopher Textbook of Surgery*, ed 2. Philadelphia, Saunders, 1977, pp 82–92.

29. Altmeier WA, Todd CA, Wellford WE: Gram-negative septicemia: A growing threat. *Ann Surg* 1967;166:530–542.

30. Fox MS, Wilk PJ, Weissmann HS, et al: Acute acalculous cholecystitis. *Surg Gynecol Obstet* 1984;159:13–16.

31. Wilson RF: Special problems in the diagnosis and treatment of surgical sepsis. *Surg Clin N Amer* 1985;65:965–989.

32. Deutschman CS, Wilton P, Sinow J, et al: Paranasal sinusitis associated with nasotracheal intubation: A frequently unrecognized and treatable source of sepsis. *Crit Care Med* 1986;14:111–114.

33. Parker MM, Parrillo JE: Septic shock: Hemodynamics and pathogenesis. *JAMA* 1983;250:3324–3327.

34. Sprung CL, Schultz DR, Marcial E, et al: Complement activation in septic shock patients. *Crit Care Med* 1986;14:525–528.

35. Shatney CH, Benner C: Sequential serum complement (C3) and immunoglobulin levels in shock/trauma patients developing acute fulminant systemic sepsis. *Circ Shock* 1985;16:9–17.

36. Olson LM, Moss GS, Baukus D, Das-Gupta TK: The role of C5 in septic lung injury. *Ann Surg* 1985;202:771–776.

37. Jacob HS, Craddock AR, Hammerschmidt DE, Moldow CF: Complement induced granulocyte aggregation: An unsuspected mechanism of disease. *N Engl J Med* 1980;302:788–803.

38. Slotman GJ, Burchard KW, William JJ, et al: Interaction of prostaglandins, activated complement, and granulocytes in clinical sepsis and hypotension. *Surgery* 1986;99:74–751.

39. Parrillo JE, Burch C, Shelhamer JH, et al: A circulating myocardial depressant substance in humans with septic shock. *J Clin Invest* 1985;76:1539–1553.

40. Groenwald AJ, Bronsveld W, Thijs G: Hemodynamic determinants of mortality in human septic shock. *Surgery* 1986;99:140–152.

41. Parker MM, Shelhamer JH, Bacharach SL, et al: Profound but reversible myocardial depression in patients with septic shock. *Ann Int Med* 1984;100:483–490.

42. Natanson C, Fink MP, Ballantyne HK, et al: Gram-negative bacteremia produces both severe systolic and diastolic cardiac dysfunction in a canine model that simulates human septic shock. *J Clin Invest* 1986;78:259–270.

43. Cunnion RE, Schaer GL, Parker MM, et al: The coronary circulation in human septic shock. *Circulation* 1986;73:637–644.

44. Thomas F, Smith JL, Orme JF, et al: Reversible segmental myocardial dysfunction in septic shock. *Crit Care Med* 1986;14:587–588.

45. Haupt MT, Gilbert EM, Carlson RW: Fluid loading increases oxygen consumption in septic patients with lactic acidosis. *Ann Rev Resp Dis* 1985;131:912–916.

46. Kaufman BS, Rackow EC, Falt JL: The relationship between oxygen delivery and consumption during fluid resuscitation of hypovolemic and septic shock. *Chest* 1984;85:336–340.

47. Sprung CL, Canalis PV, Marcial EH, et al: The effects of high dose corticosteroids in patients with septic shock: A prospective controlled study. *New Engl J Med* 1984;311:1137–1143.

48. Bone RC, Fisher CJ, Clemmer TP, et al: A controlled clinical trial of high-dose methylprednisolone in the treatment of severe sepsis and septic shock. *N Engl J Med* 1987;317:653–658.

49. Hinshaw L, Peduzzi P, Young E, et al: Effect of high dose glucocorticoid therapy on mortality in patients with clinical signs of systemic sepsis. *N Engl J Med* 1987;317:659–665.

5 | Pain Management

Ronald Kaplan, Sheldon Goldofsky, and Mathelyn Claudio

Since the first report addressing the inadequacy of postoperative pain control,[1] little has changed in rectifying the problem and up to 75% of postsurgical patients are undertreated for pain.[2] Postoperative pain control has a number of theoretical and practical aspects in addition to the humanitarian concept of relieving suffering of one's fellow human being. Surgical pain can restrict deep breathing, ambulation, and activity. This may worsen the risk for atelectasis, pneumonia, and deep vein thrombosis. The ability to manage postsurgical pain is influenced by several preoperative factors: underlying anxiety, extroversion, and depression (nonsituational); education status; prior chronic pain; and attitudes toward drug use.[3] Pain intensity is uninfluenced by demographic factors (age, sex, prior operations, and ethnicity). These factors influence analgesic administration, probably related to attitudinal biases. Health professionals prescribe or restrict analgesics based upon their belief of what a patient should receive, or how much pain a patient should be perceiving.

The placebo response must be considered in pain management. Approximately one third of a given population of patients in pain will respond to placebo. This is a physiologic response mediated via the endogenous opioid system.[4] Its effect is usually short-lived and fades with subsequent administration.

The ability of profound postoperative analgesia to effect long-term morbidity and mortality is doubtful. There is, however, growing evidence that it can reduce complications in the immediate postoperative period.[5-7] In addition, a theory that adequate early analgesic intervention for acute traumatic nociception might reduce the incidence of chronic pain[8] is gaining support from clinical studies.[9]

PAIN MECHANISMS[10-13]

Postsurgical pain is nociceptive, from clear and recognized tissue damage; facial grimaces and body muscle splinting; signs of increased autonomic activity (tachycardia, hypertension, and sweating); and emotional responses related to anxiety and sleep deprivation. As the wound heals, these diminish in their presentation and patients report less pain with time. The nociception arises from cutaneous (A delta, C), visceral (B, vagal), muscle (groups III and IV, corresponding to A delta and C), vascular (? B), and fascial and/or periosteal (A delta, C) neural receptors (Table 5-1).

Locally, algesic mediators are liberated by the injury, possibly via neurons antidromic to the axons transmitting the impulses. Some of these mediators are kinins, prostaglandins, 5-hydroxytryptamine, histamine, and substance P. Sympathetic fibers, activated via spinally mediated reflexes, release norepinephrine, which lowers the threshold to firing of mechanoreceptors.[8] Sympathetic activity will also reduce blood flow via vasoconstriction, and the acidic medium may further release or sensitize receptors to algesic substances (Fig. 5-1).

Neural activity is transmitted from peripheral receptors to the spinal cord via two categories of pseudopolar sensory neurons: (1) type A, which are large-diameter myelinated fibers; and (2) type B, which are small-diameter myelinated or unmyelinated fibers. Histologic and structural differences further distinguish these fiber types. The cell bodies are in the dorsal root ganglion. Primary afferents A delta and C (categorized by their conduction velocity) transmit cutaneous nociceptive information. Group III (corresponding to A delta) and group IV (corresponding to C) are afferents that relay muscle nociceptive information.

Afferent impulses from peripherally activated receptors enter the cord via the dorsal root entry zone; ventral root afferents have also been found. The bulk of the fibers terminate ipsilaterally in the dorsal horn; some cross directly to the other side upon entering the spinal cord. Electrical messages may be transmit-

TABLE 5-1. SOURCES OF NOCICEPTION

Nociceptor Site	Fiber Type
Cutaneous, fascia, periosteal	A delta, C
Visceral	B, vagal
Muscle	Groups III, IV
Vascular	? B

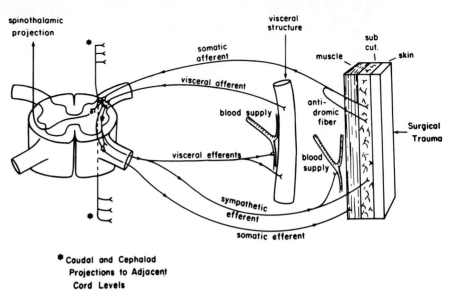

Figure 5–1. Tissue trauma releases algesic substances probably by antidromic neural stimulation. These mediators (5-hydroxytryptamine, bradykinin, kallikrein histamine) sensitize the neural receptors. Substance P promotes the release of algesic substances, and prostaglandins potentiate their effects. The spinal reflex arc initiates somatic motor and sympathetic autonomic activity. The former produces muscle splinting and guarding, and the latter vasoconstriction, acidosis from the decreased blood flow, and decreased bowel activity. The acidosis, ischemia, and sympathetic stimulation sensitize afferent receptors.

ted caudally, rostrally, or at the segmental level of the spinal cord entry.

The afferent terminals may synapse within one of several laminations in the cord. These are often referred to as *Rexed laminae,* and define anatomic zones of the gray spinal matter. Ten laminae have been defined in the cat (Fig. 5–2). Lamina I is referred to as a marginal zone. Laminae II and III comprise the substantia gelatinosa, while the nucleus proprious consists of laminae IV and V. Afferents that do not syn-

apse in the dorsal lamina may terminate in the preganglionic intermediate lateral horn cells of sympathetic fibers or sacral parasympathetic fibers. Stimulation of these and ventral somatic motor neurons (lamina IX in the cat) contribute to the immediate reflex responses of nociception.

Transmission of information cephalad occurs from primary afferent fibers synapsing with neurons in the dorsal horn; the bulk of these will then cross to form tracts in the ventrolateral spinal cord on the

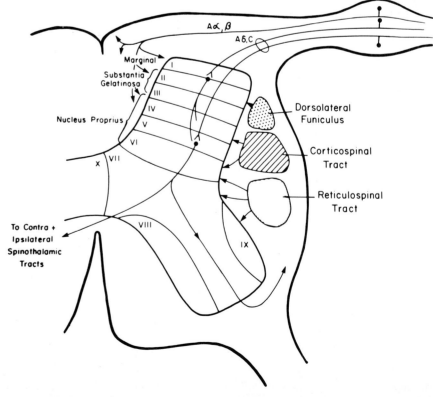

Figure 5–2. Segmental cord anatomy. Ten laminations of spinal gray matter have been identified in the cat. Laminae are also present in humans, and comprise the marginal zone, substantia gelatinosa, and nucleus proprius. Large A alpha and beta fibers traversing to the posterior columns give branches to the dorsal horn laminae. These, and descending fibers from the dorsolateral funiculus, corticospinal and reticulospinal tracts, modulate transmission of nociceptive input.

opposite side. Fibers can also project in ipsilateral tracts. A somatotopic arrangement exists, and fibers from caudal regions are more lateral, and rostral fibers are more ventral and medial. These projections are classified into the spinoreticular, spinomesencephalic (which comprise the paleospinothalamic system), and neospinothalamic tracts. These tracts may carry afferent input other than nociception, and spinal pathways other than those in the ventrolateral cord may transmit nociceptive information cephalad.

The neospinothalamic tract, also referred to as the *discriminatory* or *protopathic system*, is oligosynaptic, conducts more rapidly, and is believed to provide discrete information regarding stimulus location, intensity, and duration. It synapses with fibers in the ventrolateral and posterior thalamus before projecting to the somatosensory cortex (Fig. 5–3). The paleospinothalamic system projects to several areas of the brain stem, midbrain, hypothalamus, and medial and intralaminar thalamic nuclei. Diffuse projections are made to the reticular formation, limbic system, and areas involved in reflex responses of ventilation, circulation, and endocrine function. Because they are multisynaptic, diffuse, and slower conducting, they localize pain poorly, stimulate the affective emotional component of the pain response, probably trigger the modulation that occurs by higher centers, and initiate the behavioral response of the organism.

Afferent sensory transmission can be modulated at a number of points along the neuraxis. Descending and ascending neurons from a variety of higher structures and local intrinsic pathways can alter neuronal activity (Fig. 5–4). Major mechanisms of modulation are via monaminergic pathways involving serotonin and norepinephrine, and the endorphinergic pathways involving enkephalins. Other pathways that appear to influence nociceptive perception are gabaergic, neurotensin, and cholinergic systems. These modulatory systems are reflexly activated, and are selective on the fiber type they affect. They act as a variable gain, gain tuning, or threshold control to screen the wide amount of information being input to the system, and may be facilitory as well as inhibitory.

The response to surgical trauma can be summarized as follows. Surgical nociceptive input arises from skin, somatic structures, and visceral contents. Skin damage produces a sharp, well-localized sensation. Somatic damage manifests itself locally or in a referred area that is more diffuse and aching in perception. Visceral injury, though detectable to a local area, is typically manifest by a dull, aching, and diffuse sensation and frequently referred widely from the injured site and to referred distant areas. The tissue injury sets up responses at the spinal cord level corresponding to the site of injury. These responses

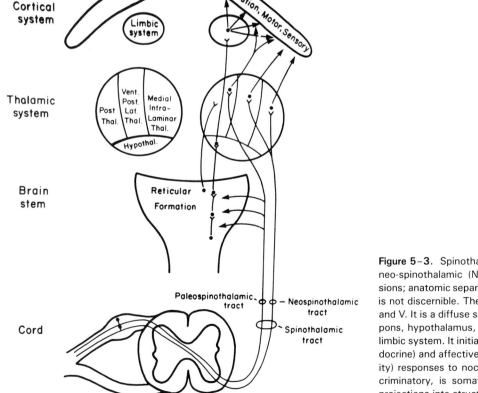

Figure 5–3. Spinothalamic projections. The paleo- (P) and neo-spinothalamic (N) tracts are functionally useful divisions; anatomic separation within the spinothalamic system is not discernible. The P is older, originating from laminae I and V. It is a diffuse system, projecting onto the brainstem, pons, hypothalamus, and thalamus with projections to the limbic system. It initiates reflex (circulatory, ventilatory, endocrine) and affective (mood, emotion, wakefulness, activity) responses to nociception. The N is referred to as discriminatory, is somatotopically arranged, and has fewer projections into structures other than thalamus and cortex.

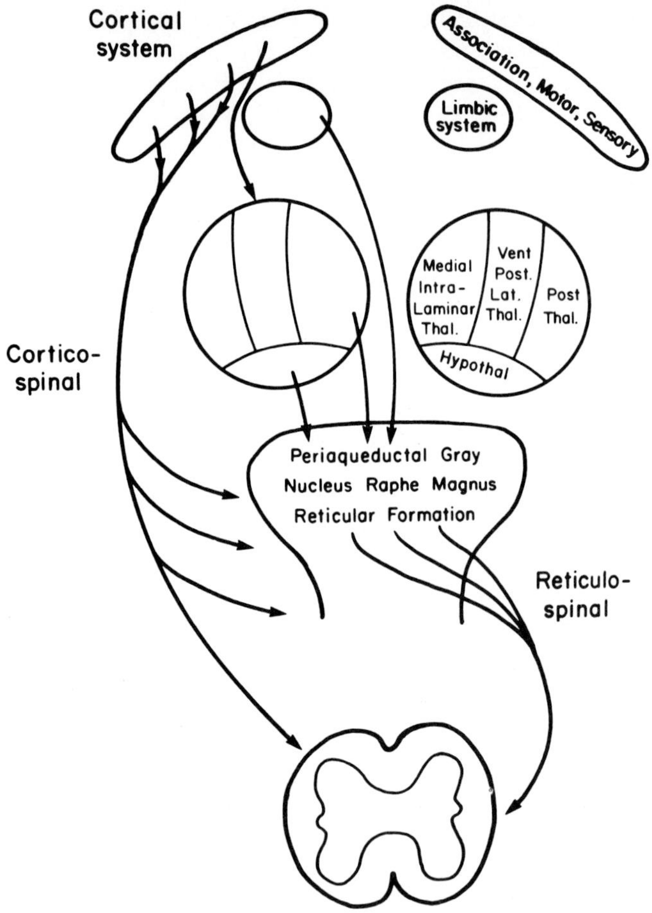

Figure 5–4. Descending modulating fibers of nociception. Cortical modulation will affect pain perception, the psychodynamic responses contributing to fear and anxiety, and behavioral responses (motivation, motor activity). Periaqueductal gray will project to serotinergic fibers of the Raphe Magnus. The latter will descend via the dorsolateral funiculus of the reticulospinal system (lateral to the corticospinal tract) synapsing with laminae I, II, and V.

are skeletal muscle spasm, vasospasm, visceral smooth muscle inhibition or contractions, with secondary nociception or nociceptive enhancement from the muscle spasm, ischemia, and the release of algesic substances. Stimulation of brainstem and diencephalon, mostly through lateral ascending spinal tracts, activates autonomic responses: ventilation; circulation; sympathetic output; and hypothalamic endocrine stimulation. Cortical projections perceive pain, and this perception initiates voluntary skeletal muscle activity, and contributes to the emotional responses. Postoperative pain is influenced by preoperative preparation; emotional, psychological, and motivational factors; the site and nature of the operation; and the type and location of the incision.

PHARMACOLOGIC CONSIDERATIONS[14-19]

The route and method of administration will influence the dose, frequency of administration, and duration of analgesic effect. The goal is to maintain a therapeutic (analgesic) level of drug, preventing sharp peaks into toxic levels, and trophs into subtherapeutic concentrations. Oral and intramuscular administration may be beset by variability of absorption, resulting in variable plasma concentrations. A drug should be administered at each half-life for four to five half-lives in order to obtain a steady state level in the analgesic range. An around-the-clock, not as needed (prn), administration of drug is required, and dosages may need adjustment to prevent peaks into toxic levels. Loading doses can shorten the time to steady state, but may lead to toxic blood levels (Fig. 5–5). Intravenous administration of drugs allows for rapid onset and titration to desired effect. Without continued infusion or repetition of frequent small amounts of drug, the effect will be short lived compared to oral or intramuscular administration. Deposition of the analgesic at the site of action would eliminate transport considerations of the drug, and uptake and distribution would be important only in its removal. This is not possible with any drug or technique to date; the administration of spinal opiates is the closest to the receptor an analgesic drug can be given.

Potentiation of analgesia by one class of drug is possible by combining it with an agent from another class. Nonsteroidal antiinflammatory drugs (NSAIDS), such as aspirin or acetaminophen; or ataractics/anti-

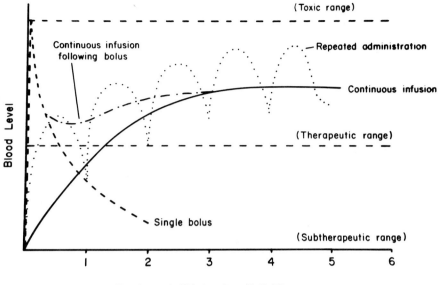

Figure 5-5. Effect of mode of administration on blood levels of analgesics.
– – – – Bolus dose
· · · · · · Repeated doses
——— Continuous Infusion
— · — · — Continuous infusion after bolus

An IV bolus dose allows a rapid onset of effect, early maximum concentrations, and relatively rapid decline of drug effect with rapid decline of concentration, minimizing the time the drug level remains in the toxic range. A larger initial bolus is required for sustained duration, but would lead to a greater risk of toxic effects.

Repeated administration of therapeutic doses at intervals equal to the half-life will eliminate the large swings from boluses and permit the blood level to remain longer in the therapeutic range. The fluctuation in blood level will be affected by the time between doses, the half-life, and by the rate of absorption. The widest fluctuations would occur with repeat IV injections, and least with oral. As the rate of absorption increases and the fluctuations widen, the likelihood for approaching toxic and subtherapeutic ranges increases. Repeated intramuscular injections are represented in the figure, but the principle is applicable to repeated oral and intravascular administration.

If the therapeutically equivalent dose is administered by continuous infusion, the wide fluctuations are avoided. An initial bolus can produce an immediate therapeutic level, avoiding delay in establishing an effect, and be sustained by the continuous infusion of the drug.

The repeated or continuous administration of drug is predicated on an unchanging elimination pattern and a therapeutic effect equal in duration to its elimination half-life. Changes in the ability to eliminate the drug (eg, decreased renal or hepatic clearance) or a drug with a short therapeutic half-life but long elimination half-life (eg, methadone) can lead to drug levels reaching and staying in the toxic range with continued administration.

histaminics/neuroleptics, such as hydroxyzine/diphenhydramine/droperidol, can markedly improve the analgesic effect of narcotics. Where one or the other is not effective alone, their combination often is, from potentiation (Fig. 5–6).

Patients exhibit pharmacodynamic variability (different responses to identical tissue levels of drug). This may relate to the stage of healing (postoperative nociception), environmental influences (noises, stimuli), and interaction with other factors noted earlier. Pharmacokinetics will also be influenced by alterations in tissue blood flow, volume status, changes in hepatic and renal clearance accompanied by the stress responses, third spacing, and metabolic alterations associated with surgery. Another phenomenon associated with oral analgesic usage is the first pass effect by the liver. Therapeutic systemic levels of

drug in some individuals are never reached because of near 100% clearance on the drug's first exposure to the liver after gastrointestinal absorption.

Binding to nonreceptor tissue, equilibration with the volume of distribution, and elimination by metabolism or excretion will influence the amount of drug available to produce a response at the receptor, regardless of the route of administration (Fig. 5–7). Distribution will be influenced by the type of membrane that the drug must pass; this can be simple capillaries or the complex multicellular structures of the blood–brain barrier. Most drugs will transfer by simple diffusion across a concentration gradient, dependent upon lipid–water partition coefficients. Other influential factors are membrane thickness and surface area; molecular size and configuration; dissociation constants and pH gradients across membranes; and

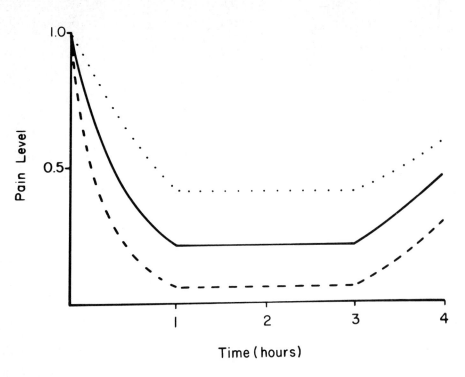

Figure 5–6. Effect of adjuvant drugs on narcotic. Pain level is normalized to 1. Administration of narcotic N lowers the pain level as depicted by · · · ·. Adding an adjuvant agent(s) with N lowers the pain level in a manner analogous to giving twice the dose of N (———). If the adjuvant is given with twice the dose of N, then the pain level is further lowered (— — —).

hydrostatic or osmotic pressure gradients. Membrane penetration and bioavailability in the brain is greatest for those drugs with the least ionization, least drug binding, and a high lipid–water partition coefficient. Removal of drug out of the cerebrospinal fluid is influenced by activity of the arachnoid villi and choroid plexus. The latter utilizes active transport for some drugs.

Intravenous administration produces rapid blood and tissue levels, allows the drug to be titrated to the desired effect, and assures systemic levels when blood flow to a site used for drug administration is compromised. These positive attributes can be offset by a greater risk of adverse effects from too high a level. Subcutaneous and intramuscular administration of aqueous preparations can produce systemic levels comparable to intravenous administration, but require a larger dose. Levels are reached at a slower rate, and last for a more sustained period of time, depending upon factors affecting uptake from the site of drug deposition. Pain and scarring at sites used for repeated injection can result, and intramuscular injection can be the source of major nerve damage, may lead to increased systemic levels of muscle enzymes, and are sometimes prohibited in the presence of anticoagulation.

Oral analgesia is the most convenient, economic, and safe method of drug administration. Its use is often precluded in the immediate postoperative period by poor patient cooperation from residual anesthetic effect or surgery on gastrointestinal function; nausea and vomiting; and the type of surgery. Some

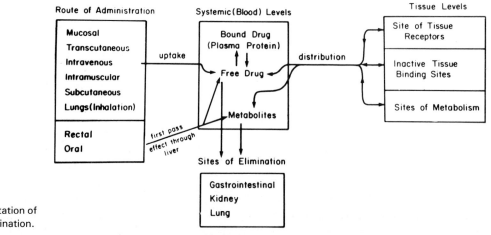

Figure 5–7. Diagramatic representation of drug uptake, distribution, and elimination.

agents are available in suppository form and can be given rectally. It should be noted that only about half of the rectally administered drug is affected by hepatic first-pass metabolism, the rest entering directly into the systemic circulation. Rectal drug administration has the problem of incomplete and erratic uptake, and rectal mucosal irritation can occur with repeated administration.

Spinal drug administration will be discussed later in the chapter.

ANALGESIC AGENTS[20-22]

There are two categories of analgesics: nonsteroidal antiinflammatory drugs (NSAID) and opiates.

The NSAIDs act at peripheral sites inhibiting the action of prostaglandins via antagonism of cyclo-oxygenase and probably immune system responses. Cyclo-oxygenase is needed to synthesize prostaglandin E2, a sensitizer of peripheral nociceptors. Although these drugs exert an antiinflammatory effect, their analgesic effects most likely involve other mechanisms, since acetaminophen, also classified with this group, has essentially no antiinflammatory action. Acetaminophen may produce its analgesia via central as opposed to peripheral mechanisms. In addition, it has no antiplatelet effects but does share antipyresis in common with other NSAIDs. All of these NSAIDs have a ceiling effect for analgesia (more drug does not produce more analgesia), but tolerance and physical and psychological dependence do not occur.

These properties are in contradistinction to agonist narcotics that have a central effect, and do not have a ceiling effect, antipyresis, antiplatelet, or antiinflammatory actions. They can produce tolerance, physical or psychological dependence, and respiratory or mental depression. The mixed agonist–antagonist agents have a ceiling effect for respiratory depression and analgesia, may cause hallucinations, and can reverse the effects of previously administered agonist narcotics. They may be used for short-term analgesia in narcotic-naive patients with mild to moderate pain.

The principles of analgesic management are several. These are described below and summarized in Table 5–2.

1. Choose the route appropriate for the patient's situation. The ambulatory patient will usually receive oral agents. However, the patient who cannot easily swallow following an oral surgical procedure might benefit from analgesics available via the rectal route. The patient with an indwelling spinal catheter for chronic narcotic administration could have a supple-

TABLE 5–2. PRINCIPLES OF ANALGESIC THERAPY

I.	Choose appropriate route
	Oral
	Intramuscular
	Intravenous
	Rectal
	Spinal
II.	Time-contingent dosing
	Patient's option to refuse
III.	Drug, dosage, and frequency adjustment
	Different drug side effect liabilities
	Variable therapeutic responses
	Individual differences in duration/elimination
	Changing analgesic requirements with time
IV.	Familiarity with several agents
	Short, intermediate, and long duration
	Different agents may affect different receptors
	Variable side effects with different agents
V.	Familiarity with oral/parenteral/rectal conversions

mental dose administered for the acute pain of surgery.
2. Administer the drug on a regular basis, not prn, allowing the patient the option to refuse. In this way, the therapeutic level of drug will be maintained (see Fig. 5–5).
3. Change the agent and/or the dosage and/or frequency of administration according to the patient's individual response. Adequate analgesia that is not sustained until the next dose may require an agent of longer duration or shortening the interval of administration.
4. Be thoroughly familiar with a few drugs to permit alternative trials of analgesics if one agent fails to relieve a patient. Although presumably acting at similar opiate receptors, one agent can be more beneficial than another, probably as a result of pharmacokinetic differences in the patient.
5. Be knowledgeable of the conversion from parenteral to oral and oral to parenteral dosing.

The importance of this last principle is illustrated by meperidine. The intramuscular (IM) to oral (PO) ratio for equivalent doses is 1:4. The postsurgical patient receiving 75 mg IM will need 300 mg PO. If the same parenteral dose is administered PO (in this example 75 mg) the patient will undoubtedly have inadequate analgesia. This may lead to a request for more pain medication or a return to the injections. The patient may then be labeled as drug-seeking or addiction-prone when in fact the amount of drug by the oral route was inadequate. Similarly, a patient chronically receiving hydromorphone PO may have respiratory and mental depression if the amount given IM is the same as the oral dose (IM:PO is 1.5:5).

The average surgical patient will rarely require analgesics longer than three to four days for severe or moderately severe pain, at which point those agents used for mild or moderate pain can be utilized. Drugs classified as useful for mild or moderate pain have a ceiling effect and dosage escalation consistently produces organ toxicity or side effects (for example, salicylates, meperidine). Drugs for severe pain may be limited by physiologic effects (for example, nausea and vomiting) in some patients, but dosage escalation to analgesic effect is generally well tolerated and does not produce toxic side effects. Tables 5–3 and 5–4 list commonly used analgesics; Table 5–5 lists those available as suppositories.

Adjuvant agents (Table 5–6) are useful in enhancing the analgesic effects of narcotics and nonnarcotic analgesics, have inherent analgesic properties of their own, or address an issue unrelated to analgesia. Reactive depression to an individual's situation (eg, diagnosis of cancer, loss of a body part through amputation) can be helped with antidepressants and support. Anxiety can interfere with the effectiveness of analgesics. Hydroxyzine (Vistaril, Atarax) is a useful agent for these circumstances because it possesses analgesic, antiemetic, and sedative properties in addition to anxiolysis. Its analgesic property can lower the requirement of narcotic agents (see Fig. 5–6). The phenothiazines and butyrophenones can be useful for more agitated patients; they also have the features noted for hydroxyzine.

The risk of producing iatrogenic addiction, manifest by psychological dependence and compulsive drug seeking for purposes other than analgesia, is very low in postsurgical patients.[22] Addiction is not the same as tolerance (a larger dose of drug is needed to achieve the same effect) or physical dependence (manifest by the abstinence syndrome). These are physiological phenomena, and are also very unlikely to occur when used for postsurgical analgesia in narcotic-naive individuals. Their development can be minimized by switching to the oral route of administration as soon as feasible, utilizing nonnarcotic agents to lower the requirements of narcotic agents, and gradually reducing the drug over several days.

PATIENT-CONTROLLED ANALGESIA

The current understanding of pain mechanisms, pharmacology, agents, and routes for their administration should make acute pain a rare problem in hospitalized patients. This is, unfortunately, not the case.[1,23] Reasons include inadequate pharmacologic knowledge and understanding, and personal biases staff members have toward pain and its management. The fear of addiction; belief that pain is ex-

TABLE 5–3. COMMONLY USED ANALGESICS[a]

Generic Name (Trade Name)	Oral Dosage[b] (mg)	Duration of Effect (h)	Comments
Salicylates			
Aspirin	650–1300	4–6	Available for rectal use often combined with other agents (eg, oxycodone, codeine).
Diflunisal (Dolobid)	250–500	8–12	Possibly more effective than aspirin. Requires loading dose and few days use for maximum effect.
Choline magnesium trisalicylate (Trilisate)	500–1500	8–12	Requires loading dose. Does not affect platelets.
Proprionic Acids			
Ibuprofen (Motrin, Advil)	300–400	8	Possibly more effective than aspirin.
Naproxen (Naprosyn)	250–500 (1500 maximum/day)	6–12	Usually taken twice a day.
Pyrole Acetic Acid			
Sulindac (Clinoril)	150–200	12	Possibly less GI and renal toxicity.
Para-Aminophenol			
Acetaminophen	650–1000 (4000 maximum/day)	4	Does not affect platelets. May cause hepatic damage. Rare GI upset. Combination with other NSAIDs may potentiate their renal toxicity. Often combined with narcotics (eg, Percoset, Tylenol with codeine). Available for rectal use.

[a]All are antipyretic and (except for acetaminophen) have the potential for GI distress/ulcers, inhibition of platelets (except choline magnesium trisalicylate), and nephritis.
[b]Recommended starting doses. Filtration required to optimize beneficial effect.

TABLE 5-4. COMMONLY USED NARCOTIC ANALGESICS[a]

Generic Name (Trade Name)	Dosage(mg)[b]		IM/PO Ratio	Duration of Effect (h)[c]		Comments
	IM/SC	PO		IM	PO	
Agonists[d]						
Morphine	5-10	30-60	1/3-1/6	4-6	1-3	Standard for comparing other narcotics. Available in suppository form. Sustained-release preparations (MS-Contin, Roxonol-SR) provide 8-12 hours duration. IM/PO ratio 1/6 for chronic users, 1/3 for opioid-naive individuals.
Meperidine (Demerol)	50-100	200-400	1/4	1-3	2-4	Toxic metabolite: normeperidine, with 24-36-hour half-life, accumulates with each dose. Proconvulsant and CNS excitation can precipitate seizures, neuropsychiatric disorders. May occur with as little as 300 mg/24 hours. Impaired renal function prolongs effect. Interacts with monoamine oxidase inhibitors.
Hydromerphone (Dilaudid)	1.5	4-8	1/5	4-5	3-6	Available for rectal use.
Methadone (Dolophine)	5-10	10-20	1/1-1/2	4-6	4-6	Duration of analgesic effect (8-12 h) shorter than sedative effect. Greater than 24-hour administration may lead to CNS and respiratory depression from cumulative doses.
Oxycodone	—	10-15	—	—	4-6	Usually given in combination form with aspirin or acetaminophen.
Codeine	120	200	2/3	3-4	4-6	Usually combined with aspirin or acetaminophen.
Agonist-Antagonists						
Pentazocine (Talwin)	60	150-200	1/4-1/3	2-3	3-4	May produce psychotomimetic effects. Do not use in narcotic-dependent individual. Irritates tissues on injection.
Butorphanol (Stadol)	2-3	—	—	3-4	—	Less likely to produce withdrawal in narcotic-dependent individual. Low incidence of abuse potential.
Partial Agonist						
Buprenorphine	0.3-0.4	—	—	6-8	—	Narcotic effects may not reverse with naloxone.

IM = intramuscular, SC = subcutaneous, PO = oral.
[a]Use with caution in patients with ventilatory difficulties (COPD, asthma), elevated intracranial pressure, compromised airway, or liver disease.
[b]Recommended starting doses; tritration required. Dosages are equianalgesic to morphine.
[c]The time to effect and duration of oral doses are generally longer than IM. Difference may arise from GI absorption and hepatic first-pass removal.
[d]Agonists are morphine or like substances that act primarily on the mu and kappa receptors. Agonists-antagonist drugs are agonist at some (kappa, sigma) and antagonist at other (mu) receptors; they can reverse the effects of pure agonists. Partial agonists partially bind when the mu receptor is empty and displace previously bound drugs, reversing their effect.

pected after surgery; concern about respiratory depression; misunderstanding of the placebo response; the belief that current analgesic regimens are satisfactory; the subjective nature of pain; the fear of patients expressing their pain; and patient variability to fixed drug regimens are identifiable reasons that contribute to an inadequate administration of analgesics for many patients.

The time from the request for medication until it has been administered and analgesia develops contributes to inadequate medication dosage, intermittent relief, and patient anxiety. The traditional approach requires the patient to call the nurse who, upon responding, makes an assessment of the pa-

TABLE 5-5. ANALGESICS AVAILABLE AS RECTAL SUPPOSITORIES

Hydromorphone
Oxymorphone
Morphine
Aspirin
Acetaminophen

TABLE 5-6. ADJUVANT AGENTS

Antidepressants
Anxiolytic/antihistaminic
Phenothiazines
Butyrophenones

tient. The orders for that patient are then checked; the appropriateness of medicating the patient is made (determining if the time interval since the previous dose has elapsed); the keys to the narcotic box are obtained; drug counts and administrative logging of dispensal are done; and the drug is prepared. Finally, the drug is administered. This process may take 10 to 30 minutes, depending on delays caused at any point in this process. The nurse must give priority to patient requests and other care may supersede requests for pain medication.

Once administered, a patient must wait until enough is absorbed into the therapeutic range. The therapeutic dose range may be exceeded by the continued absorption of drug, leading to sedation. If the drug concentration falls into subtherapeutic levels prior to the next scheduled dose, the analgesia will dissipate and the patient will be required to wait until the next ordered dose of medication can be given. The duration of time that the agent is in the therapeutic range can be as little as 30 to 50% of the time between administrations.[24] Though the minimum analgesic blood concentration can vary severalfold,[25] individualization of dosage according to each patient's response would compensate for this variable.

These inadequacies in postoperative analgesia led to the concept of allowing patients to administer their own analgesics,[26,27] or patient-controlled analgesia (PCA). Features central to PCA are defined in Table 5–7. The loading, or bolus dose, is administered until the desired analgesic effect is obtained. It is typically initiated at the time the PCA system is prepared for the patient. The incremental dose, lockout interval, and time period maximum are also defined at this time as safety features to prevent excessive dosing. After therapeutic drug levels from the loading dose fall to ineffective levels (see Fig. 5–5), the patient can deliver an incremental dose by pressing a hand-held demand button analogous to a call device for a nurse. The drug will be administered from an infusion device to the IV, raising the level back into the therapeutic range. A typical regimen using morphine for PCA is outlined in Table 5–8.

The intravenous self-administration of narcotic

TABLE 5–8. INITIATION OF PATIENT-CONTROLLED ANALGESIA[a]

Loading (bolus) dose: 1–5 mg
Incremental dose: 1 mg
Lockout interval: 6 min
Four-hour maximum: 15 mg

[a]This is a representative starting regimen in the PACU using morphine for an ASA I or II patient having completed intraabdominal or orthopedic prosthetic surgery. Settings will require modification for age, debility, prior drug usage (tolerance), individual variability, and changing analgesic requirements, wound healing, and recovery.

analgesics would not be possible without computer technology. This permits programming, storage, and retrieval of data. Printers, either built in or externally attached, allow hard copies for medical records. They can be built small and lightweight, permitting easier use for the ambulating patient. The reservoir holding the drug is a syringe or bag. Security against tampering with drug and program settings is arranged through a mechanical lock and key, electrical access codes, or both.

While PCA has come to be associated with intravenous analgesia, it can be accomplished by other techniques. PCA using oral medication has been administered with good results.[28] The epidural route has also been used.[29] It is conceivable that subcutaneous, sublingual, transnasal, and transdermal modes of PCA could be developed in the future if the features in Table 5–8 could be applied.

The advantages of PCA are outlined in Table 5–9. Studies have confirmed a greater stability of blood analgesia levels[30,31] with improved analgesia, lessened patient anxiety, and increased satisfaction.[32,33] Earlier mobilization, improved pulmonary toilet, and reduced hospital stay with PCA versus IM, alluded to in verbal reports and abstracts, require further confirmation.

The initial cost for establishing a PCA program is large. Evaluated over 5 years, however, it is only slightly more expensive than conventional analgesic therapy.[34] The expense should decrease with improved technology and competition between manufacturers. The major limitations to effective use of

TABLE 5–7. FEATURES CENTRAL TO PATIENT-CONTROLLED ANALGESIA

I.   **Loading (bolus) dose:** The administration of an adequate amount of analgesic to establish levels within the therapeutic range.

II. **Incremental dose:** Subsequent doses of analgesic to maintain levels wtihin the therapeutic range.

III. **Lockout interval:** The time between incremental doses.

IV. **Time period maximum:** The maximum amount of analgesic that can be received in a specific time.

TABLE 5–9. ADVANTAGES OF PCA OVER CONVENTIONAL IM INJECTION

Safe and simple to use
Stable analgesic levels
Less traumatic to tissues
Nursing time freed for other needs
Reduced patient anxiety
Increased patient satisfaction
Applicability to a wide age range
Possibly: Fewer pulmonary abnormalities
          Shortened hospital stay

PCA are mental disabilities in understanding the concept of its use or physical disabilities in initiating device activation.

Problems operating the PCA device can be caused by the health care team, patient, or device malfunction (Table 5–10).[35] PCA use has a very safe history. It is theoretically possible to overdose a patient if the device is programmed for a lower drug concentration than the concentration in the syringe, and the lockout interval is short, giving rise to large incremental doses in short periods. The PCA would have to be activated after each lockout interval. If this were performed with usual doses and settings as in Table 5–8, the patient would become drowsy and sedated, preventing requests for further doses of medication and minimizing respiratory depression. Shutdown of device operation with loss of stored data can occur from battery exhaustion when the battery is not required and the staff fail to utilize main outlet power.

Hypotension can occur in the hypovolemic patient from small (1 mg) morphine incremental doses. An unreported yet interesting observation by our service is an apparent psychological dependency that some patients manifest. These patients have been surprisingly reluctant to have the device removed despite resumed oral intake, reduced narcotic usage to minimal amounts, and the fact that they are ambulating. They invariably express a security in knowing it is available. Mechanical and software failure has led to inactivation of the PCA in our experience; there are no reports of "runaway" devices in which drug is continuously or repetitively administered. Anecdotal stories have been told of patient visitors pushing the demand button purposely to give more medication to the patient or accidentally in calling for the nurse. Problems from this have not been reported in the literature.

TABLE 5–10. PROBLEMS ASSOCIATED WITH PCA

Health care team
 Incorrect setup— programming, IV attachment, syringe
  reservoir placement
 Battery exhaustion
 Unfamiliarity with concept or device
 Lack of access to code or key

Patient
 Confusing PCA demand and nurses' call buttons
 Misunderstanding how to use PCA
 Hypovolemia
 Psychologic dependence

PCA device
 Mechanical failure
 Software failure

Miscellaneous
 IV infiltration
 Visitor tampering

For postoperative pain, PCA represents a milestone. The participation of patients in the management of their pain alleviates anxiety and permits the patient to deliver and maintain antinociceptive agents at therapeutic levels required for their particular needs. It addresses more capably the wide degree of pharmacokinetic and dynamic responses that cannot be matched by conventional fixed-dose, time-controlled analgesia. It should continue to have a place in postoperative analgesia for these and the other reasons noted in Table 5–9.

SPINAL OPIATES

The recent interest and new wealth of information in spinal and epidural opiate therapy in humans has evolved from work published in 1979.[36,37] The actions of spinal opiate agonists and antagonists along with their specific receptors are not completely understood and drug dosages that produce maximal pain relief with fewest side effects are still being ascertained. Thus, only guidelines as to the use of spinal opiates are presented.

Receptors

Opioid agonists interact at the spinal cord level with different classes of opioid receptors to produce analgesia and side effects. The categories of receptors are labeled by the first Greek letter corresponding to their primary agonists. Mu (μ) receptors, whose primary agonist is morphine, account for approximately 40%[38] of opioid receptors. These mu receptors may be further broken down into mu-1 receptors, which are primarily responsible for supraspinal analgesia; and mu-2 receptors, which cause bradycardia, hypoventilation, physical dependence, and euphoria (Table 5–11).

Delta (δ) receptors account for a small percentage of opioid receptors, of which D-ala^2-D-leu^5-enkkephalin (DADL) is a primary agonist. This synthetic compound is thought to modulate mu receptor activity through the activity of the delta receptors.

Kappa (κ) receptors account for approximately 50%[38] of opiate receptors and most agonist–antagonist opioids act on this receptor. Ethylketocyclazocine (EKC), a kappa primary agonist, is associated with analgesia, sedation, miosis, and minimal depression of ventilation.

Sigma (σ) receptors are thought to effect dysphoria, hypertonia, tachycardia, and tachypnea. N-allylnormetazocine (SKF 10,047), a primary agonist, has hallucinogenic properties and is able to produce abstinence in the morphine-dependent dog (partial mu antagonist effect).

Different opioid receptors appear to be effective

TABLE 5–11. CLASSIFICATION OF OPIOID RECEPTORS

	Effect	Agonist	Antagonist
Mu-1	Supraspinal	Beta-endorphine Morphine	Naloxone Pentazocine
Mu-2	Depression of ventilation Decreased heart rate Physical dependence Euphoria	Meperidine Fentanyl Sufentanil Alfentanil Leu-enkephalin	Nalbuphine
Delta	Modulate mu receptor activity	Leu-enkephalin	Naloxone Met-enkephalin
Kappa	Analgesia Sedation Depression of ventilation(?) Miosis	Dymorphin Pentazocine Butorphanol Nalbuphine Buprenorphine Nalorphine	Naloxone
Sigma	Dysphoria Hypertonia Tachycardia Tachypnea	Pentazocine(?) Ketamine(?)	Naloxone

From Stoelting RK: Opioid Agonists and Antagonists. Pharmaology and Physiology in Anesthesia Practice. *Philadelphia, Lippincott, 1987, pp 69–101.*

for distinct types of pain. Mu agonists have been effective in animal studies in relieving noxious stimulation of cutaneous thermal tests (somatic pain), and intraperitoneal administration of irritant chemicals (visceral pain). Delta agonists are only effective in cutaneous thermal tests (somatic pain), while kappa agonists are only effective in visceral pain tests.[39,40] Therefore, delta agonists may be useful for somatic pain while kappa agonists may be more effective against visceral pain.

Opiate Peptide System

There is an extensive endogenous opiate peptide system composed of precursor peptide molecules that are cleaved into active opioid peptides. Pre-proopiomelanocortin is converted into ACTH (corticotropin), and B-lipoprotein. B-lipoprotein is cleaved into alpha, beta, gamma, and delta endorphins. In situations of stressful stimuli, ACTH and B-endorphin outflow is increased. B-endorphin is a more potent analgesic agent than morphine. Methionine (met-) and leucine (leu-) enkephalins are cleaved from pre-pro-enkephalin A and also have opiate activity. Pre-pro-enkephalin B (pre-pro-dynorphin) forms leu-enkephalin and dynorphin, which is further fragmented into dynorphins A and B. Synthetic enkephalins have been produced that do not have the short duration of action characteristic of endogenous compounds. Thiorphan, an enkephalinase inhibitor, may cause analgesia by prolonging the effect of endogenous opioids.

Sites of Action

Spinal opioids probably act as inhibitory agents of nociception at the dorsal horn and particularly at the substantia gelatinosa. The mu opiate receptors in the periaqueductal gray matter of the midbrain, the raphe nucleus, and adjacent nuclei in the medulla oblongata are the most important to effect the descending dorsolateral tracts by inhibiting reception through the dorsal horn.[41] Serotonin and norepinephrine (aminergenic system) may be involved in the descending inhibition that is activated by opiates. Spinal morphine after rostral spread may have this secondary effect in the brain, as well as other interactions in the perception of pain.[41] Kappa agents appear to be less active in the descending pathway as spinal transection does not reduce the analgesic effects of kappa agonists in the distal cord.[42]

Mode of Action

Selective spinal analgesia[43] is a term that indicates that the effect of spinal opiates is more specific for antinociception as opposed to local anesthetic action that demonstrates a nonselective blockade of axonal conduction. Spinal opioids, in comparison to local anesthetics, lack sympathetic, sensory, and motor blockade. Postural hypotension and cardioaccelerator block therefore are not problems. Furthermore, spinal opiates have a slow onset, and toxic effects are easily detectable by proper monitoring. Local anesthetics that block surgical pain can result in immediate hypotension, cardiac arrest, central nervous system depression, and seizures. Surgical pain is not blocked by spinal opiates. Myelinated A-delta fibers are blocked by local anesthetics but not as readily by spinal opiates,[39] which are most effective against unmyelinated C-fibers. Spinal opiates, in contrast to local anesthetics, have minimal effect on intraoperative or postoperative neurohumeral effects. Morphine may increase antidiuretic hormone levels secondary to migration into the brain.

The fraction of morphine crossing the dura after epidural injection is approximately 3.6% in humans,[44] while approximately 0.1% of an intravenous dose of morphine penetrates the central nervous system.[45] Greater analgesia is accomplished with less opiate administrated by the epidural or spinal route than by the IV route with less sedation and enhanced postoperative recovery. The onset of analgesia is related to the agonist's lipid solubility. Molecular weight may have a role in the permeability of the dura matter when the epidural concentration gradient to spinal cord is high.[46] The more lipid-soluble an agent, the faster its removal, and if the agonist does not bind tightly to its receptor the agent will be removed more quickly (receptor dissociation). If an increased amount of a lipid-soluble agent is required to effect analgesia, systemic absorption of that substance may occur with more sedation or side effects secondary to an increased plasma level. The long duration of morphine may be secondary to its high water solubility and low lipid-solubility so that it migrates cephalad with the bulk flow of the cerebrospinal fluid. Morphine, as opposed to lipophilic opiates, has a low concentration of un-ionized drug in the epidural space and cerebrospinal fluid (CSF).

Opiates pass across the arachnoid granulations to the CSF in the un-ionized form. Once the drug is in the CSF only those particles that remain un-ionized will penetrate the spinal cord, and a drug such as morphine will be primarily ionized in the CSF. Therefore, morphine has a slow onset and long duration of action. There is a possibility that un-ionized drugs will pass directly to the spinal cord from the epidural space via the posterior radicular arteries. The subdural is a nonvascular space and opiates may be less absorbed through the posterior radicular arteries, which may account for less absorption when the subdural space is unintentionally entered.

Complications of Spinal Opiates

Respiratory Depression. Spinal opiates have a low incidence of respiratory depression, but this is nevertheless of major concern because if undetected it may be a source of major morbidity. Proper dosaging and adequate monitoring minimize these complications. Early respiratory depression may occur secondary to vascular absorption of the opiate, and late respiratory depression secondary to cephalad migration. Late respiratory depression occurs mainly after administrating water-soluble opiates such as morphine. This occurs more often with intrathecal administration with an incidence of 4 to 7%, compared to an incidence 0.1 to 0.4% in epidural administration.[47] Risk for respira-

tory depression is reduced by lower dosages. One study indicated an incidence of approximately 0.3% for intrathecal morphine 0.2 to 0.8 mg.[39] Early respiratory depression with intrathecal administration rarely occurs.

Age, poor general health, concomitant parental administration of opiates, impaired respiratory function, accidental dural puncture, thoracic epidural approach, opiate naivete, and residual effects of other depressant medications (including anesthetics) are factors implicated in the risk of respiratory depression.[39] In circumstances of increased abdominal pressure as in pregnancy, obstruction of the inferior vena cava will cause more blood flow from the epidural veins to the azygos system, increasing systemic uptake of epidural opiates. Infusion of naloxone at a rate of 5 μg/kg/h may prevent respiratory depression and other side effects.[48] A naloxone infusion may not antagonize morphine analgesia, but may antagonize the analgesia of other agents. The use of lipid-soluble agents by infusion may be associated with a smaller incidence of delayed respiratory depression as there may be less rostral spread. Posture, originally theorized to have a role in CSF spread, has not been demonstrated.[49] Hyberbaric solutions of morphine, once advocated to prevent respiratory depression, are not protective against CSF spread.

The most effective way to monitor respiratory depression is by frequent assessment of ventilation and measuring sedation. Respiratory monitors used in the postoperative period produce false alarms and patient acceptance is poor.[50] Somnolence precedes respiratory depression and decreased tidal volume often precedes a slower respiratory rate.[51] The following scale can be used for assessing sedation: 0 = none (alert); 1 = mild (occasionally drowsy, easy to arouse); 2 = moderate (frequently drowsy, easy to arouse); 3 = severe (somnolent, difficult to arouse); and S = sleep (normal sleep, easy to arouse).[52] Nurses can use this scale to rate the level of consciousness following epidural opiate administration hourly (Table 5–12).[52]

Nausea and Vomiting. Nausea and vomiting varies from 15 to 50% in patients receiving spinal opiates, and compares to an incidence of approximately 30%

TABLE 5–12. BEDSIDE SEDATION SCALE

Sedation	Description
0 (None)	Patient alert
1 (Mild)	Occasionally drowsy; easily aroused
2 (Moderate)	Frequently drowsy; easily aroused
3 (Severe)	Somnolent; difficult to arouse
S (None)	Normal sleep; easily aroused

From Ready LB, Chadwick HS, Wild LM: Additional comments regarding an anesthesiology-based postoperative pain service (letter to editor). Anesthesiology 1988; 69:139.

in patients receiving systemic opiates.[39,47] Early nausea and vomiting with epidural morphine may occur from systemic uptake, and can be seen six hours following intrathecal administration, secondary to rostral spread to the chemoreceptor trigger zone and vomiting center. Lipid soluble agents may have a lower incidence of this complication. Nausea and vomiting may be treated with metoclopramide 5 to 10 mg IV, droperidol 0.625 mg IV, or with an infusion of naloxone at 5 to 15 μg/kg/h. Transdermal scopalamine applied to the mastoid region may be used prophylactically.[53]

Pruritus. Itching occurs in 8.5% of patients receiving epidural opiates and in 46% of patients receiving spinal opiates.[54] This compares with 1% pruritus in patients receiving systemic morphine. Itch and hyperalgesia after intrathecal opiates are thought to be secondary to local excitation by opiates in the spinal cord.[54] Pruritus usually spreads segmentally and is common in the head and neck region from rostral involvement of the trigeminal nucleus. Itching may be treated with diphenhydramine 25 mg IM, hydroxyzine 25 mg IM, or with a naloxone infusion at 5 to 15 μg/kg/h.

Urinary Complications. Urinary retention occurs in 15 to 42%[47,55] of postoperative patients who received spinal opiates and has not been found to be dose related. Mammals release urine by neural transmission through the parasympathetic pathways to the detrusor muscle, and inhibition of somatic input to the external urethral sphincter. Urinary retention by spinal opiates is probably secondary to interaction with the parasympathetic outflow to the bladder.[55] Beta-adrenergic receptors are predominant in the detrusor muscle, and alpha-adrenergic receptors in the trigone and proximal urethra. In rats treated with spinal opiates, cholinergic agents caused contraction of the internal sphincter and increased bladder pressure.[55] Urinary retention may persist despite treatment with cholinergic agents such as bethanecol, and may be harmful. This corresponds with the apparent ineffectiveness of bethanecol in previous studies.[56] The rate of urinary retention secondary to epidural morphine decreased by administering 10 mg of phenoxybenzamine (an alpha blocker) orally 24 and 2 hours before caesarian section and 8 and 16 hours postpartum.[57] Lipid-soluble agents may have a lower incidence of urinary retention as studies with epidural methadone have indicated.[58] Animal studies have indicated that kappa agonists may be devoid of urinary retentive properties.[39] Urinary retention may be treated by an infusion of naloxone 5 to 15 μg/kg/h.

Hyperalgesia. Morphine can cause hyperalgesia in high dosages. High concentrations of spinal opiates may physiologically antagonize the analgesia mediated by spinal opiate receptors, possibly through nonopiate receptors. This also may be secondary to a metabolite of morphine (morphine-3-glucuronide).[59] Hyperalgesia from morphine has not been observed in therapy for acute pain.

Available Agents

Intrathecal opiate is introduced directly into the subarachnoid space with resulting high cerebrospinal fluid levels; 3.6% of epidural dosages diffuse subarachnoid. Suggested intrathecal dosages are: morphine 250 μg; sufentanil 10 to 20 μg; alfentanil 125 to 250 μg; and lofentanil 1 to 2 μg (Table 5–13).[60-62]

Epidural opiate analgesia should be achieved at the minimal possible dose. The higher dosages increase the duration of action but at the cost of more side effects. Lower extremity and abdominal surgery require 2 to 5 mg of epidural morphine. Lumbar epidural morphine for thoracic analgesia requires 2 to 6 mg, while a thoracic injection requires 1 to 4 mg. Lower dosages are needed for elderly patients. Morphine infusion at 0.1 to 0.2 mg/h after a 2-mg bolus has been utilized. The effectiveness of morphine in achieving analgesia appears equal in lumbar epidural and thoracic epidural pain control for thoracic surgery. Epidural morphine improves FEV_1 and vital capacity, but maximal inspiratory and expiratory pressures are depressed. The onset of action may be enhanced by opiates diluted into a larger volume. Volumes used have varied between 10 and 20 mL. For example, hydromorphine 1.25 mg to 1.5 mg has been diluted in 10 to 15 mL of preservative-free saline for use through a lumbar epidural catheter for relief of postthoracotomy pain.[63] Increased volume may cause a faster onset, greater potency, or respiratory depression.[64,65]

Lipid-soluble agents are associated with more sedation than morphine, and have a shorter onset and duration of action. There may be less respiratory depression or urinary retention at recommended dosages. Fentanyl 100 μg or fentanyl 50 μg with epinephrine 1:200,000 are equipotent and effective dosages. These dosages of fentanyl have been followed by continuous infusion of 0.02 mg/hr when prolonged effect is desired. Alfentanil has been used as an infusion after a bolus of 1 mg. Sufentanil 10 to 30 μg is a

TABLE 5–13. SPINAL OPIATE ADMINISTRATION

Drug	Dosage	Onset	Duration (h)
Morphine	0.1–0.5 mg	15	8–24
Sufentanil	10–20 μg		
Diamorphone	1–2 mg		20
Alfentanil	125–250 μg		
Meperidine[a]	10–30 mg		10–30

[a]Meperidine as sole anesthetic agent = 1 mg/kg.

TABLE 5–14. EPIDURAL OPIATE ADMINISTRATION

Drug	Dosage	Infusion Technique		Onset	Duration (h)
		Bolus	*Infusion*		
Morphine Lumbar catheter	2–6 mg	2 mg	0.1–0.2 mg/h	30	6–24
Morphine Thoracic catheter for thoracic surgery	1–4 mg				6–24
Sufentanil	10–30 μg	0.3 μg/kg	0.3 μg/kg/h Caution: has shown accumulation	5	4–6
Alfentanil	1 mg	1 mg	0.2 mg/h	5	
Methadone	2–6 mg			15	6–10
Hydromorphone	1–1.5 mg			15	10–16
Hydromorphone	1.5 mg with epinephrine 1:200,000				
Fentanyl	25–100 μg 50 μg with epinephrine 1:200,000 = 100 μg	1.5 μg/kg or 25–100 μg	0.5 μg/kg/h or 25–150 μg/h	5	4–6
Buprenorphrine	0.15–0.3 mg	0.15 mg	0.018 mg/h		6–12
Diamorphine	4–6 mg			5	12
Meperidine	20–60 mg			5	6–8

Use lowest dosages in the elderly or if catheter is in thoracic region.

drug with avid opiate receptor binding, which may cause sedation, particularly at the higher dosages. Sufentanil, when used in conjunction with naloxone as a prophylactic infusion shows less analgesia than dosages of naloxone, which cause fewer side effects. Therefore prophylactic naloxone infusions for sufentanil are not recommended (Table 5–14).

OTHER MODALITIES

Transcutaneous Electrical Nerve Stimulation (TENS)

The modern era of electroanalgesia followed the spinal gate control theory.[66] The simplicity of its concept had great appeal, and led to trials of controlled electricity to provide a differential stimulation of large nonnociceptive fibers in an attempt to inhibit nociceptive input. Release of endogenous opiates[67,68] as another possible mode of action has not been substantiated. It is possible that other unrecognized mechanisms contribute to the observed analgesic effect.

The initial reports of TENS providing postoperative pain relief, reduction in analgesic requirements, and decreased pulmonary morbidity, have not been universally found. Patients receiving TENS report less pain, but the demand for supplemental analgesics and the effects on ventilatory parameters are no different from those not receiving TENS for abdominal operations.[69,70] TENS may be more effective in reducing cutaneous, movement-associated incisional pain than deeper, visceral-related pain.[71,72]

Local Anesthetics

Local anesthetics can provide excellent pain relief. Their use is limited by the need for personnel knowledgeable and skilled in their administration on a continuing basis postoperatively. When used for the surgical procedure or given prior to the end of surgery, the reduced general anesthetic requirements may result in a more rapid recovery and in immediate postsurgical pain relief that can extend for several hours in some circumstances.

Local anesthetic infiltration of surgical wounds can provide hours of relief from incisional pain.[73,74] Multi-orificed catheters have been placed into incisions to permit the ongoing use of local anesthetic.[75] Twice-daily irrigation doses of 10 to 20 mL of 0.125 to 0.5% bupivacaine has been suggested for this purpose. While useful for the management of incisional or somatic pain, narcotic or other analgesic agents will be needed for deeper visceral pain.

Nerve blocks permit analgesia in a wide area often with less drug than that required for infiltration. Proximal or distal blocks of nerves innervating extremities, an incision (eg, iliohypogastric, ilioinguinal, intercostal), or a terminal structure (penis, digits) can provide many hours of relief. Extension of local analgesia is possible when a neurovascular bundle is present to permit catheter placement for intermittent or continuous instillation of drug. This has been accomplished for the upper extremity[76,77] and upper abdominal incisions.[78] Catheter placement in the paravascular space containing the femoral nerve is also possible. Continuous analgesia would require an infusion of 5 to 10 mL/h of 0.125 to 0.5% bupivacaine.

In addition to spinal opiates for analgesia (described earlier in the chapter), epidural local anesthetics can be administered for postoperative pain management.[79] While this is the most effective method of providing profound analgesia for surgical procedures of the abdomen and thorax, it may cause autonomic block affecting the cardiovascular, gastrointestinal, and bladder systems and somatic motor functions. Placing the catheter tip at a spinal level innervating the center of the surgical site will lessen the amount of anesthetic and the extent of block, reducing the risk of untoward system dysfunction. A continuous infusion of 10 to 20 mL/h of 0.1 to 0.125% bupivacaine can help maintain a narrow band of spinal analgesia following an initial loading dose. Supplemental injections of 5 to 10 mL of 0.5% bupivacaine with adjustment of the continuous infusion may be required for break through pain.

This approach requires close nursing supervision and availability of an anesthesiologist. Orthostatic vascular instability, and loss of sensory, motor, or proprioceptive function, will preclude mobilizing the patient, and may require termination of epidural local anesthetics. A possible synergism between epidural local anesthetics and narcotics may permit reducing their amounts, and hence side effects, when given as a combined infusion.[80]

Intrapleural analgesia is accomplished by local anesthetic injection into the pleural space, allowing diffusion of drug to multiple intercostal nerves. A Tuohy epidural needle is inserted at the 6th, 7th, or 8th intercostal space over the superior rib border posteriorly at approximately its angle.[81] The needle is directed posteriorly and at an angle of 30 to 40° to the skin. Once the tip is within tissue, the stylet is removed and a well-lubricated or freely moving glass syringe with air or saline is attached to the needle hub. The needle is then advanced until, in a manner analogous to the entry into the epidural space, the syringe plunger gives way as "clicking" perforation is felt upon entering the pleural space. An epidural catheter is then passed approximately 5 cm past the needle tip. Twenty mL of 0.5% bupivacaine is then injected 3 to 4 times a day. This has been reported to produce excellent anesthesia for unilateral incisions for renal, breast, and gallbladder surgery.[81-83] It is not effective after thoracotomy[84] because of loss of drug

in the pleural drainage, and poor distribution or spread from the reactive tissues and change in pleural pressure dynamics. Surprisingly, very few reports indicate that pneumothorax occurs; a preliminary report[85] has identified pneumothorax, suboptimal catheter location, and lung penetration to be significant complications with this technique. Systemic drug uptake with seizure activity has also been reported.[83]

Chemical and Cryoneurolysis

The use of neurolytic agents (alcohol, phenol) is extremely limited for postoperative pain management. It is restricted to those with inoperable cancer. In the postoperative period, it cannot usually be immediately applied, and thus becomes part of the overall plan of pain management in the cancer patient. In patients with pain from unresectable chest wall tumor, 1 to 3 mL of 6% phenol can be injected intraoperatively at each intercostal level involved with tumor. Care must be taken by the surgeon to inject as proximal to the spinal nerve as possible, but to avoid the dural sleeve of each nerve. Injection into the latter could lead to spread of the caustic substance centrally into the cerebrospinal fluid with serious consequences. Neuritis is a common problem and the resulting pain can be as devastating or worse than the pain for which it is being used.

Abdominal pain from pancreatic cancer, determined to be unresectable at surgery, can be treated with 20 to 30 mL of 50 to 75% alcohol injected into the celiac plexus at the time of exploratory surgery.[86] The results for long-term relief may not be as good as closed percutaneous injections because of loss of alcohol by evaporation from an open wound and irrigation of the wound.

In contrast, cryoneurolysis causes nerve destruction by cold thermal injury with very low risk for neuritis.[87-89] It has been reported to be very effective in reducing thoracotomy[90,91] and herniorrhaphy[87] surgical pain. The duration of analgesia from cryoneurolysis can be days to weeks. This results from damage to the myelin sheath and axonal disintegration, resulting in Wallerian-type degeneration. Recovery of nerve function occurs because the endoneurium and basic tubular architecture remain intact, permitting regeneration with minimal risk of neuroma formation.

The low temperature (-60 to $-80°C$) at the tip of the probe develops from expansion of nitrous oxide under high pressure across a narrow orifice (Joule-Thompson effect). With the cryoprobe tip situated on the nerve, the cooling by the gas expansion creates an ice ball at the tip, encompassing the nerve. The best results are obtained if a nerve is frozen for two 1- to 2-minute intervals, each interval separated by a thaw of the nerve for approximately the same time.

As all fiber types are damaged, its use on mixed or motor nerves may lead to weakness. Patients should be warned that sensory or motor deficit may last for weeks to months, and they should take precautions against injury to those areas. Some may find the anesthesia bothersome and can only be encouraged that it is expected to resolve in the time frame noted above.

Other miscellaneous techniques have limited usefulness. Acupuncture for postoperative pain requires personnel skilled and knowledgeable in its application to be frequently available for repeat administration. Its efficacy has been reported as comparable to placebo.[92] Hypnosis, which can be self-administered, can reduce pain, but is not amenable to all patients and requires preoperative teaching. The use of subliminal suggestion during anesthesia to reduce morbidity and improve analgesia[93] appears to be a simple addendum to anesthesia care; further clarification of its effectiveness is needed. Music as a therapeutic agent has also been reported.[94]

A low dose (2 mg/min) 24 hours intravenous lidocaine infusion reduces postoperative pain and narcotic requirements without adverse physiologic changes.[95] Blood concentrations were 1 to 2 $\mu g/mL$. Whether this can be safely extended beyond the first 24 hours is not known.

Although appearing attractive, nitrous oxide analgesia in the postoperative period is not advised because of (1) its adverse effects on hematologic and hepatic function[96]; (2) difficulties in instituting and monitoring its use on the ward; (3) exposure of personnel to waste nitrous oxide; and (4) its physical effects on air-filled spaces.

FUTURE DEVELOPMENTS

The future of postoperative analgesia lies in the development of better delivery systems, more potent and analgesic-specific drugs, education, and research. Delivery of analgesics other than the conventional oral, intramuscular, and intravenous, and the fairly recent spinal, routes, holds promise for simpler, easier, more readily available analgesia. Areas of current development include transdermal[97] and sublingual[98] delivery. Transnasal[99] and oral transmucosal[100] routes used for anesthetic induction could probably be extrapolated for analgesia in the postoperative period. It is also conceivable that transpulmonary inhalation of metered doses of an analgesic could be developed.

Enkephalinase is an enzyme that inactivates endogenous enkephalins.[101] Inhibitors of this enzyme have been developed and animal studies have shown analgesic activity comparable to morphine, but with no evidence of tolerance, withdrawal phenomena, or gastrointestinal, respiratory, or central nervous system depression.[102] If applicable in humans, this novel approach would utilize the endogenous opioid system to produce analgesia.

Pediatric pain management has only recently been addressed. Methods of pain assessments, techniques of drug delivery, pharmacology, and long-term psychologic effects are but a few areas that require scientific exploration. Myths and misconceptions about the lack of pain perception and lack of need for control of pain are only recently being corrected.[7]

Finally, many different analgesic regimens have been discussed separately. Studies are needed to evaluate the possible synergistic effect of combining different modalities to optimize the beneficial effects of each approach. This would be analogous to a "balanced anesthetic" technique for surgery where lesser amounts of different agents are given to minimize the side effects of each, but potentiate each other's desirable effects. One could then conceive of "balanced analgesia," where different agents (local anesthetics, narcotic and nonnarcotic drugs, adjuvant drugs, and enkephalinase inhibitors) could be administered by different techniques to minimize the total of each yet maximize any synergistic effects of the combination.

COMMENTARY

The current era of postoperative pain management concerns itself with effective ways to reduce pain and suffering in a cost-effective manner that will also decrease morbidity and promote earlier recovery and shortened hospital stays. Although the emphasis has been on the understanding of pharmacologic principles, technologic advances, and the development of better and safer analgesic agents, the basic health care team and patient relationships should not be overlooked. Patient knowledge of expected events, instruction and relaxation, suggestion in ways to minimize pain with movement, and enthusiastic and confident encouragement, have a definite effect on postoperative pain. This attention to patient care can reduce narcotic use by half, make the patients more comfortable physically and emotionally, and shorten the hospital stay by two to three days.[103] It may well be that part of the effectiveness of modern pain services for postoperative analgesia is in the increased attention provided to patients.[33] This fundamental interaction between the health care team and patient in influencing outcome should never be dismissed as technologic advances in pain management continue.

REFERENCES

1. Marks RM, Sachar EJ: Undertreatment of medical inpatients with narcotic analgesics. *Ann Int Med* 1973; 78:173–181.

2. Donovan M, Dillon P, McGuire L: Incidence and characteristics of pain in a sample of medical-surgical inpatients. *Pain* 1987; 30:69–78.

3. Taenzer P, Melzack R, Jeans ME: Influence of psychological factors on postoperative pain, mood and analgesic requirements. *Pain* 1986; 24:331–342.

4. Korczyn AD: Mechanism of placebo analgesia. *Lancet* 1978; 1304–1305.

5. Carron H, Covino BG (eds): Symposium: Influence of anaesthetic procedures on surgical sequelae. *Reg Anesth* 1982; 7(Suppl).

6. Yeager MP, Glass DD, Neff RK, Brinck-Johnson T: Epidural anesthesia in high risk surgical patients. *Anesthesiology* 1987; 66:729–736.

7. Anand KJS, Hickey PR: Pain and its effect in the human neonate and fetus. *N Engl J Med* 1987; 317:1321–1329.

8. Roberts WJ: A hypothesis on the physiological basis for causalgia and related pains. *Pain* 1986; 24:297–311.

9. Wall PD: The prevention of postoperative pain. *Pain* 1988; 33:289–290.

10. Raja S, Meyer RA, Campbell JN: Peripheral mechanisms of pain. *Anesthesiology* 1988; 68:571–590.

11. Considerations in Management of Acute Pain: A Symposium. New York, HP Publishing Company, January 1977.

12. Current Concepts in Postoperative Pain: A Symposium. New York, HP Publishing Company, January 1978.

13. Yaksh TL: Neurologic mechanisms of pain, in Cousins MJ, Bridenbaugh PO (eds): *Neural Blockade in Clinical Anesthesia and Management of Pain*, ed 2. Philadelphia, Lippincott, 1988, pp. 791–844.

14. Hug CC: Improving analgesic therapy. *Anesthesiology* 1980; 33:441–443.

15. Ghoneim M, Spector R: Pharmaco-Kinetics of drug administered intravenously, in Scurr C, Feldman S (eds): *Scientific Foundations of Anaesthesia*, ed 3. London, W. Heinemann Medical Books, 1983, pp 415–424.

16. Lant AF: Factors effecting the action of drugs. In Scurr C, Feldman S (eds): *Scientific Foundations of Anaesthesia*, ed 3. London, W. Heinemann Medical Books, 1983, pp 425–449.

17. Benet LZ, Sheiner LB: Pharmacokinetics: The dynamics of drug absorption, distribution, and elimination, in Gilman AG, Goodman LS, Rall TW, Murad F (eds): *The Pharmacologic Basis of Therapeutics*, ed 7. New York, Macmillan, 1985, pp 3–34.

18. Ross EM, Gilman AG: Pharmacodynamics: Mechanism of drug action and the relationship between drug concentration and effect, in Gilman AG, Goodman LS, Rall TW, Murad F (eds): *The Pharmacologic Basis of Therapeutics*, ed 7. New York, Macmillan, 1985, pp 35–48.

19. Blaschke TF, Nies AS, Mamelok RD: Principles of therapeutics, in Gilman AG, Goodman LS, Rall TW, Murad F (eds): *The Pharmacologic Basis of Therapeutics*, ed 7. New York, Macmillan, 1985, pp 49–65.

20. Principles of analgesic use in the treatment of acute pain and chronic cancer pain. A concise guide to medical practice. Washington, DC, American Pain Society, 1987.

21. Flower RJ, Moncada S, Vane JR: Analgesic-antipyretics and anti-inflammatory agents, in Gilman AG, Goodman LS, Rall TW, Murad F (eds): *The Pharmacologic Basis of Therapeutics*, ed 7. New York, Macmillan, 1985, pp 674–704.

22. Porter J, Jick H: Addiction rare in patients treated with narcotics. *N Engl J Med* 1980; 302:123.

23. Weis OF, Sriwatanakul, Alloza JL, et al: Attitudes of patients, housestaff, and nurses toward postoperative analgesic care. *Anesth Analg* 1980; 62:70–74.

24. Austin KL, Stapleton JV, Mather LE: Multiple intramuscular injections: A major source of variability in analgesic response to meperidine. *Pain* 1980; 8:47–62.

25. Austin KL, Stapleton JV, Mather LE: Relationships between blood meperidine concentrations and analgesic response. *Anesthesiology* 1980; 53:460–466.

26. Forrest WH Jr, Smethurst PWR, Kienitz ME: Self administration of intravenous analgesics. *Anesthesiology* 1970; 33:363–365.

27. Kerri-Szanto M: Apparatus for demand analgesia. *Can Anaesth Soc J* 1971; 18:581–582.

28. Jones L: Patient controlled oral analgesia. *Orthop Nurs* 1987; 6:38–41.

29. Sjostrom S, Hartvig D, Thompson A: Patient controlled analgesia with extradural morphine or pethidine. *Br J Anaesth* 1988; 60:351–366.

30. Tamsen A, Hartvig D, Fagerlund, et al: Patient controlled analgesic therapy, part I: Pharmacokinetics of pethidine in the pre- and post-operative periods. *Clin Pharmacokinet* 1982; 7:164–175.

31. Dahlstrom B, Tamsen A, Paalzow L, et al: Patient controlled analgesic therapy, part IV: Pharmacokinetics in analgesic plasma concentrations of morphine. *Clin Pharmacokinet* 1982; 7:266–279.

32. Bollish SJ, Collins CL, Kirking DM, Bartlett RH: Efficacy of patient-controlled versus conventional analgesia for postoperative pain. *Clin Pharmacy* 1985; 4:48–52.

33. White PF: Use of patient-controlled analgesia for management of acute pain. *JAMA* 1988; 259:243–247.

34. Hecker BR, Albert L: Patient-controlled analgesia: A randomized, prospective comparison between two commercially available PCA pumps and conventional analgesic therapy for postoperative pain. *Pain* 1988; 35:115–120.

35. White PF: Mishaps with patient-controlled analgesia (PCA). *Anesthesiology* 1987; 28:81–83.

36. Wang JK, Nauss LE, Thomas JE: Pain relief by intrathecally applied morphine in man. *Anesthesiology* 1979; 50:149–151.

37. Bahar M, Olshwang B, Majora F, Davidson JT: Epidural morphine in treatment of pain. *Lancet* 1979; 1:527–529.

38. Czlonkowkski A, Costa T, Przewlocki R, et al: Opiate receptor binding sites in human spinal cord. *Brain Res* 1983; 267:392–396.

39. Cousins MJ, Cherry DA, Gourlay GK: Acute and chronic pain. Use of spinal opioids, in Cousins MJ, Bridenbaugh PO (eds): *Neural Blockade*, ed 2. Philadelphia, Lippincott, 1988, pp 955–1029.

40. Yaksh TL, Noveihed R: The physiology and pharmacology of spinal opiates. *Ann Rev Pharmacol Toxicol* 1985; 25:443.

41. Carr DB: Opioids. *Int Anesth Clin* 1988; 26:273–287.

42. Przewlock R, Stala L, Greczek M, et al. Analgesic effects of mu-delt- and kappa- opiate agonista, and, in particular, dynorphin at the spinal level. *Life Sci* 1983; 33(suppl):649–652.

43. Cousins MJ, Mather LE, Glynn CJ, et al: Selective spinal analgesia. *Lancet* 1979; 1:1141–1142.

44. Sjostrom S, Tamsen A, Persson MP, Hartvig P: Pharmacokinetics of intrathecal morphine and meperidine in humans. *Anesthesiology* 1987; 67:889–895.

45. Stanely TH: Intrathecal opiates. A patient tool to be used with caution. *Anesthesiology* 1980; 53:523–524.

46. Moore RA, Bullingham RSJ, McQuay HG, et al: Dual permeability to narcotics: In vitro determination and application to extradural administration. *Br J Anaesth* 1982; 54:1117–1128.

47. Mather LE, Raj PR: *Spinal Opiates; Practical Management of Pain*. Chicago, Year Book, 1986, pp 709–727.

48. Rawal W, Schott V, Dahlstrom B, et al: Influence of naloxone on analgesia and respiratory depression following epidural morphine. *Anesthesiology* 1986; 64:194–201.

49. Molke Jensen F, Madsen JB, Guldager H, et al: Respiratory depression after epidural morphine in the postoperative period. Influence of posture. *Acta Anaesthesiol Scand* 1984; 28:600–602.

50. Ready LB, Oden R, Chadwick HS, et al: Development of an anesthesiology based postoperative pain management service. *Anesthesiology* 1988; 68:100–106.

51. Hammonds WD, Hord AH: Additional comments regarding an anesthesiology-based postoperative pain service (letter to the editor). *Anesthesiology* 1988; 69:139.

52. Ready LB, Chadwick HS, Wild LM: Additional comments regarding an anesthesiology-based postoperative pain service (letter to the editor). *Anesthesiology* 1988; 69:139–140.

53. Loper KA, Ready LB, Dorman BH: Prophylactic transdermal scopalamine reduces nausea in postoperative patients receiving epidural morphine. *Anesth Analg* 1989; 68:144–146.

54. Ballantyne JC, Loach AB, Carr DB: Itching after epidural and spinal opiates. *Pain* 1988; 33:149–160.

55. Durant PAC, Yaksh TL: Drug effects on urinary bladder tone during spinal morphine-induced inhibition of the micturition reflex in unanesthetized rats. *Anesthesiology* 1988; 68:325–334.

56. Bromage PR, Camporesi EM, Durant PAC, Nielsen CH: Nonrespiratory side effects of epidural morphine. *Anesth Analg* 1982; 61:490.

57. Evron S, Magora F, Sadovsky E: Prevention of urinary retention with phenoxybenzamine during epidural morphine. *Br Med J* 1984; 288:190.

58. Evron S, Samueloff A, Simon A, et al: Urinary function during epidural analgesia with methadone and morphine in post-caesarean section patients. *Pain* 1985; 23:135.

59. Yaksh TL, Harty GJ, Onofrio BM: High doses of spinal morphine produce a nonopiate receptor-mediated hyperesthesia: Clinical and theoretic implications. *Anesthesiology* 1986; 64:590–597.

60. Nordberg G: Pharmacologic aspects of spinal morphine analgesia. *Acta Anaesthesiol Scand* 1984; 79(Suppl):1–38.

61. Nordberg G, Hedner T, Mellstrand T, Dahlstrom B: Pharmacokinetic aspects of epidural morphine anesthesia. *Anesthesiology* 1983; 58:545–551.

62. Yaksh TL, Noveihed RY, Durant AC: Studies of the pharmacology and pathology of intrathecally administered 4-aminopiperidine analogues and morphine in the rat and cat. *Anesthesiology* 1986; 64:54–66.

63. Shulman MS, Wakerlin G, Yamaguchi L, Brodsky JB: Experience with epidural hydromorphone for post-thoracotomy pain relief. *Anesth Analg* 1987; 66:1331–1333.

64. Cohen SE, Tan S, White PF: Sufentanil analgesia following cesarian section: Epidural versus intravenous administration. *Anesthesiology* 1988; 68:129–134.

65. Whiting WG, Sandler AW, Lau LC, Chaven PM: Analgesic and respiratory effects of epidural sufentanil in post-thoracotomy patients. *Anesthesiology* 1986; 65:A176.

66. Melzack R, Wall PD: Pain mechanisms: A new therapy. *Science* 1965; 150:971–979.

67. Sjolund BF, Ericson MBE: The influence of naloxone on analgesia produced by peripheral conditioning stimulation. *Brain Res* 1979; 173:295–301.

68. Salar G, Gob I, Mingrino S, et al: Effective transcutaneous electrotherapy in CSF beta endorphin content in patients without pain problems. *Pain* 1981; 10:169–172.

69. Galloway DJ, Boyle P, Burns HJG, et al: A clinical assessment of electroanalgesia following abdominal operations. *Surg Gyn Obstet* 1984; 159:453–456.

70. Gibert JM, Gledhill T, Law N, George C: Controlled trial of transcutaneous electrical nerve stimulation (TENS) for postoperative pain relief following inguinal herniorrhaphy. *Br J Surg* 1986; 73:749–751.

71. Smith CM, Guralnick MS, Gelfand MM, Jeans ME: The effects of transcutaneous electrical nerve stimulation on post caesarean pain. *Pain* 1986; 27:181–193.

72. Arvidsson I, Eriksson E: Postoperative TENS pain relief after knee surgery: Objective evaluation. *Orthopedic* 1986; 9:1346–1351.

73. Owen H, Galloway DJ, Mitchell KG: Analgesia by wound infiltration after surgical excision of benign breast lumps. *Ann R Coll Surg Engl* 1985; 67:114.

74. Patel JM, Lanzufame RJ, Williams JS, et al: The effect of incisional infiltration of bupivacaine hydrochloride upon pulmonary functions, atelectasis and narcotic

need following elective cholecystectomy. *Surg Gynecol Obstet* 1983; 157:338.

75. Levack IB, Holmes JD, Robertson GS: Abdominal wound perfusion for the relief of postoperative pain. *Br J Anaesth* 1986; 58:615–619.

76. Gaumann DM, Lennon RL, Wedel DJ: Continuous axillary block for postoperative pain management. *Reg Anesth* 1988; 13:77–82.

77. Manriquex RG, Pallares VS: Continuous brachial plexus blockade for prolonged sympathectomy and control of pain. *Anesth Analg* 1978; 57:128–130.

78. Murphy DF: Continuous intercostal nerve blockade for pain relief following cholecystectomy. *Br J Anaesth* 1983; 55:521–524.

79. Scott DB: Acute pain management, in Cousin MJ, Bridenbaugh PO (eds): *Neural Blockade.* Philadelphia, Lippincott, 1988, pp 861–863.

80. Fischer RL, Lubenow TR, Liceago A, et al: Comparison of continuous epidural infusion of fentanyl-bupivacaine and morphine-bupivacaine in management of postoperative pain. *Anesth Analg* 1988; 67:559–563.

81. Reiestad F, Stromskag KE: Intrapleural catheter in the management of postoperative pain. A preliminary report. *Reg Anesth* 1986; 11:89–91.

82. Stromskag KE, Reiestad F, Holmgist ELO, Ogenstad S: Intrapleural administration of 0.25%, 0.375% and 0.5% bupivacaine with epineperhine after cholecystectomy. *Anesth Analg* 1988; 67:430–434.

83. Seltzer JL, Larjani GE, Goldberg ME, Man AT: Intrapleural bupivacaine, a kinetic and dynamic evaluation. *Anesthesiology* 1987; 67:798–800.

84. Rosenberg PH, Scheinin BMA, Lepantalo MJA, Lindfors O: Continuous intrapleural infusion of bupivacaine for analgesia after thoracotomy. *Anesthesiology* 1987; 67:811–813.

85. Gomez MN, Symreng T, Johnson B, et al: Intrapleural bupivacaine for intraoperative analgesia—Dangerous technique? *Anesth Analg* 1988; 67:S78.

86. Charlton JE: Relief of the pain of unresectable carcinoma of the pancreas by chemical splanchnicectomy during laparotomy. *Ann R Coll Surg Engl* 1985; 67:136.

87. Evans PJD: Cryoanalgesia. The application of low temperatures to nerves to produce anaesthesia or analgesia. *Anaesthesia* 1981; 36:1003–1113.

88. Myers RR, Powell HC, Heckman HM, et al: Biophysical and pathological effects of cryogenic nerve lesion. *Ann Neurol* 1981; 10:478–485.

89. Barnard D: The effects of extreme cold on sensory nerves. *Ann Royal Coll Surg Engl* 1980; 62:180–187.

90. Katz J, Nelson W, Forrest R, Bruce DL: Cryoanalgesia for post-thoracotomy pain. *Lancet* 1980; 1:512–513.

91. Glynn CJ, Llowd JW, Barnard JDW: Cryoanalgesia and the management of pain after thoracotomy. *Thorax* 1980; 35:325–327.

92. Frost E, Sadowsky D: Acupuncture therapy. Comparative values in acute and chronic pain. *NY State J Med* 1976; 76:595–597.

93. Evans C, Richardson PH: Improved recovery and reduced postoperative stay after therapeutic suggestions during general anesthesia. *Lancet* 1988; 2:491–493.

94. Locsin RG: The effect of music on the pain of selected post-operative patients. *J Adv Nurs* 1981; 6:1925.

95. Casuto J, Wallin G, Hogstrom S, et al: Inhibition of postoperative pain by continuous low-dose intravenous infusion of lidocaine. *Anesth Analg* 1985; 64:971–974.

96. O'Sullivan H, Jennings F, Ward K, et al: Human bone marrow biochemical function and megaloblastic hematopoiesis of nitrous oxide anaesthesia. *Anesthesiology* 1981; 55:645–649.

97. Caplan RA, Ready LB, Oden RV, et al: Transdermal fentanyl for postoperative pain management: A double-blind placebo study. *JAMA* 1989; 261:1036–1039.

98. Shah MV, Jones DI, Rosen M: "Patient demand" postoperative analgesia with buprenorphine—Comparison between sublingual and IM administration. *Br J Anaesth* 1986; 58:508–511.

99. Henderson JM, Brodsky DA, Fisher DM, et al: Preinduction of anesthesia in pediatric patients with nasally administered sufentanil. *Anesthesiology* 1988; 68:671–675.

100. Streisand JB, Hague B, van Vreeswijk H, et al: Oral transmucosal fentanyl premedication in children. *Anesth Analg* 1987; 66:S170.

101. Schwartz JC, Malfroy B, DeLaBaume S: Biological inactivation of enkephalins and the role of enkephalin-dipeptidyl-carboxypeptidase ("enkephalinase") as a neuropeptidase. *Life Sci* 1981; 29:1715–1750.

102. Zhang AZ, et al: Nociception, enkephalin content and dipeptidyl carboxypeptidase activity in brain of mice treated with exopeptidase inhibitors. *Neuropharmacology* 1982; 21:625–630.

103. Egbert LD, Battit GE, Welch CE, Bartlett MK: Reduction of postoperative pain by encouragement and instruction of patients. A study of doctor–patient rapport. *N Engl J Med* 1964; 270:825–827.

6 Pulmonary Complications and Respiratory Therapy

Gene Pesola, Nashaat Eissa, and Vladimir Kvetan

The incidence of postoperative pulmonary complications is extremely variable. It has been reported to be as low as 3% when patients have a variety of surgical operations and as high as 76% during upper abdominal surgery (Table 6–1 contains a partial list only). The extreme variability is due to confusion as to what constitutes a pulmonary complication; method of determining when a complication exists; as well as the differing selection of patients at risk. Previous studies focus primarily on atelectasis and/or its primary pulmonary sequelae, pneumonia, as the predominent postoperative pulmonary complications.[1-9,11,12] One recent study includes bronchospasm as a significant postoperative clinical entity.[10] We will consider postoperative pneumonia, atelectasis, bronchospasm, pulmonary embolism, and pleural effusions as significant postoperative pulmonary complications. In Table 6–2 and the discussion relating to pulmonary function, incidence, and prevention, atelectasis with and without penumonia will be inferred. The other complications are discussed separately.

The incidence of postoperative pulmonary complications, considered historically as pneumonia and atelectasis, depends to a large extent on the type of surgery. Table 6–1 clearly shows that the incidence is higher after upper abdominal surgery (6 to 76%) than when all surgery is considered together (3 to 28%). When further broken down, pulmonary complications were 0.9% of cases following extraperitoneal operations, 27% after upper abdominal laparotomies, and 9.7% after other laparotomies in one study,[3] and 0.7, 19, and 10.9%, respectively, in another study.[5]

ATELECTASIS

Atelectasis, the collapse of alveoli, was first described by Pasteur in 1910.[13] It is the most common complication seen after surgery. The pathophysiology of atelectasis is due to an abnormal pattern of breathing. In normal awake adults the respiratory pattern consists of a 400 to 500-mL tidal volume interrupted every five to ten minutes by a maximal deep breath to near total lung capacity.[14] During a normal breath a few alveoli collapse at the end of expiration and fail to expand with the ensuing inspiration. These alveoli are eventually recruited by a maximum inflation known as a sigh or yawn. The etiology of atelectasis in the postoperative state, especially after upper abdominal or thoracic surgery, is felt to be related to smaller tidal volumes and the inability to take the normal sigh due to postoperative pain, sedative drugs such as narcotics,[15] and postoperative diaphragmatic dysfunction. If the atelectasis is not reversed early, insidious complications such as hypoxemia and pneumonia can occur. A similar type of respiratory abnormality, small tidal volume breathing with no sigh, can be reproduced in healthy human subjects whose chests have been strapped tightly.[16] The resulting abnormalities of pulmonary function include decreases in functional residual capacity, inspiratory capacity, lung compliance, and arterial oxygen levels. These abnormalities did not correct themselves completely after the chest was free. The addition of a very deep breath, however, fully corrected the pulmonary dysfunction.

Postoperative Pulmonary Function and Atelectasis

Pulmonary function tests (Fig. 6–1) taken soon after upper abdominal surgery show a restrictive pulmonary deficit that lasts for greater than one week.[8,17-19] There is a 60% drop in vital capacity (VC) and forced expiratory volume in one second (FEV_1) with no change in the FEV_1/FVC ratio on postoperative day one; which improves to a 30% drop by seven days. Postthoracotomy operations not requiring pulmonary resection have a 40% drop in VC on day one with recovery by day seven.[17] Surgery of the lower abdom-

TABLE 6-1. INCIDENCE OF POSTOPERATIVE PULMONARY COMPLICATIONS (PPCs)

Method of Diagnosis		PPCs (%) by Site of Surgery						
Source	Number of Patients	Upper Abdomen	Mixed	PE	Roent	ABG	Upper Abdomen	Mixed
Whipple 1918[1]	3719		+	+	+			3
Elwyn[2] 1922	2932	+	+	+			8	3
King[3] 1933	7065	+	+	+	+		13	6
Dripps & Deming 1946[4]	1240	+		+	+		6	
Pooler[5]	5869	+	+	+	+		19	4
Thoren 1954[6]	343	+		+	+		30	
Wightman 1968[7]	785	+	+	+			21	6
Latimer et al 1971[8]	46	+		+	+	+	76	
Bartlett et al 1973[9]	150	+		+	+	+	17	
Gracey et al 1979[10]	157	+	+	+	+	+	25	19
Celli et al 1984[11]	172	+	+	+	+	+	46	28
Roukema et al 1988[12]	153	+			+	+	41	

inal cavity and outside of the abdomen causes a 35% drop in VC, and no drop, respectively, on day one. The VC recovers by day seven after lower abdominal surgery. In view of the absence of changes in pulmonary function in the nonabdominal (nonthoracic) patients, it is possible to conclude that the anesthetic used does not alter postoperative mechanical pulmonary function properties.

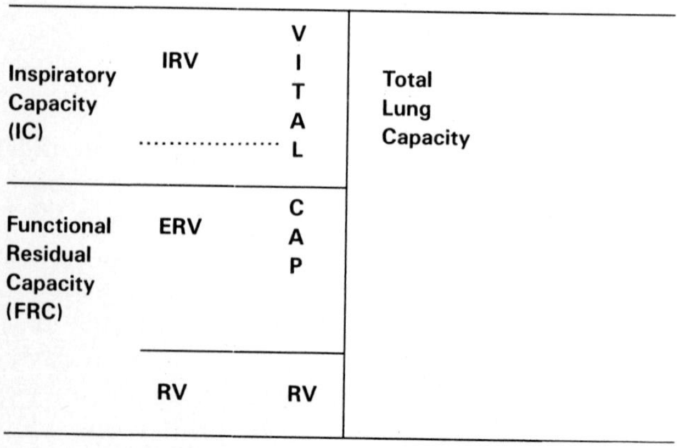

Tidal volume (TV) decreases by about 25% and respiratory frequency increases on day one after upper abdominal surgery with no significant change in minute ventilation.[17,20] By day seven the TV is normal with a persistent elevation in respiratory rate. There is a drop in TV of 25% on day one after lower abdominal surgery with no significant change in respiratory rate. The TV returns to normal on day two.

The FRC exhibits no drop immediately after operation and a subsequent 30% drop at 16 to 24 hours after upper abdominal surgery.[18] The FRC recovers to normal at about seven to ten days. There is no significant drop in FRC with thoracic surgery not requiring pulmonary resection,[17] lower abdominal, and extraperitoneal surgery.

Diaphragm activity is reduced in the immediate postoperative period after upper abdominal surgery, with a shift from predominantly abdominal to rib cage breathing.[21] The reduced diaphragm excursions during tidal and deep breathing are not suppressed

		V	
Inspiratory Capacity (IC)	IRV	I T A L	Total Lung Capacity
	....		
Functional Residual Capacity (FRC)	ERV	C A P	
	RV	RV	

Figure 6-1. Normal lung volumes

by postoperative pain relief[22] and the dysfunction appears unrelated to anesthesia.[23] The latter effect was shown by studying three groups of mongrel dogs under general anesthesia. Six dogs received no surgery (control); nine dogs underwent upper abdominal surgery (cholecystectomy); and six dogs underwent lower abdominal surgery (pseudoappendectomy). Diaphragm function was assessed by changes in transdiaphragmatic pressure swings, the ratio of changes in gastric to esophageal pressure swings, and the ratio of changes in abdominal to rib cage diameters during quiet tidal breathing. In the upper abdominal surgery group there were significant postoperative decreases in all parameters of diaphragm function. In the control and lower abdominal surgery groups there were no significant postoperative changes. This implies that anesthesia and lower abdominal surgery do not effect diaphragm function. Although the mechanism of the surgery-induced dysfunction is unknown, it may explain part or all of the cause for the restrictive postoperative pulmonary pattern and atelectasis.

Gas exchange in the postoperative period can have two temporal patterns. After minor operations in patients without prexisting lung disease, arterial hypoxemia with or without hypercarbia is often present with recovery in the first two hours.[24] Causes of the early postoperative hypoxemia are related primarily to general anesthesia. They include respiratory depression with alveolar hypoventilation from mild narcotic or anesthetic overdose; loss of pulmonary vasoconstriction reflexes after general anesthetics[25]; increased oxygen consumption due to hypertonic muscles and shivering; depressed cardiac output; increased venous admixture; and V/Q mismatch. Diffusion hypoxemia can occur during the first ten minutes after anesthesia with nitrous oxide if the patient is given a low or room air inspired oxygen fraction.[26] This is due to reequilibration of nitrous oxide in the bloodstream into the alveolus after the nitrous oxide is discontinued. This dilutes the inspired oxygen and nitrogen, causing a lower concentration of both gases, which can cause a transient hypoxemia. If nitrogen was a more soluble gas in blood than nitrous oxide this would not occur due to rapid equilibration of nitrogen in the bloodstream and maintenance of a reasonable inspired oxygen fraction in the alveolus. This latter effect is overcome by the use of supplemental oxygen in the immediate postoperative period.

A second pattern of gas exchange abnormalities is seen associated with surgery that affects the ability of the patient to breath deeply or causes immobilization in bed. The classic defect is arterial hypoxemia without hypercarbia.[24] This type of abnormality is usually seen in surgery of the upper abdomen or tho-

rax and resolves over a period of two weeks.[27] The mechanisms for the hypoxemia are V/Q mismatch secondary to disordered ventilation of aging[28] and shunting.[29] Another overlapping mechanism that causes part of the mismatching of ventilation with perfusion is related to the relationship between closing volume (CV) and FRC. Closing volume is the lung volume at which airways begin to close[30] during exhalation and is normally near residual volume in the young and healthy, but occurs at larger lung volumes with advancing age, pulmonary disease, cigarette smoking, or pulmonary edema.[31,32] Therefore, during normal tidal volume breathing, there usually is no airway collapse with subsequent V/Q mismatch or shunting. The mechanism of airway collapse during expiration is related to the gradient in pleural pressure seen in the lung, which is more negative at the top of the lung than the bottom. In an upright person at FRC, apical lung units are at 60% of their total capacity and basal units are at 30% of total capacity. The basal units are smaller due to the accumulated weight of the lung above them. At lung volumes less than FRC, pleural pressure in the base of the lung may exceed atmospheric pressure, with airway collapse and gas trapping. Closing volume is the lung volume at which this collapse occurs. Risk factors such as increased age and smoking can damage small airways (< 2 mm in diameter) with airway collapse occurring at lung volumes much greater than residual volume. This encroachment into FRC can eventually invade the tidal volume with airway closure and hypoxemia occurring during normal breathing. Factors that reduce FRC such as obesity, pregnancy, abdominal pain, supine posture, and general anesthesia, will also bring the lung volume during tidal volume breathing closer the the closing volume and predispose to hypoxemia.

The reduction in total lung volumes and the mechanisms of hypoxemia seen in the late postoperative state, V/Q mismatch, and shunting, are all compatible with the common postoperative complication, atelectasis.

Incidence and Types of Atelectasis

Micro- or miliary atelectasis involves no detectable abnormalities on chest x-ray or by clinical exam but arterial blood gas analysis reveals an increase in alveolar–arterial gradient and relative arterial hypoxemia.[33-35] It is most likely associated with a reduction in pulmonary compliance.[36,37] A more restrictive clinical definition of atelectasis, sometimes called macroatelectasis, consists of rales, fever, sputum production, and radiographic alterations.[38,39] Using this latter definition, atelectasis occurs in 20 to 30% of patients after upper abdominal surgery, 5% of patients after lower abdominal surgery, and 1% of patients undergoing surgery outside the pleural and peritoneal cavity.[3,5,35] When cardiac surgery is considered, the incidence of atelectasis in the postoperative period is the highest at 91%.[40] Acute lobar atelectasis is a third type of atelectasis that occurs infrequently and can result in severe hypoxemia.[13,41]

RISK FACTORS

The location of surgery is, as noted earlier, the most important risk factor for postoperative pulmonary complications. In descending order, the types of surgery most likely to develop postoperative pulmonary complications are upper abdominal surgery; thoracic surgery with lung resection; thoracic surgery without lung resection; lower abdominal surgery; and extrathoracic and extraabdominal surgery.

The second most important risk factor in predicting pulmonary complications is the presence of chronic obstructive pulmonary disease.[7,8,42,43] Wightman[7] showed that 53% of 455 patients had preexisting chronic respiratory disease as determined by history, physical exam, and chest x-ray. Of this group, 26.4% developed a pulmonry complication versus 8.2% without respiratory disease. Stein[39] used pulmonary function tests to determine pulmonary dysfunction and found the incidence of postoperative atelectasis to be 3% with normal values and 70% with abnormal tests.

Men have previously been thought to have a higher incidence of postoperative atelectasis than women.[3,4] But the difference disappears among patients with similar smoking histories.[7] When cigarette smoking is evaluated, patients who smoke ten cigarettes or more a day have a postoperative pulmonary morbidity rate six times that of nonsmokers.[44] This correlation with smoking occurs even when pulmonary function tests among smokers are not impaired.[45]

Obese patients are more likely to develop postoperative pulmonary complications.[6,8,46-48] In a study of over 20,000 postoperative surgical patients with an average pulmonary complication rate of 12%, the incidence of pulmonary complications in the obese was 35%.[46] Another group of morbidly obese patients undergoing jejunoileal bypass surgery had a pulmonary complication rate of 25.3%, which increased to 57.1% in a subset of patients who had underlying disease affecting pulmonary function.[47] In one study, macroatelectasis developed in 53% of obese patients compared to 9% who were of normal weight.[8] Part of the etiology of this atelectasis may be related to the larger atelectatic areas of dependent lung seen during anesthesia in the obese.[49] This compression atelectasis may be carried over into the postoperative period when expansion of the lung is difficult due to sedation and pain.

Although some studies reveal an increase in pulmonary complications with age alone,[6,12] other studies cannot detect an age-related increase.[7,8]

The type of anesthesia has little bearing on the rate of pulmonary complications.[3,4,50] In general it is felt that the duration of anesthesia is important. Anesthesia times longer than three to four hours appear to have an increased incidence of pulmonary complications.[4,46] One recent study, however, found no increased incidence with different anesthesia times.[12]

In separating out atelectasis and looking at pneumonia as the pulmonary complication, the predisposing risk factors are similar. They include low serum albumin, smoking history, prolonged preoperative stays, duration of surgery greater than four hours, and thoracic and upper abdominal surgery.[51]

PREVENTION OF POSTOPERATIVE PULMONARY COMPLICATIONS: ATELECTASIS AND PNEUMONIA

Preoperative Assessment

Preoperative pulmonary function testing is widely advocated in many departments to identify the high-risk surgical patient.[42] It is felt by the majority, however, that a good history and physical are as good as pulmonary function tests in identifying the high risk pulmonary patient.[11,39,52] In general, a history that includes smoking, recurrent pulmonary infections including tuberculosis, occupational background, asthma, exertion necessary to bring on dyspnea, and presence of chronic bronchitis (sputum production in at least three months out of at least two consecutive years) will alert the physician. When there is any doubt about significant pulmonary disease or when there is a history of significant pulmonary disease, a preopertive chest x-ray and room air arterial blood gas analysis should be obtained as a baseline and to determine the presence of hypoxemia and hypercarbia.

A multitude of different methods have been used to prevent postoperative atelectasis. The most widely used techniques are geared toward restoring the restrictive pulmonary defect with its accompanying increased work of breathing and hypoxemia. The etiology of the restriction is related to small tidal volumes with no sigh breaths, which over a period of hours results in atelectasis, which may be difficult to reverse. To prevent or at least minimize this phenomenon the sigh can be artificially introduced. This is done by encouraging the patient to inspire deeply. The deep breath will produce an increase in transpulmonary pressure and distend the lungs. Another approach toward lung inflation is the use of nonphysiologic positive force to distend the lungs with intermittant positive pressure ventilation (IPPB). This latter approach is controversial, expensive, and has a high complication rate. Studies in humans and dogs have indicated that alveoli, once inflated, remain inflated for at least one hour.[36,37] Therefore, any respiratory maneuver should be carried out hourly to maintain sustained alveolar inflation and maintenence of normal lung volumes. An additional maneuver, sitting in a chair, has been shown by Meyers and associates to promote an increase in FRC compared to lying in bed in patients who had undergone upper abdominal surgery.[19]

The measures actually used to improve postoperative pulmonary function include chest physiotherapy with coughing (with and without deep breathing); blow bottles; incentive spirometry (IS) with a number of devices; IPPB; continuous positive airway pressure (CPAP) systems; and positive end-expiratory pressure (PEEP) masks. The most popular method appears to be incentive spirometry, used in 95% of hospitals; followed by chest physical therapy in 83%; IPPB in 82%; CPAP in 25%; and blow bottles in 17%.[53] Randomized studies appear to prove that deep breathing exercises with[9,54-56] or without[6] an adjunctive breathing device (IS) are superior to no treatment,[6] conventional chest physical therapy,[9,54] and IPPB.[55,56b] One study looking only at conventional chest physiotherapy with deep breathing versus IS in 103 laparotomy patients revealed a 2% incidence of pulmonary complications with deep breathing exercises alone and a 5% incidence with IS. The general conclusion from all these studies is that deep breathing exercises of any type decrease pulmonary complications.[57] The most popular mode of deep breathing is with the quantifiable IS device. No specific IS device appears to produce better results than another.[58] It is recommended that all patients, particularly high-risk chronic obstructive lung disease patients undergoing upper abdominal or chest surgery, have preoperative instruction in deep breathing exercises prior to surgery. The ideal deep breath should be one that is held for 3 seconds. A 3-second deep breath was found to be superior to multiple deep breaths or a single unsustained deep breath.[59] Presumably, the sustained deep breath is what occurs during a normal yawn. The deep breathing maneuver used should be supervised hourly by a nurse since preoperative patient education and training alone is not effective in decreasing postoperative pulmonary complications.[60]

The use of IPPB is extremely controversial in the postoperative patient population. Five studies comparing IPPB versus a control population have been done. In one nonrandomized[61] and one randomized[11] study, treatment with IPPB four times per day decreased the incidence of pulmonary complications compared to untreated patients.[5] However, in one randomized[62] and two nonrandomized studies[63,64] in patients undergoing upper abdominal surgery, this outcome was not confirmed. When IS is compared to IPPB it is superior[55,56] or equal to[11,65] IPPB with less of a complication rate. Due to expense, complications of treatment,[11,66] and variable study results, IPPB should only be used in refractory cases of atelectasis when conventional therapy fails or is not used at all. If used, inhaled volume and not pressure should be emphasized as being the most effective for improving atelectasis. One of the reasons for the partial failure of IPPB may lie in the incorrect practice of controlling the volume inspired by the peak airway pressure. As the lung volumes decrease due to atelectasis, the volume required to reach a given pressure decreases. Thus, any maneuver regulated by pressure alone becomes self-defeating and leads to more shallow breathing. In addition, any resistance by the patient due to dressings, incision, pain, and other factors, makes the volume of inflation even smaller. If, instead, the inflating volume is measured, a large volume is used, and the alveolar inflating pressure is maintained for an adequate period of time to get the inflating volume in, then IPPB may work if complications such as pneumothorax and decreased venous return with hypotension do not intervene.

Continuous positive pressure mask systems that cover both the nose and mouth have decreased the incidence of postoperative pulmonary complications compared to no treatment[67] or IS.[68,69] The only disadvantage is related to putting together a more expensive and complex system, discomfort tolerating a tight fitting mask, and the potential for aspiration of gastric contents.[70] Use of nasogastric suction can prevent the latter complication. An interesting and possibly more feasible system in the future is nasal CPAP.[71] This apparatus fits over the nose and the patients are instructed to breathe through the nose with their mouth closed. In the four cases reported so far this system was able to clear up atelectasis resistant to chest PT, IS, and bronchoscopy. The potential advantages include better patient tolerance, decreased aspiration of oral secretions, mouth breathing with equipment failure, and oral feeding. Further studies need to be done to validate this method.

Blow bottles[56] and other expiratory maneuvers have fallen out of favor since they produce smaller lung volumes and deflation of alveoli. Deep breathing exercises and spontaneous breathing modalities, on the other hand, place primary emphasis on developing a gradient of pressure from the atmosphere to the alveoli and pleural space with expansion of alveoli. Although the study comparing blow bottles with IPPB and IS implied that blow bottles were at least as efficacious, they are not used to any great extent.

In conclusion, the prevention of postoperative atelectasis and the resultant complication of pneumonia that can follow, is only partially successful at this time in patients with upper abdominal and thoracic surgical procedures. The routine postoperative measures should include:

1. Breathing exercises that emphasize a large inspiratory effort of at least three-second duration such as incentive spirometry.
2. Supervision of breathing exercises at least once per hour while awake.
3. Encouragement when possible to be in an upright position in bed.
4. Sitting upright in a chair as soon as possible.
5. Adequate pain relief.
6. A trial of mask CPAP or nasal CPAP for refractory atelectasis.

POSTOPERATIVE PLEURAL EFFUSIONS

Historically pleural effusions are rarely present in the postoperative state with an incidence of less than 2% in those who do report it.[7,72,73] In a study that looked specifically at the incidence of pleural effusions with the use of posteroanterior, left lateral, and bilateral decubitus chest roentgenograms obtained 48 to 72 hours after abdominal surgery, the incidence was 48.5% or 97 of 200.[74] The incidence was greater after upper abdominal surgery (60%), when free peritoneal fluid was present, and in those with atelectasis. In 20 patients the effusion was deamed large enough to justify a thoracentesis. Sixteen of the 20 patients had an exudative effusion. All the effusions resolved without specific therapy except for one infected exudative effusion that resolved with antibiotic therapy and chest tube placement. Therefore, postoperative pleural effusions are more common than previously thought, and most resolve spontaneously without therapy.

POSTOPERATIVE PULMONARY EMBOLUS

Pulmonary embolus, whose origin is from the deep veins of the legs in more than 90% of cases, is a common problem in the postoperative state. The incidence of fatal postoperative pulmonary embolism, in the absence of prophylaxis, depends on the site of surgery. It varies from less than 1% in patients undergoing elective general surgery[75,76] to 3% in patients undergoing elective hip surgery.[77]

Long-term reduction in death from pulmonary embolism should emphasize prophylaxis and prevention rather than treatment since many cases of pulmonary embolus are diagnosed postmortem[78] and two thirds of patients who die from the disease do so within 30 minutes after the acute event, before therapy can be started.[79]

Risk factors for pulmonary embolus include obesity, oral contraceptive use, varicose veins, malignancy, prolonged immobility, congestive heart failure, aging and the type of surgical procedure.[80,81]

Treatment Regimens for Postoperative Prophylaxis (Table 6–2)

Low-Dose Heparin. Low-dose heparin is usually given as a dose of 5000 units two hours preoperatively and either every eight or twelve hours postoperatively. It acts by binding to antithrombin III and making it a more effective enzyme in removing activated factors II, X, IX, XI, and XII. Since it acts high in the coagulation cascade, much lower doses are needed to inhibit the initiation of a clot compared to treatment of an established thrombosis. This is because each step in the coagulation cascade amplifies the next step. Blocking steps high in the cascade prevents any amplification. With its use there appears to be no increased risk of bleeding in general surgical patients.[82] Due to its theoretical potential for bleeding it should not be used in patients undergoing cerebral, eye, or spinal surgery.[83]

Adjusted-Dose Subcutaneous Heparin. Low-dose heparin is not effective in the prophylaxis of venous thromboembolism for hip surgery or prostatic sur-

TABLE 6–2. RECOMMENDED PROPHYLAXIS DEPENDING ON THE TYPE OF SURGERY

Surgery Type	Prophylactic Regimen
Neurosurgery	Intermittant pneumatic compression[87]
Genitourinary surgery	Intermittant pneumatic compression[88]
Major knee surgery	Intermittant pneumatic compression[89]
Elective hip surgery	Adjusted-dose heparin[77] or oral coumadin[85]
Low-risk general surgery	Graduated compression stockings[84] or low-dose heparin[82]
Moderate-risk general surgery (lasting > 30 min and > 40 years old)	Intermittant pneumatic compression or low-dose heparin
High-risk general surgery (abdominal surgery for malignancy, past history of DVT or PE, orthopedic surgery of lower limbs)	Oral coumadin or adjusted-dose heparin

gery. Adjusted-dose heparin therapy given as a dose of 3500 units initially and adjusted to maintain the APTT between 31.5 and 36 seconds markedly reduced the incidence of venous thrombosis in patients undergoing elective hip surgery compared to a lower-dose heparin regimen.[77]

Graduated Compression Stockings. Graduated compression stockings apply a graded degree of compression, with the distal limb or ankle receiving the most pressure and the calf less. The stockings are inexpensive and free of significant side effects. Recent studies reveal a reduction in deep venous thrombosis in low-risk general surgical patients when compression stockings are used.[84]

Intermittent Pneumatic Leg Compression. Intermittent pneumatic leg compression of the calf and thigh prevents venous thrombosis by enhancing venous blood flow and preventing stasis. It is relatively free of complications and its use should be continued until a patient is fully ambulatory when used.

Oral Anticoagulants. Oral anticoagulants prevent venous thrombosis by inhibiting the synthesis of the vitamin-K dependent factors II, VII, IX, and X. Although not routinely used for postoperative prophylaxis, a two-step regimen of low-dose coumadin, which raises the PT between one and three seconds longer than control one week prior to surgery; and 1.5 times control postsurgery; has been shown to decrease postoperative thrombosis after hip[85] and general surgery.[86]

POSTOPERATIVE BRONCHOSPASM

Postoperative wheezing is generally seen in patients with a prior history of asthma or chronic obstructive pulmonary disease with bronchospasm. The patient is usually on a preoperative regimen of bronchodilating drugs with or without steroids. The only danger and therapeutic dilemma occurs when there is the possibility that the bronchospasm is related to cardiac disease. When there is any question and the patient is doing poorly, a Swan-Ganz catheter with determination of cardiac function and estimation of left atrial pressure is required to rule out cardiac wheezing. An elevated estimated left atrial pressure of greater than 18 cm H_2O is compatible with heart failure.

Treatment of postoperative wheezing can be started with the use of a nebulized selective B_2 agonist, which results in the formation of cyclic AMP and bronchial smooth muscle relaxation.[90] They also improve the movement of airway mucus. These agents (Table 6–3) are more desirable than epinephrine and isoproterenol due to their lack of cardiac effects at low doses and their minimal systemic effects when inhaled. The major side effect of these drugs is tremor, and it is seen more with noninhalational use. The primary differences between B_2 agents is related to their duration of action. Due to its long duration of action and recent preparations used for inhalational therapy, albuteral is becoming one of the more popular agents. If subcutaneous therapy is desired, terbutaline 0.25 mg is as effective as epinephrine with a much longer duration of action.

Intravenous theophylline, a medium-potency bronchodilator, can be used if the bronchospasm is not relieved with B_2 agonists. Intravenous theophylline is usually administered as the salt form, theophylline plus ethylenediamine or aminophylline. Aminophylline has greater solubility in water with therapeutic activity attributed solely to its theophylline content. Although it was originally felt to increase cyclic AMP through phosphodiesterase inhibition, recent evidence does not support this concept and its mechanism of action is unknown.[91] It is known to cause bronchial smooth muscle relaxation, decrease diaphragm fatigue, and improve the movement of airway mucus. The approximate volume of distribution of the drug is 0.5 L/kg. Therefore, the loading dose is 5 to 6 mg/kg to get a desired concentration of 10 μg/mL in the plasma with a 0.2 to 1 mg/kg/h maintenance infusion depending on a number of factors. If the serum level is subtherapeutic and known, the loading dose is:

Loading dose (mg/kg) = desired serum level (mg/L) − existing serum level (mg/L) × 0.5 L/kg.

TABLE 6–3. B-AGONISTS

Agent	Receptor activity	Availability	Duration of Effect (h)
Epinephrine	alpha, B_1, B_2	subcutaneous	< 1
Ephedrine	alpha, B_1, B_2	oral	4
Isoproterenal	B_1, B_2	inhalational	< 1
Isoetharine	B_2	inhalational	1
Metaproterenal	mild B_1, B_2	inhalational, oral	4
Terbutaline	B_2	subcutaneous, oral	6
Albuteral	B_2	inhalational, oral	6

TABLE 6-4. GLUCOCORTICOID PREPARATIONS

Agent	Physiologic Half-Life (h)	Potency Relative to Cortisol	
		Glucocorticoid	*Mineralocorticoid*
Cortisol (hydrocortisone)	8-12	1.0	1.0
Prednisone	12-36	4.0	0.25
Prednisolone	12-36	4.0	0.25
Methylprednisolone	12-36	5.0	not measurable
Triamcinolone	12-36	5.0	not measurable
Betamethasone	> 48	25.0	not measurable
Dexamethasone	> 48	30-40.0	not measurable

The maintenance dose should be decreased in the elderly, patients with liver disease or congestive heart failure, or patients simultaneously medicated with cimetidine, erythromycin, troleandomycin, allopurinol, rifampin, prednisone, carbamazepine, propranolol, or oral contraceptives. Maintenance doses should be on the higher side in the young and may need to be adjusted up in heavy smokers, patients on high-protein diets, or patients taking barbiturates or isoproterenal. Desired plasma concentrations are between 10 and 20 μg/mL, although lower or even higher levels are acceptable if the desired therapeutic effect is noted without toxicity. The main side effects include nausea and vomiting, restlessness and irritibility, palpitations, tachycardia, and ventricular arrhythmias.

Glucocorticoids are used when bronchospasm is not relieved with the use of traditional agents. The precise mechanism of action is unknown but possibilities include a decrease in airway inflammation and enhanced responsiveness of beta$_2$ receptors to endogenous catecholamines and administered sympathomimetic drugs.[92] The effective dose depends on the steroid used since each has its own physiologic half-life and potency (Table 6-4). The loading dose for hydrocortisone is 4 mg/kg with a 3 mg/kg bolus every six hours to give a plasma cortisol level above 100 μg/dL. Bronchospastic effects are not instantaneous but occur within six hours of therapy. Therapy is usually continued for a minimum of 48 to 72 hours and then can be tapered, stopped, or changed to oral therapy depending on the clinical indications.

Anticholinergic agents were previously of limited usefulness because of systemic side effects. The newer synthetic quaternary ammonium compounds are nonabsorbable and relatively free of side effects when used as inhalation agents. They are effective in both asthma[93] and chronic obstructive pulmonary disease.[94-96] The peak onset of action is delayed up to 60 to 90 minutes. They can be used as an alternative to or alternating with beta$_2$ agonists.

MECHANICAL VENTILATION IN THE POSTOPERATIVE SETTING

Patients with normal lung function can usually be transferred from a ventilator to a T-piece and extubated within 24 hours after any type of operation. The rate-limiting factor is the length and duration of sedation after anesthesia. If patients become alert and do not tolerate a T-piece, weaning criteria can be utilized to determine whether the problem is related to inadequate oxygenation or ventilation, neuromuscular weakness, inadequate endurance, or is due to an abnormality of ventilatory mechanics (Table 6-5).

Early extubation within five hours versus prophylactic mechanical ventilation for greater than 15 hours has been evaluated in patients after abdominal surgery[97] and CABG operations.[98] It was felt that this type of patient with abdominal or thoracic surgery, due to an element of pulmonary compromise, might benefit from more prolonged ventilation to minimize pulmonary complications. However, there was no difference in the incidence of pulmonary or cardio-

TABLE 6-5. CRITERIA FOR WEANING

Oxygenation	
PaO_2/FIO_2	> 200 mm Hg
A-a gradient ($FIO_2 = 1.0$)	< 350 mm Hg
Shunt fraction	< 15%
Ventilation	
Dead space	< 0.6
$PaCO_2$	< 50 mm Hg
Neuromuscular strength	
PNP	< -20 cm H_2O
Respiratory muscle endurance	
Minute ventilation	< 10 L/min
MVV	> 20 L or
	> 2 × minute ventilation
Ventilatory mechanics	
VC	> 10 mL/kg
TV	> 5 mL/kg

pulmonary complications in patients undergoing prolonged mechanical support versus rapid extubation. All patients undergoing prolonged ventilatory support required more sedation and pain relief with narcotics to maintain comfort on the ventilator compared to patients undergoing early extubation. Therefore, the earliest possible extubation from mechanical ventilation is recommended after operation.

Ventilator Settings and Techniques

The tidal volume in mechanically ventilated patients is recommended to be 12 to 15 mL/kg instead of the normal physiologic breath of 7 mL/kg. Lung compliance studies reveal the best lung compliance at these values with no improvement in compliance or oxygenation above 15 mL/kg.[99] No improvement in $P(A-a)O_2$ was noted in another group of patients ventilated above 15 mL/kg.[100] These large tidal volumes prevent atelectasis and sigh volumes are not needed. In patients with loss of lung volume after pulmonary resection, thoracoplasty for tuberculosis, and other restrictive diseases, reduced lung volumes need to be used. A rough guide can be the peak pressure on the ventilator. If it suddenly rises by more than 10 to 15 torr during an increase in tidal volume, the upper extent of the pressure volume curve for that lung has been reached and a smaller tidal volume should be used.

Respiratory rates above 20 with normal lungs and above 12 in patients with obstructive lung disease are associated with air trapping and increased dead space ventilation.[101,102] The initial respiratory rate should be 8 to 12 with adjustments based on arterial blood gas analysis.

Continuous positive airway pressure can be used in the postoperative setting at a pressure of 5 or less since that approximates or is slightly above physiologic PEEP (epiglottic). Zero end-expiratory pressure (ZEEP) is also acceptable if the arterial blood gases are favorable and is preferable with obstructive lung disease.

Mechanical ventilatory modes that are often used in the postoperative period are controlled mechanical ventilation (CMV), intermittent mandatory ventilation (IMV), and assisted or assist control mechanical ventilation (AC). CMV is a mode that delivers an operator selected number of mechanical breaths and does not allow the patient to breathe spontaneously between breaths. It can only be used when the patient is heavily sedated or paralyzed since its use otherwise will result in a frustrated patient who cannot breath spontaneously despite the attempt. Due to this factor CMV has fallen out of favor and either AC or IMV is used.

AC allows the patient to spontaneously make an inspiratory effort, which lowers the pressure in the breathing circuit and triggers the machine to deliver a preset tidal volume. A minimum fail safe rate of 8 to 12 is dialed in for the patient who is not spontaneously breathing. This allows a smoother transition to the spontaneously breathing state during emergence from anesthesia and is more comfortable to the patient. Disadvantages of the method include an increased mean intrathoracic pressure with hypotension, particularly if the patient is hypovolumic; and respiratory alkalosis when an increased respiratory drive is present. Fluid resuscitation and change to an IMV setting will correct each problem respectively.

IMV or synchronized intermittent mandatory ventilation (SIMV) is the other popular mode of therapy used in the postoperative state. This mode delivers a preset respiratory rate and tidal volume with each breath synchronized or designed to deliver a breath that does not interfere with the patient's own spontaneous tidal volume breathing if it is present. The minimum rate to start with should be 8 to 12 with adjustments based on arterial blood gas analysis. The patient is allowed to take a spontaneous tidal volume between breaths. The size of the spontaneous tidal volume varies with lung compliance, respiratory effort, the diameter and length of the endotrachial tube, compliance of the respiratory tubing, and the characteristics of the demand valve on the respirator used. Assuming a large diameter endotracheal tube (#8 Fr or greater), new ventilator with a sensitive demand valve, and high compliance respirator tubing, this mode of therapy should work well. The spontaneous breaths the patient takes will result in a lower mean intrathoracic pressure with more favorable hemodynamic consequences than AC. Since most patients undergoing postoperative mechanical ventilation have normal lungs, the type of ventilator and ventilator mode should not be of critical importance. The type of mode should be the one the staff is most comfortable with.

Weaning

Weaning a patient from AC ventilation is usually done when the patient is alert and consists of taking the patient off the respirator and placing the intubated patient on a T-piece. The T-piece consists of an external tube from the wall connected to an endotracheal tube with humidified air at a given fraction of inspired oxygen (FIO_2). The FIO_2 chosen is the same as or greater than that on the ventilator. If the patient is clinically stable with good arterial blood gases after one half to two hours on the T-piece he or she can be extubated.

Weaning from SIMV in the alert patient can be accomplished via T-piece but is often done by simply turning down the respiratory rate to 2 or 4. After one half to two hours on this low rate the patient is extubated if the arterial blood gases and clinical state of the patient are acceptable.

OXYGEN THERAPY

Oxygen Delivery

Oxygen delivery to the tissues can be quantitiated by the formula:

$$\text{Tissue } O_2 \text{ delivery} = \text{cardiac output (CO)} \times \text{arterial } O_2 \text{ content (CaO}_2)$$

or,

$$CaO_2 = \text{Hb sat} \times \text{Hb conc.(g/dL)} \times 10 \times 1.34 \text{ mL of } O_2/\text{g of Hb (Hb oxygen)} + 0.0031 \text{ mL of } O_2 \times \text{partial pressure of arterial oxygen (dissolved oxygen).}$$

Since the amount of dissolved oxygen in the blood at normal atmospheric pressure is a very small amount, the formula reads as:

$$\text{Tissue } O_2 \text{ delivery} = CO \times \text{Hb sat} \times \text{Hb (g/dL)} \times 13.4.$$

From the formula it can be seen that a drop in tissue O_2 delivery can occur with a decrease in cardiac function; a drop in the saturation of hemoglobin, which is directly related to a low arterial oxygen tension; or a drop in hemoglobin.

Adequate tissue oxygenation is the primary goal of oxygen therapy. When there is inadequate tissue oxygenation, hypoxia is said to have occurred. Hypoxia can be further divided into normoxemic and hypoxemic hypoxia. Normoxemic hypoxia can occur with a drop in cardiac function (circulatory hypoxia) and the inability to pump oxygenated blood to the tissues, or with a drop in hemoglobin or anemic hypoxia. Hypoxemia, on the other hand, is a low arterial partial pressure of oxygen (Po_2), which often leads to tissue hypoxia or hypoxemic hypoxia. One crude estimate of tissue hypoxia is an elevation of serum lactate in the absence of liver disease, recent seizure, or acute exercise.

Arterial hypoxemia is the result of hypoventilation, diffusion defect, ventilation–perfusion inequality, or shunt. All will respond quickly to exogenous oxygen except for large shunts of greater than 20 to 25% of cardiac output. In this latter case, increasing the inspired oxygen concentration to 100% will not significantly improve the partial pressure of oxygen.

Although the absolute level of arterial Po_2 at which supplemental oxygen is needed is unkonwn, it appears practical and reasonable to main a Po_2 of 60 or an arterial hemoglobin saturation of at least 90%. This is related to the sigmoid shape of the oxygen hemoglobin saturation curve (Figure 6–2, dashed line with saturation on the inner y axis). At an arterial

Po_2 of 60 the saturation of hemoglobin is 90%, and increasing the Po_2 any further will increase the hemoglobin saturation only to a minor degree. However, if the arterial Po_2 was 45 with a hemoglobin saturation in the 70 range, an increase in Po_2 to 60 would markedly increase the hemoglobin saturation. This is important since the primary determinant of arterial oxygen content is the level of hemoglobin. This can be seen from Figure 6–2 and the two solid lines representing two different hemoglobin levels. At a Po_2 greater than 60 the arterial oxygen content levels off for both levels of hemoglobin. The oxygen content at the same arterial Po_2 is markedly different. Once an arterial hemoglobin saturation of 90% has been reached, increasing the hemoglobin or other factors are needed to increase oxygen delivery to tissues.

Oxygen Delivery Systems

The multiple modes of oxygen delivery are summarized in Table 6–6. They can be categorized into fixed- or variable-performance modes. Fixed-performance modes deliver a predictable inspired oxygen concentration independent of variations in the patient's breathing pattern. They are large-capacitance or high-flow systems that exceed a patient's inspiratory demand, no matter how large. Fixed modes are generally considered to be the Venturi mask, partial rebreathing mask, and total rebreathing mask. The variable-performance mode is a low-capacitance system that delivers an inspired oxygen concentration which varies with the patient's breathing pattern. These systems are the nasal cannula and simple oxygen mask.

To visualize the variability of inspired oxygen concentration with a variable performance mode, a nasal cannula at 5 liters per minute of 100% oxygen

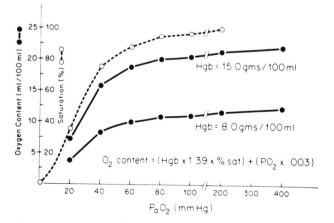

Figure 6–2. Oxygen content of the blood as a function of Po_2 at two Hb concentrations. The oxyhemoglobin dissociation curve is shown as the dashed line and is referenced to % saturation. Adapted from Murray, Nadel, (eds): *Textbook of Respiratory Medicine.* Philadelphia. Saunders, 1988, 1983.

TABLE 6-6 OXYGEN CONCENTRATIONS FOR DELIVERY SYSTEMS

Cardiac output may be decreased postoperatively due to factors that reduce preload or cardiac contractibility.

Causes of low cardiac output:

Effect	Causative Factors	
Decreased Preload	Hypovolemia	Blood loss
		Diuresis
	Vasodilatation	Rewarming
		Drug induced
Decreased Contractibility	Myocardial ischemia/infarction	
	Acid-base imbalance	
	Hypoxia	
	Drug induced	
	Mechanical ventilation	
	(decreased atrial contraction)	

From Respiratory Care: A Guide to Clinical Practice, Burton/Hodgkin, Ed, Lippincott 1984, 407.

will be used as an example. The following respiratory parameters of an imaginary patient will be used:

Tidal Volume = 500 mL
Respiratory Rate = 20 breaths per minute
Inspiratory Time = 1 sec
Expiratory Time = 2 sec with most of expiratory flow complete in 1.5 sec
Anatomic reservoir = 50 mL

The anatomic reservoir, composed of the nose, nasopharynx, and oropharynx, will be assumed to be one third of the anatomic dead space of 150 mL. If most of expiration takes place in the first 75% of expiration, 41 mL of this space will be filled by the nasal cannula during expiration, ie 5 liters/min or 83 mL/sec multiplied by 0.5 sec. A typical inspiration taken over one second will then be composed of:

41 mL of 100% oxygen taken from the anatomic reservoir
82 mL of 100% oxygen supplied by the nasal cannula
376 mL of 21% oxygen supplied by room air or 79 mL of oxygen

The resulting fraction of inspired oxygen is calculated as:

$$\frac{203 \text{ mL of oxygen}}{500 \text{ mL total}} = \frac{0.41 \text{ or } 41\% \text{ inspired oxygen}}{\text{concentration}}$$

The same patient became more uncomfortable due to early acute respiratory distress from sepsis with the following respiratory pattern:

Tidal Volume = 500 mL
Respiratory Rate = 30 breaths per minute
Inspiratory Time = 0.67 sec

Expiratory Time = 1.33 sec
Anatomic Reservoir = 50 mL

Using the same reasoning the new fraction of inspired oxygen on 5 liter/min nasal cannula is:

$$\frac{171 \text{ mL of oxygen}}{500 \text{ mL total}} = \frac{0.34 \text{ or } 34\% \text{ inspired oxygen}}{\text{concentration}}$$

Therefore, in a small-capacitance system or variable performance-mode oxygen delivery system, the faster the respiratory rate or the larger the tidal volume (not illustrated) the smaller the inspired oxygen concentration. The converse is also true.

The nasal cannula or prongs deliver 100% oxygen at flow rates of 1 to 6 L/min. There is an approximate 3% increase in FIO_2 for each L/min increase in oxygen flow. The increase is less with larger minute ventilations and smaller with small minute volumes due to the dilutional effect with room air.[103] The device is comfortable and effective for mild arterial hypoxemia provided the nasal passages are patent. Mouth breathing or nasal breathing does not change the final oxygen concentration since both require entrainment of room air. Flow rates above 6 L/min should be avoided due to drying of the nasal passages.

The Venturi or oxygen-powered air entrainment mask uses the Bernoulli principle that states that as the forward velocity of a gas increases, lateral wall pressure decreases, with a subsequent increase in forward pressure. When a tube with a narrowed downstream orifice is used (injector or Venturi tube), gas will be directed through the restriction. The same amount of gas now travels through a smaller-diameter tube with an increase in the velocity of flow and forward direction of the gas molecules. This drops the lateral pressure in the tube. If the lateral pressure becomes subatmospheric, the restriction tube can be used to entrain room air. Another theory explaining the same phenomena states that a rapid velocity of gas through a restricted orifice creates a "viscous shearing force" that entrains air.[103] In either case, the entrainment ports or openings to room air need to be located immediately distal to and contiguous with the restriction. The two factors that affect the degree of entrainment of room air are the size of the narrowed orifice or jet and the size of the lateral gas entrainment ports. The smaller the jet the faster the gas flow (due to decreased lateral pressure) and the more entrainment of room air at a given entrainment port size and vice versa. Large entrainment ports cause greater entrainment of room air and a lower fraction of inspired oxygen. The delivered FIO_2 can be as high as 50% with varying accuracy, which probably is less than the textbook claims of 1 to 2% variability from desired.[104] These masks are as efficacious as the nasal cannula in treating hypoxic–hypercapnic respiratory insufficiency.[105] As with all masks, they interfere with eating and drinking and they are often removed by the patient due to discomfort or while the patient shifts around in bed.

The simple plastic oxygen mask covers the nose and mouth and delivers oxygen in concentrations up to 50%.[103] Oxygen flow rates of up to 5 to 6 L/min are required to avoid carbon dioxide accumulation within the mask. They can be used for added humidification and aerosol therapy but suffer from the limitations of the mask system in general as well as a variable and unreliable inspired oxygen concentration.

Partial rebreathing masks can deliver an FIO_2 of up to 80%. The mask is equipped with a reservoir bag that can hold about 800 to 1000 mL of air. As long as the reservoir bag does not collapse on inspiration and the mask has a reasonably tight fit, the patient will entrain room air minimally and inspire a high concentration of oxygen. An oxygen flow rate of 5 to 6 L/min is usually required to maintain a full reservoir bag. During expiration the patient will expire the first 200 mL, which consists primarily of oxygen contained in the dead space, into the reservoir bag. When the bag is full the rest of the exhaled gas will exit through vent holes in the mask.

The main difference between the nonrebreathing mask and the partial rebreather is a one-way valve system that allows the patient to inhale only from the reservoir bag and exhale through separate valves on the side of the mask. These nonrebreather face masks can deliver an inspired oxygen concentration greater than 90%.

In the PACU after extubation most patients will be placed on a simple plastic oxygen mask or a Venturi mask initially. If oxygenation is adequate they will maintain the use of such a mask. If the mask is bothersome and/or oxygenation is more than adequate oxygen may be delivered via the more comfortable nasal cannula. When the patient with hypercarbic obstructive lung disease is extubated, low inspired oxygen concentrations are needed to maintain the arterial PO_2 of 55 to 60. The nasal cannula at 1 to 2 L or the Venturi mask at 24% would probably be the method preferred. The need for a partial or nonrebreathing mask to maintain oxygenation after extubation would imply a serious problem. The etiology of the defect in oxygenation should be investigated to try to prevent reintubation.

HUMIDIFICATION

Humidity is concerned with the amount of water in vapor form in a given amount of gas at a specified temperature. At room or body temperature water is in the form of a vapor and not a gas. A gas is technically molecules of a substance above their critical temperature. Critical temperature is defined as the energy level above which molecules have the energy of motion (kinetic energy) necessary to overcome all forces attracting them to each other. Compression can liquefy these molecules at or below this temperature but not above. A vapor is the molecular form of a substance below its critical pressure and often below its boiling temperature dispersed in a true gas. The critical temperature for water at one atmosphere is $374°C$.

Absolute humidity is the weight of water vapor in a gas volume. It usually refers to the amount of water in mg/L of the gas in question. The maximum amount of water vapor a gas volume can contain is dependent on temperature. Higher temperatures allow greater amounts of water vapor to be potentially suspended in a gas.

Relative humidity, a percentage, is the ratio of the actual amount of water vapor in the air compared to the maximum amount that could be held, multiplied by 100. The temperature needs to be specified when relative humidity is mentioned.

Normal alveolar air is 100% humidified at $37°C$ and contains 43.9 mg of water vapor per L of gas. Average ambient room air at $21°C$ with an average relative humidity of 50% has a water vapor content of 10 mg/L. By the time ambient air reaches the carina it is 100% humidified and at $37°C$. The upper airway and trachea has added about 33.9 mg of water per L of inspired gas during normal breathing conditions. This difference between water vapor content in alveolar air and inspired air is termed the *humidity deficit,* and is usually made up for by body mechanisms.

The type of humidity used for patient care depends on the goal of therapy. Patients who are not intubated and who do not have a tracheostomy generally have an intact humidification system and can humidify normal inspired gases without any problem. However, oxygen delivered to the patient is stored in cylinders or liquid tanks in anhydrous (dry with zero humidity) form. Gas delivered in this form can have a rapid drying effect on the nasal and tracheal mucosa. The goal of therapy in this group is to restore humidity to that approximating room air. Patients with a tracheostomy and those intubated have their humidification system bypassed. In this patient group, 100% humidification of inspired gas heated to body temeprature is the goal.

Humidifiers come in many different forms but basically can be thought of as coming in two types. The first is the simple humidifier that does not employ heat. It is designed to add enough water vapor to make the gas administerd comfortable to the nonintubated patient. This is done by adding 80% or more relative humidity to room air gas, or 15 mg water vapor/L. This is only about 30 to 40% relative humidity when the room air gas is warmed to body temperature. The patient's upper airway does the rest. There are at least three different forms of the simple humidifier. One is the passover or blow-by humidifier, which allows gas to pass over the water surface and flow to the patient. It is the least efficient due to the short time of gas/water exposure and the limited surface area of gas/water contact. Another more popular form is the bubble humidifier. Gas is directed below the water surface and bubbles to the top. This increases the gas/water exposure and improves efficiency. Most of these humidifiers are also equipped with a device to break up the gas into very small bubbles to increase the gas/water surface area even more, and are called bubble diffusion humidifiers. The last form, which is becoming the most popular because it is the most effective, is the jet humidifier. A jet stream of air hits the tip of a capillary tube causing a negative pressure (Bernoulli effect), which evacuates water from a reservoir up the capillary tube into the stream of air. The air stream produces particles of water that are removed or evaporate after hitting a baffle system.

The second type of humidifier is the heated humidifier. It heats the gas to body temperature or above. This heating action enhances the ability of the gas to carry water vapor, and 100% humidity at body temperature can be achieved. These humidifiers should be used with wide-bore tubing tilted at a downward angle away from the patient. This action prevents the patient from drowning due to the condensation or "rain" that occurs in the tubing as the hot air cools on its way to the patient. Heated humidifiers are used in the intubated patient to provide complete or almost complete humidification of inspired gases since the patient's own humidification system is bypassed. A review of the basic structure of the cascade heated humidification system can be found by McPherson.[106]

Nebulizers and Aerosol Therapy

Aerosols. An aerosol is a system of liquid or solid particles suspended in a gas.[107] The particles can be dust, smoke, soot, water, medication, and so on. While humidity is water in a gaslike state (vapor), an aerosol of water is water droplets suspended in air.

Deposition of an aerosol depends on a number of factors including gravity, kinetic activity, inertia, ventilatory pattern, temperature variation and humidity, and physical characteristics of the particle.[108] Gravity affects the sedimentaion of particles related primarily to the size (mass) of the particle. Larger particles, greater than 5 microns (μm), settle faster than smaller ones. Kinetic activity effects particles that are primarily smaller than 0.5 μm. These small particles approach the size of the gas molecules they are sus-

pended in. Random collisions with these gas molecules (Brownian motion) may cause deposition in the airways, which is particulary pronounced at less than 0.1 μm in diameter. The process of particle deposition due to Brownian motion is called diffusion.

Inertia is the property of a moving substance to travel in a straight line until a force changes its direction. Larger particles usually have more mass and therefore more inertia than smaller ones. These large particles, 8 μm size and greater, tend to be filtered out and impact on the upper airways and bronchi. Deposition is much greater with rapid inspirations.

Ventilatory patterns reveal deeper lung penetration of small particles with slow inspirations of less than 1 L/sec, large tidal volumes, and breath holding at the end of inspiration.[109] Breath holding should increase the time for sedimentation to act. Slow inspiratory rates decrease inertial impaction. These patterns of breathing assume mouth and not nasal breathing. Nasal breathing takes out 100% of 10 μm and greater diameter particles, while deposition in this region approaches zero as the particle size approaches 1 μm.[110]

Aerosol injection into a heated, humidified gas stream tends to make the particles grow in size due to condensation of water vapor as it moves toward the patient in the tubing. The increased particle size causes deposition in the tubing or higher in the airway than would normally occur. This defeats the purpose of bronchodilator aerosol therapy.

Solutions that are aerosolized tend to gain water if hypertonic, remain stable if isotonic, and lose water or evaporate completely if hypotonic.[111] Other particle characteristics such as adhesiveness, or the tendency for particles to stick together and for hygroscopic particles to grow in size will allow more rapid deposit in the respiratory tract.

With the above background, approximate generalizations about particle size can be made during mouth breathing. Particles over 30 μm will settle out in the upper airway above the larynx with the mechanism of depostion related to gravity and inertial impaction. Particles with a size between 5 and 30 μm will settle out in the airway below the larynx at a distance dependent on the velocity of inhalation and in relation to gravity. Particles less than 5 and greater than 1 μm will enter the distal airways and deposit secondary to sedimentation. The longer the time allowed for sedimentation (gravity), the greater the amount of deposition. When particles are between 1 and 0.1 μm they often are inhaled and exhaled with no deposition. Breath-holding can increase their deposition. Very small particles less than 0.1 μm in diameter settle out by diffusion.

The device that produces an aerosol is an atomizer. The particle size is variable with a usual range up to 100 μm in diameter. These devices are often used to spray topical anesthetics into the posterior pharynx prior to bronchoscopic or endoscopic procedures. Nebulizers are atomizers that produce an aerosol of uniform size. This is usually accomplished by adding a baffling device to an atomizer. A baffle is a device that deflects the flow of gas. Large aerosolized particles collide with the baffle and fall out of the gas suspension. Small particles deflect off the baffle and continue in the gas stream. Multiple sequential baffling devices produce smaller and smaller aerosolized particles. Nebulized particles are less than 30 μm in diameter.

The primary goals of aerosol therapy are to humidify the inspired gases or to deliver medication. Another possible goal is to promote bronchial hygiene by hydrating retained secretions in patients with inflammation of the airways. This latter goal has never been proven.[112] The general feeling is that dried secretions are due to inadequate humidification, which caused the thick inspissated secretions. However, ultrasonic short-term nebulizer therapy to bring up secretions is still used.

Nebulizers. The nebulizer is the aerosol generator used in medical respiratory therapy. It is powered either by air (pneumatic) or electricity (ultrasonic). The two types of pneumatic nebulizers are the jet and hydronamic. The jet nebulizer directs a pressurized gas source over a tube immersed in a water reservoir. This draws water from the tube (Bernoulli or jet-mixing effect) with impaction in the airstream to produce the aerosol. Particle size is adjusted with baffles. Jet nebulizers preferably with or without heating devices on the reservoir are used continuously to humidify air in intubated patients on a T-piece and tracheotomized patients who are not on a ventilator. A small reservoir jet nebulizer is often used to deliver bronchodilator medication. The reservoir size is 20 to 30 mL and a small amount of fluid and medication is added to the reservoir. Treatment is initiated until the reservoir is empty.

A specialized portable jet nebulizer called the metered dose inhaler (MDI) is used by asthmatics. It is powered by an inert flourocarbon with a boiling point well below room air. Each puff gives a measured dose of drug to the oral cavity.

The hydronamic (Babington) nebulizer is a hollow sphere fed from a pressurized gas source. The sphere has a small hole through which the gas can leave. The outside of the sphere is covered with a film of water that is poured over it. Aerosol generation occurs when the pressurized air hits the film of water. The jet nebulizer series appears to be the simpler and more popular of the two types of pneumatic devices.

Electrically driven nebulizers produce sound waves that break up water into aerosols. The power unit of the nebulizer receives standard alternating house current and converts it into an ultra-high frequency. This is connected to a piezoelectric tranducer, which changes the electric current into high-frequency vibrations through a vibrating disk. The disk sits in a water bath called a couplant, which begins to vibrate. A special thin bottom plastic container is placed in the couplant fluid. The container is filled with water that vibrates violently enough to leave as an aerosol. A blower carries the particles toward the patient.

These electrically driven ultrasonic nebulizers are the most powerful and most efficient. They supposedly generate 90% of the particles in the 0.5 to 3 μm range and can generate water contents in excess of 100 mg/L. Since 100% humidified air at body temperature carries only 43.9 mg/L of water vapor it can significantly add to airway water. Most jet nebulizers do not exceed 50 mg/L of water content.

Clinical Use of Nebulizers.

Humidification of Inspired Air. Usually large reservoir heated or nonheated jet nebulizers are used for this purpose on a continuous basis. Intubated nonventilated and tracheotomized patients are the usual groups treated.

Medication Delivery. Small reservoir jet nebulizers deliver bronchodilator medication in intubated and nonintubated patients.

Bronchial Hygiene and Thinning Thick Secretions. Although not proven, short courses of three to four hours of ultrasonic nebulizer therapy are usually tried. Water or saline solutions are used. Often, due to the bronchial irritation of saline solutions, bronchodilator solutions are administered first.

Complications of Aerosol Therapy.

Infection. Unlike humidification through vaporization aerosols can carry bacteria in droplet form and cause iatrogenic infections.[113] The large reservoir jet and ultrasonic nebulizers appear to cause the most infections. All nebulizers need to be decontaminated at least once every 24 hours.

Bronchospasm. The high-volume ultrasonic nebulizers are most prone to inducing bronchospasm. If it occurs bronchodilator therapy should temporarily interrupt treatment.

Fluid Overload. Fluid overload is an extremely rare complication of nebulizer therapy, most likely restricted to the pediatric population.

REFERENCES

1. Whipple AO: A study of postoperative pneumonitis. Surg Gynecol Obstet 1918; 26:29–47.
2. Elwyn H: Postoperative pneumonia. *JAMA* 1922; 79:2154–2158.
3. King DS: Postoperative pulmonary complications; I. A statistical study based on two years personal observation. *Surg Gynecol Obstet* 1933; 56:43–50.
4. Dripps RD, Deming M: Postoperative atelectasis and pneumonia: Diagnosis, etiology, and management based upon 1,240 cases of upper abdominal surgery. *Ann Surg* 1946; 124:94–110.
5. Pooler HE: Relief of post-operative pain and its influence on vital capacity. *Br Med J* 1949; 2:1200–1203.
6. Thoren L: Post-operative pulmonary complications. Observations on their prevention by means of physiotherapy. *Acta Chir Scand* 1954; 107:193–205.
7. Wightman JAK: A prospective survey of the incidence of postoperative pulmonary complications. *Br J Surg* 1968; 55:85–91.
8. Latimer RG, Dickman M, Day WC, et al: Ventilatory patterns and pulmonary complications after upper abdominal surgery determined by preoperative and postoperative computerized spirometry and blood gas analysis. *Am J Surg* 1971; 122:622–632.
9. Bartlett RH, Brennan MF, Gazzaniga AB, Hanson EL: Studies on the pathogenesis and prevention of postoperative pulmonary complications. *Surg Gynecol Obstet* 1973; 137:925–933.
10. Gracey DR, Divertie MB, Didier EP: Preoperative pulmonary preparation of patients with COPD. *Chest* 1979; 76:123–129.
11. Celli BR, Rodriquez KS, Suider GL: A controlled trial of intermittent positive pressure breathing, incentive spirometry, and deep breathing exercises in preventing pulmonary complications after abdominal surgery. *Am Rev Respir Dis* 1984; 130:12–15.
12. Roukema JA, Carol EJ, Prins JG: The prevention of pulmonary complications after upper abdominal surgery in patients with noncompromised pulmonary status. *Arch Surg* 1988; 123:30–34.
13. Pasteur W: Active lobar collapse of the lung after abdominal operations. A contribution to the study of post-operative lung complications. *Lancet* 1910; 2:1080–1083.
14. Bendixen HH, Smith GM, Mead J: Pattern of ventilation in young adults. *J Appl Physiol* 1964; 19:195–198.
15. Egbert LD, Bendixen HH: Effect of morphine on breathing pattern. *JAMA* 1964; 188:485–488.
16. Caro CG, Butler J, DuBois AB: Some effects of restriction of chest cage expansion on pulmonary function in man: An experimental study. *J Clin Invest* 1960; 39:573–583.
17. Ali J, Weisel RD, Layug AB, et al: Consequences of postoperative alterations in respiratory mechanics. *Am J Surg* 1974; 128:376–382.
18. Craig DB: Postoperative recovery of pulmonary function. *Anesth Anal* 1981; 60:46–52.
19. Meyers JR, Lembeck L, O'Kane H, Baue AE: Changes in functional residual capacity of the lung after operation. *Arch Surg* 1975; 110:576–583.
20. Williams CD, Brenowitz CD: Ventilatory patterns after vertical and transverse upper abdominal incisions. *Am J Surg* 1975; 130:725–728.
21. Ford GT, Whitelaw WA, Rosenal TW, et al: Diaphragm function after upper abdominal surgery in humans. *Am Rev Respir Dis* 1983; 127:431–436.
22. Simmonneau G, Vivien A, Sartene R, et al: Diaphragm dysfunction induced by upper abdominal surgery: Role of postoperative pain. *Am Rev Respir Dis* 1983; 128:899–903.
23. Road JD, Burgess KR, Whitelaw WA, Ford GT: Diaphragm function and respiratory response after upper abdominal surgery in dogs. *J Appl Physiol* 1984; 57:576:582.
24. Marshall BE, Wyche MQ: Hypoxemia during and after anesthesia. *Anesthesiology* 1972; 37:178–209.
25. Mathers J, Benumof JL, Wahrenbrock EA: General anesthetics and regional hypoxic pulmonary vasoconstriction. *Anesthesiology* 1977; 46:111–114.
26. Fink BR: Diffusion anoxia. *Anesthesiology* 1955;16:511–519.
27. Knudsen J: Duration of hypoxaemia after uncomplicated upper abdominal and thoraco-abdomenal operations. *Anaesthesia* 1970;25:372–377.
28. Kitamura H, Sawa T, Ikezono E: Postoperative hypoxemia: The contribution of age to the maldistribution of ventilation. *Anesthesiology* 1972; 36:244–252.
29. Siler JN, Rosenberg H, Mull TD, et al: Hypoxemia after upper abdominal surgery: Comparison of venous admixture and ventilation/perfusion inequality components, using a digital computer. *Ann Surg* 1974; 179:149–155.
30. McCarthy DS, Spencer R, Greene R, Milic-Emili J: Measurement of closing volume as a simple and sensitive test for early detection of small airway disease. *Am J Med* 1972; 52:747–753.
31. Buist AS, Ross BB: Predicted values for closing volumes using a modified single breath nitrogen test. *Am Rev Respir Dis* 1973; 107:744–752.
32. Rehder K, Marsh M, Roderte JR, Hyatt RE: Airway closure. *Anesthesiology* 1977; 47:40–52.
33. Hamilton WK, McDonald JS, Fischer HW, Bethards R: Postoperative respiratory complications: A comparison of arterial gas tensions, radiographs, and physical examinations. *Anesthesiology* 1964; 25:607–612.
34. Shibutani K, Hyun BS, Mahboubi R, et al: Correlation between hypoxemia and physical and radiologic examinations in atelectasis. *New York J Med* 1968; 68:1046–1054.
35. Pierce AK, Robertson J: Pulmonary complications of general surgery. *Annu Rev Med* 1977; 28:211–221.
36. Mead J, Collier C: Relation of volume history of lungs to respiratory mechanics in anesthetized dogs. *J Appl Physiol* 1959; 14:669–678.
37. Ferris B, Pollard DS: Effect of deep and quiet breathing on pulmonary compliance in man. *J Clin Invest* 1960; 39:143–149.
38. Goodman LR: Postoperative chest radiograph: Alter-

ations after abdominal surgery. *Am J Roentgen* 1980; 134:533–541.

39. Schlenker JD, Hubay CA: The pathogenesis of postoperative atelectasis: A clinical study. *Arch Surg* 1973; 107:846–850.

40. Carter AR, Sostman HD, Curtis AM, Swett HA: Thoracic alterations after cardiac surgery. *Am J Roentgen* 1983; 140:475–481.

41. Marini JJ, Pierson DJ, Hudson LD: Acute lobar atelectasis: A prospective comparison of fiberoptic bronchoscopy and respiratory therapy. *Am Rev Resp Dis* 1979; 119:971–978.

42. Stein M, Koota GM, Simon M, Frank HA: Pulmonary evaluation of surgical patients. *JAMA* 1962; 181:765–770.

43. Meneely GR, Ferguson JL: Pulmonary evaluation and risk in patient preparation for anesthesia and surgery. *JAMA* 1961; 175:1074–1080.

44. Morton HJV: Tobacco smoking and pulmonary complications after operation. *Lancet* 1944; 1:368–370.

45. Chalon J, Tayyab MA, Ramanathan S: Cytology of respiratory epithelium as a predictor of respiratory complications after operation. *Chest* 1975; 67:32–35.

46. Mircea N, Constantinescu C, Jianu E, Busu G: Risk of pulmonary complications in surgical patients. *Resuscitation* 1982; 10:33–41.

47. Tseuda K, Debrand M, Bivins BA, et al; Pulmonary complications in the morbidly obese following jejunoilial bypass surgery under narcotic anesthesia. *Int Surg* 1980; 65:123–129.

48. Hanson G, Drablos P, Steinert R: Pulmonary complications, ventilation and blood gases after upper abdominal surgery. *Acta Anaesth Scand* 1977; 21:211–215.

49. Strandberg A, Tokics L, Brismar B, et al: Constitutional factors promoting development of atelectasis during anaesthesia. *Acta Anaesth Scand* 1987; 31:21–24.

50. Colgan FJ, Whang TB: Anesthesia and atelectasis. *Anesthesiology* 1968; 20:917–922.

51. Garibaldi RA, Britt MR, Coleman ML, et al: Risk factors for postoperative pneumonia. *Am J Med* 1981; 70:677–680.

52. Cain HD, Stevens PM, Adaniya R: Preoperative pulmonary function and complications after cardiovascular surgery. *Chest* 1979; 76:130–135.

53. O'Donohue JW: National survey of the usage of lung expansion modalities for the prevention and treatment of postoperative atelectasis following abdominal and thoracic surgery. *Chest* 1987; 87:76–80.

54. Craven JL, Evans GA, Davenport PJ, Williams RHP: The evaluation of the incentive spirometer in the management of postoperative pulmonary complications. *Br J Surg* 1974; 61:793–797.

55. Van De Vater JM, Watring WG, Linton LA, et al: Prevention of postoperative pulmonary complications. *Surg Gyncol Obstet* 1972; 135:229–233.

56. Iverson LG, Ecker RR, Fox HE, May IA: A comparative study of IPPB, the incentive spirometer, and blow bottles: The prevention of atelectasis following cardiac surgery. *Ann Thoracic Surg* 1978; 25:197–200.

57. Bartlett RH: Postoperative pulmonary prophylaxis: Breathe deeply and read carefully. *Chest* 1982; 81:1–3.

58. Lederer DH, Van de Water JM, Indech RB: Which deep breathing device should the postoperative patient use? *Chest* 1980; 77:610–613.

59. Ward RJ, Danziger F, Bonica JJ, et al: An evaluation of postoperative respiratory maneuvers. *Surg Gynecol Obstet* 1966; 123:51–54.

60. Risser NL: Preoperative and postoperative care to prevent pulmonary complications. *Heart Lung* 1980; 9:57–67.

61. Anderson WH, Dosett BE, Hamilton GL: Prevention of postoperative pulmonary complications. Use of isoproterenol and intermittant positive pressure breathing on inspiration. *JAMA* 1963; 186:103–106.

62. Baxter WD, Levine RS: An evaluation of intermittent positive pressure breathing in the prevention of postoperative pulmonary complications. *Arch Surg* 1969; 98:795–798.

63. Sands JH, Cypert C, Armstrong R, et al: A controlled study using routine intermittent positive pressure breathing in the post-surgical patient. *Dis Chest* 1961; 40:128–133.

64. Becker A, Barak S, Braun E, Meyers MP: The treatment of postoperative pulmonary atelectasis with intermittent positive pressure breathing. *Surg Gynecol Obstet* 1960; 11:517–522.

65. Dohl S, Gold MI: Comparison of two methods of postoperative respiratory care. *Chest* 1978; 73:592–595.

66. Gold MI: Is intermittent positive pressure breathing therapy (IPPB Rx) necessary in the surgical patient? *Ann Surg* 1976; 184:122–123.

67. Anderson JB, Oleson KP, Eikard B, et al: Periodic continuous positive airway pressure, CPAP, by mask in the treatment of atelectasis. *Eur J Respir Dis* 1980; 61:20–25.

68. Stock MC, Downs JB, Gauer PK, et al: Prevention of postoperative pulmonary complications with CPAP, incentive spirometry, and conservative therapy. *Chest* 1985; 87:151–157.

69. Ricksten SE, Bengtsson A, Soderberg C, et al: Effects of periodic positive airway pressure by mask on postoperative pulmonary function. *Chest* 1986; 89:774–781.

70. Smith RA, Kirby RR, Gooding JM, Civetta JM: Continuous positive airway pressure (CPAP) by mask. *Crit Care Med* 1980; 8:483–484.

71. Duncan SR, Negrin RS, Mihm FG, et al: Nasal continuous positive airway pressure in atelectasis. *Chest* 1987; 92:621–624.

72. Ti TK, Yong NK: Postoperative pulmonary complications: A prospective study in the tropics. *Br J Surg* 1974; 61:49–52.

73. Stringer P: Atelectasis after partial gastrectomy. 1947; 1:289–291.

74. Light RW, George RB: Incidence and significance of pleural effusion after abdominal surgery. *Chest* 1976; 69:621–625.

75. Skinner DB, Salzman EW: Anticoagulant prophylaxis in surgical patients. *Surg Gynecol Obstet* 1967; 125:741–746.

76. Shepard RM, White HA, Shirkey AL: Anticoagulant prophylaxis of thromboembolism in post-surgical patients. *Am J Surg* 1966; 112:698–702.

77. Leyvraz PF, Richyard J, Bachmann F, et al: Adjusted versus fixed-dose subcutaneous heparin in the pre-

vention of deep-vein thrombosis after total hip replacement. *N Engl J Med* 1983; 309:954–958.

78. Dalen JE, Alpert JS: Natural history of pulmonary embolism. *Prog Cardiovasc Dis* 1975; 17:259–275.

79. Donaldson GA, Williams C, Scannell G, Shaw RS: A reappraisal of the application of the Trendelenburg operation to massive fatal embolism. *N Engl J Med* 1963; 268:171–174.

80. Kelsey JL, Wood PHN, Charnley J: Prediction of thromboembolism following total hip replacement. *Clin Orthop* 1976; 114:247–258.

81. Salzman EW, Hirsh J: Prevention of venous thromboembolism, in Coleman RW, Hirsh J, Marder V, et al (eds): *Hemostasis and Thrombosis: Basic Principles and Clinical Practice.* Philadelphia, Lippincott, 1982, pp 986–999.

82. International Multicentre Trial. Prevention of fatal post-operative pulmonary embolism by low doses of heparin. *Lancet* 1975; 2:45–51.

83. Hull RD, Raskob GE, Hirsh J: Prophylaxis of venous thromboembolism: An overview. *Chest* 1986; 89:374A–383S.

84. Scurr JH, Ibrahim SZ, Faber RG, Quesne LP: The efficacy of graduated compression stockings in the prevention of deep venous thrombosis. *Br J Surg* 1977; 64:371–373.

85. Francis CW, Marder VJ, McCollister E, Yaukoolbodi S: Two step warfarin therapy: Prevention of postoperative venous thrombosis without excessive bleeding. *JAMA* 1983; 249:374–378.

86. Hull R: Different intensities of oral anticoagulant therapy in the treatment of proximal vein thrombosis. *N Engl J Med* 1982; 307:1676–1681.

87. Skillman JJ, Collins RE, Coe NP, et al: Prevention of deep vein thrombosis in neurosurgical patients: A controlled, randomized trial of external pneumatic compression boots. *Surgery* 1978; 83:354–358.

88. Coe NP, Collins RE, Klein LA, et al: Prevention of deep vein thrombosis in urological patients: A controlled, randomized trial of low-dose heparin and external pneumatic compression boots. *Surgery* 1978; 83:230–234.

89. Hull R, Delmore TJ, Hirsh J, et al: Effectiveness of intermittent pulsatile elastic stockings for the prevention of calf and thigh vein thrombosis in patients undergoing elective knee surgery. *Thrombosis Res* 1979; 16:37–45.

90. Weinberger M, Hendeles L, Ahrens R: Pharmacologic management of reversible obstructive airways disease. *Med Clin North Am* 1980; 65:579–613.

91. Miech RF, Stein M: Methylxanthines. *Clin Chest Med* 1986; 7:331–340.

92. Ziment I: Steroids. *Clin Chest Med* 1986; 7:341–354.

93. Storms WW, Bodman SF, Nathan RA, et al: Use of ipratropium bromide in asthma: Results of a multiclinic study. *Am J Med* 1986; 81 (suppl 5A):61–66.

94. Ashutosh K, Lang H: Comparison between long-term treatment of chronic bronchitic airway obstruction with ipratropium bromide and metaproterenol. *Ann Allergy* 1984; 53:401–406.

95. Rebeck AS, Chapman KR, Abboud R, et al: Nebulized anticholinergic and sympathomimetic treatment of asthma and chronic obstructive airways disease in the emergency room. *Am J Med* 1987; 82:59–64.

96. Tashkin DP, Ashutosh K, Bleeker ER, et al: Comparison of the anticholinergic bronchodilator ipratropium bromide with metaproterenol in chronic obstructive pulmonary disease. *Am J Med* 1986; 81 (suppl 5A):81–90.

97. Shackford SR, Virgilio RW, Peters RM: Early extubation vs prophylactic ventilation for the high risk patient: A comparison of postoperative management in the prevention of respiratory complications. *Anesth Analg* 1981; 29:463.

98. Quasha AL, Loeber N, Feeley TW, et al: Postoperative respiratory care: A controlled trial of early and late extubation following coronary artery bypass grafting. *Anesthesiology* 1980; 52:135–141.

99. Suter PM, Fairley HB, Isenberg MD: Effect of tidal volume and positive end-expiratory pressure on compliance during mechanical ventilation. *Chest* 1978; 73:158.

100. Levine M, Gilbert R, Auchincloss JH: A comparison of the effects of sighs, large tidal volumes, and positive end-expiratory pressure in assisted ventilation. *Scand J Respir Dis* 1972; 53:101–108.

101. Fairley HB, Blenkarn GD: Effect on pulmonary gas exchange of variations in inspiratory flow rate during intermittent positive pressure ventilation. *Br J Anesth* 1966; 38:320–328.

102. Bergman NA: Intrapulmonary gas trapping during mechanical ventilation at rapid frequencies. *Anesthesiology* 1972; 37:626–633.

103. Scacci R: Air entrainment masks: Jet mixing is how they work; the Bernoulli and Venturi principles is how they don't. *Repair Care* 1979; 24:928–934.

104. Gibson RL, Comer PB, Beckham RW, McGraw CP: Actual tracheal oxygen concentrations with commonly used oxygen equipment. *Anesthesiology* 1976; 44:71–73.

105. Bone RC, Pierce AK, Johnson RL: Controlled oxygen administration in acute respiratory failure in chronic obstructive pulmonary disease. *Am J Med* 1978; 65:896.

106. McPherson SP: Humidifiers and nebulizers, in McPherson SP (ed): *Respiratory Therapy Equipment.* St. Louis, Mosby, 1985.

107. Lourenco RV: Inhaled aerosols. *Arch Int Med* 1973; 131:21–22.

108. Brain JD, Valberg PA: Deposition of aerosol in the respiratory tract. *Am Rev Resp Dis* 1979; 120:1325–1373.

109. Dolovich M, Ruffin RE, Roberts R, Newhouse MT: Optimal delivery of aerosols from metered dose inhalers. *Chest* 1981; 80:911–915.

110. Stuart BO: Deposition of inhaled aerosols. *Arch Intern Med* 1973; 131:60–73.

111. Scherer PW, Haselton FR, Hanna FM, Stone DR: Growth of hydroscopic aerosols in a model of bronchial airways. *J Appl Physiol* 1979; 47:544–550.

112. Wanner A, Rao A: Clinical indications for and effects of bland, mucolytic, and antimicrobial aerosols. *Am Rev Resp Dis* 1979; 120:79–87.

7 | Fluid and Electrolyte Balance

Joanne L. Floyd

Ideally, evaporative, exudative, and hemorrhagic fluid losses that occur preoperatively or intraoperatively are fully repleted before the patient arrives in the postanesthetic care unit (PACU). Even so, fluid and electrolyte disorders associated with the patient's underlying illness and surgical procedure may develope postoperatively. Continuing or recurring hemorrhage, with or without shock, predictably complicates postoperative care.

An organized approach must begin with an evaluation of the patient's volume status. Although a checklist is useful (Table 7–1), no general guidelines can be proposed for such a diverse patient population. Many unique situations present during postanesthetic care and each patient must be evaluated and treated individually. The pathology of possible cases is highlighted to illustrate concepts and controversies. Fluid therapy options are reviewed and the indications for their use outlined.

EVALUATION OF VOLUME STATUS

The initial preoperative clinical assessment of a patient's fluid status is based on historical data more than physical signs. The history of present illness may include vomiting, diarrhea, gastric drainage, diuresis, or burns causing excessive fluid losses. Significant hemorrhage or uncontrolled hypertension increase the likelihood of volume depletion. Changes in pulse rate and blood pressure caused by position change or changes in central venous or pulmonary artery pressures recorded during diagnostic fluid challenges can confirm a hypovolemic state. Our ability to reconstruct the patient's status when surgery

began depends on the adequacy and accuracy of this preoperative documentation.

Losses associated with the procedure include intraoperative hemorrhage, evaporation, and exudation. Although the "educated guess" approach to estimating hemorrhage is notoriously inadequate and frequently results in the excessive use of blood products,[1-3] measurement of blood loss[4-7] has been nearly abandoned as too cumbersome and inaccurate for clinical use. The rate of water evaporation is equally difficult to estimate as it varies with ambient temperature and humidity. Also, evaporation is more crucial to discussions of heat conservation than to fluid balance. Operative trauma alters homeostatic mechanisms that maintain intravascular volume, making exudation a major source of intraoperative volume loss. During a typical abdominal procedure, 40 grams of plasma proteins and associated fluid translocate from plasma to other body compartments.[8-10] Plasma, intracellular fluid (ICF), and functional extracellular fluid (ECF) become nonfunctional ECF (interstitial edema, ascites, and so on). This nonfunctional fluid space increases with the extent of surgical trauma, duration of the operation, degree of soft tissue injury, development of an ileus, or presence of inflammatory bowel disease.[11] The exceptional situations, such as an infant with a neural tube defect, must also be mentioned here. Loss of cerebrospinal fluid from a myelomeningocele may double or triple the expected fluid losses.

When the patient arrives in the PACU, the current deficit must be assessed and replacement fluids ordered. The intravenous solutions administered intraoperatively are balanced against the estimated losses. Historical data can be supplemented with clinical evaluation. When no diuretics and no osmotic load (glucose, angiography dye, etc) have been given, urine output above 0.5 mL per kg and hour provides some reassurance of the adequacy of intravascular volume. After other factors that alter central venous pressure (CVP) have been considered, measurement of CVP can reliably reflect intravascular volume and is useful when urine output has been iatrogenically altered.[12] A diagnostic fluid challenge (300 to 500 mL infused rapidly) uses system compli-

TABLE 7–1. FACTORS IN THE EVALUATION OF VOLUME STATUS IN THE PACU

Preoperative fluid status
Losses associated with the procedure
Type and amount of fluid administered during surgery
Current clinical assessment of volume status
Expected further sequestration of extravascular fluid into traumatized or infected tissues

ance to improve CVP interpretation. Should the CVP rise more than 2 to 4 cm H_2O, and remain above baseline for more than ten minutes, the diagnosis is relative hypervolemia or cardiac failure. An increase of less than 2 cm H_2O implies hypovolemia. In a healthy, euvolemic patient, CVP will increase 2 to 4 cm H_2O and return quickly to baseline. When the CVP reading is elevated and a fluid challenge cannot differentiate hypervolemia from cardiac failure, a pulmonary artery catheter should be used. Patients with known cardiomyopathy or pulmonary hypertension requiring pulmonary artery occlusion pressure monitoring in the PACU will generally have the catheter already in place for surgery.[13] When monitoring pulmonary artery occlusion pressure (PAOP), fluids are administered until further increases in PAOP fail to increase cardiac output.[14]

Exudation continues for 24 to 48 hours after the incision is closed and the edema space continues to expand.[15] The sequestered fluid cannot be mobilized for normal body functions for several days.[16] In nutritionally depleted patients, hypoproteinemia and decreased intracellular volume exaggerate these shifts in body water distribution.[17] Maintenance IV orders must be increased to balance these predictable alterations in body fluid compartments.

BODY COMPOSITION (FLUID COMPARTMENTS)

Water comprises 45 to 65% of the adult body weight. Nearly 60% of this total body water (TBW) is intracellular. The extracellular portion (one third of TBW) is nearly three quarters interstitial with only one quarter to one third of ECF (one twelfth of TBW) being intravascular volume (Fig. 7–1).

To illustrate, a 48-kg nonobese woman is approximately 50% water (Fig. 7–2). Therefore, her TBW is 24 L of which 16 L are ICF and 8 L are ECF. Her intra-

vascular volume is only 2 or 2.5 L. By contrast, an 80-kg nonobese man is 60% water with the same distribution of TBW. Completing the calculation reveals an intravascular volume approximately twice that of the small woman depicted above.

FLUID THERAPY

Although total fluid requirements are difficult to predict and fluid deficits impossible to measure, the effect of fluid infusion is predictable. Any administered fluid will distribute throughout all accessible compartments in the same portions discussed above for total body water.

Salt-Free Water
Five percent dextrose in water (D5W) is indicated therapeutically only in the rare instances of free water deficit. The clinically euvolemic dehydrated patient will have elevated serum sodium and serum osmolality. If the etiology is nonrenal free water loss, the urine osmolality will also be high. Etiologies of free water deficit postanesthesia include fever, large areas of deepithelialized skin, nonhumidified oxygen to a tracheostomy, and diabetes insipidus.

Maintenance fluids must replace insensible losses as well as obligatory salt and water losses in urine and gastrointestinal secretions. The insensible (evaporative) losses are normally 600 to 1000 mL/day or approximately one third of the maintenance fluids. This may be provided by hypotonic crystalloids. For example, 1 L of dextrose-half-normal saline provides 500 cc of electrolyte-free water, 100 carbohydrate calories, and 500 mL of isotonic saline.

D5W will distribute throughout the TBW. As shown in Figure 7–3, only 10% of the infused volume will remain intravascular. If salt-free solution is given to replete a volume deficit, two thirds of the infused fluid will cause intracellular edema and one third will

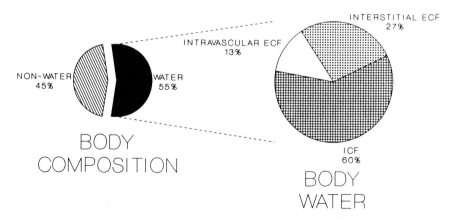

Figure 7–1. Distribution of body water.

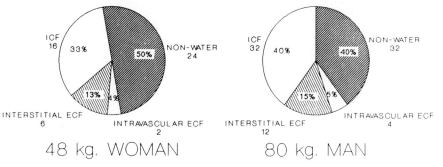

Figure 7–2. Body composition.

dilute the ECF sodium concentration. The patient will exhibit "water intoxication" (clinical signs of hyponatremia: headache, nausea, agitation, seizures), before a significant increase in intravascular volume is achieved.[18]

The nearly complete redistribution out of the vascular compartment makes D5W the first choice fluid for diagnostic fluid challenges. From 300 to 500 mL may be infused quickly to assess the compliance of the intravascular space. Using D5W, no significant harm has been done to the hypervolemic patient: only 40 mL of that fluid load will remain intravascularly. The exception is the neurosurgical patient with cerebral edema. Since redistribution of large volumes of water or crystalloid may significantly increase intracranial pressure,[18A] neither fluid can be considered safe for diagnostic challenges.

Occasionally, excessive free water is administered incidentally. During transurethral resection of the prostate, a large volume of glycine solution may be absorbed through open venous sinuses.[19] Hyponatremia will also result when D5W is administered to a patient in renal failure or with oxytocin given to induce labor and incidentally causing fluid retention.

Crystalloids

Isotonic electrolyte solutions are osmotically equivalent to body fluids, so no osmotic pressure will draw water into the intracellular space. The barrier between the interstitial and intravascular spaces is permeable to ions while the membrane protecting the ICF is not. Administered isotonic crystalloids will distribute throughout the ECF. Within 30 minutes, equilibration is complete, leaving only one quarter to one third of the infusion intravascular (see Fig. 7–3).

Crystalloids are the first-line therapy for intravascular volume depletion and to replace isosmolar losses of exudation. They are always readily available because they are inexpensive and require no special storage arrangements. Crystalloids have no allergenic

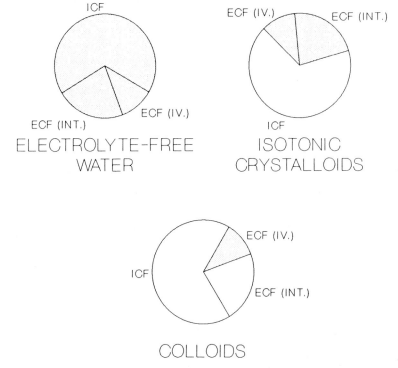

Figure 7–3. Distribution of fluids.

potential and are essentially nontoxic regardless of required quantities. For losses up to 20% of blood volume, crystalloid therapy should be three to four times the lost volume of blood.

The choice among crystalloid solutions is more often a matter of personal preference than scientific indication. Normal pH solutions were developed with concern that normal saline (NS) and lactated Ringer's (LR) solutions might cause dilutional acidosis when large volumes are used for resuscitation. Clinical studies have not substantiated this theory. In the special situation of hyperchloremia with keto- or lactic acidosis, the lower chloride content of LR or Normosol is beneficial, allowing renal tubular excretion of the organic acid. Obviously, both Normosol and LR should be avoided in hyperkalemia and the calcium in LR would be undesirable with hypercalcemia or concurrent blood transfusion.

As volume deficits are repleted with crystalloid solutions, serum protein levels fluctuate. After blood loss, plasma proteins are diluted physiologically by the influx of interstitial fluid and iatrogenically by crystalloid infusions. This decreases plasma oncotic pressure.[20]

The clinical relevance of decreased colloid osmotic pressure (COP) is still debated. Low oncotic pressure stimulates albumin synthesis, and lymph flow returns additional protein from interstitial spaces to plasma. Later, the postresuscitation diuresis ensues, rebounding serum protein concentrations toward normal. The well-publicized disadvantage of crystalloid solutions is the 750 mL of interstitial edema created by each liter infused. One touted complication is impairment of wound healing. Theoretically, edema impedes oxygen diffusion to the wound edges. This complication remains unproven because no prospective randomized study of edema and wound healing with crystalloid versus colloid has been published. Another concern is the effect of interstitial edema on the bowel, specifically, delayed healing of surgical anastomosis and return to bowel function. Again, these suggested complications have not been demonstrated.[21]

More relevant to postanesthetic care is the risk of pulmonary edema. With moderate volume replacement in hemodynamically stable patients, the choice of fluid makes no significant difference in pulmonary function.[22] Even after shock resuscitation, if the volume administered is appropriate, there is no difference in lung function between resuscitation with crystalloids or colloids.[23–27] The pulmonary edema reported after crystalloid resuscitation is more related to the quality of the resuscitation, the total volume of fluid given, and the presence of sepsis rather than to the administration of crystalloid or colloid.[28–30]

Colloids

The undamaged vascular endothelium is nearly impermeable to colloid molecules. Therefore, colloids will distribute only to the intravascular space (see Fig. 7–3). Reexpansion of plasma volume requires only liter-for-liter replacement of losses.

Colloid solutions are either isooncotic or hyperoncotic, and natural (pasteurized plasma protein solution, human serum albumin) or artificial (dextran, gelatin, hydroxyethel starch). The choice among these is more complicated than among the crystalloids. Factors for consideration include (1) the patient's TBW (interstitially depleted or edematous); (2) availability; (3) risks of that product; and (4) cost.

The 4% solutions of plasma proteins (PPS, Plasmanate R) and the 5, 20, and 25% solutions of human serum albumin are natural colloids. The 4 and 5% solutions are isotonic and will not affect interstitial or intracellular volume. They are not indicated for fluid replacement when associated interstitial depletion is expected, such as following shock. Human albumin in 20 and 25% solutions is hypertonic and may replete intravascular volume at the expense of further interstitial volume depletion. When the patient is both edematous and intravascularly volume depleted, hypertonic protein solutions might mobilize the nonfunctional ECF or prevent further transudation of fluid to that compartment. However, exogenous albumin extravasates to abdominal skin and skeletal muscle during abdominal surgery.[31] Since these colloid molecules can be expected to permeate any site of capillary endothelial disruption, their oncotic effect might paradoxically increase edema.

Human blood products, which include these natural colloids, are in limited supply. Although they require no special storage requirements, their distribution is frequently regulated and intentionally restricted by institutional blood banks. Natural colloids are several times more expensive than artificial colloids, and many times more expensive than crystalloids. As discussed in the "Crystalloids" section earlier in the chapter, there is no clear benefit to justify the additional cost except in severely hypoproteinemic patients.

The risk of human protein solutions includes a small incidence (< 0.1%) of anaphylactoid reactions. These reactions to plasma proteins range from mild histamine release with wheal and flare skin findings to profound hypotension with cardiac arrest. The mechanism may be IgE-mediated Type 1 hypersensitivity, anti-IgA,[32] or Hageman factor fragments activating the humoral amplification (kininogen–kinin) system.[33,34]

A large variety of artificial colloids are marketed in Europe and the United States, each having its own risks and benefits. Isotonic colloids include 6% solutions of dextran 70 or hydroxyethyl starch. The indications for these solutions are those already discussed for 5% albumin products. Dextran 40 is also available in a 10% solution that is potently hyperoncotic. The concern about interstitial fluid depletion during 25% albumin administration applies equally to this product.

The risks of artificial colloids may not be fully elucidated as yet. Persistant fluid overload is a greater risk with dextran and hydroxyethyl starch (HES) due to prolonged intravascular retention. Gelatins are composed of smaller molecules that easily pass the glomerular membrane, giving less prolonged complications of excessive infusion. Hydroxyethyl starch is eliminated from the plasma via uptake to the reticuloendothelial system. Storage of HES may cause reticuloendothelial dysfunction. Disturbances of hemostasis have occurred secondary to dilution of coagulation factors when any fluid is given in large quantities. Dextrans and gelatins also have an antithrombotic effect due to interference with platelet adhesiveness and improved capillary blood flow.[35] Anaphylactic reactions also occur to artificial colloids, with some types of gelatins having incidences of up to 10%.[36] Reactions to dextrans are reported in 0.07 to 1.1% of cases; HES has a much lower incidence of anaphylactoid reactions at 0.1%.[36] These vary from skin reactions to life-threatening hypotension with respiratory or cardiac arrest.

Artificial colloids are much less expensive than human protein solutions and have no limitation in availability or storage arrangements. The risks described above and the lack of demonstrable benefit of colloids limit the indications for these solutions to massive volume replacement in patients refusing transfusion of all blood-derived products.

BLOOD PRODUCTS

Fresh Frozen Plasma
Until the consensus conference in 1985,[37] the use of fresh frozen plasma (FFP) was increasing each year, most of which was used simply as a volume expander. The risk of virus transmission must be added to the risks of pasteurized plasma protein products mentioned earlier. The consensus opinion now allows no justification for the use of FFP for volume replacement. The indications for FFP are limited to treatment of specific factor deficiencies (factors II, V, VII, IX, X, XI); emergency reversal of warfarin; and provision of antithrombin III to deficient patients requiring heparin anticoagulation.[38]

Packed Red Blood Cells
Transfusion of erythrocytes is indicated only to improve oxygen-carrying capacity in a patient with anemia. Blood cells should never be used as intravascular volume expanders.

Each homologous transfusion has a 3 to 5% risk of transfusion reaction.[39] The fatal reactions are due to ABO incompatibility most commonly caused by clerical errors.[40] Homologous transfusion also carries a risk of transmitting viral disease. With current screening techniques, the incidence of transfusion-related acquired immune deficiency syndrome (AIDS) may be as low as 1 in 250,000.[41] Transmission of non-A, non-B hepatitis in blood products is common. Elimination of donors with elevated alanine aminotransferase (ALT) levels or antibodies to hepatitis B core antigen may have decreased the risk of transfusions since 1987. Prior to this, non-A, non-B hepatitis occurred in 10% of patients receiving erythrocytes from hepatitis-B-negative volunteers.[41]

Due to the risks described above, homologous transfusion is indicated only when further hemodilution would be risky and autologous blood is not available.

SAMPLE PATIENT SITUATIONS

To illustrate fluid and electrolyte abberations and rational fluid therapy, several commonly encountered patient situations are presented.

The Typical Patient
A healthy patient whose preoperative deficit and intraoperative losses have been fully repleted should arrive in the PACU in fluid and electrolyte balance. If the procedure was minor and peripheral, fluid requirements will be daily maintenance: 35 mL per kg. One third of that fluid should be "free water" to replace solute-free insensible losses (evaporation from skin and respiratory tract). For convenience, dextrose–half-normal saline (D5.45 NaCl) is frequently utilized for short-term infusions. Some authors contend that despite NPO orders intravenous fluids are not necessary for surgical procedures as significant as cholecystectomy.[42] However, the majority opinion holds that recovery is improved when maintenance fluids are provided.[43]

The Patient After Bowel Surgery
The patient having bowel surgery will start the perioperative period with a deficit unless maintenance and replacement fluids have been provided intravenously. Preparation of the bowel for elective surgery includes the restriction of oral intake and cathartics,

which usually results in volume depletion, electrolyte-free water depletion, and hypokalemia. The abdominal pathology necessitating operation may be associated with vomiting, nasogastric tube suctioning, diarrhea, massive fistula drainage, or gastrointestinal hemorrhage. Bowel obstruction may leave more than 10 L in the bowel lumen, and peritonitis causes liters of additional fluid sequestration.

Eliminating these deficits before surgery will decrease perioperative mortality in fragile patients such as the elderly and infants.[44] As optimal status is not always achieved, residual preoperative deficits must be added to several liters of intraoperative ''third spacing'' and blood loss. As previously discussed, historical information, the intravenous fluid administration records, and the clinical evaluation of the patient constitute the initial assessment in the PACU.

The obligatory expansion of ECF after injury makes a positive fluid balance essential to postoperative preservation or restoration of plasma volume.[45] Whatever the deficit on arrival, ECF will continue to redistribute to the nonfunctional edema compartment and previously infused crystalloids will continue to diffuse to the interstitial space. Infusions may remain at their intraoperative rate of 6 mL per kg and hour for several hours postoperatively. Some authors now recommend intentionally keeping elderly patients hypovolemic to minimize cardiopulmonary complications.[46] There is not adequate documentation of efficacy to make this recommendation.

When a patient arrives in the PACU after bowel surgery with a blood pressure of 105/60 mm Hg, a pulse of 120/min, CVP of 2, and oliguria, residual perioperative fluid deficits should be suspected. Following the ''Fluid Therapy'' section earlier in the chapter, a volume three to four times the deficit will be administered as isotonic crystalloid solution. Normosol, LR, or NS will support intravascular and functional interstitial volume during the postoperative redistribution of ECF. Assessment of the adequacy of intravascular volume as resuscitation progresses must include the predicted redistribution of fluids infused within the hour. For example, if 3L LR has returned the CVP to 6 to 8, the urine output to one mL/kg. and h, and the pulse to 90 within one hour of PACU arrival, 2.25 L of that LR will leave the intravascular space by the second hour. In addition to replacement for perioperative deficits, bowel surgery patients require the same maintenance infusions as the ''typical patient'' depicted above.

The Trauma Patient

Shock induces excessive reduction in functional ECF[47] that is not resolved by replacing whole blood.[48] Failure to replete the ECF space results in hemoconcentration and increased mortality.[49] Adequate

ECF replacement (approximately 4 L in the adult) in addition to returning plasma volume will reestablish circulatory stability,[50] restore acid–base balance,[51] and decrease the incidence of acute renal insufficiency.[52] Treatment of hemorrhagic shock by replacement of ECF and plasma volume with normal saline without replacement of red cell mass is adequate for full resuscitation[53] and survival despite hematocrit dilutions well below 20.

The obligatory increase in ECF after resuscitation of injury and shock is three times the shift occurring after bowel resection. Associated weight gains are 10 to 15%. The formidable size of the edema space and its complications (eg, increasing A–a gradient) stirs controversy in trauma care.

Exercising moderation in fluid resuscitation from hypovolemic shock has long been recommended.[54] Recently, a causal relationship has been implied between excessive fluids and poor prognosis. The volume infused negatively correlates with prognosis in trauma patients independent of the severity of the patient's injuries.[55] Evaluation of volume status by invasive hemodynamic monitoring as discussed earlier may prevent excessive fluid administration to the patient in shock.

The Patient with Fluid Overload

Etiologies of hypervolemic hyponatremia include congestive heart failure; renal tubular disorders; cirrhosis; syndrome of inappropriate antidiuretic hormone secretion (SIADH); and iatrogenic water intoxication.[56] The last category includes inappropriate intravenous replacement of electrolytes; infusions of oxytocin with electrolyte-free fluids; and the special situation of the transurethral resection of the prostate gland (TURP) syndrome.

Symptoms of cellular edema and altered membrane potentials occur with hyponatremia because electrolyte-free water distributes intracellularly as well as extracellularly. If the patient is alert when the serum sodium falls precipitously below 120 mEq/L, he or she may become agitated, complain of headache and nausea, or show other signs of cerebral edema and central nervous system irritability.[57] Myocardial contractility is also reduced at this level. When serum sodium falls below 110 mEq/L, seizures and/or coma are likely. Bradycardia and widening of the QRS complex, ventricular ectopic beats, and T-wave inversion are evidenced. Cardiac standstill is caused by levels below 100 mEq/L.[58] If the residual effects of a general anesthetic mask the central nervous system signs, hemodynamic instability may be the only clue to the diagnosis. A high index of suspicion must be maintained when caring for any patient at risk.

The origin of postoperative convulsions and respiratory arrest is often missed with devastating outcomes when the syndrome of inappropriate antidiuretic hormone secretion is involved.[59] Secretion of antidiuretic hormone despite hyper- or euvolemia causes excessive water retention, dilutional hyponatremia, and highly concentrated oliguria. The differential diagnosis of syndrome of inappropriate antidiuretic hormone secretion includes neurotrauma and neurosurgery, with a weak association with positive pressure ventilation. Elevated antidiuretic hormone secretion is so common in the postoperative period that it has been dubbed a "normal" metabolic response to surgery.[60] However, this is often appropriately elevated antidiuretic hormone secretion in response to missed intraoperative hypovolemia.[61]

The TURP syndrome is an example of increased intravascular volume that usually presents during recovery from anesthesia. Complications associated with absorption of irrigating fluids include circulatory overload, hyponatremia, and solute toxicity.

The amount of absorption is governed by the height of the container of irrigating solution above the surgical table, which determines the hydrostatic pressure driving fluid into prostatic veins and sinuses, and the length of time of resection. Several estimates and measurements suggest that as many as 8L of fluid may be absorbed during TURP, the average rate of absorption being approximately 20 to 30 mL/min.[62,63] The average weight gain during surgery is about 2 kg.[64] Absorption of irrigating solution is greater during resection of cancerous prostate gland than if the pathology is simple hypertrophy.

A simple method to determine the approximate amount of solution absorbed is to compare serum sodium levels before and after surgery.[58] The following equation estimates intravascular absorption:

$$\text{Volume absorbed} = [(\text{preop serum Na}/\text{postop serum Na}) \times \text{ECF}] - \text{ECF}$$

where ECF is estimated from body weight (20 to 30% of body weight in kg).

Many types of irrigating fluids have been used for TURP (Table 7–2). Although currently used solutions do not cause significant hemolysis, hyponatremia

TABLE 7–2. IRRIGATING SOLUTIONS COMMONLY USED FOR TURP

Solution	Percent	Osmolality
Mannitol	5	275 mOsm
Glycine	1.5	200 mOsm
Cytal		
Sorbitol	2.7	
Mannitol	5.4	195 mOsm
Sorbitol	3.3	165–180 mOsm
Glucose	5	280 mOsm

and circulatory overload may result. Prostatic surgery is frequently undertaken under regional anesthetic techniques. Sympathetic block increases venous capacitance and tends to work against fluid overload. When the block dissipates, venous capacitance acutely decreases and circulatory overload may occur.

Absorption of solutes in irrigating solutions also may cause problems. Glycine, mannitol, and glucose may have adverse effects. Glycine, a nonessential amino acid, is toxic to the heart and the retina of the eye, causing transient blindness when absorbed intravenously.[65,66] Glycine has a distribution similar to that of gama-aminobutyric acid (GABA), which is an inhibitory transmitter in the brain. It is postulated that glycine is also a major inhibitory transmitter, acting in the spinal cord and brain stem.[67]

Ammonia is a major metabolic byproduct of glycine; hyperammonemia is another potential complication of glycine irrigation.[68] Although blood ammonia levels remain within normal limits in most patients during TURP, glycine solutions should be avoided if encephalopathy preexists.

Diabetic patients may be particularly susceptible to side effects of absorption of sorbitol solution. This substance, although rapidly excreted by the kidneys, is metabolized to glucose, which may lead to hyperglycemia. Sorbitol solution is also metabolized to lactate from pyruvate and may compound lactic acidosis caused by sepsis, hypotension, or hypothermia.

Mannitol remains intravascular and exerts an osmotic effect causing further volume expansion. When mannitol is absorbed through prostatic venous channels, the hypervolemic changes may contribute to symptoms of the TURP syndrome.

Prompt recognition and treatment of the TURP syndrome is necessary. Several diagnostic and therapeutic steps are recommended.

1. Administer furosemide 20 mg IV.
2. Give oxygen. If pulmonary edema develops, tracheal intubation and positive pressure ventilation are indicated.
3. Monitor arterial blood gases and sodium levels.
4. If the serum sodium level is below 120 mEq/L, hypertonic saline 3% should be administered at a rate no faster than 100 mL/h. Usually, infusion of no more than 300 mL is needed to correct the dilutional hyponatremia. Often, spontaneous or induced diuresis corrects the hyponatremia within a few hours without therapy.[69] Certainly it is not necessary to replace the calculated deficit of sodium. Indeed, rapid correction of hyponatremia with hypertonic saline may lead to further complications including pulmonary edema, pantene my-

TABLE 7-3. CLINICAL FEATURES OF HYPOGLYCEMIA AND HYPERGLYCEMIA

Hypoglycemia	Hyperglycemia
Coma	Dehydration
Seizures	Hypokalemia
Tachycardia	Metabolic acidosis
Low blood pressure	Hyperventilation
Blood glucose < 70 mg/dL	Coma
	Blood glucose > 300 mg/dL

elinosis, and even death. Hypertonic saline must be given slowly after infusion of a diuretic.

5. If seizures develop, barbituates and tracheal intubation are indicated. Phenytoin (diphenyl-hydantoin) may be given slowly (50 mg/min) to a loading dose of about 10 mg/kg. The benzodiazepine derivatives (diazepam and midazolam), although effective anticonvulsant agents, have a very long half-life (24 h) in therapeutic doses in elderly patients and are best avoided. As a last resort, a paralyzing dose of an intermediate-acting muscle relaxant should be considered to protect the patient from seizure-induced trauma.

6. If pulmonary congestion or hypotension are evident, insertion of a pulmonary artery catheter is indicated to guide pharmacologic support with inotropes, vasodilators, and vasopressors.

7. Significant blood loss should be replaced with red cells to avoid circulatory overload. Coagulation profiles should be studied.

Perioperative bleeding is a common complication of TURP. Several possible causes have been suggested. Elderly patients may be confused because of dementias with pain and may pull on their catheters, traumatizing the prostatic bed. Another possible cause of perioperative bleeding is dilution of thrombocytes. When a large volume of irrigation solution is absorbed, the platelet count may decrease, increasing bleeding time and causing hemorrhage. Coagulopathies may also be causative for postoperative bleeding.

The prostate gland and, particularly, malignant prostatic tumors are rich in tissue thromboplastins.[70] The tissue thromboplastins apparently enter the circulation during surgery and trigger disseminated intravascular coagulopathy and fibrinolysis syndrome (DIC, DICF). Typically, TURP patients with a coagulopathy have a low platelet count, hypofibrinogenemia, prolonged partial thromboplastin and prothrombin times, and an increase in fibrin split products, all of which suggest a consumptive coagulopathy.

Review of the therapy of patients with coagulopathy related to TURP including heparinization, correction of platelet and clotting factor deficiencies, and ligation of hypogastric arteries, revealed no long-term survivals.[71]

The Patient with Hypokalemia

Unlike previously discussed disorders, hypokalemia is usually not associated with a volume aberration. The imbalance may be suspected by history or EKG changes and confirmed by laboratory studies. Hypokalemia is caused either by intracellular redistribution or depletion.[72]

Potassium depletion is common in the perioperative period[73] when oral intake is disrupted. Obligatory urinary potassium losses, approximately 20 mEq/day, will increase with alkalosis, diuretics, a high sodium intake, steroids, or the steroid response to injury. Losses from the gastrointestinal tract, normally 60 mEq/day, increase several-fold with vomiting, nasogastric suction, diarrhea, and cathartics; larger losses occur with fistula drainage or secretory tumors such as villus adenomas and vasoactive intestinal polypeptide-secreting tumors of the pancreas (VIPomas). When fluid balance is maintained with solutions containing little or no potassium, both ICF and ECF become depleted. With complete equilibration, a serum deficit of 1 mEq/L may reflect a total deficit of 800 mEq of potassium. Acute changes are associated with much smaller intracellular losses.[74] Hypokalemia can result from intracellular shifting of potassium without any actual loss. In the postoperative period, this is most commonly due to alkalosis (eg, inappropriate bicarbonate administration or hyperventilation).[75]

The neuromuscular effects of hypokalemia complicate recovery from anesthesia. Although rare, familial periodic paralysis is an acute electrolyte shift of special interest to anesthesiologists. It may present in the PACU as sudden hypokalemia and severe muscle weakness and potentiation of nondepolarizing muscle relaxants due to precipitous intracellular movement of potassium ion.[76] While potassium is repleted, all dextrose-containing fluids must be avoided as carbohydrate facilitates intracellular migration of potassium ions. Chronic hypokalemia is also associated with skeletal muscle weakness[77] and clinically insignificant potentiation of neuromuscular blockade.[78]

In postanesthetic care, the clinical significance of hypokalemia relates only to the cardiac effects of intracellular depletion. Acute shifts of potassium ion to the ICF are ineffectual alone.[79] Chronic hypokalemia, especially if potentiated by acute potassium shifts, will depress myocardial contractility[80] and impair cardiac conduction. However, recent studies show no correlation between the incidence of arrhythmias and the presence of hypokalemia.[81,82] ECG signs of hypokalemia include prolongation of PR and QT intervals, flattening of the T-wave, and appearance of prominent U-waves.

The Patient with Diabetes Insipidus

Although diabetes insipidus (DI) has many etiologies, the differential diagnosis in the PACU is usually quite limited (Table 7–3). Hypophysectomy or incidental destruction of the posterior pituitary gland during craniotomy generally presents as DI several hours to days postoperatively. Lesser intracranial trauma may cause a transient syndrome of DI that commonly presents in the early postoperative hours. Nephrogenic DI also complicates postanesthetic care when the etiology is postobstructive uropathy, postrenal transplantation, severe potassium depletion, or drug-induced unresponsiveness to ADH.

When a patient developes DI in the PACU, the first sign is likely to be polyuria of a specific gravity below 1.010. The serum sodium will quickly exceed 155 mEq/L, while progressive volume depletion develops. If untreated the patient becomes febrile with alterations of mental status, and death may result.

Diabetes insipidus differs from the previous cases by demonstrating an extreme free water deficit. Accordingly, the fluid therapy is large quantities of D5W with replacement of electrolytes only as they are lost in the urine. However, the danger of hyperglycemia in neurosurgical patients has been well emphasized.[83] Moreover, large amounts of dextrose may cause nonketotic hyperglycemic coma to develop.[84] The syndrome is characterized by sudden loss of consciousness, focal tonic–clonic seizures, and even respiratory arrest. Laboratory values show serum sodium levels in the range of 145 to 155 mEq/L, serum osmolarity of 350 to 380 mOsm/kg, and serum glucose around 1000 mg/dL.

When urine volume is 0.5 to 1.0 L/h, fluid therapy alone cannot adequately manage the syndrome. Vasopressin (5 to 10 units subcutaneously every three hours) should be given for centrally induced DI. Control can also be obtained within five to ten minutes in cooperative patients by nasal insufflation of 1-desamino-8-D-arginine vasopressin (DDAVP). Nonketotic hyperglycemic coma requires withdrawal of dextrose-containing solutions, and administration of regular insulin, in addition to vasopressin therapy.

REFERENCES

1. Hill ST: Blood ordering in obstetrics and gynecology: Recommendations for type and screen. *Obstet Gynecol* 1980;62:2336–2340.
2. Czer LSC: Optimal hematocrit in critically ill postoperative patients. *Surg Gynecol Obstet* 1978;147:363–368.
3. Tartter PI: Unnecessary blood transfusions in elective colorectal surgery. *Transfusion* 1985;25:114–115.
4. Gatch WD: Amount of blood loss during some surgical operations. *JAMA* 1924;83:1075–1079.
5. Baronofsky ID: Blood loss in operations: A statistical comparison of losses as determined by the gravimetric and colorimetric methods. *Surgery* 1946;19:761–769.
6. Bonica JJ: Blood loss during surgical operations. *Anesthesiology* 1951;12:90–99.
7. Underwood PS: Serial blood volume determinations associated with major cancer surgery. *Anesth Analg* 1966;45:797–803.
8. Ariel IM: The internal balances of plasma proteins in surgical patients. *Surg Gynecol Obstet* 1951;92:405–414.
9. Jarnun S: Plasma protein exudation in the peritoneal cavity during laparotomy. *Gastroenterology* 1951;41:107–118.
10. Rustad H: Changes in blood volume and red cell volume following gastric resection. *Acta Chir Scand* 1966;357(suppl):127–132.
11. Shires T: Acute changes in extracellular fluids associated with major surgical procedures. *Ann Surg* 1961;154:803–810.
12. Otto CW: Central venous pressure monitoring, in Blitt CD (ed): *Monitoring in Anesthesia and Critical Care Medicine*. New York, Churchill Livingstone, 1985, pp 125–126.
13. Yang SC, Puri VK: Role of preoperative hemodynamic monitoring in intraoperative fluid management. *Am Surg* 1986;52:536–550.
14. Hesdorffer CS, Mile JF, Myers AM, Botha R: The value of Swan-Ganz catheterization and volume loading in preventing renal failure in patients undergoing abdominal aneurysmectomy. *Clin Nephrol* 1987;28:272–276.
15. Shires GT: Postoperative, posttraumatic management of fluids. *Bull NY Acad Med* 1979;55:248–256.
16. Ariel IM: The internal balances of plasma protein in surgical patients. *Surg Gynecol Obstet* 1951;92:405–414.
17. Elwyn DH: Nutritional aspects of body water dislocations in postoperative and depleted patients. *Ann Surg* 1975;182:76–85.
18. Berry FA: Fluid and electrolyte therapy in the pediatric patient, in American Society of Anesthesiologists: *1979 Annual Refresher Course Lectures*. Chicago, American Society of Anesthesiologists, 1979, p 105.
19. Giesecke AH, Jenkins MT: Fluid therapy. *Clin Anesth* 1976;2:57–69.
20. Hauser CJ, Shoemaker WC, Turpin I: Oxygen transport responses to colloids and crystalloids in critically ill surgical patients. *Surg Gynecol Obstet* 1980;150:811–816.
21. Zetterstrom H: Albumin treatment following major surgery: Effects on plasma oncotic pressure, renal function and peripheral oedema. *Acta Anaesth Scand* 1981;25:125–132.
22. Zetterstrom H: Albumin treatment following major surgery: Effects on postoperative lung function and circulatory adaptation. *Acta Anaesth Scand* 1981;25:133–141.
23. Hauser CJ, Shoemaker WC, Turpin I: Oxygen transport responses to colloids and crystalloids in critically ill surgical patients. *Surg Gynecol Obstet* 1980;150:811–816.
24. Lowe RJ, Moss GS, Jilek J, et al: Crystalloid vs colloid in the etiology of pulmonary failure after trauma; a randomized trial in man. *Surgery* 1977;81:676–683.

25. Moss GS, Lower RJ, Jilek J, et al: Colloid or crystalloid in the resuscitation of hemorrhagic shock. A controlled clinical trial. *Surgery* 1981;89:434–438.

26. Moss GS, Siegel DC, Cochin A, et al: Effects of saline and colloid solutions on pulmonary function in hemorrhagic shock. *Surg Gynecol Obstet* 1971;133:53–58.

27. Virgilio RW, Rice CL, Smith DE: Crystalloid vs colloid resuscitation: Is one better? A randomized clinical study. *Surgery* 1979;85:129–139.

28. Rowe MI, Arango A: Colloid vs crystalloid resuscitation in experimental bowel obstruction. *J Pediatr Surg* 1976;11:635–643.

29. Shoemaker WC, Hauser CJ: Critique of crystalloid vs colloid therapy in shock and shock lung. *Crit Care Med* 1979;7:117–124.

30. Virgilio RW, Smith DE, Zarino DK: Balanced electrolyte solutions: Experimental and clinical studies. *Crit Care Med* 1979;7:98–106.

31. Smith PC, et al: Albumin deposition in human lung, skin, and skeletal muscle during surgery. *Surg Forum* 1975;26:91–92.

32. Wells JV, King MA: Adverse reactions to human plasma proteins. *Anaesth Intens Care* 1980;8:139–144.

33. McMillin RD, Hood TR, Griffen WO: Systemic anaphylaxis secondary to the use of 5 per cent plasma protein fractions. *Am J Surg* 1978;135:706–707.

34. Alving BM, Hojima J, Pisano JJ, et al: Hypotension associated with prekallikrein activator (Hageman factor fragments) in plasma protein fraction. *N Engl J Med* 1978;299:66–70.

35. Gruber UF: Dextran and the prevention of postoperative thrombotic complications. *Surg Clin North Am* 1975;55:676–696.

36. Ring J, Messmer K: Incidence and severity of anaphylactoid reactions to colloid volume substitutes. *Lancet* 1977;1:466–469.

37. Consensus Conference: Fresh frozen plasma. Indications and risks. *JAMA* 1985;253:551–553.

38. Stehling L: New concepts in transfusion therapy. IARS Review Course Lectures, 1989, pp 24–28.

39. Gettinger A: Rational use of blood products and alternative fluids. ASA Annual Refresher Course Lectures, 1988, p 112.

40. Myhre BA: Fatalities from blood transfusion. *JAMA* 1980;244:1333–1335.

41. Bove JR: Transfusion-associated hepatitis and AIDS. What is the risk? *N Engl J Med* 1987;317:242–244.

42. Blair SD, Janvrin SB: Is a drip necessary for a cholecystectomy? *Ann R Coll Surg Engl* 1986;68:61.

43. Keane PW, Murray PF: Intravenous fluids in minor surgery. Their effect on recovery from anaesthesia. *Anaesthesia* 1986;41:635–637.

44. Zeidan B, Wyatt J, Mackersie A, Brereton RJ: Recent results of treatment of infantile hypertrophic pyloric stenosis. *Arch Dis Child* 1988;63:1060–1064.

45. Lyon RP, Stranton JR, Freis ED: Blood and available fluid (thiocyanate) volume studies in surgical patients. Part 1: Normal patterns of response of blood volume, available fluid, protein chloride and hematocritin postoperative surgical patient. *Surg Gynecol Obstet* 1949;89:9–19.

46. Nishim Y, Hioki K, et al: Risk factors in relation to postoperative complications in patients undergoing esophagectomy or gastrectomy for cancer. *Ann Surg* 1988;207:148–154.

47. Bergstrom J, Furst P, Holstram B: Influence in injury on muscle water and electrolytes: Effects of operation. *Ann Surg* 1987;193:134–136.

48. Shires T, Cohn D, Carico J: Fluid therapy in hemorrhagic shock. *Arch Surg* 1964;88:688–695.

49. Wiggars MD, Ingraham RC: Hemorrhagic shock: Definition of criteria for its diagnosis. *J Clin Invest* 1946;25:30–35.

50. Carrico CJ, Canizaro PD, Shires GT: Fluid resuscitation following injury, rationale for the use of balanced salt solutions. *Crit Care Med* 1976;4:46–48.

51. Canizaro PC, Prager MD, Shires GT: The infusion of Ringer's lactate solution during shock. *Am J Surg* 1974;108:349–352.

52. Saltz NJ: Shock and the extracellular fluid space. *Am J Surg* 1969;117:603–604.

53. Reynolds M: Cardiovascular effects of large volumes of isotomic saline infused intravenously in dogs following severe hemorrhage. *Am J Physiol* 1949;158:418–420.

54. Roth E, Lax LC, Maloney JV Jr: Changes in extracellular fluid volume during shock and surgical trauma in animal and man. *Surg Forum* 1967;18:42–47.

55. Vassar MJ, Moore J, Perry CA, et al: Early fluid requirements in trauma patients. A predictor of pulmonary failure and mortality. *Arch Surg* 1988;123:1149–1157.

56. Narins RG, Jones ER, Strom MC, et al: Diagnostic strategies in disorders of fluid, electrolyte and acid base hemostasis. *Am J Med* 1982;72:496–520.

57. Rowntree LG: Water intoxication. *Arch Intern Med* 1923;32:157–174.

58. Henderson DJ, Middleton RG: Coma from hyponatremia following transurethral resection of prostate. *Urology* 1980;15:267–271.

59. Arieff AI: Hyponatremia, convulsions, respiratory arrest, and permanent brain damage after elective surgery in healthy women. *N Engl J Med* 1986;314:1529–1535.

60. Traynor C, Hall GM: Endocrine and metabolic changes during surgery: Anaesthetic implications. *Br J Anaesth* 1981;53:153–160.

61. Judd BA, Haycock GB, Dalton N, Chantler C: Hyponatremia in premature babies and following surgery in older children. *Acta Paediatr Scand* 1987;76:385–393.

62. Mazze RI: Anesthesia for patients with abnormal renal function and genitourinary operations, in Miller RD (ed): *Anesthesia.* New York, Churchill Livingstone, 1986, pp 1651–1659.

63. Oester A, Madsen PO: Determination of absorption of irrigating fluid during transurethral resection of the prostate by means of radioisotopes. *J Urol* 1969;102:714–719.

64. Taylor RO, Maxson ES, Carter FH, et al: Volumetric gavimetric and radioisotopic determination of fluid transfer in transurethral prostatectomy. *J Urol* 1958;79:490–499.

65. Ovassapian A, Joshi CW, Brumer EA: Visual disturbances: An unusual symptom of transurethral prostatic resection. *Anesthesiology* 1982;52:332–334.

66. Wang JM, Wong KC, Creel DJ, et al: Effects of glycine

on hemodynamic responses and visual evoked potentials in the dog. *Anesth Analg* 1985;64:1071–1077.

67. Apreson MH, Werman R: The distribution of glycine in cat spinal cord and roots. *Life Sci* 1965;4:2075–2083.

68. Hoelestra PT, Kahnoski R, McCamish MA: Transurethral prostatic resection syndrome: A new perspective: Encephalopathy with associated hyperannonemia. *J Urol* 1983;130:704–705.

69. Osborn DE, Rao PN, Green MJ, et al: Fluid absorption during transurethral resection. *Br Med J* 1980;281:1549–1550.

70. Marx GF, Orkin LR: Complications associated with transurethral surgery. *Anesthesiology* 1962;23:802–813.

71. Friedman NJ, Hoag MS, Robinson AF, et al: Hemorrhagic syndrome following transurethral prostatic resection for benign adenoma. *Arch Intern Med* 1969;124:341–349.

72. Boelhouwer RU, Bruining HA, Ong GL: Correlations of serum potassium fluctuations with body temperature after major surgery. *Crit Care Med* 1987;15:310–312.

73. Bruining HA, Boelhouwer RU, Ong GL: Unexpected hypopotassemia after multiple blood transfusion during an operation. *Neth J Surg* 1986;38:48–51.

74. Hilgenberg JC: Water and electrolyte disturbances, in Stoelting RK (ed): *Anesthesia and Co-Existing Disease.* New York, Churchill Livingstone, 1988, pp 461–465.

75. Edwards R, Winnie AP, Ranamurthy S: Acute hypocapneic hypokalemia and iatrogenic anesthetic complications. *Anesth Analg* 1977;56:786–792.

76. Melnick B, Chang J-L, Larson CE, Bedger RC: Hypo-

kalemic familial periodic paralysis. *Anesthesiology* 1983;58:263–265.

77. Hill GE, Wong KC, Shaw CL, Blatnick RA: Acute and chronic changes in intra- and extracellular potassium and responses to neuromuscular blocking agents. *Anesth Analg* 1978;57:417–421.

78. Miller RD, Roderick LL: Diuretic-induced hypokalemia, pancuronium neuromuscular blockade and its antagonism by neostigmine. *Br J Anaesth* 1978;50:541–544.

79. Wong KC, Wetstone D, Mortin WE: Hypokalemia during anesthesia: The effects of d-tubocurarine, gallamine, succinylcholine, thiopental, and halothane with or without respiratory alkalosis. *Anesth Analg* 1973;52:522–528.

80. Abbrecht PH: Cardiovascular effects of chronic potassium deficiency in the dog. *Am J Physiol* 1972;223:555–559.

81. Papademetriou V, Burris JF, Notargiacomo A, et al: Thiazide therapy is not a cause of arrhythmia in patients with systemic hypertension. *Arch Intern Med* 1988;148:1272–1276.

82. Hirsch IA, Tomlinson DL, Slogoff S, Keats AS: The overstated risk of preoperative hypokalemia. *Anesth Analg* 1988;67:131–136.

83. Sieber FE, Smith DS, Traystman RJ, et al: Glucose; a reevaluation of its intraoperative use. *Anesthesiology* 1987;67:72–81.

84. Friedenberg GF, Kosnik EJ, Sotos JF: Hypoglycemic coma after surgery. *N Engl J Med* 1980;303:863–865.

8 | Parenteral Nutrition

Olli Kirvelä, Vladimir Kvetan, and Jeffrey Askanazi

Protein–calorie depletion is a frequent finding in surgical patients as well as in the critically ill.[1,2] Patients with malnutrition have been shown to be at an increased risk for infections and mechanical complications in the postoperative period. Malnutrition has been associated with increased abdominal wound disruption, delayed gastric emptying, increased surgical infection rates, and poor wound healing.[3-11] Total parenteral nutrition (TPN) can be used to correct the nutritional abnormalities and thus decrease the risk of postoperative morbidity and mortality with a shortening of the hospital stay.[12]

Although the effectiveness of TPN is well established in treating malnutrition, the use of parenteral nutrition during the immediate postoperative period in patients not previously malnourished (albumin greater than 3.5) is still debated. Although nitrogen loss and energy requirements are increased in the postoperative period, it is not yet known whether the provision of nutrients that will correct these deficits will also improve postoperative convalescence. TPN initiated early in the postoperative period, before the patient is able to receive complete enteral nutrition, improves nitrogen balance and restores the plasma levels of transferrin and prealbumin. As with the use of preoperative TPN, there is still some question as to whether the observed improvement in nutritional indices correlates with an improved postoperative course. The studies by Hill and associates[13-15] on patients with abdominoperineal resections compared the effects of routine intravenous fluid therapy, sole amino acid (4.25%) infusion delivering 0.23 g N/kg/day, and TPN with glucose and amino acids providing the same amount of nitrogen plus 36.5 kcal/kg/day. TPN and amino acid infusions were begun on the second or third postoperative day and continued for approximately 13 days. Compared with the amino acid and control groups, the TPN group showed a significantly shorter healing time for perineal wounds and also a significant decrease in the length of hospital stay. Plasma proteins, which were decreased in all three groups postoperatively, returned to normal only in the TPN group. Similarly, TPN spared more body protein and fat and restored plasma amino acids to normal levels. These studies show the beneficial effects of administering adequate postoperative TPN, which not only improved abnormal nutritional parameters, but also enhanced clinical outcome.

A study by Askanazi and colleagues[12] reviewed the effect of nutritional support on duration of hospitalization in patients undergoing radical cystectomy. Thirty-five patients were randomly assigned to either 5% dextrose solution plus electrolytes or TPN following operation. The assigned nutritional regimen was continued for 1 week after operation until oral intake resumed. The group receiving immediate postoperative TPN had a median duration of hospital stay of 17 days, while median hospital stay for the group receiving 5% dextrose solution was 24 days. All other patient characteristics, such as age, sex, state or grade of tumor, and extent of preoperative radiotherapy, were similar. The results of these studies demonstrate that immediate postoperative institution of nutritional support reduces hospitalization time, and indicate that the routine use of 5% dextrose as postoperative nutrition should be reevaluated.

GENERAL PRINCIPLES

The metabolic support for the acutely ill or the surgical patient requires an understanding of the basic changes in body composition and metabolic responses to surgical trauma and stress.

Body Composition and Fuel Stores

Definitions. The body is composed of fat and lead body mass (LBM). The latter is subdivided into extracellular fluid (ECF), body cell mass (BCM), and extracellular supportive structures such as skeleton, cartilage, and tendons. The sum of the lean body mass and adipose tissue is equal to total body weight (TBWt). The fat functions as the energy storage area. It is a relatively anhydrous mass with water representing only about 5% by weight, whereas in skeletal muscle total water content is 80% by weight. Since fat provides 9.5 calories per gram and fat tissue is only 5% water, this is a very compact storage area.

Metabolic use of 1 kg of fat yields 9000 kcal whereas 1 kg of muscle yields only 800 kcal.

Extracellular mass consists of plasma, interstitial water, transcellular water (cerebral spinal fluid, pericardial fluid, and the fluid in the joint spaces), and the supporting structures such as skeleton, tendons, and cartilage. Body cell mass is the metabolically active portion of lean body mass. It consists of skeletal muscle (60%), viscera (30%), and the cells of the supporting structure of the extracellular mass such as red blood cells and the cellular component of adipose tissue. The standard 70-kg man has about 20 kg of fat and about 50 kg of LBM which is about equally divided by weight as ECF and BCM. These parameters vary with sex, body build, and age. Females tend to have decreased LBM and increased adipose tissue. The ratio of LBM to TBWt also decreases with age. Very muscular individuals will have a LBM:TBWt ratio that is greater than normal. These relationships remain constant as long as caloric intake equals expenditure. With excess caloric intake, there will be an increase in the adipose tissue unless a vigorous exercise program is undertaken, in which circumstances an increase in skeletal muscle mass will occur if adequate protein is supplied. Excess energy is stored as fat; there are no storage deposits of protein and glycogen cannot be stored in any significant amount.

Fuel Stores. To maintain adequate metabolism during periods with enhanced energy needs or reduced dietary intake, expenditure of endogenous tissue stores is required. The energy available from circulating substrates is negligible. Carbohydrate is stored as glycogen in liver and muscle. The average healthy adult stores 200 to 300 g of carbohydrate, which gives a total available energy of approximately 900 kcal. This can fulfill energy requirements for 8 to 10 hours; thus the glycogen stores become depleted within 24 hours during starvation.

Fat contributes to about 15 to 30% of the body weight. The average adult man has about 140,000 kcal stored as fat. This constitutes 85% of the total body energy stores and is the major energy source during periods of prolonged starvation. Fat is stored as triglyceride.

Protein is present in lean body tissue; the major part is in skeletal muscle and visceral organs. Fourteen to 20% of body weight is protein, giving a total amount available of about 24,000 kcal. Although protein breakdown provides some energy, this is by no means its main function. Some degree of function loss always accompanies the use of lean body mass for energy generation.

An individual's total caloric storage could potentially sustain life for about 2 months; in practice most persons would be at the point of death after having burned about 140,000 kcal, or about 75% of the fat and 50% of the protein.

Clinical Implications of Body Composition in Postoperative Patients. Body composition changes in postoperative patients can result from various combinations of starvation, injury, sepsis, different substrate infusions, and other factors that may be less well defined.

The rate of LBM loss increases with the severity of surgical trauma.[16] Both surgical and accidental trauma will often necessitate the administration of large quantities of fluid, causing an acute increase in the ECF compartment.[17,18] These fluids are not usually retained in normal patients, but underlying complications such as sepsis may cause a failure in diuresis. After initial fluid resuscitation, sepsis has been shown to be associated with further increases in ECF volume and decreases in serum Na concentration.[19]

Infusions of glucose alone will cause an absolute and a relative increase in the ECF. One week of carbohydrate feeding can produce the fully developed kwashiorkor syndrome (marked expansion of ECF with pitting edema, ascites, and anasarca) in an undernourished child.[20] In adults the normal 5% dextrose infusion (100 g glucose/day) results in marked sodium retention with little effect on potassium losses; that is, carbohydrate administration exacerbates the increased ECF/BCM when used as the only nutrient.[21] The use of D5 saline has been found to abolish the sodium loss completely while potassium loss exceeds that of a complete fast, thus resulting in a greater ECF/BCM ratio than total starvation. Carbohydrates can also increase the ECF when given in greater excess even if protein is given simultaneously.[22]

Typically, patients who have lost weight experience an increase in ECF and a decrease in BCM. Recent weight losses of less than 10% of normal body weight may not require urgent nutritional treatment. Losses of 10 to 30% represent a serious complication, and failure to provide nutritional therapy will almost certainly interfere with recovery despite treatment that is optimum in other respects. Losses greater than 30% are life-threatening. Nutritional therapy must be administered immediately, but with caution, since overfeeding in these conditions can cause severe complications.[23]

An expanded ECF volume is generally considered undesirable because it is correlated with postoperative complications and undesirable effects on pulmonary and cerebral function.[24] Adequate nutrition will result in a relative decrease of the ECF when the water retention has occurred for nutritional reasons alone. If the expanded ECF results from trauma or sepsis, however, nutritional support alone may not be sufficient.

Protein depletion will affect the protein content of all organs. The liver and gut are rapidly depleted while the brain is well protected against protein depletion. In severe protein depletion the gut may be unable to tolerate or digest food, presumably because protein is needed to produce digestive enzymes. The skeletal muscle is most affected and may lose as much as 70% of its protein.

Diagnosis of Malnutrition in Surgical Patients. An evaluation of nutritional status in surgical patients is important both in identifying the patient who needs nutritional support pre- and postoperatively and in assessing the efficacy of the nutritional therapy. The lack of a specific test for protein–calorie malnutrition makes the diagnosis difficult in many cases.

Nutritional assessment begins with a medical history and physical examination, including the recording of height and weight. In the chronically malnourished patient with underlying disease, extracellular volume is expanded with a relatively increased total body water and exchangeable sodium, and a decreased exchangeable potassium.[18] The body weight may thus underestimate the degree of malnutrition. On the other hand, nutritional repletion may be associated with a diuresis and contraction of the extracellular fluid compartment, so that early weight loss may occur even though body cell mass is increasing. Nevertheless, the best single index of malnutrition is evidence of weight loss from the patient's normal level of weight.

Practical clinical tools of anthropometric measurement of body composition include the triceps, skinfold thickness, and midarm circumference as indicators of body fat and muscle and, thereby, of lean body mass. Both measurements have a wide range of normal values and are rather insensitive to early changes in nutritional status.

Creatinine excretion is directly related to muscle mass and expected creatinine excretion can be calculated based on sex and height.[25] The creatinine/height index is thus a useful indicator of muscle mass.

The biochemical parameters used most often to assess nutritional status are the visceral proteins synthesized in the liver: albumin, transferrin, retinol-binding protein, and prealbumin. Serum albumin appears to be most useful in the initial assessment of chronic malnutrition. Transferrin has a shorter half-life (approximately eight days), however, it is also an acute-phase reactant and is affected by the status of iron stores. This lack of specificity limits the clinical usefulness of transferrin. Retinol-binding protein and

prealbumin turn over more rapidly, with half-lives of 12 and 36 hours, respectively. They may be potentially more sensitive and specific indicators of nutritional status, but their clinical utility has not yet been established.

Decreased humoral and cellular immunity is a serious consequence of protein–calorie malnutrition. Total lymphocyte count and cutaneous reactivity are used in some clinical settings. However, sepsis and carcinoma also cause anergy independent of nutritional status. This lack of specificity limits their use in the clinical setting.

At present, there is no single best indicator of nutritional status or the efficacy of nutritional support. The prognostic nutritional index[26] and the protein-energy malnutrition scale[27] attempt to develop more objective measures to predict outcome based on a combination of parameters. However, clinical judgment has been reported to be as good as any of the objective measurements in predicting morbidity and mortality.[28]

Metabolism

Energy Generation. By metabolism of carbohydrate, lipid and protein energy is released for mechanical work, synthesis, membrane transport, and thermogenesis. Glucose, amino acids, fatty acids, triglycerides, lactate, and ketones all, under different circumstances, play a role in energy generation. Glucose metabolism generally occurs along the glycolysis and the oxidative phosphorylation pathways. Glycolysis produces a small amount of ATP as compared to oxidative phosphorylation; since it can proceed anaerobically, however, it becomes important during anoxic and hypoxic conditions. Fatty acids and amino acids are metabolized aerobically and use slightly more oxygen per kcal of energy generated than does glucose.

Metabolic Responses to Trauma and Surgical Stress

Classically the metabolic response to trauma is divided into the early "ebb" or shock phase and the subsequent "flow" phase.[29] The shock phase is associated with an early period of weight gain due to fluid sequestration. The metabolic rate is depressed, body temperature is lowered, and the circulating blood volume reduced. The "ebb" phase is followed after a day or two by the "flow" phase with increased metabolic activity. In this phase body energy stores are mobilized to meet increased needs. Weight is lost as the retained fluid is mobilized along with fat and lean body mass. Maximal N loss generally occurs between the fourth and eighth day after injury. N-excretion and resting energy expenditure (REE) are increased as a function of the severity of the trauma.[30,31] However, uncomplicated elective operations do not significantly increase REE.

The degree of catabolic response depends on the severity and duration of the trauma or stress. After an uncomplicated surgical procedure in an otherwise healthy patient, the catabolic response persists for about a week with a net nitrogen loss. These mild N-losses are well tolerated and readily replaced by subsequent oral feeding. By contrast, a patient who is fasting after severe trauma or stress catabolizes considerable amounts of lean body tissue and fat.

The catabolic response can be seen as a mobilization of body glycogen, protein, and fat stores to ensure adequate circulatory levels of substrate (glucose, fatty acids, and amino acids) when dietary intake is limited. The increased available amino acid pool occurs predominantly at the expense of skeletal muscle. These amino acids may be oxidized directly for fuel but are mainly used for gluconeogenesis; this process also makes more precursors available for synthesis of visceral protein and the proteins of tissue repair.

In response to injury, gluconeogenesis is increased despite high circulating levels of glucose.[32] This hyperglycemia, referred to as the "diabetes of injury," reflects the urgent nature of the healing tissues' requirement for glucose.[33] Fat is mobilized to obtain high circulating levels, and is used for the energy needs of cardiac, skeletal, and respiratory muscles; this allows glucose to be spared for tissues that specifically require it, such as the central nervous system (CNS), the cellular immune system, and the healing wound. There is an increased body metabolism in response to trauma that is characterized by fever and enhanced oxygen consumption. The hormonal changes include increased release of adrenal glucocorticoid, glucagon, and catecholamines. These changes contribute to the mobilization of energy stores and provide gluconeogenic substrates.

INDICATIONS AND GOALS FOR POSTOPERATIVE PARENTERAL NUTRITION

Goals of Parenteral Nutrition

Nutritional therapy has three main goals. The first is to maintain body tissue. This is a prophylactic support in which TPN is given to prevent the development of malnutrition. The second is to replete body tissues in the already malnourished patient. The third goal is the prevention and correction of specific micronutrient deficiencies (vitamins, trace elements, and so on).

The first step in planning any nutritional regimen is to identify the need for nutritional support. The next step is to prescribe the amounts of macronutrients and micronutrients based on the clinical setting and nutritional assessment of the patient. The last step is to determine the route of delivery.

Indications

Patients who are well nourished and require intravenous fluids for less than five days may receive conventional hypocaloric fluid therapy postoperatively. If the patient is depleted, TPN or enteral feeding should be considered even if a return to normal oral diet is anticipated within a few days. TPN or enteral nutrition should always be considered if the postoperative semistarvation time is likely to be greater than four or five days. In general, one should begin TPN early, based on this estimation, rather than waiting in anticipation of a return of gastrointestinal function.

Critically ill patients are often hypermetabolic and hypercatabolic and are at high risk for rapidly developing malnutrition, even though their premorbid nutritional status was adequate. The goal is to meet their increased nutritional requirements in order to minimize the loss of lean body mass and function during the catabolic phase. Patients with severe injury, major burns, or sepsis fall into this group.

Patients with all kinds of chronic diseases will often require artificial nutrition. Patients with short gut syndrome, gastrointestinal fistula, severe malabsorption, or inflammatory bowel disease will require intravenous nutrition. Often, nutritional debilitation is seen in chronic diseases even though the gastrointestinal tract is not directly involved—for example, in patients with chronic renal failure.

Malnutrition is common in patients with cancer. There is evidence that TPN may improve patient tolerance to chemotherapy and radiation.[34,35] However, no significant long-term benefit has been demonstrated to date. In our opinion TPN should be given to cancer patients with the same criteria as to other surgical patients as long as they receive other treatments.

NUTRITIONAL REQUIREMENTS

The different nutrients required vary considerably depending on the type of operation and underlying disease. Therefore the specific needs of each patient should be carefully defined and the changes in them, which may be quite dramatic in the critically ill, should be monitored and responded to accordingly. For this reason, we will give only guidelines for designing postoperative TPN.

Energy

Energy expenditure should be evaluated to prevent insufficient caloric intake as well as overfeeding. Overfeeding, particularly with glucose, may lead to hypermetabolism, hepatic steatosis, and elevated CO_2 production. Energy requirements can be measured using indirect calorimetry. The introduction of new machines that are smaller and easy to use has made this method available for clinical practice. Their use is recommended in critically ill patients where predicting the requirements is very difficult.

When exact measurement cannot be obtained, the resting energy expenditure can be calculated from the Harris-Benedict equation.[36] The equation is based on the patient's sex, weight (W), height (H), and age (A):

$$Female: 655 + 9.6(W) + 1.7(H) - 4.7(A)$$
$$= kcal/day$$

$$Male: 66 + 13.7(W) + 5(H) - 6.8(A)$$
$$= kcal/day$$

In clinical practice the calorie requirements are often estimated on the basis of the patient's weight: 25 to 40 kcal/kg/day.

Depending on the clinical condition of the patient, the energy intake may be increased. If the patient has fever, the energy expenditure will increase by approximately 7% for each degree F of body temperature above normal. Major surgery, sepsis, and burns increase energy expenditure (Fig. 8–1). Intake must be adjusted upward if urinary and fecal calorie losses are increased. On the other hand, semistarvation, which is often seen in surgical patients, may reduce energy expenditure by as much as 30%. In a nutritionally depleted patient a greater intake than calculated expenditure is necessary for repletion and synthesis of tissue. For nutritional repletion, energy intake should exceed resting energy expenditure (REE) by 50%. For maintenance, only 20% above REE is necessary. In the previously malnourished individual with more than 10% weight loss one should aim for repletion, while the previously healthy individual requires maintenance only.

Nonprotein Calories

Normally, carbohydrates contribute 40 to 60%, protein 10 to 15%, and fat 30 to 40% of the total energy intake. The amount of protein intake used for energy varies since parts of the amino acids are used for protein synthesis. Nitrogen balance is sensitive to protein intake as well as to total energy (calories) intake; for comparative calories the effect of protein exceeds that of nonprotein calories. Optimal nutritional support first maximizes protein intake and only then

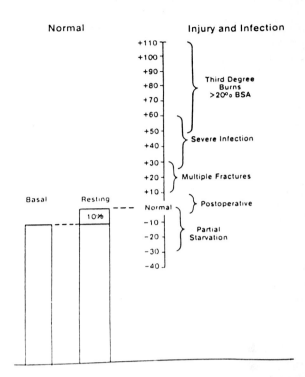

Figure 8–1. The effects of injury, sepsis, and nutritional depletion on resting energy expenditures. (From Kinney JM: The application of indirect calorimetry to clinical studies, in Kinney JM (ed): *Assessment of Energy Metabolism in Health and Disease.* Columbus, OH, Ross Laboratories, 1980, pp 42–48.)

adds sufficient calories in the form of glucose and fat.[37] In surgical patients, positive nitrogen balance cannot be achieved by giving amino acids alone, without other calories. Nonprotein calories can reduce N excretion, but only to a minimum level in the absence of protein intake.[38] Thus both protein and nonprotein energy are required. However the effects of nitrogen and energy intake on N balance are not independent of one another; their interaction is complex. If N intake is adequate, zero N balance is achieved when caloric intake meets caloric expenditure. Similarly, increasing caloric intake above requirements in normal individuals increases N retention and results in net positive N balance.[39] Changes in body composition that occur with hyperalimentation have been found to consist of approximately two parts fat to one part lean body mass,[40,41] but will depend on the kind of nutritional composition.

The large N loss that occurs during the first six days of fasting can be halved by daily ingestion of only 100 g of glucose.[21] The N-sparing effect of a relatively small (400 kcal/g) caloric load occurs with carbohydrates only; fat does not produce the same suppression of N excretion during fasting in normal individuals.[42] On the other hand, restriction of either fat or carbohydrate in the diet increases N output, although N loss is greater than carbohydrate restriction,[43] while adding either back improves N retention.[44] The ability of fat as compared to glucose to spare nitrogen has been studied extensively. At low dosages, glucose is clearly superior to fat. When carbohydrate is administered in amounts of more than 600 kcal/day, however, the nitrogen-sparing effects of fat and carbohydrate are equal,[44] while fat has only a small N-sparing effect in the absence of 600 kcal/day of carbohydrates.[45,46] However, no differences in N-balance have been detected in studies comparing groups receiving nonprotein calories in the form of glucose with those whose nonprotein calories were supplied as half fat and half glucose.[47,48] When the lipid-based system is administered, a lesser calorigenic response and a decreased norepinephrine excretion have been found, as compared to the "glucose system."[49] A reduction in carbon dioxide production has also been observed in patients receiving the "lipid system."[50] Liver function tests have shown fewer abnormalities when lipid was used to replace one third of the glucose calories.[51] These studies provide evidence of the efficacy of 20%-fat emulsion as a concentrated nutrient source that allows provision of calories without overhydration and hemodilution. General use of fat as a calorie source in TPN in the United States has developed only gradually even though fat emulsions represent a logical alternative to glucose loading, especially in patients with an exaggerated caloric requirement and a diminished ability to clear exogenous glucose (eg, in metabolic stress), as well as in those with hepatic or pulmonary dysfunction. Fat emulsions also serve as a source of essential fatty acids, and therefore fat emulsions should be provided to prevent essential fatty acid deficiency syndrome.

Once the minimal intake for glucose (approximately 500 kcal/day to supply carbohydrate for the brain, bone marrow, and injured tissue) and fat are met, the additional nonprotein calories may be provided as either of these substrates. The optimum balance of fat and glucose is not yet determined. TPN systems with 50% of nonprotein calories delivered as fat are as effective in maintaining nitrogen balance as those with 100% glucose and seem to minimize complications.

Protein

Negative N balance is associated with resorption and positive with deposition of cellular protoplasm. In healthy adults an N equilibrium is established when daily protein intake is above 1.0 g/kg/day. Surgical stress and postoperative complications increase protein breakdown and nitrogen intake has to be increased accordingly. As a simple guide to make up for the increased protein needs after major surgery and postoperative complications, protein must be increased in proportion to energy (calorie/nitrogen ratio) to about 100 to 125 kcal per gram of N. When a nutritional program is aimed at repleting lean body mass, protein intake must be increased above maintenance protein requirements.

Severe Injury and Major Surgery

Metabolic and hormonal derangements seen in severe injury and major surgery do not easily respond to nutritional manipulation. As a result, hypertonic glucose administration is usually ineffective in these patients and may add stress by increasing oxygen consumption, carbon dioxide production, and noradrenaline excretion, and by inducing hepatic complications and hyperosmolar states. These findings do not indicate that glucose infusion is contraindicated in stressed patients; a certain amount of carbohydrate intake is essential to meet obligatory glucose requirements. The importance of glucose has been underscored by data associating the administration of amino acids alone (without supplementary glucose) with reduced cellular energy levels in injured patients.[52] A nutritional regimen appropriate for a patient under metabolic stress would therefore consist of a relatively modest amount of glucose administered with amino acids and other essential nutrients. Fat emulsions represent the logical alternative to glucose loading in patients with an increased caloric requirement. The fat emulsion allows provision of the calories without overhydration and hemodilution. It seems therefore that a regimen supplying nonprotein calories in the form of both glucose and fat may be particularly appropriate for the stressed patient.

Branched-chain amino acid (BCAA) enriched solutions have been advocated for hypercatabolic patients. The rationale arose from the fact that BCAAs are chiefly metabolized in muscle, as well as from the evidence pointing to muscle as the major site of the increased postinjury breakdown of protein. Due to the abnormal peripheral utilization of glucose and fat under these conditions. BCAA supplementation was expected to provide useful energy for peripheral tissues, despite the already elevated plasma levels of BCAA. It was expected that improving the nutrition of peripheral tissues might improve the nutrition of the viscera.

There were three rationales for the BCAA enrichment in TPN: to serve as a caloric substrate; to stimulate protein synthesis; and to reduce protein catabolism.[53-57] All of these effects may be beneficial in controlling protein losses in states with metabolic stress.

Despite the theoretical advantages of BCAA in the

support of critically ill patients, the numerous clinical studies have failed so far to show any benefits when compared to balanced amino acid solutions.[58-60] Increasing the BCAA content of the amino acid solution leads to a decrease in the amount of other essential amino acids and nonessential amino acids in the amino acid solution. This can lead to deficient intakes of these important elements of protein metabolism. BCAAs are also rather insoluble and thus require more diluted solutions, which makes their use difficult in patients with fluid restriction.

Electrolytes, trace-elements, and vitamins are important in maintaining normal metabolic functions. They are essential and therefore have to be supplied with the nutrition (Tables 8–1 and 8–2). The supply should cover the basal requirements and the extra needs and losses caused by surgery, drainage, and so on. When the patient begins to become anabolic additional supplementation of potassium and phosphate will be needed as these shift into the intracellular space. Hypophosphatemia may reduce cardiac and muscle contraction, as well as CNS, red blood cell, and leucocyte function.[61] Based on clinical experience, the use of large amounts of glucose increases potassium requirements by approximately 40 mmol/1000 kcal.

In Table 8–3 we have outlined a nutritional program based on a glucose/lipid system, for an average 70-kg male who has suffered a weight loss of 10 kg

TABLE 8–1. RECOMMENDED DAILY INTAKES OF ELECTROLYTES AND MICRONUTRIENTS BY PARENTERAL ROUTE

Natrium	(mmol)	1–1.4
Kalium	(mmol)	0.7–0.9
Calcium	(mmol)	0.11
Phosphorus	(mmol)	0.15
Magnesium	(mmol)	0.04
Iron	(μmol)	20
	(mg)	1.1
Zinc	(μmol)	100
	(mg)	6.4
Copper	(μmol)	20
	(mg)	1.3
Iodine	(μmol)	1.0
	(mg)	127
Manganese	(μmol)	5
	(mg)	0.27
Fluoride	(μmol)	50
	(mg)	0.95
Chromium	(μmol)	0.2
	(mg)	0.01
Selenium	(μmol)	0.4
	(mg)	0.03
Molybdenum	(μmol)	0.2
	(mg)	0.02

Adapted from Shenkin A: Vitamin and essential trace element recommendations during intravenous nutrition: Theory and practice. Proc Nutr Soc 1986; 45:383–390.

TABLE 8–2. RECOMMENDED DAILY INTAKES OF VITAMINS IN PARENTERAL NUTRITION

		AMA	GRI$_2$
Retinol	(μg)	1000	1000
	(IU)	3300	3300
Ergocalciferol	(μg)	5	5
	(IU)	200	200
A-Tocopherol	(mg)	10	10
Vitamin K	(μg)	–	150
Ascorbic acid	(mg)	100	100
Thiamin	(mg)	3.0	3.0
Riboflavin	(mg)	3.6	3.6
Pyridoxine	(mg)	4.0	4.0
Niacin	(mg)	40	40
Vitamin B$_{12}$	(μg)	60	60
Pantothenic acid	(mg)	15	15
Biotin	(μg)	60	60
Folic acid	(μg)	400	400

From Shenkin A: Vitamin and essential trace element recommendations during intravenous nutrition: Theory and practice. Proc Nutr Soc 1986; 45:383–390.

due to stress and illness. Formulas for nutrition for specific disease states will be discussed later in the chapter.

TYPES OF PARENTERAL NUTRITION USED DURING THE POSTOPERATIVE PERIOD

Several systems for postoperative parenteral nutrition have been developed. The route of administration will divide the treatment into two subgroups—peripheral and central parenteral nutrition.

Short-term intravenous nutrition can be administered by peripheral vein. The limiting factor in peripheral nutrition is the osmolality of the solution, because peripheral veins do not tolerate hyperosmolal liquids. Solutions consisting solely of diluted amino acids were suggested for postoperative parenteral nutrition by Blackburn and associates.[62] This kind of

TABLE 8–3. NUTRIENT REGIMEN FOR THE STANDARD 70-KG MALE FOLLOWING WEIGHT LOSS AIMING FOR NUTRITIONAL REPLETION

Nutrient Mixture

Protein	110 g
Nonprotein calories	1000–2000
Distribution	50% glucose and 50% fat

Parenteral Solutions

1.000 mL	11% amino acids
1.000 mL	20% glucose
500 mL	20% fat emulsion

The parenteral solutions can be mixed in one bag and infused over 24 hours at 100 mL/h. Electrolytes, trace elements, and vitamins are added to the TPN mixture.

treatment is unfortunately still widely used even though it is both ineffective and expensive.[63]

In central European countries, the use of diluted amino acid solutions together with fructose, sorbitol, or xylitol as nonprotein caloric source is widespread in postoperative nutritional support. These products usually contain electrolytes and even trace elements in varying compositions and are meant to be used as basic postoperative fluid therapy. A commercial mixture of glycerol and amino acids with electrolytes is also available. It is meant for nutritional maintenance in the postoperative period and may have some advantages over conventional solutions for diabetic patients.[64] All the presented therapies are essentially hypocaloric if given in near iso-osmolal concentrations and cannot therefore contain enough calories to cover the postoperative needs. Consequently their use is mainly restricted to patients recovering from uneventful surgery, and their benefits thus remain limited.

There are several reasons for the use of xylitol, sorbitol, and glycerol instead of glucose in these mixtures. The first is purely technical: a mixture of amino acids and glucose is difficult to manufacture. It cannot be sterilized by autoclaving because of caramelization and discoloring during heating. The nonglucose carbohydrates and glycerol do not have this problem. The second reason is their supposed metabolic efficiency in posttraumatic metabolism. Fructose does not require insulin for phosphorylation and conversion to glucose and thus may be more efficiently metabolized even by patients with insulin deficiency or resistance. It is more readily converted to glycogen and it produces lower serum glucose levels and less glucosuria than similar doses of dextrose. Its use as a single energy source is limited by total dose and infusion rate. Fructose is contraindicated in patients with fructose intolerance and also should not be used in the therapy of acute hypoglycemia. Side effects of fructose administration, including uricemia, lactic acidosis, and hypophosphatemia, are related to total dose and infusion rate. A maximum delivery of 1 g/kg/hour should not be exceeded in either infants or adults.[65]

Sorbitol has a similar fate to that of fructose. Like fructose, it does not cause increased insulin production or hyperglycemia upon administration. However, its use does not offer any advantage over fructose.[66]

Xylitol offers several of the same metabolic advantages as fructose; the initial step has little or no insulin dependence, glycogen formation occurs independent of plasma glucose levels, and it has an antiketogenic effect. However, its toxicity at hyperosmolal concentrations or at high infusion rates limits its use in parenteral nutrition.[67]

Glycerol is a naturally occurring sugar alcohol. Small amounts of glycerol are contained in fat emulsions, but glycerol has not commonly been utilized as an energy source and its introduction as a single energy source in parenteral nutrition is relatively recent. It has a caloric value of 4.32 kcal/g and appears to have the same metabolic effect on protein breakdown as assessed by urinary nitrogen loss that glucose does. This is believed to be due to its gluconeogenic activity. It also has antiketogenic effects.[68]

When lipids are added to peripheral nutrition, the caloric content can be substantially higher without raising the osmolality of the solution. An example of such a mixture would be 500 mL of a 20% fat emulsion, 1000 mL of 8.5% amino acid solution, and 1000 mL of 10% dextrose. This provides nearly 1800 kcal/day. The use of an "all-in-one system" makes this system very simple and safe. The final concentration of dextrose is less than 5%, hence the phlebitis rate is quite low and comparable with that observed with 5% dextrose and saline solution. The results with this kind of nutritional support are good because the amounts of nutrients are sufficient for most patients recovering from uneventful surgery. The therapy can be started on the first postoperative day with full concentration. The water load of the regimen is enough to cover most patient's needs. In patients with fluid restriction, the use of more concentrated solutions and the central route is recommended. The vein puncture site should be rotated every 2 to 3 days.

The central venous line is still the most commonly used route for administering parenteral nutrition. Many of the patients who need nutritional support have a central venous line for other reasons and the use of this line for delivering nutrition is then a rational approach. However, in long-term TPN, a separate line for nutrients is recommended. The central line is necessary if a high concentration of glucose or other carbohydrates, amino acids, or electrolytes is needed.

The administration of high-concentration glucose should be started gradually. On the first postoperative day we recommend the use of a mixture similar to that used in peripheral parenteral nutrition with lipid emulsion. On the following days the glucose concentration can be increased according to blood glucose levels. If the blood glucose levels cannot be controlled by changing the glucose concentration, insulin can be given with the mixture.

Delivery of Nutrients

Cyclic administration of nutrients has been suggested, alternating dextrose-containing with dextrose-free solutions. This method has the theoretical advantage of avoiding prolonged hyperinsulinemia and allowing release of endogenous fatty acids from adipose tissue, and may also optimize visceral protein preservation and avoid alterations in hepatic function.[69]

Mixing of all the components for TPN in one mix ("three-in-one system") before administration simplifies procedures for nursing personnel and may also reduce the risk of infection. Until now the most common mode of delivery has been to give separate infusions of amino acids, fat, and carbohydrate, and add electrolytes, vitamins, and trace elements into the solutions before infusion ("bottle system"). The nursing personnel have to mix the components, monitor infusion rate of more solutions given at the same time, and change bottles several times during the day. In addition to the work for the nursing staff, the mixing of solutions on the floor may not be satisfactory from a hygienic point of view, considering the frequently required manipulations with infusion sets and connections.

Complications

The most common metabolic complications are hyperglycemia and glucosuria. These are dependent on the rate of infusion and carbohydrate source. Frequent monitoring of glucose in urine and serum is required during TPN. If the patient becomes hyperglycemic (blood glucose > 250 mg/dL) the infusion rate of glucose should be reduced[70] and insulin may be administered. The requirement for insulin often decreases rapidly when the patient's stress resolves and the patient shifts from the catabolic to the anabolic state. The need for insulin should be reevaluated daily by close monitoring of blood and urinary sugars. The discontinuing of glucose–insulin mixtures should be done with caution, to avoid hypoglycemia, since the effect of the insulin lasts longer than that of glucose. The tendency towards hyperosmolarity can be prevented if the plasma osmolarity, Na, BUN, acid–base balance, and blood sugar are carefully monitored. A metabolic complication described in the literature is hyperchloremic acidosis, which can be prevented by decreasing the ratio of chloride to acetate in the TPN.[71] Rapid infusion of amino acid solutions has been associated with nausea, headache, and a warm sensation. When the patient begins to become anabolic, large amounts of K^+ and phosphate shift into the intracellular space; to avoid a deficit of these supplementation will be needed. Hepatic dysfunction has been reported. However, replacement of part of the TPN glucose calories with fat leads to better glucose tolerance and fewer hepatic complications.[51]

The mechanical catheter-related complications are outlined in Table 8–4. Of these complications sepsis deserves special mention. Strict antiseptic conditions should prevail during catheter placement, and

TABLE 8–4. MECHANICAL COMPLICATIONS OF TPN

Central Venous Catheter
Malposition
Catheter embolism
Air embolism
Thrombosis and thromboembolism
Sepsis
Cardiac dysrhythmias
Myocardial perforation

Subclavian or Internal Jugular Venipuncture
Arterial puncture
Pneumothorax, hemothorax, chylothorax
Brachial plexus injury
Mediastinal hematoma

Peripheral Venipuncture
Pain
Hemotoma
Thrombosis
Phlebitis
Extravasation

the catheter should be, if feasible, used only for the infusion of TPN. The frequency of the induction of sepsis is increased with the use of multilumen catheters for TPN.[71,72]

Patient Monitoring

Table 8–5 gives guidelines for monitoring the patient for the development of infection or metabolic complications. When the patient is stable and tolerating a particular regimen, most of these determinations can be performed less frequently.

TABLE 8–5. SUGGESTED MONITORING SCHEDULE DURING TPN

Parameter	Suggested Frequency	
	Early	*After Stable*
Volume in (IV and oral)	Daily	Daily
Volume out (urine and drainage)	Daily	Daily
Body temperature	Daily	Daily
Urine S&A	qid	bid
Electrolytes	Daily	Biweekly
BUN/creatinine	Biweekly	Biweekly
Ca^{++}, P, Mg^{++}	Biweekly	Weekly
CBC, platelets	Weekly	Weekly
Glucose	Daily	Biweekly
PT, PTT	Weekly	Weekly
Triglycerides, cholesterol	Weekly	Weekly
Liver profile	Biweekly	Weekly
ABGs, urine electrolytes, drainage analysis, blood cultures, serum insulin, ketones, plasma amino acids, plasma fatty acids		
Weight	Biweekly	Biweekly

IV = intravenous; S&A = sugar and acetone; BUN = blood urea nitrogen; CBS = complete blood count; PT = prothrombin time; PTT = partial thromboplastin time; ABGs = arterial blood gases.
From: Robin AR, Greig PD: Clin Chest Med 1986;

Weight should be measured daily; acute changes reflect changes in water and sodium.

POSTOPERATIVE PARENTERAL NUTRITION IN DIFFERENT DISEASE ENTITIES

Liver Disease

Several metabolic alterations caused by liver disease affect the design of postoperative TPN in this patient group. These patients often are malnourished, but at the same time their protein tolerance is low. However, protein metabolism in other tissues is not necessarily changed. Therefore, rather than starting special hepatic formulations in all patients with hepatic insufficiency, the first step in a patient with moderate hepatic impairment is to try cautious administration of standard amino acid formulas without exceeding 50 to 60 g of protein. For those patients who do not tolerate such an approach or who become encephalopathic, a special solution with a modified amino acid composition may be tried.

In hepatic failure the plasma levels of aromatic amino acids (AAA) (phenylalanine, tyrosine, and tryptophan) and methionine increase due to decreased hepatic metabolism. Simultaneously the branched chain amino acid (BCAA) levels are decreased because of peripheral utilization.[73,74] In hepatic encephalopathy (HE) there may be a derangement of the blood–brain barrier,[75] which results in a selective increase in transport of the neutral amino acids. It is hypothesized that within this group the transport of aromatic amino acids is preferentially increased due to their elevated plasma levels as well as decreased competition for the transport system due to decreased plasma concentrations of BCAA.[74,76] According to this theory,[77] a decrease in the BCAA:AAA plasma ratio would be responsible for an imbalance of central aminergic neurotransmitters. The AAAs are precursors of neurotransmitters, and an increase in brain concentrations of serotonin and false neurotransmitters has been found in HE.[78] Therefore, special BCAA-enriched amino acid solutions have been developed. They have a high concentration of BCAA and low concentrations of AAA and methionine. Some have elevated concentrations of arginine to feed the urea cycle.

These solutions are theoretically attractive in hepatic failure because of their ability to provide usable calories that can be utilized by peripheral conversion, to arrest protein catabolism and promote protein synthesis, and to normalize BCAA:AAA plasma levels.[79] Clinical studies of the benefits of BCAA solutions have very conflicting results.[80-86] The other treatments given, the amount of other amino acids infused simultaneously, the role of fat emulsions, and the very unhomogenous patient groups make the interpretation of these results very difficult.

During TPN, blood glucose and serum FFA levels should be monitored carefully and the regimen adjusted accordingly. There is a persistent elevation of glucagon and insulin and increased lipolysis, probably because of diminished degradation of circulatory hormones and portal systemic shunting.[87-90]

Respiratory Disease

The effects of nutrition on respiration involve respiratory drive, respiratory muscle function, and pulmonary parenchyma as well as increased metabolic demand. In general, nutritional support increases the respiratory workload by increasing metabolic demand and ventilatory drive, but it seems that improvements in respiratory muscle and lung function also occur if nutrition is given over a longer period.

When hypertonic glucose is used as the sole source of nonprotein calories in TPN, a marked rise in CO_2 production occurs.[91,92] As substrates shift from fat oxidation to glucose oxidation, an increase in RQ occurs; if sufficient glucose is given, lipogenesis occurs, with a further rise in the level of CO_2 production.[93] This increase in CO_2 production, with its increase in ventilatory demand, can lead to respiratory distress in patients with impaired lung function. Substitution of fat emulsions for nonprotein calories lowers the RQ and reduces minute ventilation and ventilatory demand.[50] Thus, administration of the nonprotein calories as a mixture of fat and carbohydrate is important in patients with pulmonary disease.

A series of studies has demonstrated that amino acids stimulate ventilation.[94-96] Solutions that are high in the branched-chain amino acids seem to have a greater stimulatory effect than the standard amino acid solutions.[96] This would suggest that part of this phenomenon is an effect of amino acids on neurotransmission as precursors for neurotransmitter production. This will be discussed in more detail under ''Future Possibilities'' later in the chapter.

Cardiac Disease

Acute Effects of Nutrients. The effect of nutrition on myocardial protein synthesis and degradation is important in the postoperative period. During the immediate postoperative period the parenteral nutrients can alter the substrate supply (glucose, fat, lactate, etc) for myocardium.

Cardiac muscle is capable of using a wide variety of substrates as sources of energy.[97-99] Glucose and plasma-free fatty acids are the primary fuels but lactate, pyruvate, ketone bodies, triglycerides, and to a lesser extent amino acids, can all serve as sources of energy under varying conditions. Utilization of these substrates by the heart is a function of their plasma concentrations, availability of alternate competing substrates, mechanical activity of the heart, supply of oxygen, and plasma levels of certain hormones. Under normal circumstances, oxidative phosphorylation accounts for almost all of the ATP produced. In a well-oxygenated heart all substrates are completely oxidized in the citric acid cycle. The importance of fatty acids in myocardial metabolism is well known. Their oxidation normally accounts for 60 to 70% of oxidative metabolism, but may under some conditions account for as much as 100%.[100,101] Under most conditions free fatty acids are utilized in preference to carbohydrates. This is particularly true at high levels of cardiac work, where fatty acids are the main substrate utilized.[102,103] Although fatty acids appear to be the preferred fuel under most circumstances, glucose represents an important fuel for respiration in hypoxic hearts. Its metabolism through glycolysis is a major source of ATP in hypoxic tissue. The acceleration and alterations of substrate utilization under various conditions involves a complicated system of regulatory interactions in various metabolic pathways—the glucose fatty acid cycle.[97] This cycle controls substrate utilization and adjusts rates to match substrate supply with energy needs.

Experimental and clinical observations of infusion of free fatty acids during ischemia have demonstrated a depression of the contractile myocardial function and an increase in the frequency of serious rhythm disturbances[104–106] and in O_2 consumption.[107] Therefore the administration of fat emulsions in patients who presented ischemic symptoms during anesthesia should be made cautiously.

Experimental data have demonstrated a preservation of function and structure of hypoxic myocardium with increased perfusion of glucose.[108,109] With early infusion of GIK (glucose, insulin, potassium) during experimental acute coronary occlusion, the predicted size of the myocardial infarction was reduced.[110] In human studies GIK solutions have been found to stabilize ischemic myocardium[111]; to improve ventricular function[112]; to reduce the infarction size[113]; and to reduce hospital mortality in acute myocardial infarction.[114]

Nutrition in Cardiac Cachexia. The heart has often been considered to be protected from chronic protein–energy starvation. Undernutrition, however, also affects the myocardium, and nutritional support can prevent or partially reverse the heart disease associated with undernutrition. The undernourished state characteristic of severe heart disease is usually called *cardiac cachexia*.[115] There are two types of cardiac cachexia; (1) the "classic" type, which occurs in patients suffering from severe heart failure; and (2) the "nosocomial" type, which develops in the postoperative state when complications develop preventing a resumption of normal eating after surgery. One third of the patients with class III or IV heart disease have been found to suffer from cardiac cachexia.[116] A study has estimated that 1 out of every 15 patients in the surgical intensive care unit is suffering from nosocomial cardiac cachexia.[117] One half of the patients admitted with cardiac disease have been found to have clinically significant undernutrition as diagnosed by serum albumin and anthropometric measurements.[118]

In nosocomial cardiac cachexia the preoperative nutritional status is usually adequate. The cachexia develops in days or weeks postoperatively because of complications; intake is sharply reduced and nutrient losses are excessive. Frequently, the cachexia is clinically deceptive, since many patients will appear to be normally nourished according to standard assessment techniques, despite severe depletion of lean body tissue. If large amounts of carbohydrates but little or none of the other essential nutrients are infused, the glucose-induced insulin response prevents breakdown of adipose tissue without completely stopping lean tissue breakdown. Nutritional support is indicated when the underlying surgical complication cannot be corrected in three to five days.

Although some studies conclude that the undernutrition of cardiac cachexia can be at least partially corrected, the available reports about the beneficial effects of nutritional support on cardiac performance are incomplete and further controlled studies are needed to resolve these questions. Postoperative complications following cardiac surgery often lead to rapid depletion of lean body mass, and therefore nutritional therapy using nutrient solutions is indicated.

Acute Renal Failure

Most patients with acute renal failure (ARF) have some degree of net protein breakdown and disordered fluid, electrolyte, or acid–base status. There is often excess total body water, azotemia, hyperkalemia, hyperphosphatemia, hypocalcemia, hyperuricemia, and a large anion gap metabolic acidosis. The net protein degradation in ARF can be massive.[119] Patients are more likely to be catabolic when the ARF is caused by shock or sepsis. These patients quite frequently require surgery, which further increases protein breakdown. It is likely that the profound catabolic response of many patients with ARF may increase the risk of infection and delayed wound healing, prolong convalescence, and increase mortality. The net protein catabolism may accelerate the rate of rise in the plasma levels of potassium, phosphorus, nitrogenous metabolites, and acids.[120]

The aim of nutritional therapy in ARF is to reduce protein breakdown and to maintain protein stores. This goal should be accomplished without an increase in the production of uremic toxins—for example, without worsening azotemia. This can only be achieved by frequent hemodialysis. Ultimately, improved nutritional status in ARF patients should improve recovery, renal function, and survival.

Clinical studies performed in the 1960s suggested that amino acid therapy hastened recovery and lessened mortality in ARF.[121,122] Patients with ARF who received an essential amino acid solution and hypertonic glucose had an improved recovery of renal function but no significant improvement in overall hospital survival.[122] In a more recent study three treatment regimens were compared: hypertonic dextrose alone; dextrose in combination with essential amino acids; and dextrose in combination with essential and nonessential amino acids.[119] They found no improvement in the recovery of renal function or in patient survival among the three groups, and the patients in the amino acid groups did not show an improvement in nitrogen balance. Increasing the nitrogen intake of patients with ARF does not seem to improve nitrogen balance.[123] It has been suggested that a different formulation of amino acids might be required for patients with ARF. Histidine and tyrosine are considered as essential amino acids in this patient group and therefore they should be added to conventional essential amino acid solutions. It has also been suggested that ketoanalogues of BCAA may be beneficial in chronic renal failure patients, but so far the results from clinical studies remain contradictory.

In experimental ARF, amino acid solutions have been reported to increase the rapidity and severity of ARF and to increase the severity of postischemic ARF.[124,125] Lysine has recently been suggested to cause the nephrotoxic effects in rats,[126] but it is not known whether the lysine in standard amino acid solutions exerts a nephrotoxic effect in humans.

Adequate calorie intake in nonuremic patients is correlated with positive nitrogen balance and better outcome. Since the provision of adequate calories in many patients requires an infusion of 1 to 1.5 L of fluid daily, an increased frequency of dialysis may be needed if dealing with oligoanuric renal failure. Those patients undergoing dialysis usually tolerate standard amino acid solutions, but special attention should be given to monitoring fluid and electrolyte balance. Those who are nonoliguric and require less

or no dialysis tolerate standard amino acid formulations poorly, and administration of an essential amino acid formula with adequate amounts of carbohydrate may result in better utilization of endogenous urea by conversion to nonessential amino acids.[127]

FUTURE POSSIBILITIES

Respiratory depression is a common problem in the postanesthetic care of surgical patients. The reasons are many and are not the focus of this review. The pharmacological effects of BCAA may offer a new alternative for the prevention and treatment of some types of postanesthetic hypoventilation.

An alteration in plasma amino acids may play a role in neurotransmission and fatigue.[97] Tryptophan is a precursor of 5-hydroxytryptomine (5HT, serotonin), and the resulting decrease in brain serotonin activity may be responsible for the central effects observed with BCAA-enriched infusions on fatigue, ventilation, food intake, and gastric emptying. Elevated plasma BCAA levels may decrease the transport of tryptophan across the blood–brain barrier (BBB). In experimental animals, the brain serotonin content is related to the brain content of its precursor, tryptophan,[128] and tryptophan competes with other large neutral amino acids of the same transport system into the brain.[129] An increased rate of transport of tryptophan across the BBB increases the rate of synthesis of 5HT in the brain, thereby increasing the cerebral concentration of 5HT. There is evidence that an increase in this latter neurotransmitter can result in sleep; consequently it might also cause a decrease in mental alertness or cause fatigue, or both. In a recent study in healthy volunteers during sustained exercise, the plasma levels of BCAA decreased significantly while there was no change in total tryptophan.[130] The plasma concentration of free tryptophan was found to rise 2.4-fold during prolonged exercise (1.5 hours). This increase in probably due to pronounced elevation in the concentration of plasma-free fatty acids during exercise, since these are known to displace tryptophan from albumin. The observed increase in plasma tryptophan concentration, together with the decrease in plasma BCAA concentration, gives rise to a marked increase in the plasma concentration ratio of free tryptophan: BCAA. This should lead to an increase in the rate of transport of tryptophan across the BBB and hence to an increase in the rate of synthesis of 5HT in the brain. An elevated concentration of 5HT in specific areas of the brain may be responsible, at least in part, for the development of physical and/or mental fatigue during prolonged exercise.

Diaphragm muscle fatigue has been demonstrated in humans[131] and may be responsible for some of the symptoms experienced by patients with respiratory diseases,[132] especially upon exertion.[133] Diaphragmatic fatigue refers to the inability of the muscle to maintain an expected force with continued or repeated contraction.[134] Studies have also demonstrated that there is an increased incidence of ventilatory fatigue under conditions of undernutrition.[135]

Increasing the amino acid content of total parenteral nutrition increases the ventilatory demand by increasing both oxygen consumption and ventilatory drive.[95] The study of Takala and associates,[96] where an 85% BCAA solution was compared to standard amino acid solution, showed that not only the quantity of amino acids but also the composition of the amino acid solution affects the ventilatory response. There was a major increase in the ventilatory response to CO_2 inhalation during administration of the BCAA solution but not the standard solution. Serotonin and its precursors depress both resting ventilation and the ventilatory responses to CO_2 in experimental animals, evidently via serotoninergic activation in the brain.[136,137] If the same is true for human beings, an increase in the plasma ratio of the large neutral amino acids to tryptophan may well contribute to increasing respiratory drive during the high BCAA supply. The accentuation of the respiratory effects of amino acids by BCAA may have important clinical relevance. Increasing respiratory drive will further increase the work of breathing and make fatigue of respiratory muscles more likely to ensue. On the other hand, recovery of normal ventilatory responsiveness may be enhanced in patients with decreased ventilatory drive due to anesthesia, medication, surgery, prolonged administration of 5% dextrose, or apneas due to different origins. The combined effect of decreasing central fatigue in respiratory muscles and increasing ventilatory drive may prove to be beneficial in postoperative patients. However, no clinical data are yet available and therefore no proposals for their clinical use can be made.

REFERENCES

1. Bistrian BR, Blackburn GL, Hallowell E, et al: Protein status of general surgical patients. *JAMA*, 1974; 230:858–860.
2. Bistrian BR, Blackburn GL, Vitale J, et al: Prevalence of malnutrition in general medical patients. *JAMA* 1976;235:1567–1570.
3. Mullen JL: Consequences of malnutrition in the surgical patient. *Surg Clin North Am* 1981;61:465–487.
4. Mullen JL, Gertner MH, Buzby GP, et al: Implications of malnutrition in surgical patients. *Arch Surg* 1979; 114:121–125.
5. Buzby GP, Mullen JL, Matthews DC, et al: Prognostic nutritional index in gastrointestinal surgery. *Am J Surg* 1980;139:160–167.
6. Studley HO: Percentage of weight loss, a basic indicator of surgical risk in patients with chronic peptic ulcer. *JAMA* 1936;106:458–460.
7. Tweedie FJ, Long RC: Abdominal wound disruption. *Surg Gynecol Obstetr* 1954;99:41–47.
8. Efron G: Abdominal wound disruption. *Lancet* 1965; 1:1287–1290.
9. Rhoads JE, Alexander CE: Nutritional problems of surgical patients. *Ann NY Acad Sci* 1955;63:268–275.
10. Cannon PR, Wissler RW, Woolridge RL, et al: The relationship of protein deficiency to surgical infection. *Ann Surg* 1944;120:514–525.
11. Mecray PM, Barden RP, Raudin IS: Nutritional edema: Its effect on the gastric emptying time before and after gastric operation. *Surgery* 1937;1:53–64.
12. Askanazi J, Hensle TW, Starker PM, et al: Effect of immediate postoperative nutritional support on length of hospitalization. *Ann Surg* 1986;203:236–239.
13. Young GA, Collins JP, Hill GL: Plasma proteins in patients receiving intravenous amino acids or intravenous hyperalimentation after major surgery. *Am J Clin Nutr* 1979;32:1192.
14. Young GA, Hill GL: A controlled study of protein sparing therapy after excision of the rectum. *Ann Surg* 1980;192:183.
15. Collins JP, Oxby CB, Hill GL: Intravenous amino acids and intravenous hyperalimentation as protein sparing therapy after major surgery. A controlled clinical trial. *Lancet* 1978;1:788.
16. Kinney JM, Long CL, Gump FE, et al: Tissue composition of weight loss in surgical patients. *Ann Surg* 1968;168:459–474.
17. Ariel IM, Kremen AJ: Compartmental distribution of sodium chloride in surgical patients pre- and post-operatively. *Ann Surg* 1950;132:1009–1026.
18. Elwyn DH, Bryan-Brown CW, Shoemaker WC: Nutritional aspects of body water dislocations in postoperative and depleted patients. *Ann Surg* 1975;182:76–85.
19. Insel J, Elwyn DH: Body composition, in Askanazi J, Starker P, Weissman C (eds): *Fluid and Electrolyte Management in Critical Care*. Stoneham, MA, Butterworths, 1986, pp 3–31.
20. Viteri F, Behar M, Arroyave G, Scrimshaw NS: Clinical aspects of protein malnutrition, in Munro HN, Allison JB (eds): *Mammalian Protein Metabolism*. New York, Academic Press, 1969, pp 325–390.
21. Gamble JL: Physiological information gained from studies on the life raft ration. *Harvery Lect 1946–1947*;42:247–273.
22. Schutz Y, Acheson K, Bessard T, Jequier E: Effects of a 7-day carbohydrate hyperalimentation on energy metabolism in healthy individuals. *JPEN* 1982; 6:351(abstr).
23. Keys A, Brozek J, Henschel H, et al: *The Biology of Human Starvation*. Minneapolis, University of Minnesota Press, 1950.
24. Abrams JS, Deane RS, Davis HJ: Adverse effects of salt and water retention on pulmonary functions in

patients with multiple trauma. *J Trauma* 1973;13:788–798.

25. Kudsk KA, Sheldon GF: Nutritional assessment, in Fisher JE (ed): *Surgical Nutrition*. Boston, Little, Brown, 1983, pp 407–420.

26. Mullen JL, Buzby, GP, Waldman MT, et al: Prediction of greater morbidity and mortality by preoperative nutritional assessment. *Surg Forum* 1979;30:80–82.

27. Linn BS: A protein energy malnutrition scale (PEMS). *Ann Surg* 1984;200:747–752.

28. Baker JP, Detsky AS, Wesson DE, et al: Nutritional assessment. A comparison of clinical judgment and objective measurements. *N Engl J Med* 1982;306:969–972.

29. Cuthbertson DP: Post-shock metabolic response. *Lancet* 1942;1:433–437.

30. Cuthbertson DP, Tilstone WJ: Metabolism during the post injury period. *Adv Clin Chem* 1969;12:1–55.

31. Kinney JM, Duke JH Jr, Long CL, et al: Tissue fuel and weight loss after injury. *J Clin Pathol* 1970;4(suppl 23):65–72.

32. Long CL, Spencer JL, Kinney JM, et al: Carbohydrate metabolism in man: Effect of elective operations and major surgery. *J Appl Physiol* 1971;31:110–116.

33. Chen RW, Postlethwart RW: The biochemistry of wound healing. *Monogr Surg Sci* 1964;1:215–276.

34. Copeland EM, MacFayden BV, Lanzotti VF: Intravenous hyperalimentation as an adjunct to cancer therapy. *Am J Surg* 1975;129:167–173.

35. Dematteis R, Herman RE: Supplementary parenteral nutrition in patients with malignant disease. *Cleveland Clin* 1973;40:139–145.

36. Blackburn GL, Bistrian BR, Miani BS, et al: Nutritional and metabolic assessment of the hospitalized patient. *JPEN* 1977;1:11–22.

37. Calloway DH, Spector H: Nitrogen balance as related to calorie and protein intake in active young men. *Am J Clin Nutr* 1954;2:405–412.

38. Wolfe BM, Culebras JM, Sim AJ, et al: Substrate interaction in intravenous feeding. Comparative effects of carbohydrate and fat on amino acid utilization in fasting man. *Ann Surg* 1977;186:518–540.

39. Cutbertson DP, McCutcheon A, Munro HN: A study of the effect of overfeeding on the protein metabolism of man. *Biochem J* 1937;31:681–693.

40. Calloway DH: Nitrogen balance of men with marginal intakes of protein and energy. *J Nutr* 1975;105:914–923.

41. Keys A, Anderson JT, Brozek J: Weight gain from single overeating. Character of tissue gained. *Metabolism* 1955;4:427–432.

42. Cathcart ED: The influence of carbohydrates and fats on protein metabolism. *J Physiol (Lond)* 1909;39:311–330.

43. Werner SC, Habif DV, Randall HT, et al: Postoperative nitrogen loss; comparison of effects of trauma and of caloric readjustment. *Ann Surg* 1949;130:668–702.

44. Munro HN: General aspects of the regulation of protein metabolism by diet and by hormones. In Munro HN, Allison JB (eds): *Mammalian Protein Metabolism*. New York, Academic Press, 1964, vol 1, pp 381–481.

45. Brennan MF, Fitzpatrick GF, Cohen KH, et al: Glycerol: Major contributor to the short term protein sparing effect of fat emulsions in normal man. *Ann Surg* 1975;182:386–394.

46. Long JM III, Wilmore DW, Mason AD Jr, et al: Effect of carbohydrate and fat intake on nitrogen excretion during total intravenous feeding. *Ann Surg* 1977;185:417–422.

47. Nordenstrøm J, Askanazi J, Elwyn DH, et al: Nitrogen balance during total parenteral nutrition: Glucose vs fat. *Ann Surg* 1983;197:27–33.

48. MacFie J, Smith RC, Hill GL: Glucose or fat as a non-protein energy source. *Gastroenterology* 1981;80:103–107.

49. Nordenstrøm J, Jeevanandam M, Elwyn DH, et al: Increasing glucose intake during total parenteral nutrition increases norepinephrine excretion in trauma and sepsis. *Clin Physiol* 1981;1:525–534.

50. Askanazi J, Nordenstrøm J, Rosenbaum SH, et al: Nutrition for the patient with respiratory failure: Glucose vs fat. *Anesthesiology* 1981;54:373–377.

51. Meguid MM, Akahoshi M, Jeffers S, et al: Amelioration of metabolic complications of conventional TPN: A prospective randomized study. *Arch Surg* 1984;119:1294–1298.

52. Liaw KY, Askanazi J, Michelson CB, et al: Effect of postoperative nutrition on muscle high energy phosphates. *Ann Surg* 1982;195:12–18.

53. Sakamoto A, Moldawer LL, Usui S, et al: In vivo evidence for the unique nitrogen-sparing mechanism of branched-chain amino acid administration. *Surg Forum* 1979;30:67–69.

54. Odessey RK, Khairallah EA, Goldberg AL: Origin and possible significance of alanine production by skeletal muscle. *J Biol Chem* 1974;249:7623–7629.

55. Blackburn GL, Moldawer LL, Usui S, et al: Branched chain amino acid concentrations and metabolism during starvation, injury, and infection. *Surgery* 1979;86:307–315.

56. Freund HR, Yoshimura N, Fischer JE: The effect of branched chain amino acids and hypertonic glucose infusions on post injury catabolism in the rat. *Surgery* 1980;87:401–408.

57. Blackburn GL, Desai SP, Keenan RA, et al: Clinical use of branched chain amino-acid enriched solutions in the stressed and injured patient. In Walser M, Williamson JR (eds): *Metabolism and Clinical Implications of Branched Chain Amino and Ketoacids*. New York, Elsevier, 1981, p 521.

58. Van Way CW, Moore EE, Allo M, et al: Comparison of total parenteral nutrition with 25 percent and 45 percent branched chain amino acids in stressed patients. *Ann Surg* 1985;51:609.

59. Wounde PV, Morgan RE, Kosta JM: Addition of branched-chain amino acids to parenteral nutrition of stressed critically ill patients. *Crit Care Med* 1986;14:685–688.

60. Daly JM, Mihranian MH, Vehoe JE, et al: Effects of post operative infusion of branched chain amino acids on nitrogen balance and forearm muscle substrate flux. *Surgery* 1983;94:151–158.

61. Knochel JP: Hypophosphatemia. *West J Med* 1981;125: 15–19.

62. Blackburn GL, Flatt JP, Glowes GNA, et al: Peripheral intravenous feeding with isotonic amino acid solutions. *Am J Surg* 1973;125:447–454.

63. Elwyn DH, Gump FE, Iles M, et al: Protein and energy sparing of glucose added in hypocaloric amounts to peripheral infusions of amino acids. *Metabolism* 1978;27:325–331.

64. Lev-Ran A, Johnsson M, Hwang DL, et al. Double-blind study of glycerol vs glucose in parenteral nutrition of postsurgical insulin-treated diabetic patients. *JPEN* 1987;11:271–274.

65. Trissel LA. *Handbook of Injectable Drugs*, 2nd ed. Bethesda, MD, Am Soc Hosp Pharm, 1980, p 583.

66. Ahnefeldt EW, Bassler KH, Bauer BL, et al. Suitability of non-glucose carbohydrates for parenteral nutrition. *Eur J Intensive Care Med* 1975;1:105.

67. Thomas DW. Complications following intravenous administration of solutions containing xylitol. *Med J Aust* 1972;1:1238.

68. Tao RC. Glycerol: its metabolism and use as an intravenous energy source. *JPEN* 1983;7:4779.

69. Miani B, Blackburn GL, Bistrian BR, et al: Cyclic hyperalimentation: An optimal technique for preservation of visceral protein. *J Surg Res* 1976;20:515–525.

70. Parsa MH, Habif DV, Ferrer JM, et al: Intravenous hyperalimentation: indications, technique and complications. *Bull NY Acad Med* 1972;48:920–942.

71. Wolfe BM, Ryder MA, Nishikawa RA, et al: Complications of parenteral nutrition. *Am J Surg* 1986;152:93–99.

72. Maki DG, Goldman DA, Rhame FS: Infection control in intravenous therapy. *Ann Intern Med* 1973;79:867.

73. James JH, Freund H, Fischer JE: Amino acids in hepatic encephalopathy. *Gastroenterology* 1979;77:421–423.

74. Rosen HM, Yoshimura N, Hodgman JM, et al: Plasma amino acid patterns in hepatic encephalopathy of differing etiology. *Gastroenterology* 1977;72:483–487.

75. Cangiano C, Cascino A, Fiaccadori F, et al: Is the blood-brain barrier really intact in portal-systemic encephalopathy? *Lancet* 1981;20:1:1367.

76. James JH, Escourrou J, Fischer JE: Blood-brain neutral amino acid transport activity is increased after portacaval anastomosis. *Science* 1978;200:1395–1397.

77. Shaw W, Lieber CS: Plasma amino acid abnormalities in the alcoholic: respective role of alcohol, nutrition, and liver injury. *Gastroenterology* 1978;74:677–682.

78. Fischer JE, Rosen HM, Ebeid AM, et al: The effect of normalization of plasma amino acids on hepatic encephalopathy in man. *Surgery* 1976;80:77–91.

79. Cardelli-Cangiano P, Cangiano C, James JH, et al: Uptake of amino acids by brain microvessels isolated from rats after portocaval anastomosis. *J Neurochem* 1981;36:627–632.

80. Michel H, Pomier-Layrargues G, Duhamel O, et al: Intravenous infusion of ordinary and modified amino acid solutions in the management of hepatic encephalopathy (controlled study of 30 patients). *Gastroenterology* 1979;79:1038–1042(abstr).

81. Rossi-Fanelli F, Riggio O, Cangiano C, et al: Branched-chain amino acids vs lactulose in the treatment of hepatic coma. A controlled study. *Dig Dis Sci* 1982;27:929–935.

82. Gluud C, Dejgaard A, Hardt F, et al: Preliminary treatment results with balanced amino acid infusion to patients with hepatic encephalopathy, abstracted. *Scan J Gastroenterol* 1983;18 (suppl 86):19.

83. Wahren JJ, Denis J, Desurmont P, et al: Is intravenous administration of branched chain amino acids effective in treatment of hepatic encephalopathy? A multicenter study. *Hepatology* 1983;3:475–480.

84. Fiaccadori F, Ghinelli F, Pedretti G, et al: Branched chain amino acid enriched solutions in the treatment of encephalopathy: A controlled study. In Capocaccia L, Fischer JE, Ross-Fanelli F (eds): *Hepatic Encephalopathy in Chronic Liver Failure*. New York, Plenum, 1984; pp 311–321.

85. Cerra FB, Cheung NK, Fischer JE, et al: Disease-specific amino acid infusion (F080) in hepatic encephalopathy: A prospective, randomized, double-blind, controlled trial. *JPEN* 1985;9:288–295.

86. Michel H, Bories P, Aubin JP, et al: Treatment of acute hepatic encephalopathy in cirrhotics with a branched-chain amino acids enriched versus a conventional amino acids mixture. *Liver* 1985;5:282–289.

87. Sherwin R, Joshi P, Hendler R, et al: Hyperglucagonemia in Laennec's cirrhosis. The role of portal-systemic shunting. *N Engl J Med* 1974;290:239–242.

88. Striebel JP, Holm E, Lutz H, et al: Parenteral nutrition and coma therapy with amino acids in hepatic failure. *J Parent Ent Nutr* 1979;3:240–246.

89. Soeters PB, Fisher JE: Insulin, glucagon, amino acid imbalance, and hepatic encephalopathy. *Lancet* 1976;2:880–882.

90. Fischer JE: Current concepts of pathogenesis of hepatic encephalopathy. In Preisig R, Bircher J (eds): *The Liver*. Bern, Edito Cantor Aulendorf, 1979; pp 374–385.

91. Askanazi J, Carpentier YA, Elwyn DH, et al: Influence of total parenteral nutrition on fuel utilization in injury and sepsis. *Ann Surg* 1980;194:40–46.

92. Askanazi J, Rosenbaum SH, Hyman AL, et al: Respiratory changes induced by the large glucose loads of total parenteral nutrition. *JAMA* 1980;243:1444–1447.

93. Askanazi J, Elwyn DH, Silverberg PA, et al: Respiratory distress secondary to a high carbohydrate load: A case report. *Surgery* 1980;87:596–598.

94. Weissman C, Askanazi J, Rosenbaum SH, et al: Amino acids and respiration. *Ann Intern Med* 1983;98:41–44.

95. Askanazi J, Weissman C, LaSala P, et al: Effect of protein on ventilatory drive. *Anesthesiology* 1984;60:106–110.

96. Takala J, Askanazi J, Weissman C, et al: Changes in respiratory control induced by amino acid infusions. *Crit Care Med* 1988;16:465–469.

97. Newsholme EA, Leech AR: *Biochemistry for the Medical Sciences*. New York, John Wiley and Sons, 1983.

98. McGinty DA. Blood lactic acid and coronary circulation. *Proc Soc Exper Biol and Med* 1931;28:451–453.

99. Bing RJ. Myocardial metabolism. *Circulation* 1956; 12:635–47.

100. Miller HI, Yum KY, Durham BX. Myocardial free fatty acid in unanesthetized dogs at rest and during exercise. *Amer J Physiol* 1971;220:589–596.

101. Most AS, Brachfeld N, Gorlin R, et al: Free fatty acid metabolism of the human heart at rest. *J Clin Invest* 1969;48:1177–1188.

102. Neely JR, Bowman RH, Morgan HE. Effects of ventricular pressure development and palmitate on glucose transport. *Amer J Physiol* 1969;216:804–811.

103. Crass MF 3rd, McCaskill ES, Shipp JC. Effect of pressure development on glucose and palmitate metabolism in perfused heart. *Amer J Physiol* 1969;216:1569–1576.

104. Henderson AH, Most AS, Parmley WW, et al: Depression of myocardial contractility in rats by free fatty acids during hypoxic periods. *Circ Res* 1970;26:439–449.

105. Kjekshus JK, Mjos OD. Effect of free fatty acids on myocardial function and metabolism in the ischemic dog heart. *J Clin Invest* 1972;51:1767–1776.

106. Oliver MF, Kurien VA, Greenwood TW. Relation between serum free-fatty-acids and arrhythmias and death after acute myocardial infarction. *Lancet* 1968;1:704–710.

107. Oram JF, Bennetch SL, Neely JR: Regulation of fatty acid utilization in isolated rat hearts. *J Biol Chem* 1973;248:5299–5309.

108. Rogers WJ, Russell RO Jr, McDaniel HG, et al: Acute effects of glucose-insulin-potassium infusion on myocardial substrates, coronary blood flow and oxygen consumption in man. *Am J Cardiol* 1977;40:421–428.

109. Ahmed SS, Lee CH, Oldwurtel AH, et al: Sustained effect of glucose-insulin-potassium on myocardial performance during regional ischemia. *J Clin Invest* 1978;61:1123–1135.

110. Opie LH, Bruyneel K, Owen P: Effects of glucose, insulin and potassium infusion on tissue metabolic changes within first hour of myocardial infarction in the baboon. *Circulation* 1975;52:49–57.

111. Rackley CE, Russell RO Jr, Rogers WJ, et al: Morcardial metabolism in coronary artery disease. In CI Rackley, RO Russell Jr, (eds): *Coronary Artery Disease: Recognition of Management.* Mt. Kisco, NY, Futura, 1979, pp. 261–298.

112. Gwata T, Edwards IR: Glucose, insulin, potassium (GIK) in the treatment of congestive cardiomyopathy. *Cent Afr J Med* 1980;26:249–250.

113. Whitlow PL, Rogers WJ, Smith LR, et al: Enhancement of left ventricular function by glucose-insulin-potassium infusion in acute myocardial infarction. *Am J Cardiol* 1982;49:811–820.

114. Rogers WJ, Stanley AW, Breinig JB, et al: Reduction of hospital mortality rate of acute myocardial infarction with glucose-insulin-potassium infusion. *J Am Heart* 1976;92:441–454.

115. Pittman JG, Cohen P: The pathogenesis of cardiac cachexia. *N Eng J Med* 1964;271:403–409.

116. Heymsfield SB, Bleier J, Wenger N: Detection of protein-calorie undernutrition in advanced heart disease. *Circulation* (suppl III) 1977;56:102.

117. Abel RM: Parenteral nutrition for patients with severe cardiac illness. In Greep JM, Soeters PB, Wesdorp RIC, et al (eds): *Current Concepts in Parenteral Nutrition.* The Hague, Martinus Hijnoff Med Div, 1977, pp 147–158.

118. Blackburn GL, Gibbons GW, Bothe A, et al: Nutritional support in cardiac cachexia. *J Thoracic Cardiovasc Surg* 1977;73:480–496.

119. Feinstein EI, Blumenkrantz MJ, Healy H, et al: Clinical and metabolic responses to parenteral nutrition in acute renal failure. A controlled double-blind study. *Medicine* 1981;60:124–137.

120. Kopple JD: Altered metabolic and nutritional status in acute renal failure. American Society for Parenteral and Enteral Nutrition, Eleventh Clinical Congress, New Orleans, 1987; pp 27–30.

121. Abel RM, Beck Jr CH, Abbott WM, et al: Improved survival from acute renal failure after treatment with intravenous essential amino acids and glucose. Results of a prospective double-blind study. *New Engl J Med* 1973;288:685–699.

122. Toback FG: Amino acid enhancement of renal regeneration after acute tubular necrosis. *Kidney Int* 1977; 12:193.

123. Feinstein EI, Kopple J, Silberman H, et al: Total parenteral nutrition with high or low nitrogen intakes in patients with acute renal failure. *Kidney Int* 1983;26:S-323.

124. Solez K, Stout R, Bendush B, et al: Adverse effect of amino acid solutions in amino glycoside-induced renal failure in rabbits and rats. In Eliahou H (ed): *Acute Renal Failure,* Libbey, London, 1982, pp 241–247.

125. Zager RA, Venkatachalam MA: Potentiation of ischemic renal injury by amino acid infusion. *Kidney Int* 1983;24:620.

126. Racusen LC, Whelton A, Solez K: Effects of lysine and other amino acids on kidney structure and function in the rat. *Am J Pathol* 1985;120:436–442.

128. Abel RM, Shih VE, Abbot WM, et al: Amino acid metabolism in acute renal failure. *Ann Surg* 1974;180:350–356.

128. Fernstrom JD, Wurtman RJ: Brain serotonin content: Physiologic dependence on plasma tryptophan levels. *Science* 1971;173:149–152.

129. Fernstrom JD, Larin F, Wurtman RJ: Correlations between brain tryptophan and plasma neutral amino acid levels following food consumption in rats. *Life Sci* 1973;13:517–524.

130. Blomstrand E, Celsing F, Newsholme EA: Changes in plasma concentrations of aromatic and branched chain amino acids during sustained exercise in man and their possible role in fatigue. *Acta Physiol Scand* 1988;133:115–121.

131. Juan GP, Calverley C, Talamo J, et al: Effect of carbon dioxide on diaphragmatic function in human beings. *N Engl J Med* 1984;310:874–879.

132. Aldrich TK, Arora NS, Rochester DF: The influence of airway obstruction and maximal voluntary ventilation

in lung disease. *Am Rev Respir Dis* 1982;126:195–199.

133. Aldrich TK, Adams JM, Arora NS, et al. Power spectral analysis of the diaphragm electromyogram. *J Appl Physiol* 1983;54:1579–1584.

134. Roussos C, Moxham J. Respiratory muscle fatigue. In Roussos C and Maklem PT (eds): *The Thorax.* New York, Marcel Dekker, 1985, pp 829–870.

135. Arora NS, Rochester DF. Respiratory muscle strength and maximal voluntary ventilation in undernourished patients. *Am Rev Respir Dis* 1982;126:5–8.

136. Armijo JA, Florez J: The influence of increased brain 5-hydroxytryptamine upon the respiratory activity of cats. *Neuropharmacology* 1974;13:977–986.

137. Lunberg DB, Mueller RA, Breese GR: An evaluation of the mechanism by which serotonergic activation depresses respiration. *J Pharmacol Exp Ther* 1980;212:397–404.

9 | Medicolegal Considerations

Thomas J. DeKornfeld

The postanesthetic recovery period may be the most dangerous time of the entire hospital stay.

The preexisting pathology, the stress of anesthesia and surgery, the shifts in fluids and electrolytes, and the drugs used in anesthesiology, all conspire to make the immediate postanesthetic period a challenge to both the patient and to the health care providers. The problems are further compounded in many recovery rooms by divided lines of authority, acute and chronic staffing problems, and a general applicability of Murphy's law.

In theory the postanesthetic care unit (PACU) should be under the overall management of the anesthesia care team. In fact both anesthesiologists and surgeons feel that they have a proprietary right to the patients in the PACU. In many hospitals neither surgeons nor anesthesiologists are present or immediately available in the unit and hence the patient is truly dependent on the PACU nursing staff, who may or may not be adequately trained to assume this responsibility. This can lead to very serious problems, since the complications that are likely to appear in the immediate postanesthetic period are rarely trivial, usually serious, and not infrequently life-threatening.

While the principles largely remain the same, there is a substantial difference in the conditions that prevail in a PACU dedicated to this single activity and an intensive care unit, serving as a recovery area for some patients in all hospitals and for all patients in some hospitals.

The subjects that will be discussed in this chapter include the legal theories of negligence, the problems of legal responsibility, the ethical and legal issues of the ''do not resuscitate'' order, withholding and withdrawing life support, the right to die and, lastly, a few simple techniques that can significantly reduce the likelihood of a malpractice suit and simultaneously increase the likelihood of a successful outcome should a suit be filed.

THE LEGAL THEORIES OF MALPRACTICE

Medical ''malpractice'' is generally a civil offense, known as a tortuous act. It is rarely of a criminal nature and is almost always tried on the legal theory of negligence under the general rules of tort.

In order for negligence to be found, four criteria must be met:

1. There has to be a physician–patient relationship—that is, there has to be a duty.
2. There has to be a breach of that duty—that is, the physician must perform below the prevailing standards of care.
3. There have to be damages—that is, the patient must be harmed in some fashion.
4. The damages must be the proximate result of the breach of the standard or care—that is, there must be a causal relationship between the physician's substandard care and the patient's injury.

The physician–patient relationship is practically never an issue in anesthesiology. If the anesthesiologist assumes the responsibility for any part of the anesthetic management, this relationship is established and remains in effect until (1) the need for anesthesia services is terminated; (2) the patient is turned over to another health care provider, competent and willing to assume this responsibility; or (3) the patient dies.

The second item, the breach of the standards of care, is much more difficult to define and to evaluate. Standards are practically never written down and are thus subject to individual interpretation and dispute. Generally, in law, the standards are defined as the behavior (level of competence) that can be expected from a prudent anesthesiologist under the same or similar circumstances. Since a jury of laypersons can not be expected to know what this level of care may be, it usually depends on an expert to explain to the jury what the applicable standards are and in what way the anesthesiologist deviated from these standards. The expert need not be local, but should have a reasonable familiarity with the type of practice and type of location where the alleged negligence has taken place. It is now well accepted in law, that specialists are being held to national standards and all anesthesiologists must perform at the same level of competence regardless of location, type of hospital, geographic region, and so on.

It is possible to have local standards, but only if these are more stringent than the national ones. It is for this reason that policies for an institution or for a PACU must be written very carefully. The policies accepted by the medical staff organization become the standards for the hospital, and if they are breached it will not serve as an excuse that they were more demanding than the national standards. It is also well to remember that the standards change over time. Once the national professional organization publishes "recommendations" or "advisories," these become the standard in spite of the disclaimer made by the national organization. Similarly, once a certain new drug, procedure, or technique receives fairly wide publicity in the appropriate medical literature, in the form of either recommendation or condemnation, using it (or not using it) becomes the standard. When the magic moment arrives that the new technique becomes the standard depends on a variety of factors. These include availability, cost–benefit ratios, potential complications, and other features. A standard does not really become a standard until a jury decides that it is the standard in a contested case in court.

The requirement for damages is also relatively simple to meet. In most cases they are obvious and do not even require an expert to explain them to the jury. The noneconomic damages—such as pain and suffering, loss of consortium, and loss of parental guidance or filial love—are much more difficult to determine and to translate into dollars and cents.

Proximate causation is also usually easy to establish. There are a number of situations, however, where it is very difficult to determine a causal relationship and where a post hoc, propter hoc, that is "event A occurred after event B and therefore A was the cause of B", argument of the plaintiff may be very difficult indeed to counter by the defendant. The "bad baby" cases are a good example for this point. There is very little scientific evidence for the relationship of fetal distress, time, and the presence of certain central nervous system (CNS) deficits found in the newborn. Yet juries will consistently find for the plaintiff if it can be shown that there was fetal distress and that there was a delay in delivering the distressed fetus.

There are several exceptions to the general principles discussed above. Some malpractice cases are tried under the "Res Ipsa Loquitur" doctrine. This translates into "the case speaks for itself"—that is, the facts of the matter are so obvious that the lay jury does not need an expert to explain them. In Res Ipsa cases the assumption is made that the damages could not have happened in the absence of negligence and thus the burden of proof shifts to the defendant. It is the defendant who has to prove that he or she was not negligent. The classic cases are the sponge or instrument left in the abdomen, the procedure done on the wrong patient, or the wrong medication or the wrong dose given to the patient. Courts generally do not like Res Ipsa cases, since they do appear to be contrary to the traditional basis of Anglo-Saxon jurisprudence, according to which the defendant is innocent until proven guilty. In some states, such as Michigan, Res Ipsa, as such, cannot be pled at all.

Other areas that are generally subsumed under "malpractice," but which do not fall under the theory of negligence, include abandonment, assault and battery, invasion of privacy, breach of confidentiality, breach of promise, fraud, and intentional torts. The first four are of considerable importance in the postanesthesia period and deserve a more thorough discussion.

Abandonment is defined as the unilateral severance of a professional relationship without adequate notice and while there was still a need for continuing professional service.

In a PACU context a nurse who does not adequately monitor a patient may be said to have abandoned the patient, and an anesthesiologist who becomes unavailable by virtue of the hour of the day or the demands of the remainder of the surgical schedule may also have "abandoned" the patient, if it can be shown that the patient continued to require medical services that could not be provided by a nurse.

Assault and battery simply mean anything done to the patient without the patient's consent. A person's body is held inviolate in law and any touching thereof is considered unlawful unless it is done with the person's knowledge and approval. This being the case, the patient's consent must be obtained before anything is done to the patient. Ordinarily, the preanesthetic consent should cover the immediate postanesthetic period, provided that nothing unexpected happens, in which case consent must be obtained all over again. In order for consent to be legally correct, three conditions must be met: the consent must be (1) valid; (2) free; and (3) informed.

For the consent to be valid it must be given by the patient, provided that the patient is of legal age and legally competent to do so. Legal age varies, but in most jurisdictions it is 18 to 19 years of age. Being of sound mind is more difficult to define and it is usually defined in a negative way. A patient is of sound mind unless he or she has been declared to be of unsound mind by a court. This becomes important since some patients behave in a very bizarre way and would certainly be considered to be of unsound mind by the ordinary person. Yet, in law, such a person should be regarded as competent and his or her wishes should be respected. The patient obviously may be incompetent when unconscious or when under the influence of psychoactive drugs, such as anesthetics, hypnotics, centrally acting analgetics, or alcohol. In such a case *and* in the presence of a life-threatening situation the physician may proceed without the patient's consent. It is general practice to get "consent" under such circumstances from the patient's next of kin. This may be good public relations but is legally meaningless, since no persons, even a relative, can "consent" for another adult in the absence of specific authority granted by a court. There are a few exceptions to this rule. In Michigan a legal spouse can give consent for a temporarily incapacitated spouse, but this is not the case in most jurisdictions. In an emergency situation the health care provider has the right to proceed to do whatever is deemed to be in the best interest of the patient. The assumption is that any reasonably prudent person would have consented, had they had the opportunity to do so.

In the case of minors, only a parent or legal guardian can give consent. Any person under legal age is considered to be a minor, except for those who have been legally declared to be of age, are members of the armed forces, are self-supporting and living away from the parental home, are married, or are exempted by statute. The last of these usually applies to problems in the realm of reproduction and sexually acquired diseases.

The freedom of consent is usually not an issue in anesthesiology. This area is important in experimental medicine and has little relevance in clinical practice, unless the patient is also asked to serve as an experimental subject in a clinical study. In this situation it is important that the patients clearly understand that they have the absolute right to refuse to participate in the study and that such refusal will in no way effect the quality of care that they will receive.

The most difficult area of consent is the one dealing with being "informed." No layperson, and even some health care providers, can possibly comprehend all the possible complications of even a relatively very simple procedure in anesthesiology. Fortunately it is not required that the patient be given *all* possible complications. Courts have consistently held in such situations that the information that must be given to the patient has to include only those matters that may reasonably influence the patient's decision to proceed with the proposed procedure. In other words the patient must be given an opportunity to know what is planned, why it is planned, what the likely outcome is going to be, and what may be expected in the way of major complications. Any procedure that may result in sterility or disfigurement, or that may permanently affect the quality of life, must

be explained in considerable detail. Alternative treatment modalities must be offered and the patient must be given a full opportunity to ask questions. Under no circumstance should the patient be intentionally misled. It is legally not necessary for the patient to sign a consent form. The form is a hospital requirement and only shows that the patient has had a discussion on consent. It does not guarantee that the patient in fact gave informed consent. There are few cases in which the informedness of the consent played a significant role. The burden of proof is on the patient to satisfy the jury that the consent would have been withheld, had the patient known about the complication that did happen and the likelihood of it happening.

The patient must also be informed of the risks of refusing a procedure.

Doing anything to the patient without consent is technical assault, and this includes such things as incidental appendectomies, going beyond the proposed procedure, or doing a different procedure than the one the patient consented to.

Invasion of privacy is common in the postanesthetic period, but fortunately is only very rarely the subject of litigation. Exposing a patient's body to view by other persons is an invasion of privacy and should be avoided whenever possible. In the average PACU the patients are not separated from each other by more than a few feet of space. There are curtains available, but they are rarely used. Attending personnel also tend to forget that not all patients in the unit are recovering from general anesthesia. Some patients, after regional anesthesia, are wide awake and can observe what is going on in the entire unit. The health care providers in the unit must be sensitive to this issue and protect each patient's privacy as much as is consistent with safe and efficient care.

A special area of privacy is the taking of unauthorized photographs. Plastic and ENT surgeons are the most common offenders. The fact that the patient cannot be identified on the photograph is not a valid excuse for taking an unauthorized photograph and thus invading the patient's privacy. Consent must be obtained from the patient and the patient must be told how the photograph is going to be used.

Confidentiality is another area that is regularly breached in all health care facilities. All of us have been guilty of relating an "interesting case" or a "funny thing" that happened in the hospital to colleagues, friends, and members of our own family. Even if it is done with the best intentions, and even if no names are mentioned, it is still a breach of the confidential relationship that exists between the patient and the health care provider. Especially in a teaching context all efforts must be made to maintain the anonymity of the patient. There is no excuse for discussing a patient's problems with any person who does not "need to know" as part of his or her responsibilities for the patient's care. Even the patient's family is not "entitled" to know and there are certain conditions that the patient may not wish to have divulged to a spouse, parent, or child.

Breach of contract is a rare and totally avoidable legal dilemma in medicine. All of us have been guilty of telling a patient: "Don't worry, everything is going to be all right." Technically this is a contractual guarantee for which the patient may hold us legally accountable if "everything is not all right." Plastic surgeons have been particularly vulnerable in this context and indeed have been sued successfully under this theory. What makes this matter even more interesting is that the insurance policy may not cover a breach of contract suit and the insurance company may not provide for the legal defense of the suit. Fortunately, courts have held that in order for a promise of a successful outcome to be considered a breach of contract, it must be made in writing or under conditions that make the contractual nature of the obligation obvious.

LIABILITY

It is a fundamental rule in common law that the tort feasor—that is, the person who commits the tort—is liable for the results of his or her actions. In a medical malpractice situation this is true only for those health care providers who are independent contractors and have thus a personal provider–consumer relationship. All health care providers who are employed have only a very limited liability since it is another and overriding principle of common law that the employer (master) is liable for the negligence of the employee (servant), provided that the "servant" acted within the general scope of his or her employment and did not commit the negligent act with malice and with intent to injure. This is known in law as "respondent superior," and this is one of the reasons why the hospital is almost always a defendant in a malpractice case in which the alleged negligence took place in the hospital. The other reason, of course, why the hospital is brought into the case whenever possible, is that the hospital usually represents the deepest pocket.

There is a further exception to the "respondent superior" doctrine. If the employee was under the complete control of another person, not the employer, then the "borrowed servant" doctrine may be applied and the employer is not liable. This may well be the situation in the PACU but even more so in the operating room, where the nurses are generally considered to be under the control of the surgeon under the old and now largely abandoned "captain of the ship" doctrine.

The situation in the PACU is confusing. The anesthesiologist or nurse anesthetist is responsible for the patient in the PACU. Yet in the normal course of events the anesthesiologist cannot be present in the unit during the entire recovery period and may be unavailable at a moment's notice. This places a heavy burden on the nurses in the unit, who become the primary providers during the patient's stay. It has been my experience in several cases involving PACU patients that, provided certain conditions were met, the anesthesia personnel were not held liable for a disaster that occurred after the physician or nurse/anesthetist had left the unit. Most units have policies and procedures dealing with this matter and these must be followed rigidly. The person responsible for the anesthetic management should be the person taking the patient to the unit. It is this person's responsibility to turn the patient over to a PACU nurse. The turnover must consist of a report that gives all necessary details about the patient; the anesthetic and surgical procedure; the drugs used, with special reference to narcotics and muscle relaxants and their antagonists; any complications that may have occurred in the operating room; and any special instructions that may be pertinent to that particular case. The anesthesia personnel must remain with the patient while the nurse takes the vital signs, evaluates the patient, and in effect accepts responsibility for the patient. If this is done, the anesthesia personnel can leave the patient and return to their usual duties.

Assuming that there are no problems that arise in the PACU, the patient is discharged either back to his or her hospital room or, in the case of outpatients, to some discharge area. In theory the discharge of a patient is a medical responsibility that should be performed by the person who originally assumed the responsibility for the patient's anesthetic care. In practice this is rarely the case. Most PACUs have standing orders that specify the condition of the patient that must be present before the patient can be discharged. In other words, the responsibility is shifted from the physician to the nurse and in the vast majority of cases this is quite satisfactory. If the nurse makes an error in judgment or does not follow the regulations, he or she and, vicariously, the hospital are liable.

If a complication occurs in the PACU, the nurse has to provide emergency care and must call the appropriate physician. If the physician is not immediately available, the nurse must continue in her or his efforts to obtain medical assistance. If no assistance is obtained and irreversible damage is suffered by the patient, liability will lie with the hospital and also with the original attending physician. Some cases illustrating these matters will be described in the next section.

The liability situation with nurse-anesthetists is one of several unresolved issues in the arena of legal medicine. Few states have regulated this relationship and in most malpractice cases involving both nurse-anesthetists and anesthesiologists the courts have made widely varying decisions. If the nurse is employed by the anesthesiologist the situation is simple and the doctrine of vicarious liability is in effect. If the nurse is employed by the hospital, the hospital has the liability under the same doctrine. If the nurse is an independent practitioner, the surgeon may be held liable. Some states have determined by statute or by legal precedent that anesthesiology was the practice of medicine and thus could be performed only by a licensed physician or under the supervision of a licensed physician. If there is no anesthesiologist on the scene, this responsibility devolves on the surgeon, even though the surgeon may have very little knowledge about the current standards in anesthesia care.

An Ohio Supreme Court decision in the case of *Baird* vs *Sickler*[1] upheld the decision of the Ohio Court of Appeals and ruled that even though there was an anesthesiologist on the staff of the hospital, the surgeon was the only physician present in the room and thus bore the medical responsibility for the injury suffered by the patient. The court went out of its way to deny any attempt to resuscitate the Captain of the Ship doctrine, but stated that:

> We make no attempt to impose upon the operating physician the duty of overseeing all that occurs in the high technical milieu in which he works. Instead we wish only to ensure that where in the operating room the surgeon does control or realistically possesses the right to control events and procedures, he does so with a high degree of care.

It is evident from the above that this area of the law requires attention by the legislatures that will ultimately have to decide whether anesthesiology is the practice of medicine or not.

In the same general area is the special concern of teaching hospitals, where much if not all of the actual hands-on care is delivered by a trainee under the nominal supervision of a faculty member anesthesiologist. Even though the trainee is almost always a hospital employee, in this situation the attending physician has the right to control and thus the doctrine of the borrowed servant may well be in effect. In fact there are several cases on record where the attending physician or the head of the department was found liable for the resident's negligence when the attending physician was not even physically present in the

hospital. This latter situation is quite pertinent to the PACU, where in most teaching hospitals a resident is frequently assigned at the first level of support available to the nurses.

It is not the intent of this section to raise unnecessary apprehension among the faculty and staff. These are all problems, however, that need urgent and careful attention by administration, the medical and nursing staff, and the hospital attorney.

Although it is not specifically related to the PACU, there is one other area of the liability issue that is so important that it must be discussed in some detail.

In the past hospitals were considered to be free from any liability for any act of malpractice committed by a member of the medical staff who was not an employee of the hospital. The hospital and its governing body was supposed to provide only a safe and salubrious environment for the physicians to perform their duties. Furthermore, many hospitals were immune from suit under the theory of charitable or governmental immunity.

This is no longer true and the precedent-setting case of *Darling* vs *Charleston Community Hospital*[2] has completely changed the legal liability of the hospital as a corporate entity. It was the Darling case that established the principle that the hospital and its governing body were liable for the negligence of a nonemployee physician if they knew or should have known that the physician was incompetent. Since the Darling case there have been several cases in other jurisdictions, such as Misevch in Arizona[3] and Gonzales in California,[4] which have upheld the validity of the Darling decision.

Even more alarming is the *Corleto* vs *Shore Memorial Hospital*[5] case, which carried the Darling doctrine to its ultimate conclusion. In this case a New Jersey court found that not only was the hospital liable for the incompetent acts of a medical staff physician, but that the medical staff itself, collectively and individually, shared in this liability.

The Darling and Corleto decisions impose a heavy responsibility on every member of the hospital family. If any members of the staff—physicians, nurses, technicians—know that a member of the staff is incompetent or impaired, they have the responsibility to report this through the regular channels to the appropriate hospital medical or administrative authority. Nobody likes to "blow the whistle" on a colleague or coworker, but the court in the Gonzales case quoted the famous saying of Edmund Burke: "The only thing necessary for the triumph of evil, is for good men to do nothing." It is also a very real possibility that a staff member who does not report an incompetent or impaired colleague may be held personally liable for injury caused to a patient by the incompetent or impaired health care provider. In a Missouri case (*Burns* vs *Durus*)[6] the physician was held liable for the mistake of the hospital-employed nurse, since, in the opinion of the court, the physician knew or should have known that the nurse was incompetent.

THE MAJOR DANGER AREAS

The medicolegal cases centered on the PACU fall into relatively few categories. These can be identified rather clearly and must be recognized by all who work in the PACU. They can be listed as follows: (1) inadequate monitoring; (2) equipment failure; and (3) administrative and staffing problems.

Inadequate monitoring is by far the most important area and, with few exceptions, all cases in my experience have fallen into this category. Inadequate monitoring simply means a lack of timely recognition of a developing problem and the lack of timely and adequate response to the incipient emergency. The reason for inadequate monitoring may be a lack of adequate or adequately trained personnel, unrecognized monitoring equipment failure, and lack of equipment.

The staffing requirements for a good PACU are discussed in other chapters of this book and need not be repeated here. Suffice it to say that in law, adequate monitoring means that the personnel charged with the responsibility for the patient will be familiar with the patient under their care, and will not only be sufficient in number and training to recognize changes in the physiologic parameters, but will also know when to call for medical assistance and be able to provide emergency care efficiently and effectively while a physician is being summoned. This rather all-encompassing statement can be broken down into the following components:

1. Each patient must be assigned to a nurse who then becomes responsible for that patient.[7]
2. The PACU nurse must not assume responsibility for a patient until and unless the person responsible for administering anesthesia gives a full report and is present for the initial assessment.[8]
3. The nurse must remain in essentially continuous visual contact with the patient and the electronic monitors, so that changes in circulation and respiration will be recognized almost immediately and before they progress to the stage of imminent catastrophe.[9]
4. The nurse responsible for more than one patient must remain in contact with all patients under his or her care to note any deterioration in mental status, awareness, and so on.
5. The nurse assuming responsibility for a patient must be adequately trained to assume this responsibility.[10]
6. Adequate and appropriate records must be kept on each patient.

ILLUSTRATIVE CASES

Beauchamps vs Sparrow Hospital et al[7]

This case illustrates the importance of proper PACU organization and the need for individual accountability. Beauchamps was a healthy young college student who was in a motor vehicle accident and suffered a ruptured kidney. She had a nephrectomy under general anesthesia and was taken to the PACU following reversal of the muscle relaxant and extubation. She was responding only to painful stimulation. The turn-over was done appropriately, but there were no policies written for the PACU and the nurse who accepted Beauchamps into the unit did not assume any specific responsibility for her. According to the traditions of the unit, all nurses were responsible for all patients, which of course translates that no nurse took responsibility for any patient.

Another complicating factor in this case was the unfortunate coincidence that a going-away party was held for one of the nurses and all nurses went to a back room from time to time for coffee and cake. Much was made of this at the trial, although it probably played little if any role in the events.

Since no nurse was specifically responsible for Beauchamps, monitoring was at best intermittent. Whether the curare antagonist wore off and the patient became recurarized, or whether she just obstructed and was too depressed to overcome this, will never be known. The fact is that Beauchamps was found to be in cardiorespiratory arrest and the resuscitative effort was ineffective and unsuccessful.

The jury awarded the family a large sum of money and the hospital has since established more sensible policies for the PACU.

Bronson vs Sisters of Mercy et al[8]

Bronson was a middle aged woman who had a series of steroid epidurals for "backache." The first one was uneventful. Following the second procedure, there was no anesthesia chart and no evidence of monitoring before, during, or after the epidural. She was taken to the PACU about seven minutes after the epidural had been administered (lidocaine 50mg plus steroid). The anesthesiologist who gave the epidural took her to the unit and, in essence, pushed her through the door and left. When the nurse tried to take the vital signs, she found that the patient was not responsive, apneic, and without detectable peripheral pulses or blood pressure. Resuscitation was ''successful'' but Bronson was severely damaged and ultimately died.

The anesthesiologist settled out of court for a relatively very small sum, since he had no insurance coverage.

An interesting side issue of this case is that the plaintiff's attorney omitted to sue the hospital and is now the target of a legal malpractice suit by the estate of Bronson.

Goldsby vs Deaconess Hospital et al[9]

The issue was simple. Goldsby, a 36 year old male, was mugged on the street in Detroit and was taken to Deaconess Hospital with a fractured mandible. Two days later his mandible was reduced under general, nasotracheal anesthesia, arch bars were placed on the mandible and maxilla, and the mouth was wired shut. The nasotracheal tube was removed in the OR and Goldsby was taken to the PACU by the attending anesthesiologist. The turn-over was entirely appropriate and the admission vital signs were normal even though Goldsby was not responsive. The postoperative orders included instructions that the patient be in a head-up position and that wirecutters be at the bedside.

As soon as the anesthesiologist left to take care of his next patient, both PACU nurses also left to attend an ''in-service'' lecture. The unit was left to a circulating nurse, borrowed from the OR, who had some experience in recovery work but who was given no report on Goldsby. All she was told was that everybody was ''fine.'' When she went to take vital signs, some five minutes later, she discovered that Goldsby had suffered a cardiorespiratory arrest. Resuscitation was not successful. Considering Goldsby's age, the jury award of $350,000 was surprisingly modest.

Incidentally, Goldsby was flat on his back and there was no wirecutter in the PACU.

The anesthesiologist was found to be ''not negligent,'' even though he was nominally the medical director of the PACU. In fact he had no say in selecting, training, and supervising the nurses, who reported directly to the OR supervisor.

Blandings vs Richland Memorial Hospital[11]

A 17-year-old man died in the PACU room after a relatively minor plastic procedure. The patient appeared to be in good condition on admission to the unit. Turn-over was appropriate and the anesthesiologist

left after the nurse took the vital signs and formally accepted the patient.

There was no electronic monitoring and the nurse was clearly not as attentive as she should have been. Airway obstruction developed and was not recognized until too late. Resuscitation was done promptly and well, but the patient did not recover and died a few days later.

Three anesthesiologists and the hospital were sued. All three anesthesiologists were ''no caused,'' but the hospital was held vicariously liable for damages of $500,000.

Fayson vs Saginaw General Hospital et al[10]

This patient required respirator support while recovering from adult respiratory distress syndrome (ARDS) that occurred as a sequel to the aspiration of vomitus. The background is interesting inasmuch as the patient was a 38-year-old male who was receiving shock therapy for depression. Several of these therapies were performed under thiopental-succinylcholine anesthesia without any problems. The last scheduled shock therapy was administered and the patient vomited and aspirated. The nurses had made a mistake and fed the patient, and the anesthesiologist had omitted to check.

The management of the ARDS was very skillfully done and the patient had every chance of recovery, when one evening he was left in the care of an LPN who had less than one week of experience and no particular instruction in monitoring a ventilator-dependent patient. The respirator became disconnected from the tracheotomy tube, the alarm was turned off, and the LPN did not recognize that anything was amiss until the patient's wife walked into the room and noticed that there was something radically wrong. At this point the LPN ran out of the room in search of the RN. By the time the RN arrived and reconnected the ventilator, severe and irreversible brain damage had occurred and the patient was essentially decerebrate.

The hospital settled out of court for a large sum and the anesthesiologist was tried and ''no caused.''

An interesting feature of this case is that the jury recognized the lack of proximate causation between the anesthesiologist's obvious negligence and the ultimate outcome.

ETHICAL CONSIDERATIONS

Ethical considerations cannot be separated from legal considerations. There is inevitably a considerable overlap even though there may be things that are unethical but legal, just as there may be things that are illegal even though they are ethically unobjectionable. The area is a very large one and much of it is outside the scope of this chapter. There are three areas within the broad field of ethics, however, that are of considerable practical importance in the PACU: (1) the "do not resuscitate" order; (2) the withholding or withdrawing of life support; and (3) care of the patient with acquired immune deficiency syndrome (AIDS).

The "do not resuscitate order," also known widely as the "no code" order, is considered a legitimate medical decision. Its legal foundation is the Dinnerstein[12] case. A Massachusetts court held that treatments, including cardiorespiratory resuscitation, had to serve a positive purpose and could not be a "mere suspension of the act of dying." In other words, unless the resuscitative effort had a reasonable chance of reestablishing an acceptable quality of life, the physician was at liberty to decide not to resuscitate.

This decision has far-reaching effects on the practice of medicine, particularly in the major tertiary-care hospitals where the house staff considers it a personal affront if a patient does not respond to therapy. All of us have seen patients subjected to extensive resuscitative efforts, including major invasive procedures, even though the patient was terminally ill and the most successful resuscitation could only prolong the dying process.

"Do not resuscitate" orders should be written, just like any other order. They should be entered in the order book and should be seen and understood by the attending nursing personnel. It is not necessary, but may be prudent to discuss it with the next of kin. If the patient is competent, the "do not resuscitate" order obviously has to be discussed with, and must have the consent of, the patient.

In the large teaching hospitals we occasionally see a patient who has a written "do not resuscitate" order and who is brought to the operating room for a penultimate, quasipenultimate, or ultimate "try." The propriety of operating on a patient under these conditions is a surgical decision and as anesthesiologists we have to cooperate, except in the most outrageous cases, where it may be entirely proper to refuse any participation. It is my opinion that a decision to take the "DNR" patient to the operating room automatically cancels the DNR order. In our institution, where this is a not uncommon occurrence, we consider the patient in the operating room to be a candidate for resuscitation.

I believe the same principles apply to the PACU. Unless the surgeon rewrites the DNR order and includes it in the postoperative orders, the nurses in the unit have the obligation to start resuscitation and maintain it until a physician pronounces the patient dead. There may be perfectly valid reasons for not trying to resuscitate a patient, but there can be no excuse for deliberately resuscitating at less than full vigor. There is no such order as "do not resuscitate effectively."

Once resuscitation is started it must be continued until the patient either resumes vital functions or is pronounced dead. The first case is simple, but the second is not. In recent years many states have defined death by statute, but there are still some states where death is a medical decision issue that has few, if any, meaningful and well-defined parameters. In its simplest terms death can be defined as the complete and irreversible cessation of all vital functions. Under this definition death cannot be established unless both electroencephalographic and evoked potential studies indicate a complete absence of any CNS activity. In most jurisdictions such rigid criteria are not required. In fact most states follow the recommendations of the ad-hoc committee established at the Massachusetts General Hospital–Harvard Medical School at the time of the introduction of single-organ transplant technology, where the line between declaring a person dead and being able to harvest viable organs is a very thin one.

Closely allied to the DNR issue is the problem of withholding life support. There is a distinction that must be made clearly: withholding life support is a vastly different problem from withdrawing life support. The legal situation and the ethical concerns are distinct and must be considered individually. While the distinction may appear to be an artificial one, there is a very real difference between "omission" (not starting something) and "commission" (taking something away that has been started).

The classic situation in withholding life support is where the physician must decide whether to start a patient on a ventilator or not. This is a medical treatment decision and thus subject to consent on the part of the patient or the patient's legal guardian. If the patient is incompetent, the decision has to be based on the assumption of what the patient may have wished to do, had he or she been competent to make the choice. In some cases there is a clear indication concerning the patient's wishes. Many thoughtful persons will discuss these matters with their family and leave precise instructions. In some states there is statutory support for this form of delegation of authority. California has led the country in this regard by enacting the "Natural Death Act" of 1977. This is called "living will" legislation. A number of other states have followed suit, but the laws vary from state to state and, indeed, some states have been entirely unsuccessful in passing such eminently reasonable legislation. In the states that as yet have no such legislation, a similar result can be obtained by giving a durable power of attorney to a third party, who will then be able to make the proper decisions.

Withdrawing life support—turning off the ventilator or stopping parenteral fluids or alimentation—is one of the very major issues in contemporary medico-legal-ethical circles. If the patient is conscious and competent the situation is usually simple. The Perlmutter[13] case has well established the principle that a patient has the constitutional right to demand that his or her artificial life support be terminated. Perlmutter was an elderly man who was suffering from amyotrophic lateral sclerosis and had required ventilatory support for many months. He wanted the ventilator disconnected. The attending physicians refused and Perlmutter applied to the Florida courts. The court had no difficulty in backing up Perlmutter's wish.

The situation is much more difficult in patients who are not competent, but who are irreversibly committed to life support in the form of respirator care, parenteral nutrition, or nutrition by any means other than normal feeding. As far as the respirator is concerned, the precedent-setting case was the one in which a New Jersey Court authorized the physicians of Karen Quinlan[14] to terminate her respiratory support.

Numerous other cases confirm the Quinlan court's opinion and it has been generally accepted that respirators could be discontinued if indeed there was no hope for recovery. The matter of discontinuing parenteral nutrition or nutrition via a nasogastric tube or gastrostomy tube have been very hotly debated, and for some time it appeared that withholding fluids and alimentation was not ethically permissible. Most recently there has been a dramatic change in the approach to this problem and several courts have ruled that alimentation other than by oral feeding were subject to the same considerations as artificial ventilation. Rather than detailing these court decisions it might be best to quote the opinion of the AMA Council on Ethical and Judicial Affairs, issued on March 15, 1986, that states the view of organized medicine clearly and concisely:

> *Withholding or Withdrawing Life-Prolonging*
> *Medical Treatment*
>
> The social commitment of the physician is to sustain life and relieve suffering. Where the performance of one duty conflicts with the other, the patient's wishes should prevail, if the patient is incompetent to act in his own behalf and, in the absence of a durable power of attorney (living will), the physician must act in the best interest of the patient.
>
> For humane reasons, and with informed con-

sent, a physician may do what is medically necessary to alleviate severe pain, or cease or omit treatment to permit a terminally ill patient, whose death is imminent, to die. However, he should not intentionally cause death. In deciding whether the administration of potentially life-prolonging medical treatment is in the best interest of the patient who is incompetent to act on his behalf, the physician should determine what the possibility is for extending life under humane and comfortable conditions and what are the prior expressed wishes of the patient and attitudes of the family or those who have the responsibility for the custody of the patient. Even if death is not imminent but a patient's coma is beyond doubt irreversible and there are adequate safeguards to confirm the accuracy of the diagnosis and with the concurrence of those who have responsibility for the care of the patient, it is not unethical to discontinue all means of life-prolonging medical treatment. Life-prolonging medical treatment includes medication and artificially or technologically supplied respiration, nutrition or hydration. In treating a terminally ill or irreversibly comatose patient, the physician should determine whether the benefits of treatment outweigh its burdens. At all times the dignity of the patient should be maintained.

AIDS

This is a relatively new issue in the ethical–legal arena. In spite of the fact that the likelihood of transmitting AIDS in the PACU is extremely small, there have been cases where nurses have refused to care for AIDS patients. Whether patients with AIDS or other communicable diseases are admitted to the PACU or taken back to their room for recovery is a matter for hospital policy. It is my belief that modern PACUs should have isolation facilities and that AIDS and other infectious patients should have the same skilled and competent care as any other patient. It is ethically indefensible and legally at best doubtful to refuse to care for an AIDS patient. Obviously appropriate precautions must be taken, but to refuse care is no different from the medieval approach to lepers and for even poorer reasons.

PREVENTIVE MEASURES

The legal situation is not a cheerful one, and the prophets of doom and gloom blame everyone but themselves, and despair of any remedy except special legislation immunizing the physician against liability litigation. In fact, there are a number of steps that can be taken by every physician, other health care providers, and by the health care facility that could and would substantially reduce the likelihood of litigation and that would and could make the suits that are filed very much more defensible.

First and foremost is the requirement of practicing good and careful medicine. This is rather obvious and I do believe that most practitioners honestly try and truly believe that they are indeed practicing good medicine. Unfortunately there is a considerable amount of very poor medicine practiced. Many physicians do not keep abreast of current developments and practice according to standards that were in effect 10 to 20 years ago. Medicine has grown so rapidly that it is virtually impossible to keep up with the developments in one's own specialty, and it is absolutely beyond all reasonable expectations to keep current outside one's specialty or subspecialty. It is therefore of critical importance for every health care provider to recognize his or her limitations and not to try to practice beyond them. The law does not expect a physician to be all-knowing in all areas, but it does expect that every health care provider recognize the limits of his or her knowledge and ability and obtain assistance from colleagues. Many suits have as one of their primary allegations the failure to seek consultation, or the failure to refer.

It is a sign of professional maturity to realize early that a patient's problems are baffling, out of the ordinary and falling into the area of another specialty or subspecialty. To ask for a consultation is not an admission of ignorance, but evidence of good and thoughtful care.

A point very important to consider: a consultant's recommendations need not be followed, but if the primary physician decides to ignore the consultant's advice, this decision and the reasons for it must be documented in the record.

The second and almost equally important fact in preventing liability litigation is to establish the best possible relationship with the patient, the patient's family, or both. It is axiomatic in malpractice circles that only an angry patient or family sues. A bad result by itself may be the reason for a suit, but usually it takes a combination of a bad result and anger with the physician or the hospital to trigger the litigation.

Patients can be angry for many reasons, but by far the most common is a feeling that the physician was not interested in the patient as a person or as a human being. Comments such as: ''the doctor would not talk to me,'' ''he would not answer my questions,'' ''he would not explain anything to me,'' ''he was always in a hurry,'' ''he seemed to be mad at me,'' ''he yelled at me,'' and so on, are heard with distressing frequency. If the resulting feeling of frustration on behalf of the patient is combined with an unsatisfactory or unexpected outcome, the components of a malpractice suit are at hand and are most likely to blossom into the filing of a Complaint and Request for a Jury Trial.

Patients can also be angry because of rudeness on the part of nurses, secretaries, receptionists, and other ancillary personnel. Bad telephone manners have been a contributor to more than one lawsuit. During a hospital stay, there are frequently reasons to be angry. The call bell is not answered for a long period of time, the food is terrible, the registration and discharge processes are excessively time-consuming, or the entire experience is dehumanizing. All of these can serve as the primum mobile (first cause) of the litigation, which in this case usually tries to involve the hospital as well.

The conclusion is obvious. Every effort must be made to establish good relationships with the patient. The patient must feel that he or she is an integral part of the entire health care system and is not relegated to playing the part of a parcel in the post office. Five or ten minutes spent in talking to the patient, answering questions, allaying apprehension, and making the patient feel important, can save many hours in the court room and many thousands of dollars. The entire health care team must be acutely aware of this problem, and a nurse or receptionist must not uncommonly make up for the interpersonal shortcomings of the physicians.

The matter of informed consent, discussed earlier, is an integral part of this physician–patient relationship. If the patient feels that he or she is a partner in the decision-making process, is aware of the options and the major hazards and benefits of each, and is reasonably convinced that the physician is truly concerned, then the likelihood of a suit is very substantially reduced, even if the result is unsatisfactory.

In anesthesiology the establishment of a good physician–patient relationship is a very difficult problem. The involvement is episodic and usually limited to a single event. It is therefore even more important that the preanesthetic visit be conducted with the utmost concern for this matter. The practice of having one member of a group see the patient, while another member or a nurse-anesthetist provides the care on the following day, is hallowed by tradition but must be condemned in the strongest terms. Except in emergency situation or in cases of unexpected illness or other unfortunate circumstances, there is little if any excuse for not seeing one's own patients. In most instances the preanesthetic visit need not take more time than 10 to 15 minutes. With most patients this is sufficient to establish an interpersonal bond, gather the necessary information, perform the indicated physical examination, obtain informed consent, and lay the foundation for a smooth and problem-free relationship.

Since in many instances the patient's family is not present during this visit and since the patient may not be able to participate postoperatively in any discussions, it is particularly important to make the best possible record of the preoperative visit. This again need not take much time, and it is definitely one of the important items looked for by the plaintiff's expert. In a distressingly large number of cases there is either no preanesthetic note at all, or it is limited to a cryptic ''OK for GA'' and an illegible signature.

A good and legally helpful note should be dated and timed. It should include the gist of the discussion, briefly summarize the history and the physical findings, previous anesthetic history and complications, expected problems, ASA classification, the anesthetic plan, and the major complications that were discussed with the patient.

While this may sound like a formidable task, a preprinted form makes it relatively quite simple and it should not take more than five to ten minutes. A point frequently overlooked and yet of major importance is the drug history of the patient. The surgical record is usually quiet on this subject and many preanesthetic notes also ignore this important matter. It should be remembered that many patients, even when queried about drug usage, will not report the use of ''over the counter'' medications, eye drops, or nose drops since they do not consider these to be ''medications.'' Yet some of these drugs can significantly affect the anesthetic management and must be a part of the patient's evaluation.

In the PACU the physician–patient relationship has relatively little meaning except in the context of continuing care. Again, the practice hallowed by tradition, and perhaps inherent in the nature of the specialty, is a major contributor to the legal entanglements based on PACU misadventures. The anesthesiologist who gave the anesthetic may be involved with another patient in the operating room, may be making rounds, or may have gone home by the time trouble develops, leaving the emergency call to be answered by a colleague who knows nothing about the patient and who is forced to make critical decisions at a moment's notice and with only minimal information.

It is easy to raise these questions and indicate why these practices are fraught with legal hazards. It is very much more difficult to suggest an acceptable and practical answer, short of a complete revision of current anesthetic practices. Nevertheless, and at the risk of considerable opprobrium, I take the liberty of suggesting that, as a specialty, we could make substantial improvements in our legal exposure, by seeing our own patients preoperatively, and by trying to establish better relationships with the patient and the patient's family.

The matter of patient and family relationship is equally important in an ICU setting and easier to obtain. Here there is usually ample opportunity to talk to the family and to keep them fully apprised of the reasons for the intensive care, the treatment plan, and the prognosis. Most families are appreciative of the efforts made on behalf of the patient in the ICU and it is not surprising that relatively few lawsuits are based on ICU care. Having reviewed literally hundreds of malpractice cases, I found only a tiny number where the alleged malpractice took place in the ICU, and all but one of them were problems of equipment failure.

The third component in the prevention of litigation is the keeping of appropriate records. This is somewhat less of a problem in the ICU, where records are usually kept well. In fact, ICU records tend to be so voluminous that it takes considerable expertise to find one's way through the maze. In the PACU the records are also generally quite good, although several of the cases based on postanesthetic care did show considerable gaps in the record. This usually makes the case very difficult if not impossible to defend.

Good records are among the most important factors in both preventing and winning a malpractice suit. If the record permits the outside expert to reconstruct precisely the events preceding and following the questioned incident, it is very likely that the expert will advise the plaintiff's attorney not to initiate litigation. If litigation is started regardless, the defendant's expert should have a relatively easy time in showing the jury the course of events and guiding them through the case. Under these conditions the jury almost always concludes that there was no negligence, that the standards were not violated, and that there was no cause for action against the defendant.

It is appalling that in spite of considerable publicity on this subject, many records are still grossly unsatisfactory. While this is perhaps less important in the context of postanesthetic care, it is of sufficient general significance to warrant a brief discussion.

The purpose of the record is to enable a subsequent treating physician or a potential plaintiff's expert to reconstruct precisely the patient's progress from initial contact to discharge or death. There must be a reasoned sequence of events with each step properly planned and justified. The observations and findings must be evaluated and positive findings must be followed or explained. The invasive diagnostic and therapeutic manipulations must be justified and documented, and their outcome must be evaluated. The patient's participation in the decision-making process must be documented.

The record need not be long, but the entries must be legible, dated, and timed. The discharge summary must accurately reflect the events and must also include the instructions given to the patient and the prognosis.

The record is not the place for witticisms, for critique of earlier care, or for disparaging remarks about the patient or the patient's family. Corrections of erroneous entries must be made properly and retrospective alterations must never be allowed.

It must always be kept in mind that the medical record is a legal document. The paper that it is written on belongs to the physician or the hospital, but the information contained in the record belongs to the patient. The patient has the right to view and has the right to a copy. The physician or hospital has the right to charge a reasonable amount for copying, but does not have the right to refuse to provide the patient with a copy. The fact that the patient may not have paid his or her bill is not sufficient grounds for withholding the record. In fact there is no legitimate reason why the patient should not be provided with his or her record. Refusing to release the record automatically raises the patient's suspicions that the physician or the hospital is trying to hide something. Refusing a patient's request for the record is a very dangerous practice that almost invariably leads to highly undesirable results.

The worst possible feature of a record is a willful alteration that is made with the apparent intent to cover up an untoward event. I have personally seen records where there were obvious and rather crude alterations, and I have also seen a record where the anesthesia sheet had been completely rewritten after the fact and in order to hide a major error. Needless to say, such a record when introduced in court is a devastating indictment, making the case completely indefensible and even raising the possibility of an additional suit for fraud. How seriously a legislature may view an intentional alteration is clearly shown in the Michigan Public Health Act, which makes a conviction for alteration or destruction of a medical record the only violation for which revocation of the license is the sole permissible sanction. I have also seen PACU records that revealed long gaps in observations. It is of no use to claim afterwards that the observations were made but not recorded; juries will be inclined to doubt this. In an emergency situation it is most desirable that records be kept, at the time, and as accurately as possible. If shortage of personnel does not permit that this task be assigned to somebody as an exclusive task, the physician in charge of the resuscitation and the nurse responsible for the patient in the PACU must sit down as soon as the patient is stabilized or dead and reconstruct the events as accurately as possible. This must be entered into the body of the chart and therefore must be clear, concise, and factual. If hospital policy also requires that an incident report be prepared, this should be done at the same time. Incident reports are usually protected from legal discovery, but this may not be the case in some situations, and therefore incident reports have to be written as carefully as entries in the chart. The only way to have an absolutely protected document is to write it in the form of a letter to the hospital attorney, indicating that it is written in view of possible litigation. This letter then functions as an attorney–client communication, which is privileged.

Should the case result in litigation, many months and even several years may elapse before the participants will be asked, under oath, to reconstruct and relate the events. There is no way in which the average person can recall with any degree of precision a sequence of events and time them accurately, sometimes to the minute, after a span of months or years. For this reason the written record will ''speak for itself'' and the case is likely to stand or fall on the basis of what was entered into the record at the time of, or immediately after, the event.

Care must be taken to keep the record factual. Self-serving speculations should be avoided. They do more harm than good. A frank admission of an error and a plan to remedy the situation are helpful in convincing the jury of the sincerity of the defendant.

Only a small minority of the medical liability cases reach the jury and most of these are decided in favor of the defendant physician. In these cases a good record usually plays an important or even decisive part.

The principal reasons why relatively few cases reach the jury is that a very large number of cases have significant underlying negligence and that if the damages are minor, it is cheaper to settle the case than to try it and even to win.

The statement that underlying negligence is common will undoubtedly raise considerable arguments among readers. Nevertheless it has been documented by studies done by insurance carriers and by a state regulatory agency. The one notable area of exception is in obstetrics. The ''bad baby'' cases are usually settled out of court or are decided in favor of the plaintiff. The reason for this is that the economic and noneconomic damages tend to be enormous, the jury has a great and very natural empathy with the damaged child and its parents, the obstetrical records are frequently less than ideal, and as already stated above, there is very little good scientific evidence that can be used to show that there is probably little if any relationship between intrauterine distress and at least some forms of congenital CNS involvement.

In April 1987 the Commonwealth of Virginia enacted legislation taking some of the "bad baby" cases out of the tort system and instituting a form of "no fault insurance" in its stead. As of this writing there is no information about the cost, success, or failure of this approach. If it is successful it would make a highly significant contribution towards reducing the malpractice problem. Up to May 1989, no "bad baby" case had been resolved by this procedure in Virginia.

The last component in the protection against liability litigation can be subsumed under the term of "risk management." This is a relatively new concept that assumed a major role in claims prevention. A risk manager is a person knowledgeable in medical matters, whose responsibility is to act as the representative of the physician or institution while also functioning as an ombudsman and contact-person for the patient. The risk manager must be informed as soon as an "incident" takes place that is unexpected, damaging to the patient, and likely to lead to dissatisfaction with the services rendered. The risk manager then reviews the event, discusses the case in great detail with all the participant physicians and other health care providers, and contacts the appropriate hospital administrator and the hospital attorney. The hospital attorney and the insurance carrier(s) may not be consulted for all incidents, but where indicated, their involvement should be early in the course of events. The risk manager reviews the record and makes sure that the appropriate entries are made, that all reports (laboratory, x-ray, pathology, etc) are entered sequentially, and that the entire record is correct and complete. The risk manager also orchestrates the communications with the patient or the patient's family and serves as a two-way communication channel between the hospital and its personnel on one side and the patient and patient's family on the other. It is usually the risk manager's responsibility to advise the insurance carrier and to cooperate with the insurance investigator.

A good risk manager can save the physicians and the institution untold grief and vast sums of money. This fact has been recognized by insurance carriers, and insurance premiums may be lower for those institutions that can show a good risk management team. Legislatures have also recognized the contributions that good risk management can make and have built it into many tort reform acts of recent years.

An additional component of risk management is quality control. This is mandated by the Joint Commission on the Accreditation of Hospitals. When done properly, quality control can identify problem areas early and can also prove that the problem areas have been eliminated. Space does not permit an in-depth discussion of this important component of risk management. The reader is referred to the JCAH standards and to the considerable literature on this subject.

It is extremely unlikely that medical liability litigation will ever be eliminated. State legislatures are not going to pass laws immunizing health care providers against the legitimate claims of patients harmed by negligent or ignorant care. There will always be irresponsible attorneys as well, just as there will always be health care providers who practice below minimal acceptable standards. Alternative routes to conflict resolution, such as binding arbitration and no-fault insurance, may be helpful in limited areas but are extremely unlikely to replace the tort system entirely. Arbitration has been tried repeatedly and has not made an appreciable impact. No-fault insurance, other than perhaps in the "bad baby" cases, is far too expensive.

Whether a national health service type arrangement, with all physicians on a salary and all health care governmentally administered and funded, would resolve the malpractice situation is an interesting question. There are certainly theoretical arguments that suggest that such an arrangement would eliminate the need for litigation since the welfare state would take care of the patient and the police power of the state and federal government would discipline the careless and incompetent physician. Whether very many people would wish to practice medicine under those circumstances is another question to which there is no ready answer.

SUMMARY AND CONCLUSION

The PACU and the intensive care unit are high-risk areas both medically and medicolegally. All health care providers working in these areas should be thoroughly familiar with the legal theories of negligence and should be exquisitely sensitive to the requirements of sound, efficient, and safe care. While there is no way in which malpractice litigation can be eliminated, its current, significant impact on the individual practitioner and on the health care system in general can be substantially mitigated by following the few precepts outlined above. The fundamental truth underlying all safe and effective health care is embodied in the biblical injunction: "Do unto others . . ."

REFERENCES

1. *Baird vs Sickler*, 69 Ohio st 2d 625, 1982.
2. *Darling vs Charleston Community Hospital*, 200 NE 2d 149, Ill 1975.
3. *Tucson Med Center vs Misevch*, 520 p 2d 958 Ar 1976.
4. *Gonzales vs Nork et al*, 131 Cal Reporter 717, Cal 1976.

5. *Corleto vs Shore Mem Hospital*, 350 Atl 2d 534, 1975, 138 NJ Sup Ct 1975.
6. *Burns vs Durus*, 459 F 2d 489 (6th Circuit 1974).
7. *Beauchamps vs Sparrow Hospital*, Ingham Co, Mich Circuit Ct 1982.
8. *Bronson vs Sisters of Mercy et al*, (85-508747 NM) Wayne Co Mich Circuit Ct 1984.
9. *Goldsby vs Deaconess Hospital et al*, (74-004-754 NM) Wayne Co Mich Circuit Ct 1978.
10. *Fayson vs Saginaw General Hospital et al*, Saginaw Co, Mich Circuit Ct 1978.
11. *Blandings vs Richland Memorial Hospital et al*, (86-CP-40-2769) Court of Common Pleas, Richmond Co, SC.
12. In re Dinnerstein, 380 NE 2d 134, Ma 1978.
13. *Satz vs Perlmutter*, 362 So 2d, Fla 1978.
14. In re Quinlan, 70 NJ 10, 355 A 2d 647, 1976.

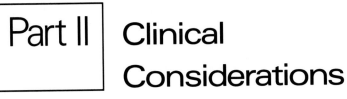

Part II Clinical Considerations

10 The Patient After Local and Regional Anesthesia

Michael D. Umanoff

The recent increase in the use of regional and local anesthetic techniques may be linked to the greater number of procedures now considered suitable for ambulatory and day care surgery. Although outpatient anesthetic recovery may be facilitated when these types of anesthetic techniques are used, postanesthetic care must be no less diligent than that afforded to patients who have undergone general anesthesia.

The successful completion of a regional anesthetic necessitates a thorough understanding of anatomic, physiologic, and pharmacologic variables, and their associated complications and management. This chapter deals with the perioperative management of regional anesthetics with emphasis on the care of potential complications.

GENERAL CONSIDERATIONS

To successfully manage a regional anesthetic, care must be taken in (1) selecting the appropriate candidate for this form of anesthesia; (2) choosing a suitable technique; (3) opting for the proper anesthetic agent or combination of agents; and (4) allowing an adequate amount of time for the performance of the chosen block.

Patient refusal is generally deemed an absolute contraindication to the selection of a particular form of anesthetic intervention (with exceptions, such as the mentally impaired patient with a history of an extremely difficult airway problem in whom guardian or administrative consent is legal). This is of paramount importance in regional anesthesia where patient cooperation is essential for a safe and favorable outcome. The apprehensive patient requires reassurance and should be informed with regard to intraoperative management and postoperative expectations. Potential sequelae deserve prudent discussion.

Choice of a specific nerve block and anesthetic agents requires consideration of (1) the surgery to be performed and the needs of the surgeon; (2) the physical capabilities and anatomical peculiarities of the patient; and (3), the anticipated hospital stay.

Another factor, often overlooked, is that of availability of sufficient time to satisfactorily administer and establish the nerve block. When insufficient time is allocated, the incidence of failed block increases and the morbidity rate escalates. In addition, an untoward degree of patient apprehension may ensue.

Ideally an induction room or a patient holding area with adequate facilities should be available for the performance of blocks.

PERIOPERATIVE VIGILANCE

Current standards for anesthetic practice dictate that the same basic levels of perioperative monitoring and vigilance be applied to all patients, despite the choice of anesthetic technique. There is a tendency towards laxity of these safeguards in regional anesthetics. Despite the oft-used phrase, "no such thing as a minor anesthetic," there is a general inclination to treat regional techniques as such. This unfortunately has also been shown to hold true for those patients requiring potent narcotic and sedative/hypnotic supplementation during surgery performed under local or regional anesthesia.[1-3]

PACU ADMISSION

Not all patients undergoing regional anesthesia require admission to the postanesthetic care unit (PACU). The decision to send a patient to the unit should be dealt with individually considering such variables as the patient's general condition; past history; the type of neural blockade utilized; the use of adjunctive sedation; and the occurrence of adverse reactions or complications. It is safe to say, however, that all patients who have received either subarachnoid or epidural anesthesia deserve PACU admittance. The decision to admit the patient to the PACU or return him or her to the ward lies with the anesthesiologist or the surgeon if the latter performed the field block and no anesthesiologist was in attendance.

DURATION OF PACU STAY

Once the decision to admit the patient has been made, the issue of length of stay should be addressed. Most would agree that it is inappropriate to admit an ASA I patient with a purely local anesthetic to the unit. In the same light it would be equally inappropriate to have a patient with a bupivacaine-based nerve block remain in the PACU until fully recovered.

Scoring systems have been developed over the years to help assess a patient's overall condition to determine readiness for discharge. These scores generally focus on the anesthetized patient (general anesthetics), rather than the anesthetized region.[4,5]

Discharge criteria for regional blocks should recognize both the well being of the patient and the smooth operation of the PACU. All that is necessary to consider discharge of a patient with a peripheral nerve block (other than systemic factors), is the demonstration of some degree of block regression. After subarachnoid and epidural blocks the commonly accepted criteria for discharge are the regression of sensory level and the ability of the patient to move the toes. However, no data have correlated this ability with the return of hemodynamic stability. Recently, new criteria based on orthostatic hemodynamic stability have been utilized with good results in patients having received intrathecal anesthetics.[6] The discharge criteria proposed are less than a 10% fall in mean arterial pressure on two successive orthostatic determinations 30 minutes apart; or supine hemodynamic stability with toe movement. Autonomic function frequently returns long before the sensory level recedes or toe movement occurs. Thus the time in the PACU may be shortened by approximately one hour.

Whatever criteria are selected, there must be an established system of postanesthetic evaluation for all patients having had regional anesthetics, especially those discharged prior to complete recovery.

POSTOPERATIVE PRECAUTIONS

It must always be kept in mind that the patient after a successful regional anesthetic, as opposed to the patient subjected to general anesthesia, has no source of continued stimulation (pain). Absence of pain can easily lead to respiratory depression in the sedated patient. Thus, constant vigilance as to adequacy of ventilation must be maintained.

If central neural blockade has been implemented,

abrupt changes in position (supine to upright or lithotomy to supine) should be avoided. Patients remain effectively sympathectomized to a variable degree, despite some regression of sensory and motor block.

Injury to the patient or to a blocked extremity is not an uncommon occurrence in the perioperative period. This may result from improper positioning, inadequate padding, or uncontrolled movement of the extremity. It is wise to restrict range of motion until sensation and motor control have returned to preoperative levels.

AMBULATORY DISCHARGE CRITERIA

Peripheral Blockade
Ambulatory surgical patients present a special situation. Under ideal circumstances a patient would be discharged home after demonstrating complete recovery from the regional block. At times a case will present itself in which recovery is incomplete after an appropriate amount of time. Flexibility is important. If patients are discharged they should be reassured that nothing is wrong and that normal function will return shortly. They must be warned about the possibility of injuring the insensate extremity (eg, told to refrain from smoking or avoid getting close to sources of heat or intense cold).[7]

Central Regional Blockade
The generally accepted sequence of return of neural function is (1) motor; (2) sensory; and (3) sympathetic. However, several studies have demonstrated earlier sympathetic recovery and thus earlier hemodynamic stability.[8]

Suitable criteria for discharge after subarachnoid and epidural anesthesia include normal perianal sensation, plantar flexion of the feet, and proprioception of the big toe. In addition, the patient must be hemodynamically stable and able to void spontaneously (construed as adequate return of sympathetic tone.)[9]

It is essential that a fine-tuned system of postdischarge follow-up be established including a checklist of what the patient might expect and a telephone number where medical advice may be obtained. Telephone follow-up by the PACU staff is also highly desirable. In addition, a protocol should be developed for the treatment of anesthetic-related complications.

COMPLICATIONS OF REGIONAL ANESTHESIA

Most regional anesthetics are straightforward and complications are rare. When complications do occur they may present a therapeutic dilemma requiring an in-depth knowledge of local anesthetic drugs, pathophysiology of nerve blocks, and treatment modalities.

Local Anesthetics

Systemic Toxicity. Appropriate use of local anesthetics rarely results in overt toxic levels. Systemic toxicity usually occurs because of either intravascular injection or use of an extravascular overdose. Certain blocks are associated with a high degree of absorption (Fig. 10–1). The addition of a vasoconstrictor or an agent such as hyaluronidase markedly alters this absorption. Systemic toxicity is manifest by actions on the cardiovascular system and the central nervous system. Generally the cardiovascular system is more resistant. A phenomenon of early profound cardiovascular collapse has been noted to occur with the more lipid-soluble and highly protein-bound local anesthetic agents such as etidocaine or bupivacaine.[10-12] Cardiovascular toxicity stems from dose-dependent blockade of the sodium channels, thus depressing cardiac conduction. Bupivacaine, because of a slower dissociation from the sodium channels, is approximately 70 times as potent as lidocaine at blocking cardiac conduction.[13] Cardiac slowing, dysrhythmias, and hypotension result. Rarely, cardiac arrest follows.

Central nervous system toxicity is biphasic with depression occurring at low levels (often therapeutic), and excitation occurring at higher levels.[14,15] Tonic clonic movements and seizures may develop. Factors decreasing the central nervous system toxic threshold include increasing $PaCO_2$, acidosis, or administration of drugs that adversely effect elimination. Conversely, the threshold may be increased by maintenance of adequate ventilation, benzodiazepines, barbiturates, and the use of inhalation agents.

Treatment of Systemic Toxicity. The treatment of cardiovascular system toxicity in humans requires general cardiac and respiratory support. Animal studies indicate successful use of epinephrine, atropine, bretyllium, and defibrillation.[16] Also evident is that cardiopulmonary resuscitation should be carried out for an extended period of time.

Following central nervous system toxicity a vicious cycle can develop quickly. With seizure activity, hypoxia, hypercarbia, and acidosis ensue, thus decreasing the toxic threshold. An adequate airway and ventilation must be established and the seizures controlled. Succinylcholine has been advocated by some (facilitates ventilation, ablates muscular activity)[17]; however, neuronal electrical activity remains unaffected. Benzodiazepines (diazepam is more efficacious than midazolam) and thiobarbiturates are useful anticonvulsants,[18-20] and when used in conjunction with oxygen and muscle relaxation, round out the therapy of central nervous system toxicity.

Allergic Response. Most reports of allergic responses to local anesthetics stem from the use of the ester-linked agents (tetracaine, procaine, and chloroprocaine), derivatives of para-aminobenzoic acid. The hypersensitivity reaction results in variable degrees of histamine release causing wheezing, dyspnea, erythemia, edema, hypotension, tachycardia, headache, and loss of consciousness. Treatment is aimed at support of the airway and circulation, and at control of the effects of histamine release by giving diphenhydramine (10 to 50 mg) intravenously or epinephrine (0.1 mg) subcutaneously.

Local Tissue Toxicity. Neurotoxicity may represent a multitude of factors that interact to effect damage (high concentrations, chemical contaminants, trauma, pressure, and ischemia). Toxic damage tends to involve the smaller nerve fibers, resulting in anesthesia, analgesia, hypesthesia, hypalgesia, hyperalgesia, paresthesias, and sympathetic disturbances.[21] Patients complaining of persistent postoperative neurologic deficits should undergo early and comprehensive neurologic, electromyographic, and evoked potential studies. It is important to note that the

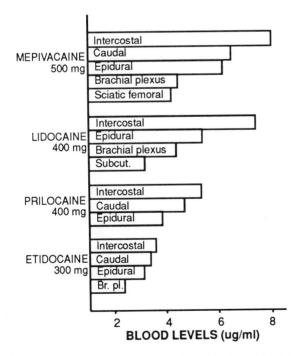

Figure 10–1. Peak serum levels of local anesthetics attained during the performance of various types of regional anesthetic procedures. (From Covino BG, Vassallo HG: Local Anesthetics: Mechanisms of Action and Clinical Use. New York, Grune & Stratton, 1976, by permission.)

symptoms may not appear immediately and can be experienced first after approximately two weeks. Electromyographic analysis is invaluable, as it enables accurate dating of the insult, determination of the level of the injury, and precise identification of the nerves involved.[22,23] Careful documentation of drugs and dosages used and the type, severity, and duration of symptoms is essential. Early, frank, and complete discussion with the patient may help to decrease medicolegal problems.

Central Regional Blockade

Epidural and subarachnoid anesthesia remain two of the most commonly used and reproducible blocks today. Nevertheless, in the mind of the public, numerous complications of a devastating nature—including permanent paralysis, persistent crippling backache, and lifelong headaches—may occur. In fact, properly performed and managed, these techniques are safe, and the potential complications can be decreased to close to zero.

Cardiovascular Complications. Hypotension is a direct result of blockade of preganglionic sympathetic fibers with an ensuing decrease in cardiac output. The drop in cardiac output is secondary to peripheral venodilation and decreased venous return. The degree of hypotension is directly proportional to volume status and the level of sympathetic blockade (Fig. 10-2). In adequately hydrated patients, blocks below the fifth thoracic dermatome (sympathetic level) rarely result in hypotension, due to compensatory vasoconstriction in unblocked segments. Blockade above the fourth thoracic dermatome, in addition to preventing compensatory vasoconstriction, blocks sympathetic outflow to the heart.[24] Patients with central neural blockade are susceptible to venous pooling and therefore prone to hypotension with abrupt changes in position.

Aside from hydrational status and degree of block, other factors contribute to hypotension including rapidity of onset such as is observed with the use of 2-chloroprocaine and alkalinized local anesthetics.[25] Also, a greater degree of hypotension is associated with the use of epinephrine-containing solutions in the epidural space. This is believed to be secondary to absorbed epinephrine stimulating beta-2 adrenergic receptors in peripheral vascular beds, leading to an enhanced state of vasodilation.[26]

As has been well described in third-trimester and term pregnant patients, profound hypotension may result from aortocaval compression.[27] This phenomenon can also be observed to occur in other patients with large intraabdominal masses such as ovarian tumors. In these patients some degree of left or right uterine displacement should be implemented.

Treatment, or better still prevention, of hypotension begins preoperatively by ensuring an adequate intravascular volume prior to performing the block. Intravenous fluids should be administered via large-bore catheters. It is also wise to have available a pressure bag to increase infusion rates if necessary. Despite these measures, if hypotension should ensue it can be treated with rapid intravenous fluids, leg elevation (NOT TRENDELENBURG POSITION), and the use of vasopressors such as ephedrine, mephentermine, or phenylephrine.

Respiratory Complications. Numerous studies have demonstrated that there is minimal effect on ventilatory mechanics, even with high spinal anesthetics. However, it must be remembered that with this degree of blockade the patient's ability to clear secretions is impaired.[28,29] Respiration may be compro-

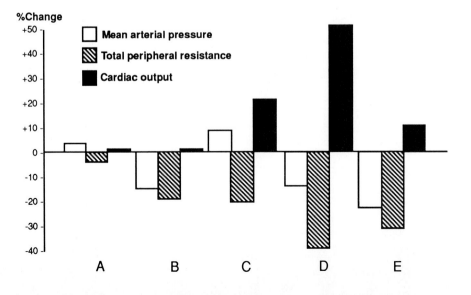

Figure 10-2. Cardiovascular effects of epidural anesthesia as influenced by analgesic dermatomal level, epinephrine, and presence of hypovolemia. The sensory level of anesthesia was T5 at A, D, and E; T1 at B; and T2-3 at C. Epinephrine was present at D and E. Hypovolemia was present at E. (Modified and reproduced with permission: Covino BG, Vassallo HG: Local Anesthetics: Mechanism of Action and Clinical Use, p 137. New York, Grune & Stratton, 1976.)

mised when there is intercostal muscle paralysis in association with certain surgical maneuvers such as use of the Trendelenburg position, the open abdomen with packs, or the use of abdominal retractors. Also of note and probably more of a theoretical concern, is the development of bronchospasm in the asthmatic patient with high levels of sympathetic block. However, a certain inconsistency is noted, as epidural and high spinal anesthesia have been reported to alleviate severe bronchospasm.[30]

Subdural Block. In recent years reports have appeared describing the development of a somewhat rapid extensive block with associated hypotension during epidural anesthesia.[31] Subsequent radiographic studies have demonstrated positioning of the catheter in the subdural space, a potential space that exists between the dura and the arachnoid mater. The onset of blockade is inconsistent with that of an intrathecal injection and the spread of solutions within the space favors a cephalad direction. Of utmost concern, aside from the development of intraoperative hypotension, is the possibility of catheter migration to the subdural space over a period of time. This is important in light of the increasing use of postoperative instillation of narcotics for pain relief through what are considered to be epidurally placed catheters. Due to the unpredictable nature of this problem and the variety of responses to injection, if there is concern or suspicion of migration, it is best to remove the catheter and reinsert it at another level.

Postdural Puncture Headache (PDPH). Probably the most common complication related to central neural blockade is postdural puncture headache. It is the direct result of dural puncture (intentional or unintentional) with a concomitant cerebrospinal fluid leak that decreases the cerebrospinal fluid pressure. With the ensuing caudal displacement of the brain there is traction upon pain-sensitive structures such as the blood vessels, falx, and tentorium cerebelli.

The headache is classically postural-aggravated upon rising and improves upon reclining. Other reported symptoms include nausea, vomiting, dizziness, and auditory and visual disturbances. Typically it occurs after 12 to 24 hours and can last more than two weeks. If enough time elapses, almost all PDPHs resolve spontaneously. Overall the incidence of headaches is greatest in pregnant patients and the young, and it is lowest in the elderly. The classic study by Vandam and Dripps demonstrates the importance of sex, age, and needle size on the incidence of PDPH (Table 10–1).[32] There is a direct relationship between needle diameter and incidence of headache. This is true for single dural puncture; however it is believed by some that the number of dural punctures is in-

TABLE 10–1. RELATION OF SEX, AGE, AND NEEDLE GAUGE USED FOR LUMBAR PUNCTURE TO INCIDENCE OF 'SPINAL' HEADACHE

	Number of Spinal Anesthetics	Number of 'Spinal' Headaches	Percent
Sex			
Male	4063	302	7
Female	5214	709	14
Vaginal delivery	938	220	22
Other procedures	4276	489	12
Totals	9277	1011	21
Age (Years)			
10–19	537	51	10
20–29	1994	321	16
30–39	1833	261	14
40–49	1759	192	11
50–59	1736	133	8
60–69	1094	45	4
70–79	297	7	2
80–89	27	1	3
Totals	9277	1011	11
Needle Gauge			
16	839	151	18
19	154	16	10
20	2698	377	14
22	4952	430	9
24	634	37	6

From Vandam LD, Dripps RD: Long-term follow up of patients who received 10,098 spinal anesthetics: III. Syndrome of decreased intracranial pressure (headache and occular and auditory difficulties). JAMA 1956; 161:586.

creased with higher-gauge needles such as 25 and 26 gauge,[33] probably due to sluggish and unobserved flow of cerebrospinal fluid through the small-bore needles.

Conflicting reports have appeared in the literature concerning attempts at decreasing the severity of complications of dural puncture. Some studies report lower rates of PDPH if the bevel of the needle is oriented longitudinally in the *purported* direction of the dural fibers.[34] However, histologically the dural fibers are arranged multidirectionally rather than in a parallel pattern. This has been demonstrated in a recent study where the use of a Whittacre (pencil-point) needle resulted in a statistically significant decrease in fluid leak across human cadaveric dura.[35]

Aside from needle design, alternative approaches to the spinal canal have been suggested in an attempt to reduce PDPH. One such approach is the paramedian route.[36]

The diagnosis of PDPH can be made on the basis of symptoms and by demonstrating the postural nature of the headache and the ability to alleviate the headache by applying firm pressure to the patient's abdomen in the upright position. If one is aware of accidental dural puncture or if subarachnoid anesthesia was intended, multiple prophylactic measures can be taken including ensuring adequate hydration perioperatively, preventing straining, and avoiding the supine position for extended periods of time. There is no benefit in keeping the patient bedridden.[37,38]

The use of prophylactic blood patches, condemned by many, has gained interest and support in cases of accidental dural puncture.[39-42] Other studies have utilized "saline patches," but with inconsistent results.[43-45] A novel approach, implemented when epidural anesthesia is used, involves intrathecal placement of the epidural catheter at the puncture site, thus resulting in an intermittent spinal technique. The catheter is left in situ for a period of a few hours. Occurrence of PDPH in patients treated in this manner appears to be reduced.[46]

Another simpler method of reducing the occurrence of PDPH is to use smaller-diameter Tuohy needles. Both 20- and 24-gauge Tuohy needles with accompanying 24- and 28-gauge catheters have been designed and will soon be generally available.

If a PDPH develops and persists despite 24 hours of rest, fluids, analgesics, and caffeine-containing products (intravenous caffeine is no longer manufactured in the United States), the patient should be offered an epidural blood patch (Figure 10-3). This technique is extremely safe and a highly effective mode of therapy. No permanent adverse effects have

been reported and transient backache, paresthesias, or radicular pain occur only in a small percentage.[47] The success rate for epidural blood patching (nonprophylactic) has been reported to be 91 to 100%.[48]

A blood patch is accomplished by depositing 10 to 20 mL of aseptically obtained autologous blood (unheparinized) at the site of the prior dural puncture. The patient should assume the supine position for 30 to 60 minutes. Thereafter the patient may ambulate freely. Attempts should be made to prevent the patient from coughing or straining. If the headache should fail to respond with the first patch, a second patch can be administered. If the headache persists despite these maneuvers, the diagnosis of PDPH should be suspected and a neurologic consultation sought.

Backache. Backache after spinal and epidural anesthetics is not an uncommon complaint. It has been found to be just as frequent an occurrence after general anesthesia and pudendal block.[49,50] It is generally accepted that the underlying problem is alteration of the lumbosacral curvature secondary to relaxation of the paraspinous muscles. This problem is compounded by patient positioning with additional stress placed upon the lumbar spine.

Another consideration is the tendency of most patients to focus on having received an injection and

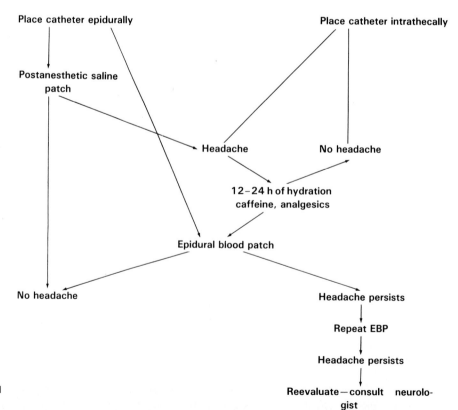

Fig. 10-3. PDPH Management; Accidental Dural Puncture.

to associate any back pain with that injection. The best way to contend with this issue is through preoperative teaching.

For a brief (one- to two-day) period may patients complain of a sharp, well-localized pain at the site of injection. Point tenderness can be demonstrated on examination. This pain is most likely secondary to needle trauma. One study has promoted the use of a field block prior to placement of an epidural needle. The researchers reported a significant reduction in complaints of local tenderness.[51]

Neurologic Sequelae. Probably the worst complications of central regional blockade are those related to neural damage. Fortunately these cases are few and far between. In one major review covering a span of ten years, a zero incidence of permanent motor dysfunction was reported out of 582,190 cases of spinal anesthesia.[52] Other comprehensive reviews of epidural and spinal anesthetics have failed to demonstrate significant numbers of neurologic complications.[53]

With any neurologic sequelae, a question that must be addressed is whether the neural damage is secondary to the anesthetic itself or due to a multiplicity of associated factors (preexisting neurologic disease, surgical intervention, patient positioning, or birth trauma). When injury does occur, objectivity must be maintained. This is not the time for pointing a finger in an effort to lay blame. The patient's well-being should be the only concern, and the objective should be early recognition, diagnosis, and effective therapy for the problem.

Mechanical trauma may result from direct injury to the cord, cauda equina, or nerve roots. Severe paresthesias are generally the rule. These are dramatically worsened with attempted injection of anesthetic agent, often resulting in loss of consciousness with subsequent onset of transient or permanent neural deficits. However, paresthesias are not uncommon, even in skillful hands. The vast majority are of a benign, transient nature and do not result in any neurological damage.

Most local anesthetic agents are devoid of neurotoxic effects in the concentrations commonly implemented in subarachnoid and epidural anesthesia.[54] Accidental intrathecal injection of 2-chloroprocaine has raised some concern because of reports of arachnoiditis and neurologic deficits.[55] Some experts believe the problem is secondary to the combination of low pH and the presence of sodium metabisulfite, rather than the 2-chloroprocaine itself.[56] Others claim that the concomitant use of epinephrine may have contributed to the damage.[57] Whatever the etiologic factor or factors, the concern generated has prompted the manufacturer to alter the formulation of the drug

to a more physiologic solution. If an accidental dural puncture has occurred and a catheter is subsequently placed at a different level, it is probably preferable to select an agent other than 2-chloroprocaine.

Infection. With acceptance of the widespread use of disposable spinal and epidural equipment the incidence of infection has been extremely low. A major concern among some anesthesiologists has been whether to use central regional blockade in febrile patients. Our policy is that these techniques can be safely implemented in selected patients (eg, patients with chorioamnionitis). Patients in septic shock with hemodynamic instability are not candidates for regional techniques. Patients with infectious processes involving the lower back are also better treated with general techniques. We have not seen any infectious complications over a span of many years.

Hematoma. Epidural hematoma is an extremely rare complication in patients not receiving anticoagulant therapy. The complication has, however, been reported in heparinized or coumadinized patients.[58] However, more than 100 cases of spontaneous epidural hematoma formation have been reported in anticoagulated patients unassociated with epidural block.[58]

Controlled epidural anesthesia has been used extensively in heparinized patients undergoing vascular surgery. No cases have been reported of epidural hematoma formation.[59,60] It has been our practice to place spinal or epidural catheters prior to heparinization and to remove them when either the effects of heparin have been adequately reversed or enough time has elapsed (6 to 12 hours) after cessation of the effects of heparin.

An area of controversy has to do with the safe use of epidural and spinal anesthesia in patients receiving antiplatelet therapy such as aspirin, persantine, or low-molecular-weight dextran. We have successfully used regional anesthesia in patients receiving these medications. The risk–benefit ratio to the patient must be assessed.

Catheter Complications

Multiple problems have been encountered with the use of continuous catheter techniques, including migration, shearing, catheter retention, and kinking. Many of these difficulties are related to poor technique or to the placement of an excessive length of catheter. When inserting a catheter, the black distance markings should be noted. All that is required both intrathecally and epidurally is 3 to 4 cm of catheter length. Other methods for determining the amount of catheter placed have been suggested. For example, advancing the catheter until initial resistance is met, represents the orifice of the needle. Then by grasping the catheter at a predetermined distance from the hub, the catheter can be advanced till the hub is contacted. An alternate approach is to use a styleted catheter. With this method the stylet is pulled back approximately 3 to 4 cm from the end of the catheter. Upon insertion, the sensation of resistance should be elicited twice, once as the catheter emerges from the needle orifice and then as the stylet within the catheter emerges from the orifice. At this point the desired amount of catheter is in place and further advancement should cease. In obese patients placement of an inadequate amount of catheter may result in a failed epidural block because of shifting of the patient's skin at the point where the catheter is fixed.

The temptation to pull back a catheter once it is beyond the bevel should be resisted. However, if an attempt is made it should be accomplished gently. If the slightest resistance is met, then further attempts should cease and the needle and catheter removed as one. Most modern Tuohy needles are designed with a blunted upper orifice edge to help prevent catheter shearing. If a portion of catheter is sheared, the patient should be informed of the event and of its essentially benign nature. It is probably in the best interest of the patient that the catheter remains be left in situ since attempted removal (unless superficial) may do more harm than good.[61]

Catheter retention can be a major problem, and in the worst of circumstances surgical intervention may be necessary. Calcification of the ligamentum, narrowed interspaces, knot formation, and entanglement about nerve roots have been reported.[62] If initial attempts at gentle removal prove difficult, further action can be taken using fluoroscopy. Epidural catheters are generally quite difficult to visualize radiographically. By injecting contrast through the catheter it can be demonstrated and its course determined. If the catheter appears knotted or entangled, removal may be facilitated by the use of a guidewire or stylet. Alternatively, sterile saline may be injected through the catheter as gentle attempts at withdrawal are made. Surgical intervention is indicated if knotting around nerve roots is causing pain.

Peripheral Regional Blockade

Selective regional neural blockade, when properly performed, is relatively painless, provides optimal conditions for surgical intervention, suppresses the neuroendocrine responses to surgical stimuli, and provides adequate postoperative pain relief.[63]

Due to the invasive nature of peripheral blocks there are several associated complications. Many of these are similar to those that are seen with central regional blockade. Other complications unique to peripheral nerve blocks include tourniquet paralysis

syndrome, pneumothorax, and trauma secondary to needle placement.

Tourniquet Paralysis Syndrome. A term coined by Moldaver in the 1950s, tourniquet paralysis syndrome relates to the development of postanesthetic neuropathy and paralysis after the use of arm tourniquets.[64] Nowadays, with the use of *properly functioning* and modern tourniquets, its occurrence is quite rare. It is due to prolonged and excessive pressures causing crush injuries of nerves.

Pneumothorax. The incidence of pneumothorax in association with nerve blocks is variable.[65,66] Stellate ganglion, brachial plexus, cervical plexus, intercostal, thoracic paravertebral, and interpleural blocks have all been linked to the occurrence of pneumothorax.

As reported by de Jong the majority of pneumothoraces are unrecognized unless by routine examination of all patients.[67] He demonstrated a 25% pneumothorax rate in patients undergoing supraclavicular brachial plexus block, a block that is reported to have a 0.2 to 6% symptomatic pneumothorax rate. Thus, extreme concern and a move to immediate action may be unwarranted on the part of the anesthesiologist if a small pneumothorax is found incidentally. Documentation, follow-up radiographs, and avoidance of the use of nitrous oxide should a general anesthetic technique be required over the next 3 to 6 weeks constitutes judicious care of the patient.

Generally a pneumothorax is the direct result of disruption of the visceral pleura with subsequent entrainment of inspired gases. The extent of the pneumothorax is usually governed by the size and number of rents, the degree of pleural scarring (which can prevent collapse of lung), the underlying condition of the lung parenchyma, and whether or not nitrous oxide was used intraoperatively for analgesia. In addition, the size of the pneumothorax is limited by blood clot formation within the pleural puncture site. As the lung collapses upon itself the disrupted area is occluded.

Routine use of postoperative radiographs in uneventful blocks is not indicated. Clinically, if the possibility of a pneumothorax is suspected by sudden coughing, chest pain, decreased ipsilateral breath sounds, onset of dyspnea, or a rise in peak airway pressure, an end-expiratory chest film (PA or AP) should be obtained. As the lung is essentially a cylinder, when pleural separation is greater than 3 cm the patient may have a 50% pneumothorax by volume (Figure 10–4). A simple pneumothorax usually does not result in hemodynamnic instability or respiratory embarrassment except in the patient with diffuse underlying lung disease or in the patient who develops a tension pneumothorax. The latter is generally the

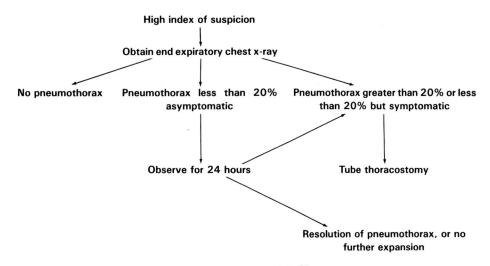

Figure 10–4. Management of Pneumothorax.

result of a one-way flap valve mechanism (air is trapped under pressure) and is an emergency that requires immediate attention. The ensuing mediastinal shift can rapidly lead to cardiovascular collapse. It can be alleviated by needle decompression followed by tube thoracostomy.

As noted above, all pneumothoraces do not require tube thoracostomy. A large number can be managed conservatively if they are not increasing. These will be reabsorbed at the rate of approximately 1.25% per day, and will be fully reabsorbed within 3 to 6 weeks.[68]

Numerous steps can be taken to minimize the chances of incurring a pneumothorax. Careful, unrushed technique in a willing, cooperative patient is essential. Secondly, awareness of the anatomical landmarks and hand-controlling of the needle braced against the patient at all times are important.

Needle Trauma. The same factors that contribute to neural damage in other regional techniques contribute to nerve damage related to peripheral blocks. Paresthesias are often an integral part of the performance of many nerve blocks. In addition, the training of many anesthesiologists focused on eliciting paresthesias prior to injection of local anesthetic solution as a prerequisite for the successful completion of blocks. Despite this fact, needle-induced trauma has remained a rare occurrence. The incidence of postanesthetic neuropathy ranges from approximately 0.1 to 5.6%.[69] Rapid injection of local anesthetic solution can increase the number and severity of these neuropathies.

Through the use of peripheral nerve stimulators and specially designed needles (blunt, pencil-point, short bevel), the problem of needle-induced nerve injury can be diminished. As previously stated, neuro-

logic exam and electromyographic studies are of utmost importance in achieving an early diagnosis.

Intravenous Regional Anesthesia

Intravenous regional anesthesia (Bier block) technique has demonstrated its efficacy even in the most unskilled hands. It has had an impressive safety record (until the widespread use of high concentrations of bupivacaine) despite the large volume of agent required for successful anesthesia.

Complications with the technique are directly related to the local and systemic effects of the anesthetic agent used. A sterile chemical thrombophlebitis can result from the use of 2-chloroprocaine (one of the least systemically toxic agents). Systemic toxicity is the result of absorption of a bolus of local anesthetic agent.

If certain precautions are taken the chances of systemic loading can be minimized. Safety measures include documenting integrity of the tourniquet prior to injection, maintaining tourniquet pressure at least 100 mm Hg above the patient's systolic blood pressure, sustaining tourniquet inflation for at least 20 minutes, and utilizing slow periodic deflation at the completion of surgery. With this technique there is minimal protracted postoperative analgesia, thus lessening the early use of analgesics.

SUMMARY

Regional and local anesthesia, like general anesthesia, are safe methods of relieving intraoperative pain. Lasting complications after any anesthetic technique are rare. However, postoperative problems associated with regional anesthetics are more likely to be associated with poor technique or incomplete understanding of the drugs used. The best therapy is prevention of complication by initial performance of a careful, unhurried block.

REFERENCES

1. Caplan RA, Ward RJ, Posner K, Cheney FW: Unexpected cardiac arrest during spinal anesthesia. A closed claims analysis of predisposing factors. *Anesthesiology* 1988;68:5–11.

2. Whitcher C, Ream AK, Parsons D, et al: Anesthetic mishaps and the cost of monitoring. A proposed standard for monitoring equipment. *J Clin Monit* 1988;4:5–15.

3. Eichorn JH, Cooper JB, Cullen DJ, et al: Standards for patient monitoring during anesthesia at Harvard Medical School. *JAMA* 1986;256:1017–1020.

4. Aldrete JA, Kroulik D: A post anesthetic recovery score. *Anesth Analg* 1970;49:924–934.

5. Steward DJ: A simplified scoring system for the postoperative recovery room. *Can Anesth Soc J* 1975;22:111–113.

6. Alexander CM, Teller LE, Gross JB, et al: New discharge criteria decrease recovery room time after subarachnoid block. *Anesthesiology* 1989;70:640–643.

7. Daos FG, Virtue RW: Sympathetic block persistence after spinal or epidural analgesia. *JAMA* 1963;183:285–287.

8. Pflug AE, Aasheim GM, Foster C: Sequence of return of neurological function and criteria for safe ambulation following subarachnoid block. *Can Anaesth Soc J* 1978;25:133–139.

9. Wetchler BV: Postoperative management, discharge, and follow up; Outpatient anesthesia. *Anesth Clin N Am* 1987;131–132.

10. Albright GA: Cardiac arrest following regional anesthesia with etidocaine or bupivacaine. *Anesthesiology* 1979;51:285–286.

11. Prentiss JE: Cardiac arrest following cardiac anesthesia. *Anesthesiology* 1979;50:51–53.

12. Marx GF: Cardiotoxicity of local anesthetics—The plot thickens. *Anesthesiology* 1984;60:3–5.

13. Clarkson CW, Hondeghem LM: Mechanism for bupivacaine depression of cardiac conduction: Fast block of sodium channels during the action potential with slow recovery from block during diastole. *Anesthesiology* 1985;62:396–405.

14. DeJong RH, Robles R, Corbin RW: Central actions of lidocaine—Synaptic transmission. *Anesthesiology* 1969;30: 19–23.

15. Wagman IH, deJong RJ, Prince DA: Effects of lidocaine on the CNS. *Anesthesiology* 1967;28:155–172.

16. Kasten GW, Martin ST: Successful cardiovascular resuscitation after massive intravenous bupivacaine overdose in anesthetized dogs. *Anesth Analg* 1985;64:491–497.

17. Moore DC, Bridenbaugh LD: Oxygen: The antidote for systemic toxic reactions from local anesthetic drugs. *JAMA* 1960;174:842–847.

18. DeJong RH, Heavner JE: Diazepam prevents local anesthetic seizures. *Anesthesiology* 1971;34:523–531.

19. DeJong RH, Heavner JE: Local anesthetic seizure prevention: Diazepam vs pentobarbital. *Anesthesiology* 1972;36:449–457.

20. Gotta AW, O'Malley T, Stucker-Beat MS, Hartung J: Diazepam vs midazolam in the prevention of lidocaine toxicity in rats. *Anesth Analg* 1989;68:S107.

21. Winnie AP: *Plexus anesthesia: Perivascular techniques of brachial plexus block; neural complications.* Philadelphia, W.B. Saunders Co. 1983:253.

22. Marinacci AA, Courville CB: Electromyogram in evaluation of neurological complications of spinal anesthesia. *JAMA* 1958;168:1337–1345.

23. Marinacci AA: *Applied Electromyography.* Philadelphia, Lea & Febiger, 1968, pp 163–180.

24. Greene NM: *Physiology of Spinal Anesthesia,* ed 3. Baltimore, Williams & Wilkins, 1981, p 95.

25. Parnass SM, Curran MA, Becker GL: Comparative hypotensive responses of the carbonated and hydrochloride salts of lidocaine in epidural blocks. *Anesth Analg* 1987;66:S134.

26. Bonica JJ, Akamatsu TJ, Berges PU, et al: Circulatory effects of peridural block: II. Effect of epinephrine. *Anesthesiology* 1971;34:514–522.

27. Eckstein KL, Marx GF: Aortocaval compression and uterine displacement. *Anesthesiology* 1974;40:92–96.

28. Askrog VF, Smith TC, Eckenhoff JE: Changes in pulmonary ventilation during spinal anesthesia. *Surg Gyn Obstet* 1964;119:563–567.

29. Egbert LD, Tamersoy K, Deas TC: Pulmonary function during spinal anesthesia. The mechanism of cough depression. *Anesthesiology* 1961;22:882–885.

30. Katz J, Renck H: *Handbook of thoraco-abdominal nerve block. Debatable applications.* Philadelphia, Grune and Stratton, 1987, 5:190.

31. Stevens RA, Stanton-Hicks M: Subdural infection of local anesthetic: A complication of epidural anesthesia. *Anesthesiology* 1985;63:323–327.

32. Vandam, LD, Dripps RD: Long term follow up of patients who received 10,098 spinal anesthetics: III. Syndrome of decreased intracranial pressure. *JAMA* 1956;161:586–591.

33. Flaatten H, Rodt SA, Vamnes J, et al: Postdural puncture headache. A comparison between 26- and 29-gauge needles in young patients. *Anaesthesia* 1989;44:147–149.

34. Norris MC, Leighton BL, DeSimone CA: Needle bevel direction and headache after inadvertent dural puncture. *Anesthesiology* 1989;70:729–731.

35. Cuplin SR, Ready LB, Haschke RH: Influence of spinal needle tip design and bevel orientation of fluid leak across human dura. *Anesthesiology* 1988;69:3A A340.

36. Yeager MP, Glass DD, Neff RK, et al: Epidural anesthesia and analgesia in high risk surgical patients. *Anesthesiology* 1987;66:729–736.

37. Corbatt P, Van Crevel H: Lumbar puncture headache. Controlled study of the preventive effect of 24 hours bedrest. *Lancet* 1981;2:1133–1135.

38. Jones RJ: The role of recumbency in the prevention and

treatment of postspinal headache. *Anesth Analg* 1974;53:788–797.

39. Palahniuk RJ, Cumming M: Prophylactic blood patch does not prevent post lumbar puncture headache. *Can Anesth Soc J* 1979;26:132–133.

40. Loesser EA, Hill GE, Bennett GM, et al: Time vs success rate for epidural blood patch. *Anesthesiology* 1978;49:147–148.

41. Anderson EF: Immediate blood patching after inadvertant dural puncture. *Anesth Rev* 1985;12:2,49–55.

42. Ackerman WE, Colclough GW: Prophylactic epidural blood patch. The controversy continues. *Anesth Analg* 1987;66:913–922.

43. Rice GG, Dabbs CH: The use of peridural and subarachnoid injections of saline solution in the treatment of severe postspinal headache. *Anesthesiology* 1950;11:17–23.

44. Craft JB, Epstein BS, Carkley CS: Prophylaxis of dural puncture headache with epidural saline. *Anesth Analg* 1973;52:228–231.

45. Shnider SM, Levinson G: Anesthesia for Cesarean section, in Shnider SM, Levinson G (eds): *Anesthesia for Obstetrics*. Baltimore, Williams & Wilkins, 1987, p 165.

46. Cohen S, Daitch JS, Goldiner PL: An alternative method for management of accidental dural puncture for labor and delivery. *Anesthesiology* 1989;70:165–166.

47. Abouleish E, de la Vega S, Blendinger I, et al: Long term follow up of epidural blood patch. *Anesth Analg* 1975;51:459–463.

48. Digiovanni AJ, Galbert MW, Wahle WM: Epidural injection of autologous blood for post lumbar-puncture headache. *Anesth Analg* 1972;51:226–232.

49. Moore DC: Complications of regional anesthesia, in Bonica JJ (ed): *Clinical Anesthesia, Regional Anesthesia: Recent Advances and Current Status*. Philadelphia, Davis, 1969, pp 217–251.

50. Moir DD, Davidson S: Postpartum complications of forceps delivery performed under epidural and pudendal nerve block. *Brit J Anaesth* 1972;44:1197–1199.

51. Peng ALC, Behar S, Blancato LS: Reduction of post lumbar puncture backache by the use of field block anesthesia prior to lumbar puncture. *Anesthesiology* 1985;63:226–228.

52. Lund PC: *Principles and Practice of Spinal Anesthesia*. Springfield, IL, Chas C Thomas, 1971, pp 504–601.

53. Kane RF: Neurologic deficits following epidural or spinal anesthesia. *Anesth Analg* 1981;60:150–161.

54. Gilman AG, Goodman LS, Rall TW, et al: *The Pharma-* cological Basis of Therapeutics: Local Anesthetics, New York, Macmillan, 1985, p 318.

55. Reisner LS, Hochman BN, Plumer MH: Persistent neurological deficit and adhesive arachnoiditis following intrathecal 2-chloroprocaine injection. *Anesth Analg* 1980;58:452–454.

56. Gissen AJ, Datta S, Lambert D: The chloroprocaine controversy: II. Is chloroprocaine neurotoxic? *Reg Anesth* 1984;9:135–145.

57. Marx GF: Maternal complications of regional anesthesia. *Reg Anesth* 1981;6:3,104–107.

58. De Angelis J: Hazards of subdural and epidural anesthesia during anticoagulant therapy: A case report and review. *Anesth Analg* 1972;51:676–679.

59. Odoom JA, Sih IL: Epidural analgesia and anticoagulant therapy. Experience with 1000 cases of continuous epidurals. *Anaesthesia* 1983;38:254–259.

60. Rao TLK, El-Etr AA: Anticoagulation following placement of epidural and subarachnoid catheters: An evaluation of neurologic sequelae. *Anesthesiology* 1981;55:618–620.

61. Bromage PR: *Epidural Analgesia: Complications and Contradictions*. Philadelphia, Saunders, p 665.

62. Kaufman RD, Reynolds RC: Occlusion of an epidural catheter secondary to osteoarthritis. *Anesthesiology* 1976;44:253–255.

63. Kehlet H: The modifying effect of general and regional anesthesia on the endocrine-metabolic response to surgery. *Reg Anesth* 1982;7:S38.

64. Moldaver J: Tourniquet paralysis syndrome. *Arch Surg* 1954;63:136–144.

65. Winnie AP: *Plexus Anesthesia: Pervascular Techniques of Brachial Plexus Block*. Philadelphia, Saunders, 1983, p 227.

66. Orkin FK, Cooperman LH: *Complications in Anesthesiology: Neural Complications*. Philadelphia, Lippincott, 1983, p 176.

67. De Jong RH: Axillary block of the brachial plexus. *Anesthesiology* 1961;22:215–225.

68. Schwartz SI, Shires GT, Spencer FC, et al: *Principles of Surgery: Chest Wall, Pleura, Lung and Mediastinum*, ed 3. New York, McGraw-Hill, 1979, p 654.

69. Selander D, Dhuner KG, Lundborg G: Peripheral nerve injury due to injection needles used for regional anesthesia. An experimental study of the acute effects of needle point trauma. *Acta Anaesth Scand* 1977;21:182–188.

11 The Cardiovascular Patient

Claudia Komer

Patients now being referred for cardiovascular surgery are often older with more extensive atherosclerosis, impaired ventricular function, and coexisting subsystem organ impairment. Technical advances, however, have resulted in improved preoperative assessment, more complete revascularization, better myocardial protection, and more comprehensive postoperative monitoring, contributing to an overall decrease in operative risk and perioperative mortality.[1]

To optimally manage the postoperative cardiovascular patient, the anesthesiologist must have a thorough understanding of the surgical procedure and anticipate likely postoperative complications. Monitoring techniques should provide detailed information regarding changes in organ function and guide specific therapeutic intervention. In addition, physiologic alterations including hypoventilation, hypoxia, acidosis, and electrolyte imbalance, represent dangers that may produce serious dysrhythmias, low cardiac output, and sudden death, and should be aggressively treated.

Lastly, the physician caring for such patients must maintain a sound understanding of hemodynamic and ventilatory function as well as of the pathophysiology of extracorporeal circulation and its ill-defined systemic effects.

TRANSPORT

The transport of the postoperative cardiac patient occurs during a period of physiologic instability. Prior to preparing the patient for transfer, the cardiovascular system must be stabilized utilizing the intraaortic balloon pump and/or ventricular assist device if necessary.

Stability of the respiratory and hemostatic system must be assessed. Arterial blood gases should be optimized and coagulation status normalized. Blood samples to assess partial thromboplastin time (PTT), prothrombin time (PT), thrombin time (TT), platelet count, and fibrinogen level should be sent from the operating room in order for results to be readily available upon patient arrival in the postanesthetic care unit (PACU) or cardiac surgery intensive care unit (CSICU).

In preparing for transfer, adequate anesthesia and muscle relaxation must be assured. Right- and left-sided filling pressures should be reevaluated and optimized. If an external pacemaker is being used, it should be set on the demand mode, particularly in the presence of underlying competing rhythms. Drugs being administered should be reviewed, rate of infusion reassessed, and left ventricular response confirmed.

Intravenous infusions should be placed in an orderly fashion, and their function confirmed. The endotracheal tube should be secured properly, secretions suctioned and equal breath sounds verified.

The presence of a transport monitor with capability of both ECG and arterial pressure monitoring and a full oxygen E cylinder should be noted. If the intraaortic balloon pump is being used, optimal augmentation as well as adequacy of battery power should be assured. The patient should be provided an FIO_2 of 1.0, which can be accomplished by using a modification of the Ayre's T-piece with a flow rate of 10 to 12 L/minute.

The move should be effected slowly and smoothly in an effort to minimize vascular volume shifts and changes in cardiac rhythm. Above all, the anesthesiologist's attention must not be diverted from the patient.

The receiving unit should be notified at least 30 minutes in advance regarding the patient's status and any special needs.

ADMISSION

Upon arrival, the ventilatory parameters found optimal in the operating room during the postbypass period should be instituted at an FIO_2 of at least 0.6 The chest should be auscultated and adequate breath sounds verified. Vital signs, including heart rate, rhythm, arterial pressure, and filling pressures, should be noted. Infusion rates of administered drugs should be verified and cardiovascular response confirmed. Crystalloid as well as blood should be available.

A complete patient report should be conveyed, including the transmission of significant preoperative, intraoperative, and specific postbypass data. End points regarding hemodynamic parameters and inotropic and vasoactive drug administration should be communicated to the nursing staff.

PULMONARY FUNCTION

Several organ systems are at particular risk after cardiac surgery and require individual assessment and specific therapy. Gibbon reported in 1959 that postoperative pulmonary dysfunction contributed more than any other complication to the morbidity of cardiac surgery with extracorporeal circulation.[2] In the 1960s, a frequently fatal pulmonary complication known to follow prolonged cardiopulmonary bypass (CPB) was identified as the ''post perfusion syndrome.''[3] It is manifest clinically as generalized weakness, anorexia, fever, respiratory insufficiency, hypoventilation, dyspnea, and sometimes cyanosis. Pulmonary function is disturbed as revealed by a definite impairment of blood gas diffusion, including hypercapnia and hypoxemia. Microscopically, diffuse atelectasis and severe congestion with perivascular and intraalveolar hemorrhage are present.[3,4] With improved technology and surgical methodology, including the use of the membrane oxygenator, this once-frequent complication is rarely seen today.

Extracorporeal circulation alters pulmonary function in nearly all patients undergoing cardiac operations.[5] The pathophysiology of the cellular injury that occurs in the lungs is not fully understood; however, interaction between cellular and humoral components of blood with the foreign surfaces of the extracorporeal circulation circuit has been described.[6] In fact, changes in plasma proteins including those of the coagulation system have been shown to result after the contact of blood with foreign surfaces, including blood–gas interfaces during bypass.[7,8]

Evidence suggests a role for complement activation and associated neutrophil sequestration. Complement levels fall and complement degradation products C3a and C5a are elaborated during CPB. C5a is rapidly bound to circulating neutrophils, which are sequestered in the pulmonary circulation during reperfusion of the lungs.[9] Mediated by the alternate complement pathway, lysosomal enzymes are released from these leukocytes. Microaggregates of these injured leukocytes form, and when filtered lodge in the alveolar microcirculation.[10] In addition, oxygen-free radicals are generated, which contribute to lipid peroxidation and damage the alveolar capillary membrane. This in turn leads to interstitial hemorrhage, engorgement of the pulmonary vascular bed, and miliary atelectasis.[11-13]

Antonsen and associates[14] studied neutrophil enzyme release and complement activation, measuring plasma concentrations of complement factor C4, complement split product C3D, elastase, and fibronectin in adult patients undergoing bypass. He found that complement was activated by the alternate pathway. Plasma concentrations of elastase, a protease released from activated neutrophils, rose exponentially during bypass implying extensive destruction of neutrophils, accelerating during the course of CPB. In addition, Antonsen found that the change in elastase concentration paralleled complement activation.

It is the hypothesis that pulmonary membrane damage is secondary to protease enzyme release that has prompted investigation regarding the use of antiproteases such as aprotinin in an attempt to attenuate the damaging affects of CPB.[15]

Complement activation has also been shown to result in a generalized increase in microvascular permeability. This assumption is based on determination of an increased interstitial fluid volume a few hours after cardiac surgery, and of the direct relationship between the durations of CPB and fluid flux.[16] Boldt and associates[17] studied elderly patients undergoing cardiac surgery to evaluate the effects of age on extravascular lung water content. They found that increasing age is associated with greater changes in extravascular lung water content after CPB, presumably due to more pronounced fragility of the pulmonary endothelial membrane and/or depressed left ventricular performance.

It is now understood that both membrane and bubble oxygenators activate the alternate pathway of complement, whereas in addition bubble oxygenators activate the classical pathway.[6]

Clinically, maximal pulmonary impairment is seen 24 hours postoperatively, gradually improving over the following seven to eight days. Braun and coworkers[18] studied the effects of cardiac surgery on various ventilatory parameters. They reported vital capacity to be 50% of control by postoperative day three, and 60 to 70% of control on the seventh postoperative day, not returning to preoperative values for 2 weeks.[19] Schramel and associates[20] reported a 25 to 40% reduction in diffusion capacity postoperatively, which remained abnormal 2 weeks postoperatively. Total lung capacity, inspiratory capacity, and functional residual capacity (FRC) are also reduced in the postoperative period.[18,19]

The reduction in functional residual capacity is further exacerbated by poor lung reexpansion after CPB; small tidal volumes; fixed tidal volumes not interrupted by sighs or PEEP; extravascular lung water; spontaneous ventilation under the effects of anesthesia or narcotics; inadequate clearance of secretions; decreased surfactant production; alveolar hypoventilation; regional hypoperfusion of the lung; and direct pressure by pleural fluid, chest tubes, or blood.

Clinical manifestations of postoperative pulmonary impairment include an increase in tracheobronchial secretions, increased A–aDo$_2$ gradient and intrapulmonary shunting, and decreased compliance. Decreased FRC further increases both intrapulmonary shunt and ventilation perfusion mismatching.[22] If the FRC remains low at the time of extubation, the withdrawal of positive pressure support facilitates alveolar collapse so that gross atelectasis and hypoxemia become evident. With atelectasis, surfactant is lost and lung reexpansion is then not possible with normal tidal volumes. Lung stiffness and work of breathing increase, and a vicious cycle results.[21]

Factors critical to the development of respiratory insufficiency after bypass have been identified. A CPB pump time greater than 120 to 150 minutes is reported to result in an increase in the severity of damage sustained by the lung. Sequestration of polymorphonuclear leukocytes in alveolar vasculature, and the normality of the lung prior to surgery, are key factors. Ratliff and associates[5] clearly demonstrated that a healthy lung is much more resistant to the trauma of cardiopulmonary bypass than is a previously injured lung.

Management

Atelectasis occurs in 62 to 84% of patients undergoing open heart surgery secondary to the effects of CPB, anesthesia, secretions, excessive fluid loading, and preexisting lung disease. This results in a reduction in FRC, increase in intrapulmonary shunt and ventilation perfusion mismatching, widening the alveolar-aterial oxygen gradient, and causing hypoxemia. Hypoxemia may subsequently lead to myocardial ischemia and dysrhythmias if not aggressively treated.[21]

In the PACU, the respiratory system is mechanically assisted to ensure adequate gas exchange during a phase of metabolic and hemodynamic instability. Initially the patient should be provided an FIo$_2$ of 0.6 or greater to avoid hypoxemia, as transport may be associated with ventilatory deterioration (Table 11–1).

Tidal volumes of 12 to 15 cc/kg should be provided with the goal of maximizing oxygenation and FRC. Initial ventilatory requirements may be as low as 80 to 90 mL/kg/min as CO$_2$ production is reduced secondary to the patient's hypothermic state. However, as the patient rewarms, CO$_2$ production will increase and ventilatory adjustments must be made. Minute ventilation should be reduced by 10% for each degree below 37°C; otherwise the postoperative patient may initially be hyperventilated and predisposed to ventricular irritability. In addition, hyperventilation can predispose the patient to coronary artery spasm.

To ensure a more laminar flow, inspiratory flow rates should be maintained at about 30 L/min. Peak inspiratory pressures should also be monitored. If the peak inspiratory pressure exceeds 35 cm H$_2$O, inadequate analgesia, chest wall rigidity, shivering, or excessively large tidal volumes, may be causative.

Arterial blood gas analyses are necessary to appropriately adjust ventilatory parameters in the early rewarming period and to allow weaning. Although helpful, endtidal CO$_2$ (ETCO2) is in itself inadequate in evaluating ventilation in the post-cardiac-surgery patient.[23]

Mechanical Ventilation   There has been much debate regarding the most appropriate mode of mechanical ventilation for the post-cardiac-surgery patient. Historically, following cardiac surgery, controlled mechanical ventilation (CMV) was used until patients met the clinical criteria for extubation (Table 11–2). Following a T-piece trial, their tracheas were extubated if the clinical criteria were satisfied.

Controlled mechanical ventilation provides respiratory stability during a potentially unstable hemodynamic interval, allows for maximum sedation and analgesia, and reduces increased work of breathing.[24]

The use of CMV has potential disadvantages. Increased airway and pleural pressures associated with

TABLE 11–1. GUIDELINES FOR INITIAL VENTILATOR PARAMETERS

F$_1$O$_2$	(Inspired oxygen concentration)	0.6
V$_T$	(Tidal volume)	12–15 mL/kg
f	(Frequency)	8/min
V$_E$	(Minute ventilation)	90 mL/kg/min (34°C)
PEEP	(Positive end-expiratory pressure)	5 cm H$_2$O
I:E ratio < 1:2	(Inspiratory/expiratory ratio)	
Peak inspiratory flow		30 LPM
PIP	(Peak inspiratory pressure)	< 35 cm H$_2$O
P$_{plat}$	(Plateau pressure)	< 3 cm H$_2$O
Cs	(Static compliance)	> 60 mL/cm H$_2$O

TABLE 11-2. CRITERIA FOR EXTUBATION

1. Patient alert, responsive to verbal stimuli, able to protect airway
2. Resolution of the effects of narcotics and neuromuscular blockers
3. Normal gas exchange
   pH > 7.35, $PaCO_2$ < 45 mm Hg, PaO_2 > 60 @ FIO_2 < 0.4
   Respiratory rate of < 28/min
4. Forced vital capacity > 15 mL/kg
   Maximum inspiratory force > −25 cm H_2O
5. $A-aDO_2$ < 250 and Qs/QT > 0.20
6. Hemodynamically stable
   Normothermic
   Low dose or no ionotrope
   Absence of dysrhythmias
   Absence of bleeding

CMV can decrease cardiac output by impeding venous return and altering diastolic volume pressure characteristics of the left ventricle.[25] Hypocapnia, which frequently occurs during the CMV mode, increases venous admixture, decreases compliance and cardiac output, and shifts the hemoglobin dissociation curve to the left. These changes combine to decrease PaO_2 and O_2 delivery to the tissues. With regards to weaning, some patients may be able to sustain spontaneous respiration who are unable to fulfill T-piece trial, unnecessarily prolonging controlled ventilation. In addition, CMV is useful only in the sedated or paralyzed patient.

Intermittent mandatory ventilation (IMV) has potential advantages.[26] It allows patients to set their own $PaCO_2$ levels preventing respiratory alkalosis. In addition, the IMV mode maintains respiratory muscle function, and reduces the cardiovascular effects of mechanical ventilation associated with positive end-expiratory pressure (PEEP) by maintaining lower mean intrapleural pressures.[27] Ventilation without sedation or paralysis is possible, offering a smoother, and perhaps more rapid, transition from mechanical to spontaneous ventilation.

The effect of ventricular function on airway pressure changes was reported by Mathru.[28] Those individuals who had normal ventricular function preoperatively had a large increase in cardiac index and stroke volume index when changed from CMV to IMV, presumably because of increased venous return. Conversely, patients with left ventricular dysfunction preoperatively had a paradoxical decrease in cardiac index associated with a significant increase in right atrial pressure (RAP) and pulmonary artery occlusion pressure (PAOP) with the institution of IMV, perhaps due to the increased venous return associated with reduced airway pressures. This autotransfusion effect is not well tolerated by an already com-

promised left ventricle. These hemodynamic changes were reversed by adding 5 cm H_2O of PEEP to IMV, or returning to the CMV mode. Thus, depending on the cardiac status, the ventilatory pattern used may have differing effects on hemodynamics, and should be tailored to each patient based on individual need and cardiac reserve.[24]

PEEP. Since most evidence suggests that arterial hypoxemia following CPB results from airway collapse rather than pulmonary microvascular injury, the application of PEEP following open heart surgery has been widely advocated and its efficacy in reducing atelectasis and right-to-left intrapulmonary shunting documented. Many studies have shown that in those cardiac surgery patients who receive PEEP as part of their postoperative ventilatory management, reversal of atelectasis is more rapid.[29] Good and associates[30] demonstrated that PEEP significantly increased PaO_2/PAO_2 during the first 15 hours after CPB. Marvel and co-workers[31] more recently, however, reported that the absence of a sustained benefit from the routine application of PEEP is consistent with the theory that PEEP can reverse arterial hypoxemia but does little to reverse underlying pathophysiologic mechanisms responsible for arterial hypoxemia.[25] Early administration of PEEP to patients at risk for ARDS has been reported to have no effect on the incidence of pulmonary dysfunction, and PEEP does not decrease lung water content.

Methods of selecting the optimal level of PEEP are varied. Many investigators routinely administer 3 to 9 cm of H_2O, while others advocate a level of PEEP that produces the highest level of static thoracic compliance. Unless chest wall rigidity is increasing, static chest compliance will improve after a PEEP increment if it reverses atelectasis and decreases lung stiffness. A widening of inspiratory pressure-plateau pressure (PIP–Pplat) infers that PEEP is increasing airway resistance and dead space rather than decreasing shunting.[21]

In a PEEP trial, the goal is to reach a level that achieves a PaO_2 of greater than 100 mm Hg at an FIO_2 of 0.4 or less, with hemodynamic stability. Oxygen delivery should be calculated and SvO_2 determined to ensure that PEEP does not adversely affect oxygen transport and extraction.[32]

The hemodynamic consequences of PEEP include a decrease in cardiac index (CI) and stroke volume index (SVI). These changes are thought to be secondary to a decrease in left ventricular end-diastolic volume (LVEDV), which is probably the result of a decrease in transpulmonary blood flow, direct pulmonary compressive effects, abnormal septal shifting, autonomic alterations, and increased pulmonary vascular resistance.[33] The magnitude of airway pressure transmitted to the heart, central circulation, and pleural space determines the magnitude of hemodynamic change. Vascular pressures measured during mechanical ventilation with PEEP may seem normal or slightly increased, but in fact may be inadequate to maintain ventricular filling pressures dependent on attendant pressure transmitted to the pleural space. Once PEEP has been implemented, the hemodynamic consequences of excessive volume administration may become manifest only after discontinuation of PEEP. With this abrupt decrease in airway pressure, there is acute redistribution of intravenous volume from the capacitance bed to the central circulation, which may result in a sudden increase in cardiac filling pressures.[28]

Although PEEP can be utilized for optimizing oxygenation, careful monitoring of hemodynamic variables and pulmonary gas exchange is essential. Obvious contraindications to its use include bronchospasm, emphysema, suspected pneumothorax, and cardiovascular instability.[21]

Controversy Regarding Early Extubation

In the early decades of cardiac surgery, assisted mechanical ventilation usually lasted until at least the first postoperative morning. Recent concerns regarding lengthly intensive care unit stays, and risks of mechanical ventilation, have provided impetus for investigations demonstrating the practicality of early extubation.

Midell and associates[34] in 1974 and Prakash and associates[35] in 1977 published the first reports challenging conventional methods of care. In each of these studies, 90% of patients were extubated successfully within several hours of operation without significant incidence of reintubation or morbidity. Quasha and co-workers[36] randomly studied early versus late extubation in 38 patients receiving an inhalation anesthetic for coronary revascularization. They found that early extubation did not adversely affect hemodynamic or pulmonary performance, and in fact was associated with a reduced incidence of postoperative hemodynamic morbidity. Gall and associates[37] studied the effects of endotracheal extubation on ventricular performance and concluded that postoperative patients with stable cardiopulmonary physiology respond to endotracheal extubation with improved cardiac performances as a result of enhanced ventricular filling. These benefits may be derived earlier in the postoperative period if mechanical ventilation is discontinued as soon as extubation criteria are met. Numerous studies concur that early extubation should be a standard of current care after uncomplicated elective cardiac operations.

Although the major limiting factor in evaluating a patient for early extubation is the anesthetic technique used, good preoperative physical status including both ventricular and pulmonary function are important selection criteria.[35,36]

Principles of weaning from assisted ventilation involve progressively decreasing the inspired oxygen fraction, as an FIO_2 of greater than 0.6 for greater than 24 hours can result in lung damage secondary to oxygen toxicity. When the patient is able to maintain an arterial PO_2 of 80 to 100 mm Hg at an FIO_2 of 0.4 to 0.5, the IMV rate is lowered in decrements of two breaths per minute. The rate is progressively decreased, while maintaining a pH of 7.35. Once the IMV rate has been lowered to four breaths per minute, PEEP is gradually decreased and ultimately the patient is placed on continuous positive airway pressure (CPAP) for one hour prior to evaluation for extubation.

Indications for extubation include an awake, alert, normothermic, and hemodynamically stable patient (Table 11-2). Normal arterial blood gases, including a pH of greater than 7.35, $PaCO_2$ of less than 45 mm Hg, PaO_2 of greater than 60 mm Hg, and an FIO_2 of less than or equal to 0.4. In addition, a forced vital capacity of greater than 15 mL/kg and a maximum inspiratory force of at least -28 cm H_2O have been found to correlate with successful weaning.[32]

Following extubation the patient should be provided with supplemental humidified O_2 by mask. Coughing, deep breathing, and incentive spirometry should be encouraged to maximize FRC, mobilize secretions, and prevent transient hypoxemia.

MYOCARDIAL FUNCTION

Low Cardiac Output State

The most frequent cause of poor outcome after cardiac surgery is low cardiac output, which may lead to organ dysfunction (Table 11-3).[38] The mortality rate in patients with low cardiac output who require mechanical ventilation over 24 hours is about 20%, in the

TABLE 11-3.   EVALUATION OF LOW CARDIAC OUTPUT

Effect	Causative Factors
Decrease preload	Hypovolemia
	Blood loss
	Diuresis
	Vasodilatation
	Rewarming
	Drug induced
Decreased contractibility	Myocardial ischemia/infarction
	Acid–base imbalance
	Hypoxia
	Drug induced
	Mechanical ventilation (decreased atrial contraction)

absence of acute lung injury. A combination of acute lung injury with low cardiac output increases the mortality rate to 40%.[39] In a study of 34 patients after open heart surgery, 15 of the patients had cardiac indices of less than 2.0 1/min/m². This low-output group had a higher mortality and more frequent occurence of sudden death.[40] Mortality associated with low cardiac output is further increased if it is associated with left ventricular failure.

In the case of difficult or incomplete revascularization, prolonged cardiopulmonary bypass and aortic cross-clamp time and difficulty in cardiopulmonary bypass weaning, postoperative ventricular dysfunction should be anticipated. Central cyanosis, cold and poorly perfused extremeties despite normal core temperature, weak peripheral pulses, hypotension, tachycardia, oliguria, and systolic hypotension suggest a poor prognosis.

Low cardiac output can be diagnosed by using thermodilution, dye dilution techniques, or by using the Fick principle, which necessitates the determination of oxygen uptake and mixed venous oxygen difference. The most commonly used technique is thermodilution, which offers the advantage of being able to obtain output values at frequent intervals while simultaneously monitoring filling pressures. It has been found to be more accurate at low cardiac outputs as there is no recirculation.

Two-dimensional transesophageal echocardiography (TEE) can also be used to differentially diagnose the low cardiac output state (Fig. 11–1). Matsumato and co-workers[41] have reported the validity and reproductibility of TEE in evaluating left ventricular

performance in the cardiac surgical patient. Terai and associates[42] confirmed TEE to be a valid, reliable technique for assessing cardiac performance in the intensive care setting. This device enables continuous cardiac evaluation of wall motion, ventricular dimensions, and cardiac output, and allows ready assessment of therapeutic intervention.

A systematic evaluation of cardiovascular parameters should be performed in an effort to appropriately direct therapeutic intervention in the patient with a low cardiac output state. Inadequate left ventricular end-diastolic volume due to hypovolemia frequently occurs in the early postoperative period, resulting in reduced cardiac output. Bleeding must be aggressively treated and hemostatic parameters evaluated. Fluid and blood balance should be followed closely as concealed hemorrhage in the absence of tamponade can occur, especially after internal mammary artery dissection. Vasodilation from rapid rewarming, vasodilator therapy, excessive diuresis, and increased capillary permeability may contribute to hypovolemia. The use of hemodilution prime in the CPB pump circuit promotes postoperative diuresis secondary to reduced colloid osmotic pressure. This effect is further enhanced if an osmotic diuretic such as mannitol is used in the pump prime. The hemodynamic affects of hypovolemia can be further exacerbated by increased intrathoracic pressure as seen with PEEP. In addition, the loss of atrial contribution to ventricular filling, particularly in patients with reduced ventricular compliance, will further reduce left ventricular preload, possibly resulting in marked hypotension.

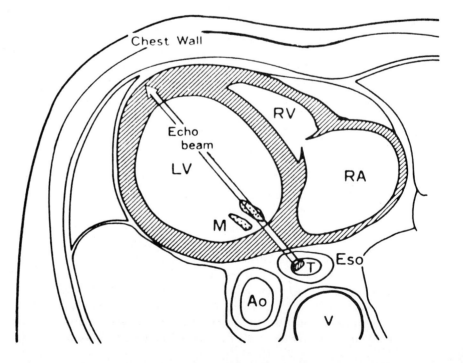

Figure 11–1. Schematic representation of two-dimensional transesophogeal echocardiogram. From the probe in the distil esophagus (Eso), the echo beam transverses the left ventricle (LV), permitting assessment of ventricular parameters, without interference from chest wall structures. RV = right ventricle; RA = right atrium; Ao = aorta; V = Inferior Vena Cava; M = mitral valve.

TABLE 11–4. DOSAGES OF COMMONLY USED VASOPRESSOR DRUGS

Drug	Dose	Effect
Epinephrine	1–2 mg/min	Primarily beta
	2–10 mg/min	Mixed alpha, beta
	10–20 mg/min	Primarily alpha
Norepinephrine	2.5–5 mg/min	Alpha, beta
Isoproterenol	1–5 mg/min	Beta
Dopamine	0.5–2.5 mg/kg/min	Dopaminergic receptor
	5–10 mg/kg/min	Primarily beta
	10–20 mg/kg/min	Primarily alpha
Dobutamine	2–20 mg/kg/min	Beta
Amrinone	1–3 mg/kg bolus	+ Inotrope, vasodilator
	5–15 μg/kg/min	
Phenylephrine	10–50 mg/min	Alpha

The diagnosis of hypovolemia is easily made since both RAP and PCWP are reduced. There has been no reported benefit of colloid administration over crystalloid infusion in restoring volume. Therefore, once blood losses have been replaced by the appropriate products, fluid replacement is a matter of preference.

Despite the use of cold potassium cardioplegia and hypothermia, myocardial dysfunction is commonly seen in the postoperative period. The cause of this dysfunction is often multifactorial and may involve myocardial ischemia, infarction, coronary vasospasm, emboli, hypoxia, acid–base abnormalities, and depressant agents such as beta blockers and calcium channel blockers.[39] Right and left ventricular failure may occur separately; however, fulminant left ventricular failure usually results in right ventricular dysfunction. Decreased cardiac output due to a hypocontractile state may require higher levels of preload inotropic agents and/or vasodilators. (Table 11–4).

In the face of suspected ischemia, empiric therapy with intravenous nitroglycerin can potentially improve regional ischemia. Concomitant inotropic support may be necessary to maintain adequate perfusion pressure.

If a low cardiac index persists and is associated with elevated ventricular filling pressures, despite aggressive pharmacologic intervention, insertion of an intraaortic balloon pump may be indicated. Particularly when ischemia is suspected as the etiology of pump failure, an IABP should be considered as it will increase coronary perfusion while reducing myocardial oxygen requirements and systemic afterload (Table 11–3).

The Hyperdynamic State

Excessive myocardial contractility characterizes the hyperdynamic state, which is particularly common in patients with preexisting left ventricular hypertrophy—for example, in patients with long-standing persistent hypertension, aortic stenosis, and idiopathic hypertrophic subaortic stenosis. These patients demonstrate normal to high cardiac output in the face of high systemic vascular resistence. The syndrome is more readily revealed when these patients are anesthetized with nondepressant narcotics. This increased inotropic state requires treatment with calcium channel antagonists or beta blockers to reduce myocardial oxygen demand. Care should be exercised when initiating vasodilator therapy as myocardial ischemia may ensue if diastolic hypotension is induced.

CORONARY SPASM

Use of the internal mammary artery (IMA) in coronary artery bypass grafting has been advocated because of its superior record of long-term patency. However, spasm of the graft has been recognized to be a potentially lethal postoperative phenomenon.

Blanche and Chaux[43] reported an episode of graft spasm occurring five hours postoperatively and resulting in acute left ventricular failure, circulatory collapse, and acute ischemic changes in the area supplied by the graft. Sarabu and associates[44] reported on the often-intractable nature of native coronary artery spasm, stating that many patients required direct intracoronary infusions of nitroglycerin or papaverine, and the majority required sublingual administration of nitroglycerin for resolution. They recommend immediate reoperation for acute refractory hemodynamic collapse in the early postoperative period to accurately assess the nature of the pathology.

Although coronary and systemic arteries differ in their degree of dilatative response to calcium channel blockers, nifedipine appears to be the most potent vasodilator on an equimolar basis. Currently it is recommended that calcium channel blockade be provided for those patients who experience such acute episodes.

In addition to the considerations of vasospasm, pharmacologic intervention has been found to modify internal mammary artery blood flow. Jett and associates[45] evaluated the relative effects of vasoactive drugs on IMA and saphenous vein graft blood flow in the canine model. Phenylephrine decreased blood flow in the IMA graft, while epinephrine administration resulted in an isolated increase in flow. Norepinephrine was found to increase graft flow; however, dP/dT also increased markedly, suggesting that this increase in flow was predominantly due to an increase in myocardial oxygen consumption.

HYPERTENSION

Postoperative hypertension occurs in approximately 30 to 60% of patients undergoing aortocoronary bypass operations and represents a major hemodynamic stress during a period when functional and metabolic recovery is incomplete.[46,47] Hypertensive episodes have been associated with cardiac ischemia and depressed ventricular performance, and certainly may induce a possibly fatal postoperative myocardial infarction. Potential predisposing factors include hypothermia, elevated plasma renin and angiotensin levels, elevated plasma epinephrine and norepinephrine levels, or pressor reflexes originating from the heart, great vessels, or coronary arteries.[42] Postoperative hypertension requires aggressive intervention to avoid progressive ischemia and left ventricular dysfunction. Several drugs have been used for this purpose (Table 11-5).

Vasodilators
Over the past decade sodium nitroprusside (SNP) has assumed a primary role in the treatment of postoperative hypertension. A known potent arteriolar vasodilator, it has less effect on venous tone, and a short half-life, permitting effective titration of blood pressure. It does not, however, reduce the tachycardia or increased inotropic state associated with postoperative hypertension.

TABLE 11-5. DOSAGES OF COMMONLY USED VASODILATOR DRUGS

Drug	Dose
Nitroglycerine	50–300 mg/min
Nitroprusside	25–100 mg/min (maximum 8 mg/kg/min and total dose < 1 mg/kg/min)
Phentolamine	50–500 mg/min
Trimethaphan	0.3 mg/min–6 mg/min

Concern regarding the use of SNP has been raised. Patel and colleagues[48] reported a 2.4% incidence of SNP toxicity after bypass in 292 patients. Three of seven patients died despite withdrawal of SNP when toxicity was recognized. Seltzer and associates[49] reported decreased arterial oxygenation associated with hypertension treated with SNP, which subsequently was found to be secondary to inhibition of adaptive hypoxic pulmonary vasoconstriction.

Nitroprusside results in a decrease in coronary perfusion pressure, which can reduce coronary flow to the vulnerable subendocardium.[50] In fact, Kaplan and Jones[51] reported that SNP improves hemodynamics without improvement of ECG changes. Mullin and associates[52] demonstrated that SNP therapy for postoperative hypertension is associated with a reversal to myocardial lactate production, without a decrease in coronary sinus blood flow, suggesting intracoronary steal. Nitroprusside may also decrease myocardial oxygen supply and regional blood flow, as well as flow to ischemic regions in patients with stable angina. In fact, ST segments may be further elevated in patients with acute myocardial infarction with SNP use.[53] Although SNP has been considered accepted therapy, it may well not be the ideal agent for postrevascularization hypertension.

Nitroglycerin (NTG) is a potent venodilator and mild arterial dilator. It has been effectively used in the treatment of postoperative hypertension; however, in patients with severe hypertension, NTG alone is not a satisfactory vasodilator and it is not as effective as SNP in restoring adequate left ventricular function in the transiently hypertensive patient with low cardiac output. NTG does decrease myocardial oxygen demand and relieves ischemia presumably by decreasing diastolic volumes. It may increase oxygen delivery to ischemic regions by dilating coronary arteries and collateral vessels and decreasing vasospasm. Myocardial blood flow is reported to be better preserved with the administration of nitroglycerin than with nitroprusside (Fig. 11-2).[50]

Calcium Channel Blockers
Calcium antagonists offer theoretical advantages in the treatment of postoperative hypertension, and may be important adjuncts when increased contractility accompanies postoperative hypertension. Nifedipine decreases blood pressure and systolic function but does not decrease heart rate. Although initial therapy with nifedipine does not improve myocardial metabolism, continued therapy has beneficial effects.[52] Diltiazem produces a more profound decrease in heart rate and systolic function and appears to have the most beneficial effect on myocardial metabolism. As sinus arrest has been reported, diltiazem should only be used postoperatively when pacing is

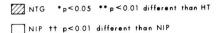

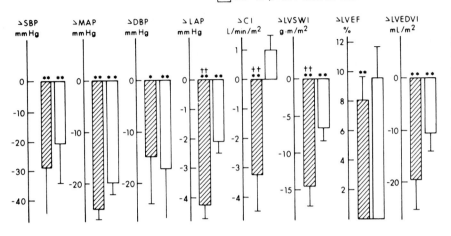

Figure 11–2. Comparative effects of nitroglycerin and nitroprusside on hemodynamic parameters. SBP = systolic blood pressure; MAP = mean arterial pressure; DBP = diastolic blood pressure; LAP = left atrial pressure; CI = cardiac index; LVSWI = left ventricular stroke work index; LVEF = left ventricular ejection function; LVEDVI = left ventricular end-diastolic valve index. From Fremes SE, Weisel RD, Mickel MD: A comparison of nitroglycerin and nitroprusside: I. Treatment of postoperative hypertension. *Ann Thorac Surg* 1985;39:53–59.

available. Donegani and colleagues[54] found that diltiazem decreased ECG evidence of ischemia and postoperative elevations of creatine kinase MB isoenzyme, when given as an infusion. Verapamil, which may reduce afterload, has markedly negative chronotropic and ionotropic effects, limiting its use postoperatively.

A new calcium antagonist, nicardipine, potentially offers many advantages as an antihypertensive agent in the cardiac surgical patient. Preliminary data have documented easy titratability and effectiveness as an antihypertensive.[55] In addition, initial results have demonstrated a decrease in myocardial lactate production. Nicardipine does not appear to inhibit hypoxic pulmonary vasoconstriction or effect AV node conduction. In addition, this drug may also be useful in the treatment of coronary vasospasm.

Beta Blockers

Beta blockers are often useful in the treatment of hypertension associated with the hyperdynamic ventricle. SNP unmasks the underlying excessive ionotropism of the hyperdynamic ventricle, which results in an increase in stroke volume and heart rate, further impairing myocardial oxygen balance. Propanolol, metoprolol, labetolol, or esmolol may be administered in conjunction with an arterial vasodilator or ganglion blocker such as trimethaphan to optimally reduce heart rate as well as blood pressure. Doses should be carefully titrated to avoid myocardial depression. Several recent studies have indicated that myocardial ischemia is less prevalent preoperatively in cardiac patients treated chronically with beta blockers than in those who receive nothing or calcium entry blockers.[56-58] Gray and co-workers[59] compared esmolol with SNP in the treatment of postoperative hypertension and found that both were equally effi-

cacious in controlling blood pressure, allowing rapid easy titratibility. Esmolol, however, resulted in a decreased heart rate and cardiac index while increasing right atrial pressure, while SNP increased heart rate and cardiac index and reduced RAP, reflecting their different mechanisms of action. Esmolol should not then be used in patients with a depressed myocardium. Esmolol therapy did not significantly change PaO_2 or oxygen saturation, while SNP administration was associated with a decrease in these parameters most probably due to intrapulmonary shunting.

The effectiveness of labetolol, an alpha and beta adrenoreceptor blocking agent, was reported by Leslie and associates.[60] They found it was effective in controlling both systolic and diastolic blood pressure with minimal change in heart rate. None of the patients in this study experienced untoward side effects such as hypotension, bradycardia, bronchospasm, or electrocardiographic changes. However, myocardial depression can occur as with any beta blocking agent.

CARDIAC TAMPONADE

The reported incidence of pericardial tamponade ranges from 3 to 6%.[61] It is characterized by a state in which blood and clot occupy space within the pericardial sac, compressing the heart and ultimately preventing normal ventricular filling. The actual hemodynamic consequences of impaired diastolic filling will depend on the rate of fluid accumulation. With tamponade, filling pressures continue to rise as stroke volume and blood pressure fall. As diastolic blood pressure decreases in the face of increasing LVEDP, the transmyocardial gradient for coronary perfusion is jeoparized, and myocardial oxygen balance altered. The shortened diastolic time interval associated with accompanying tachycardia further increases myocardial oxygen consumption, while the increase in wall tension increases myocardial oxygen demand. The diagnosis of pericardial tamponade often requires a high index of suspicion. Echocardiography may be helpful. Most suggestive are the clinical signs of a falling pulse pressure with tachycardia, rapidly rising CVP, and equalization of right- and left-sided filling pressures (Fig. 11–3). Therapy requires immediate surgical evaluation and possibly reexploration.

DYSRYTHMIAS

The incidence of dysrhythmias in the postoperative period following cardiac surgery is reported to be 25 to 40%,[62] contributing significantly to morbidity and mortality (Table 11–6).

Baerman and associates[63] studied the natural history and determinants of conduction defects, and found that the occurrence of new conduction defects is directly related to (1) the number of vessels bypassed; (2) the cardiopulmonary bypass pump time; and (3) the aortic cross-clamp time. In addition, trauma to the AV node—particularly seen in aortic and mitral valve surgery and reconstructive surgery—may further predispose the cardiac patient to dysrhythmias. Residual cold as well as myocardial cellular edema associated with the use of cold cardioplegia with hyperkalemic arrest has led to an increased incidence of conduction defects.[64] Resolution of these conduction defects, however, is high, and third-degree heart block is rare.

The most common dysrhythmia seen in the postoperative period is sinus tachycardia. Predisposing factors such as pain, anxiety, hypovolemia, hypercarbia, hypoxemia, low cardiac output, and hyperdynamic response, should be considered, and therapeutic interventions directed appropriately.

Ventricular dysrhythmias are seen most frequently in the first 24 to 48 hours. Hypokalemia and acid–base imbalance are the most common causes. Hypokalemia, which frequently occurs in the postoperative period, is exacerbated by postbypass diuresis and the accompanying alkalosis. This metabolic alkalosis may be exacerbated by the metabolism of citrate in transfused blood to bicarbonate. The incom-

TABLE 11-6. COMMON DYSRHYTHMIAS FOLLOWING CARDIAC SURGERY

Sinus Tachycardia
Sympathetic stimulation
Pain
Hypovolemia
Hypoxemia
Hypercarbia
Hyperdynamic syndrome
Low cardiac output
Drug induced

Ventricular Dysrhythmias
Sympathetic stimulation
Myocardial ischemia
Hypoxemia
Hypokalemia
Acid–base imbalance
Drug induced

Supraventricular Dysrhythmias
Sympathetic stimulation
Chronic pulmonary disease
Chronic atrial fibrillation
Preexcitation syndromes
Atrial cellular edema
Hypoxemia
Drug induced

pletely rewarmed patient with reduced CO_2 production can be easily hyperventilated, further contributing to this acid–base imbalance.

Ventricular irritability may also be the first indication of myocardial ischemia. Myocardial ischemia may be precipitated by myocardial oxygen imbalance secondary to coronary spasm, coronary embolization, incomplete coronary revascularization, and inadequate intraoperative myocardial protection. Finally, pharmacologic intervention with various inotropes and vasoactive drugs such as epinephrine, dopamine, calcium, digoxin, and aminophylline, may precipitate ventricular dysrhythmias.[21]

After the first two to three postoperative days, supraventricular irritability is the most common dysrhythmia. Precipitating factors include pain, hypovolemia, hypoxemia (which is commonly secondary to postextubation atelectasis), resolving atrial edema, and rapid atrial distention and contraction associated with fluid management. Patients with COPD have a high incidence of multifocal atrial tachycardias and those patients with chronic atrial fibrillation, al-

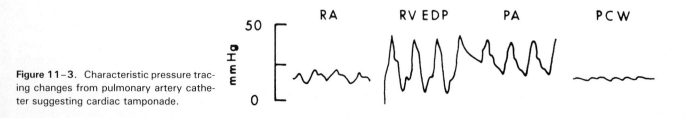

Figure 11–3. Characteristic pressure tracing changes from pulmonary artery catheter suggesting cardiac tamponade.

though they may be in sinus rhythm at the end of surgery, often revert to atrial fibrillation after the first 24 hours. Atrial fibrillation and atrial flutter in this period is frequently associated with a rapid ventricular response, which may lead to hypotension and or myocardial edema. Sympathomimetic drugs have also been implicated as predisposing agents to supraventricular dysrhythmias.

Although controversy exists regarding the use of digitalis for prophylaxis of supraventricular dysrhythmias, propranolol has been shown by various groups to be effective in reducing the incidence of supraventricular and ventricular dysrhythmias.[65] Mohr and associates[66] found that postoperative administration of propanolol was more effective in diminishing the incidence of supraventricular dysrhythmias in patients who had received propanolol preoperatively than in patients who had never received beta blockers. Abrupt discontinuation of propanolol was also noted to be associated with an increased incidence of postoperative dysrhythmias, tachycardia, and hypertension. Daudon and colleagues[67] reported that the cardioselective betablocker acebutolol was effective in preventing supraventricular tachyarrhythmias after coronary surgery.

COAGULATION ABNORMALITIES

Hematologic abnormalities following the use of extracorporeal circulation for open heart surgery have been extensively described, and contribute to the morbidity of the postsurgical cardiac patient.[68-69] Due to the multiplicity of identifiable patient variables, limitations of investigative tools, and conflicting reported observations, successful prevention, adequate diagnosis, and efficacious control of hemostasis following CPB is often met with frustration by the cardiac anesthesiologist.

Specific factors that have been identified as causative in postsurgical bleeding include: (1) inadequate heparin neutralization; (2) protamine excess; (3) heparin rebound; (4) thrombocytopenia and platelet dysfunction; (5) hypofibrinogenemia; (6) primary hyperfibrinogenolysis; (7) disseminated intravascular coagulopathy (DIC); (8) coagulation factor deficiencies; (9) transfusion reactions; (10) hypocalcemia; and (11) hypothermia.[68]

Inadequate Heparin Neutralization

The correct amount of protamine to remove heparin anticoagulation following CPB remains controversial.[70] The most commonly used protocol is based on the in-vitro capacity of protamine to neutralize heparin in a 1.3 to 1.0 ratio. Some investigators have demonstrated that a much lower protamine-to-heparin ratio is efficacious, while other authorities have recommended up to four times the original dose of heparin.[71,72] Perhaps the differences in suggested protamine dosages reflect differences in the kinetics of heparin in individual patients.[72] In addition, the heparin level at the time of neutralization is variable, reflecting the amount of heparin added to the pump prime, supplemental doses, duration of bypass, body temperature, and additional heparin given in the form of heparinized blood.

Although heparin neutralization utilizing a reversal ratio of less than 1:1 is more likely to be associated with bleeding, probably the more important issue is not the initial protamine dose selected but the adequate monitoring of heparin neutralization. The activated clotting time (ACT) is the mainstay in monitoring of heparin neutralization; however, its limitations should be recognized. ACT is dependant on hemodilution, hypothermia, platelet function, clotting factors, and fibrinogen.[73,74] More sensitive tests for heparin detection include the tri-F titer, protamine titration, and thrombin/reptilase time; however, the results take longer to obtain.

Heparin Rebound

Kolff and associates first described heparin rebound in 1956 as a ''treacherous phenomenon in which heparin is neutralized by protamine sulfate and the clotting time becomes normal in a matter of minutes. However, protamine seems to be eliminated from the blood before heparin is, thus leaving the heparin uncovered as demonstrated by protamine titration.''[75] The pharmacodynamics of an acutely administered drug undergoing redistribution, protamine, compared with a completely redistributed drug, heparin, appear sufficient to explain the phenomenon of heparin rebound. Although seldom a documented reason for excessive postoperative bleeding, heparin rebound is reported to occur in as many of 50% of patients undergoing CPB.[76] The time at which this rebound occurs varies. Most cases have been reported to occur within eight or nine hours following neutralization; however rebound has been known to develop as long as 18 hours after neutralization of heparin.[77] A possible explanation for this includes incomplete rewarming with a sustained toe–nasopharyngeal temperature gradient, resulting in a delay in heparin release from the tissues into the circulation.

Failure to consider heparin rebound in the presence of clinical bleeding after initial neutralization is unfortunate, as it is an easily treated entity. One should recheck the ACT, as reheparinization is often accompanied by an ACT elevation. If this is seen, additional protamine should be administered. Small amounts of heparin are more accurately detected by tri-F titer and protamine titration, as well as thrombin/reptilase time.

Red Blood Cells

Red blood cell damage also occurs during CPB, primarily as a result of sheer stresses producing either immediate hemolysis or shortened red cell life span with delayed hemolysis. Intracardiac suction devices are particularly damaging, partly because of the high sheer stress and deceleration injury, and partly because of the negative suction pressures applied. Thus there is a progressive loss of red cell mass during the first several days following open heart surgery, reflecting a rate of sequestration of red blood cells in excess of regenerative capacity.[78]

Thrombocytopenia and Platelet Dysfunction

Extracorporeal circulation has been identified as a major source of platelet injury. Factors contributing to this include hemodilution, adhesion of platelets to foreign surfaces of the perfusion system,[79,80] aggregation of platelets by ADP released from hemolyzed red blood cells,[81] mechanical damage, aggregation of platelets by heparin, consumption of platelets due to limited DIC, and aggregation of platelets by protamine sulfate, or heparin–protamine sulfate complexes.[82] At the conclusion of bypass many authors have described a 30 to 50% reduction in platelet count from preoperative values, with normal levels not being regained for six to seven days.[83]

Once it became clear that little correlation exists between the incidence of postoperative bleeding and the degree of thrombocytopenia, multiple investigations were undertaken to evaluate alterations in platelet function. Karpatkin[84] reported a marked selective decrease in the number of large platelets, leaving intact the remaining medium and smaller platelets, after CPB. Evidence suggests that these large platelets are the younger, more adherent ones.[85] Other investigators have shown that no patient has normal platelet adhesion during bypass, representing an average drop of 50% from preoperative measurement.[86] At one hour postbypass, adhesion began to improve slowly. McKenna and coworkers found, in their prospective study of hemostasis and extracorporeal circulation, the frequent occurrence of a qualitative platelet defect that did not correlate with the length of bypass, decrease in platelet count, or concentration of circulating fibrin split products.[87]

Functional platelet abnormalities have also been stated to be more commonly seen following the use of the bubble oxygenator than after circulation through the membrane oxygenator, especially after a prolonged bypass greater than two hours. Additional disturbances in platelet function can be affected by preoperative medications with antiplatelet activity, further excerbating postoperative bleeding.

Recent work has been directed to the pharmacologic protection of platelets. Teoh and colleagues evaluated the use of preoperative dypyridamole and found that thrombocyte count was preserved.[88] Becker and associates reported better platelet aggregation in response to ADP following dipyridamole administration.[89] The potency of dipyridamole is insufficient however to completely prevent platelet reactivity during extracorporeal circulation, and its duration cannot be controlled. Iloprost, an analogue of prostacyclin, inhibits platelet activation, and may in the future provide a means of preserving platelet function following extracorporeal circulation.[90]

Hypofibrinogenemia and Hyperfibrinogenolysis

Most studies have shown that a hyperfibrinolytic state occurs after bypass. Activity of the fibrinolytic system alters hemostasis by the conversion of plasminogen into plasmin. The hypofibrinogenemia, plasminogen depletion, and plasmin degradation of Factors V, VIII, and IX compromise coagulation. The resultant fibrinolytic degradation products further damage hemostasis by interfering with thrombin activity and fibrin monomer polymerization, altering platelet function.[91] If the physiological defenses that normally control hypercoagulability are impaired or if the magnitude and duration of the coagulation system are excessive, disseminated intravascular coagulopathy (DIC) may result. Hyperfibrinogenolysis is detected by a prolonged reptilase test, TT, and increase in fibrin degradation products.

Clinical Implications

Management of hemorrhage seen in the cardiac surgery patient can be extremely difficult secondary to the many surgical and nonsurgical variables involved, and thus it is essential the anesthesiologist have a working knowledge of hemostasis and be capable of initiating the appropriate laboratory workup, and therapy when indicated. Certainly when managing complex bleeding disorders a hematologist should be consulted.

Although "shot-gun" therapy in the treatment of postoperative bleeding is deplored, the lack of specificity of evaluative tests and delay in serial lab results creates an empiric management style. Unfortunately it becomes all too easy to treat while paying insufficient attention to long-term transfusion hazards.[92]

Postoperative bleeding—which necessitates transfusion in 20% of patients and requires reexploration of 3 to 4%—should be assessed by the measurement of chest tube drainage, inspection of surgical wounds, and the results of immediate postoperative PT, aPTT, fibrinogen, TT, and platelet count.[92] It is important that the laboratory parameters be repeated as necessary so that the smallest quantities of blood components be transfused. Clinical findings must be correlated with laboratory results.

Platelets

Thrombocytopenia alone is not an indication for platelet transfusion, as it is unlikely that bleeding will occur until the platelet count is below 50,000 to 60,000.[93] However, thrombocytopenia in the bleeding patient is the only clearly agreed upon indication for platelet administration. Platelet transfusion may also be considered in the bleeding patient, post-CPB, who has a bleeding time of greater than 20 minutes after administration of protamine, even if the platelet count is greater than 100,000.

A lack of benefit and increased risks associated with the prophylactic administration of platelets has led most authorities to caution against empiric therapy. In fact, the Consensus Statement of the National Heart, Lung and Blood Institutes Conference on Platelet Transfusion Therapy explicitly states;

Controlled prospective studies examining postoperative blood loss and outcome have demonstrated no correlation between platelet counts and bleeding, following CPB, and no detectable benefit from the prophylactic administration of platelets to such patients. The vast majority of such patients have some degree of thrombocytopenia, prolongation of bleeding time, and continued slow bleeding. With an expected pattern of bleeding, thrombocytopenia is not an indication for platelet transfusion. There is no justification for prophylactic platelet administration in patients undergoing open heart surgery.[94]

Pharmacologic manipulation of platelet activation with DDAVP and Iloprost have suggested reduced need for transfusion; however, additional studies need to be performed.[95]

Fresh Frozen Plasma

The Center for Disease Control reports that fresh frozen plasma (FFP) is the most frequently misused blood product. Indications for FFP include (1) replacement of isolated factor deficiencies; (2) reversal of warfarin effect; (3) massive blood transfusion; (4) antithrombin III deficiency; (5) treatment of immunodeficiencies; and (6) treatment of TTP. Defining the magnitude of laboratory abnormalities justfying FFP transfusion in the presence of bleeding is difficult. In the presence of generalized bleeding a PT 1.3 times control, PTT 1.3 times control, TT 1.3 times control,

fibrinogen 100mg/dL, and ACT greater than 150 seconds, indicate that FFP should be administered.[96]

Cryoprecipitate

Cryoprecipitate (CP) contains a concentrated solution of Factor VIII, Factor XIII, and fibronectin. Cryoprecipitate is indicated in the treatment of hemophilia A, von Willebrand's disease, types II and III, and deficiencies of Factor XIII or fibrinogen.[96] Excessive use of CP can produce elevation of fibrinogen levels, and increase the risk of intravascular thrombosis. There is no indication for transfusing CP in the absence of supportive laboratory data.

Desmopressin

Desmopressin acetate is a synthetic analogue of L-arginine vasopressin and has been shown to shorten the bleeding time in certain forms of hemophilia, von Willebrand's disease, uremia, and in other conditions, presumably by inducing release of von Willebrand factor (vWF), a glycoprotein required for normal platelet adhesion and normal bleeding time.[97] Another mechanism also appears to involve a nonspecific enhancement of platelet function, which is probably independant of vWF. Although it has now been established that desmopressin acetate reduces the blood loss in patients undergoing more complex cardiac operations, its usefulness in patients undergoing primary uncomplicated CABG has not been tested.[97] Its use in routine cardiac operations may have an important effect on the national requirements for blood.

The ability of DDAVP to reverse aspirin-induced platelet defect is important in patients pretreated with platelet-inhibiting agents. Ware and others[98] recommend the use of desmopressin in all complicated cardiac surgery cases in which more than minimal blood loss is expected. Doses at 0.3 μg/kg are given intravenously. The most common side effect is tachyphlaxis, which appears to occur if repeated doses are given every 12 to 24 hours. Also one may see a mild vasodilation, manifesting as facial flushing, clinically insignificant drop in systolic blood pressure, or a 10 to 20% increase in heart rate.[99]

Epsilon Aminocaproic Acid

Excessive fibrinolysis can be successfully treated with epsilon aminocaproic acid (EACA) (10 to 20 g) alone or in combination with FFP of CP. This approach markedly reduces transfusion requirements and rates of surgical reexploration and infection. EACA is a potent inhibitor of fibrinolysis and when administered in the wrong setting may predispose one to widespread thrombosis. Deep vein thrombosis and pulmonary thrombosis have not been reported as problems.

Coagulation Monitoring

The activated clotting time (ACT) test is the most commonly used test today to evaluate the adequacy of protamine reversal of heparin, and is really a refinement of the Lee–White whole blood coagulation time. However, the limitations of the ACT are well known, and no longer is it considered sufficiently sensitive to evaluate bleeding disorders. It is used almost exclusively to monitor heparin therapy.

More recently there has been a resurgence of interest in thromboelastography (TEG).[100] TEG provides a qualitative measure of viscoelastic clot strength. Blood specimen is placed in a crucible and as fibrin strands form between the wall of the crucible and a suspended piston, rotational motion of the crucible is transferred to the piston. An electronic amplification system translates the piston motion into a characteristic TEG tracing. This tracing represents the shear elasticity over time of the blood clot as it forms and eventually lyses.[100] A number of parameters (Fig. 11-4) can be measured from the TEG tracing, which in turn may be used to differentiate various bleeding disorders (Fig. 11-5).

Spiess and colleagues[101] reported that TEG monitoring accurately predicted 80% of postoperative bleeding episodes. The predictive accuracy of the ACT and the coagulation profile, either together or

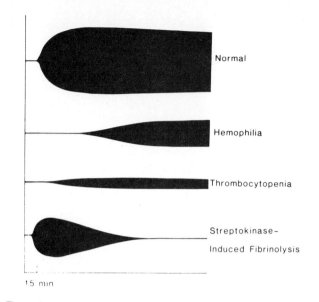

Figure 11-5. Characteristic thromboelastograph tracings seen in various clinical settings.

separately, was 50% or less. The TEG produced false positives in 20% of cases and no false negatives.

TEG is not a new monitoring technique, and anesthesiologists are now becoming accepting of its use. It has proved invaluable in the operating room where clot strength, speed of clot formation, and clot lysis provide us with critical information, guiding our therapy. It is a rapid on site qualitative test which has extensive application in other surgical procedures as well (Fig. 11-6).

THERMOREGULATION

Patients often arrive in the PACU after cardiac surgery with a temperature of 34 to 35°C. Vasoconstriction increases systemic vascular resistance and ventricular afterload, which increases myocardial oxygen consumption and reduces cardiac output.

Sladen[102] demonstrated that the time to peak temperature following cardiac surgery was about eight hours. As temperature rose, CO_2 production and O_2 consumption increased, often contributing to respiratory alkalosis, dysrhythmias, and electrolyte imbalance. As the postoperative cardiac surgery patient is routinely ventilated mechanically, it is essential that ventilatory parameters and arterial blood gases be monitored closely. Ventilator settings early in the rewarming period may not provide adequate mechanical ventilation for gas exchange later in the postoperative period. For each degree Celsius under 37, CO_2 production is reduced by 10%.

Postoperative rewarming is often accompanied by shivering, a physiologic stress that may result in

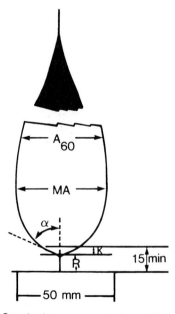

Figure 11-4. Standard measurements from a TEG tracing normal values: R = 10–15 min, K = 6–12 min, α = 45, MA = 50–60 min, A_{60} = MA − 5. (Adapted from Tuman K, Spiess B, McCarthy R, Ivankovich A: Effects of progressive blood loss on coagulation as measured by thromboelastography. *Anesth Analg* 1987; 66:856–861).

Normal-Post Bypass TEG

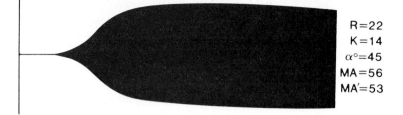

R=22
K=14
$\alpha°$=45
MA=56
MA'=53

Post-Bypass TEG Diagnostic of Fibrinolysis

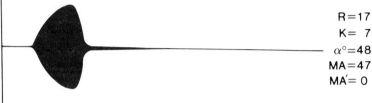

R=17
K= 7
$\alpha°$=48
MA=47
MA'= 0

Figure 11-6. Characteristic changes are seen in the thromboelastogram after bypass that may suggest fibrinolysis.

a marked increase in both metabolic and circulatory demand. Oxygen consumption has been shown to increase 500%. Michenfelder and co-workers[103] demonstrated while investigating the hemodynamic and metabolic effects of hypothermia that the anesthetized mechanically ventilated patients allowed to shiver midway through the rewarming period had an increase in O_2 uptake and decrease in right atrial O_2 saturation. These values returned to preshivering levels once muscle relaxation returned.

Rodriquez[104] demonstrated that although mechanical ventilation held constant and FIO_2 unchanged, there was a fall in PaO_2 as shivering progressed, suggesting that either shunt fraction increased or metabolic demands increased at a proportionately greater rate than cardiac output. He then demonstrated that suppression of shivering was associated with a lower VCO_2, HR, MVO_2, and MAP. Therefore prevention of shivering results in lower myocardial work.

In addition, this rewarming period is hemodynamically precarious, necessitating frequent adjustments in therapy and fluid management. Vasodilators may be effectively titrated to enhance rewarming, recognizing that this process is not uniform and may be prolonged. Vigilance is necessary to avoid a decrease in blood pressure secondary to a reduced SVR and CO. A normal RAP, PCWP, and CO should be meticulously maintained with combined volume and vasodilator therapy. The primary goal in hemodynamic management is to maintain optimal cardiac output, systemic vascular resistance, and venous capacitance.

THORACIC AORTIC SURGERY

The postoperative management of the patient undergoing thoracic aortic surgery for traumatic rupture of the aorta, thoracic aortic aneurysm, thoracic dissection, or coarctation is most challenging for the anesthesiologist. The high incidence of coexisting hypertension, coronary artery disease, chronic obstructive pulmonary disease, and prior aortic vascular surgery contributes to surgical morbidity and mortality.

Aortic dissection has been recognized as a more common lesion. DeBakey and associates[105] classified thoracic aortic dissection into three basic types: type I, intimal tear in the ascending aorta with extension of the dissection to the descending aorta; type II, ascending intimal tear with dissection limited to the ascending aorta; type IIIA, intimal tear in the descending aorta with dissection to involve the ascending aorta; and type IIIB, intimal tear in the descending aorta with dissection limited to the descending aorta.

Currently, any involvement of the ascending aorta is treated surgically. Controversy does continue to exist regarding the optional management of dissections involving the descending aorta. Many favor initial medical therapy with early elective repair while others favor aggressive surgical management. Aneurysms are classified according to shape, location, and etiology. Ascending aortic aneurysms are proximal to the origin of the inominate artery; aortic arch aneurysms are located between the origin of the inominate and origin of the left subclavian artery, and descending aortic aneurysms range from the origin of left subclavian artery to the diaphragm. These patients may present with hoarseness from recurrent laryngeal nerve involvement, atelectasis, or pneumonia secondary to compression of the tracheal bronchial tree, hemoptysis, dysphagia, and hematemesis.[106]

Thoracic artery rupture is usually due to nonpenetrating trauma, necessitating surgical intervention. In a large study, 90% of patients presented with aortic tear at the isthmus, just distal to the origin of the left subclavian artery.[107] Surgical techniques include patching, use of prosthesis, or excision with end-to-end anatomosis.

Several concerns may affect postoperative management; these are described in the following sections.

Stress of Cross-Clamping

Cross-clamping of the descending thoracic aorta results in a 40% increase in mean arterial pressure above the cross-clamp, while arterial pressure below the cross-clamp is decreased by 85%.

Marked elevations in plasma epinephrine, norepinephrine, and renin levels have been reported.[108] A direct artery vasodilator such as sodium nitroprusside is often necessary to control hypertension above the cross-clamp; however, special consideration must be given to the region below the clamp, as perfusion pressure to vital organs including the kidney and spinal cord can be compromised.

Ventilation

Isolated single-lung ventilation is used in surgical repair of the descendary thoracic aorta for improved surgical visualization, facilitation of surgical resection, and reduction of trauma to the lung. If pulmonary trauma does occur with intrapulmonary bleeding, a double-lumen ETT allows for protection and isolation of the lungs. Complications may occur, including airway trauma hypoxemia and increased intrapulmonary shunting.[109] Following completion of the surgical procedure the double-lumen ETT should be replaced with a single-lumen ETT to allow for better suctioning. Due to the large third-space losses and multiple hemodynamic alterations occurring perioperatively, the patient should be transported to the PACU intubated, ventilated via ambu, and adequately sedated.

Blood Loss

Massive blood loss can occur during the initial dissection as well as during repair of the aortic lesion. In a report from Baylor surgical group, the average blood product utilization in repair of the descending thoracic aorta was 10 units of prbc's, 7.2 units of FFP, and 13 units of platelets.[110] With continued postoperative bleeding one should also consider incomplete heparin reversal as well as dilutional coagulapathy.

Rapid autotransfusion devices presently available have markedly decreased the amount of blood product transfusion necessary.

Renal Function

In evaluating renal dysfunction it is necessary to temporally define its onset with regards to pre- or post-aortic cross-clamp, as cross-clamping is known to alter renal flow. The use of partial bypass or shunt may maintain renal perfusion more optimally. To maintain vital organ reserve it is necessary to monitor distal perfusion pressures after clamping. Crawford and associates[111] reported a 10% incidence of postop dialysis required in patients over 70 years of age undergoing aneurysm resection. These patients all had a history of ASHD and preexisting cerebral vascular disease, factors that have been found to correlate with the need for postoperative dialysis.

Following unclamping, the maintenance of adequate filling pressures is essential in maintaining renal function.

Spinal Cord Injury

The incidence of paraplegia has been reported by Cooley and co-workers[112] to range from 37% for proximal descending aneurysms to 89% for aneurysms involving the entire descending aorta. Emergency operations and cross-clamp time exceeding 30 minutes was associated with increased risk of spinal cord injury.

The gray matter of the spinal cord appears particularly vulnerable to ischemic damage, and thus the patient may present with a loss of motor function with preservation of vibratory and position sense.

Evidence suggests that damage to the vascular supply is possibly more harmful than intrinsic injury to the cord. The value of shunting procedures in preventing paraplegia has remained controversial, and probably the need for such depends on how rapidly the anastomoses can be completed.

Somatosensory evoked potential (SSEP) are used to monitor spinal cord function during surgery. SSEP are affected by the type and depth of anesthesia, temperature, hematocrit, hemodynamics, and arterial O_2 tension. Although there are reports of normal SSEPs in patients developing postoperative paraplegia, evoked potentials do appear to have value in monitoring spinal cord function in thoracic aortic surgery. Controversy exists regarding the direction of therapeutic intervention once diminution of SSEP is noted. It is also possible that alteration in the anterior spinal cord is not reflected in the posterior columns monitored by SSEP.[113]

HYPERTENSION

Hypertension is very common postoperatively secondary to preexisting hypertension, vasoconstriction from hypothermia, or inadequate analgesia. Treatment usually involves an arterial vasodilator such as SNP. Postoperative hypotension can also occur, and one must consider inadequate volume replacement.

AORTIC STENOSIS

Aortic stenosis may be congenital, rheumatic, or the result of calcification of a congenitally abnormal valve. The pleussed valve results in outflow obstruction. The subsequent increase in intraventricular pressure is a stimulus for left ventricular hypertrophy, which results in ventricular electrical instability and a tendency to ventricular dysrhythmias. This concentric hypertrophy is associated with increased filling pressures predisposing these patients to subendocardial eschemia. It may also produce left atrial distention and atrial fibrillation.

Although aortic valve replacement normalizes impedance to left ventricular ejection, compliance remains impaired due to left ventricular hypertrophy and subendocardial ischemia.

Postoperatively these patients are often hypertensive and hyperdynamic. Maintenance of normal sinus rhythm postoperatively is imperative to optimize cardiac output, in a stiffened, poorly compliant, ventricle.

AORTIC INSUFFICIENCY

Aortic insufficiency (AI) may be acute or chronic in origin, resulting from failure of the aortic cusps to align and co-opt correctly. Left ventricular failure may develop very quickly in the acute setting. As there is no time for compensatory ventricular dilatation and hypertrophy, LVEDP increases with resultant pulmonary congestion. This elevated LVEDP increases subendocardial diastolic pressure as well.

With chronic AI, a minimally elevated LVEDP exists despite an enormous increase in diastolic volume. Stroke volume and ejection fraction are preserved.

Following AVR these patients frequently require vasodilators. In addition, patients with impaired ventricular function as seen with acute AI may require inotropic support to maintain a systolic perfusion pressure while minimizing retrograde flow during diastole.

MITRAL STENOSIS

Mitral stenosis (MS) is usually the result of rheumatic heart disease, which results in thickening and calcification of the mitral valve leaflet. This stenotic mitral valve obstructs blood flow, generating a pressure gradient between the atrium and ventricle. Left atrial dilatation and hypertrophy gradually occur. Left atrial hypertension will eventually cause pulmonary venous congestion, and if severe and prolonged, pulmonary hypertension and edema will result. These changes may be reversed with mitral valve surgery, and normalization of left ventricular ejection and filling occurs. In those patients with pulmonary hypertension, their postoperative course may be more complicated, often requiring somewhat more prolonged ventilatory support as well as pulmonary vasodilator therapy.

Patients with preoperative atrial fibrillation will usually revert to atrial fibrillation postoperatively; thus adequate digitalization and avoidance of hypokalemia is necessary.

MITRAL REGURGITATION

Mitral regurgitation (MR) may be caused by disease affecting the valve leaflets or may occur secondary to abnormalities of the papillary muscles or chorda tendinae.

With chronic MR a chronic volume overload is imparted on the left ventricle. The left ventricle dilates and a cardiomyopathy eventually develops.

Mitral valve replacement eliminates the low impedance path to left ventricular ejection but does not improve left ventricular contractility. Therefore, left ventricular ejection is improved with inotropic support and afterload reduction. In addition the intraaortic balloon pump may be necessary to provide additional afterload reduction and enhance left ventricular performance.

ABDOMINAL AORTIC ANEURYSM

Patients with abdominal aortic aneurysms (AAA) are usually in the sixth to ninth decade of life and often have many other medical problems.

Vascular pathology in the aorta is often associated with similar pathologic changes in other parts of the vascular system (Table 11-7).

The high prevalence of coexisting coronary artery disease, hypertension, renal disease, diabetes, and chronic obstructive pulmonary disease, in patients with acquired vascular disease is well documented.[114]

TABLE 11–7. PREVALENCE (%) OF COEXISTING DISEASE IN PATIENTS WITH ABNORMAL AORTIC ANEURYSM, 1984–1988

Hypertension	47
Angina	9
Congestive heart failure	5
Previous myocardial infarction	15
Presence of dysrhythmias	4
Renal failure	4
Chronic obstructive pulmonary disease	5

Data provided by Gupta S, Department of Vascular Surgery, Montefiore Medical Center, Bronx, NY.

Cardiovascular Considerations

Myocardial infarction is the most common cause of death following intact aortic aneurysm repair—40 to 60% of perioperative deaths, and 3 to 9% of immediate deaths (intraoperatively or during the first 48 hours postoperatively).[114,115] Nearly 35% of patients undergoing abdominal aortic surgery develop congestive heart failure in the postoperative period, either as a consequence of myocardial infarction or exposure of the myocardium to excessive workload—such as persistent hypertension, aortic stenosis, or regurgitation.[116] The high incidence of perioperative infarction is related to advanced age, stress, prolonged duration of surgery, and large fluid shifts. Although patients with obvious coronary artery disease usually undergo bypass grafting as a first procedure, in rare, extreme situations both aneurysmal surgery and myocardial grafting procedures are performed simultaneously.

Postoperatively, dysrhythmias are not infrequent. Supraventricular dysrhythmias, including premature atrial contractions, usually do not require therapy if vital signs are stable. Paroxysmal atrial tachycardia may be treated with verapamil, esmolol, or propanolol. Digoxin is administered as second-line therapy. Atrial flutter responds to verapamil and electrocountershock of 10 to 20 watt-seconds, especially if the dysrhythmia is of recent onset.

Ventricular dysrhythmias that are more than 6/min, are multifocal, or appear three or more times consecutively, should be treated with procainamide 20 mg/min intravenously to a loading dose of 1 g, or with lidocaine.

Monitoring for patients undergoing AAA surgery requires pulmonary artery catheter and arterial cannulation. Measurement of hemodynamic parameters may be continued into the postoperative period, to appropriately guide management.

Fluid Management

As part of the operative management, the aorta is cross-clamped. Vascular resistance is increased by about 40% and stroke volume and cardiac output are decreased by 15 to 35%.[117-119] Large fluid and blood losses occur during AAA surgery due to tissue trauma, dissection, exposure of the abdominal cavity, and retroperitoneal edema. Blood loss is variable and depends on the technical difficulty encountered during surgery—poor vascular integrity, inadequate hemostasis, and anticoagulation. The aim of fluid therapy should be to maintain adequate filling pressure (as determined by PCWP), adequate urine output (1 mL/kg/h), and a hematocrit of 30% or above. If urine output falls below 40 mL/h in the presence of normal PCWP, a dopamine infusion at 2 mg/kg/h or a furosemide bolus should be used. If a decreased urine output is associated with lowered cardiac filling pressures, then the fluid status should be optimized. If the reduction in urine output is small, simply increasing the hourly intake will suffice. If the decrease is more dramatic, a fluid challenge such as 250 mL of a balanced salt solution over 20 minutes is indicated. If the PCWP increases more than 7 mm Hg, no more fluid should be given. Cardiac output should be measured and systemic vascular resistance calculated.

In some instances urine output may not reflect intravascular volume. For example, during hypothermia, reabsorption of sodium is decreased and a cold diuresis results. Osmotic diuresis from glucose or mannitol may also increase output. Patients with sickle cell disease or renal insufficiency may be unable to concentrate urine and again, output is increased. Rarely urethral obstruction may occur after insertion of an aortic bifurcation graft, especially if the graft is placed anterior to the ureter. Urinary output may be decreased.

Renal Complications

Intrarenal aortic cross-clamping is accompanied by a 75% increase in renal vascular resistance and 38% decrease in renal blood flow.[119] Plasma levels of renin and angiotensin are elevated postoperatively. Renal hemodynamic deterioration persists for at least one hour after release of the aortic clamp. Hypertension must be controlled, preferably with beta blockers. Acute renal failure occurs in 2 to 8% of patients after elective aneurysm surgery,[120] with a mortality rate of 25 to 80%. After emergent surgery the incidence increased to 20 to 40% and death supervenes in 50 to 90%.[121] Stenotic arterial supply makes the kidneys especially vulnerable to ischemic insult. Cross-clamping above the renal arteries increases the incidence of renal failure.[122] Following release of the aortic cross-clamp, glomerular filtration rate decreases—an effect that cannot be prevented either by dopamine or mannitol.[123]

Therapy is aimed at prevention of ischemia by

avoiding hypotension and hypovolemia. Causes of oliguria must be rapidly identified and appropriate therapy given.

Differentiation between prerenal and renal azotemia is important. A urinary sodium concentration less than 20 mEq/L occurs in prerenal azotemia. Levels above 30 mEq/L signify renal disease. Urinalysis must be made prior to diuretic or vasopressor therapy.

Oliguric renal failure requires restricted fluid replacement to prevent overload, especially as volume is redistributed from the third space. The role of diuretics in acute renal failure is controversial.

Aggressive dialysis therapy for acute renal failure is indicated. Hemodialysis controls uremia, volume overload, hyperkalemia, and platelet dysfunction, and may be indicated daily. If cardiovascular instability is problematic or venous access is limited, peritoneal dialysis may be required. This technique increases the risk of graft infection. Continuous arteriovenous hemofiltration may be used to control volume in patients with marked hemodynamic instability.[124] Death after postoperative renal failure is usually due to abdominal infection.[125]

Surgical Complications

Neurologic. In an attempt to decrease the risk of ischemic damage to the cord, perfusion pressure may have been increased by drainage of cerebrospinal fluid intraoperatively. This system is usually terminated at the end of the procedure. In rare instances of large aneurysms or if somatosensory evoked potential monitoring has indicated deterioration of neuronal transmission, drainage may be continued into the postoperative period. Strict asepsis must be maintained in dealing with the drainage catheter and collection bag. Neurologic evaluation should be performed routinely in the PACU.[126]

Hemorrhage. Bleeding may occur at the graft artery anastomoses. A clot developing around a superficial anastomosis may be recognized quickly and direct pressure applied. Hypotension, tachycardia, and increasing abdominal size may herald retroperitoneal hemorrhage. Immediate reexploration is indicated.

Slower hemorrhage may be due to venous disruption or coagulopathy. Coagulation parameters should be checked.

Lower Limb Ischemia. Ischemia of the lower extremities occurs in 23 to 25% of cases.[127] The major causes are embolization of mural thrombi or atheroma during aneurysm manipulation and clamping. The complication is exacerbated by distal occlusive disease.

Thrombosis is caused by hypotension, hypercoagulability, or inadequate intraoperative heparinzation. Ischemia may also be caused by kinking or twisting of grafts and intimal dissections.

Extremities should be examined at least every four hours initially for the presence of ischemia. Atheromatous embolism is recognized by mottling and discoloration of the feet and toes in a few hours. Similar changes on the buttocks are due to hypogastric or profundo femoral embolization. Large emboli are removed by embolectomy.

Gastrointestinal

Although gastrointestinal complications are not common, they are associated with high mortality.[128] Ileus and colonic ischemia (due to ligation of an inferior mesenteric artery) have been described. The diagnosis of ischemic bowel is suspected by bloody diarrhea, distension, abdominal pain, persistent lactic acidemia, sepsis, and fever. Confirmation is obtained by demonstration of muscosal duskiness and friability on sigmoidoscopy. Angiography and inferior mesenteric artery reimplantation or aorto-superior mesenteric artery bypass may be indicated.

Small bowel ischemia occurs in 0.1% of cases due to obstruction of the superior mesenteric artery, and carries a very high mortality.[129]

Infection

Graft infection has a mortality of 50 to 88%.[130] Infection is minimized with antibiotic prophylaxis with a first-generation cephalosporin (eg, cefazolin). It is given preoperatively and for 12 to 48 hours after surgery.[131]

Pain Control

After thoracic surgery, pain and muscle splinting are major determinants of decreased FRC.[132]

Parenteral narcotics are usually given in small, divided doses to decrease pain. As long as ventilation is assisted, the risks of respiratory depression are minimal.

Regional techniques, specifically intercostal nerve blocks and epidural analgesia, are more effective in preventing pulmonary complications. However, although subjective outcome may be improved, there is little documentation of improvement in FRC.[133]

Effective analgesia and objective improvement in pulmonary function (increased FEV_1) have been obtained with epidural narcotics.[134] These techniques are receiving increasing acceptance (Chapter 5).

Transcutaneous electrical nerve stimulation as an adjunct to analgesic regimens has a limited place.[135] Less depression of vital capacity and FRC has been shown in patients receiving combination therapies than in those receiving narcotics alone.

A recent study comparing pain relief obtained with intrapleural bupivacaine instilled at four-hour intervals and intramuscular injection of oxycodane failed to demonstrate superior effects with the former technique.[136]

REFERENCES

1. Marsh HM, Abel MD; Postoperative management of the adult cardiac surgical patient, in Tarhan S (ed): *Cardiovascular Anesthesia and Post Operative Care.* Chicago, Year Book, 1989, pp 609–630.
2. Gibbon JH Jr: The Lewis A. Conner memorial lecture: Maintenance of cardiorespiratory functions by extracorporeal circulation. *Circulation* 1959;19:646–656.
3. Baer DM, Osborn JJ: The post perfusion pulmonary congestion syndrome. *Am J Clin Pathol* 1960;34:442–445.
4. Pennock JL, Pierce WS, Waldhausen JA: The management of the lungs during cardiopulmonary bypass. *Surg Gynecol Obstet* 1977;145:917–927.
5. Ratliff NB, Young WG, Hackel DB, et al: Pulmonary injury secondary to extracorporeal circulation. *J Thorac Cardiovasc Surg* 1973;65:425–432.
6. Westby S: Aspects of biocompatibility in cardiopulmonary bypass. *Crit Rev Biocompat* 1987;3:193–234.
7. Leewitt J, Krumbhaar D, Fonkalsrud EW, et al: Deviation of plasma proteins as a cause of morbidity and death after intracardiac operations. *Surgery* 1961;50:29–39.
8. Kalter RD, Saul CM, Wetstein L, et al: Cardiopulmonary bypass; associated hemostatic abnormalities. *J Thorac Cardiovas Surg* 1979;77:427–435.
9. Chenoweth DE, Cooper SW, Hugle TE, et al: Complement activation during cardiopulmonary bypass: Evidence for generation of C_3a and C_5a anaphylatoxins. *N Engl J Med* 1981;304:497–503.
10. Kirklin JW, Westaby S, Blackstone EH, et al: Complement of the damaging effects of cardiopulmonary bypass. *J Thorac Cardiovasc Surg* 1983;86:845–857.
11. Asada S, Yamagucki M: The structural change in the lung following cardiopulmonary bypass. *Chest* 1971;S9:478.
12. Sobonya RE, Kleinerman J, Primuno F, Chester EH: Pulmonary changes in cardiopulmonary bypass: Short term effects on granular pneumocytes. *Chest* 1972;61:154–158.
13. Westby S: Postoperative organ system dysfunction. *Curr Opin Anesthesiol* 1989;2:40–51.
14. Antonsen S, Brandslund I, Clemensen S, et al: Neutrophil lysosomal enzyme and complement activation during cardiopulmonary bypass. *Scand J Thorac Cardiovasc Surg* 1987;21:47–52.
15. Van Oeveren W, Jansen NG, Bidstrup BP, et al: Effects of aprotinin on hemostatic mechanisms during cardiopulmonary bypass. *Ann Thorac Surg* 1987;44:640–645.
16. Smith EEJ, Naftel DC, Blackstone EH, Kirklin JW: Microvascular permeability after cardiopulmonary bypass: An experimental study. *J Thorac Cardiovasc Surg* 1987;94:225–233.
17. Boldt J, Von Bormann B, Kling D, et al: Age and cardiac surgery: Influence of extravascular lung water. *Chest* 1987;91:185–189.
18. Braun SR, Birnbaum ML, Chopra PS: Pre and postoperative pulmonary function abnormalities in coronary artery revascularization surgery. *Chest* 1973;73:316–320.
19. Peters, RM, Welton HE, Howe TM: Total compliance and work of breathing after thoracotomy. *J Thorac Cardiovasc Surg* 1969;57:348–355.
20. Schramel RJ, Cameron R, Ziskind MM, et al: Studies of pulmonary diffusion after open heart surgery. *J Thorac Cardiovasc Surg* 1959;38:281–290.
21. Sladen RN: Management of the adult cardiac patient in the intensive care unit, in Ream AK, Fogdall RP, (eds): *Acute Cardiovascular Management.* Philadelphia, Lippincott, 1982, pp 481–548.
22. West JB: *Ventilation/Blood Flow and Gas Exchange,* ed 2. Philadelphia, Davis, 1970.
23. Sladen RN, Renaghan D, Ashton JP, Wyner J: Reliability of end-tidal CO_2 monitoring after cardiac surgery. *Anesthesiology* A142 63:1986.
24. Peters RM, Wellons HA, Howe TM: Total compliance and work of breathing after thoracotomy. *J Thorac Cardiovasc Surg* 1969;57:348–355.
25. Downs JB, Mitchell LA: Pulmonary effects of ventilatory pressure following cardiopulmonary bypass. *Crit Care Med* 1976;4:295–300.
26. Luce JM, Pierson DJ, Hudson LD: Intermittent mandatory ventilation. *Chest* 1981;79:678–685.
27. Downs JB, Douglas ME, Sanfelippo PM, et al: Ventilatory pattern, intrapleural pressure and cardiac output. *Anesth Analg* 1977;56:88–96.
28. Mathru M, Rao TLK, El-Etr AA, et al: Hemodynamic response to changes in ventilatory patterns in patients with normal and poor left ventricular reserve. *Crit Care Med* 1982;3:423–426.
29. Feeley TW, Klick JM, Suamarez R, et al: Positive end-expiratory pressure in weaning patients from controlled ventilation. *Lancet* 1975;2:725–728.
30. Good JT, Wolz JF, Anderson JJ, et al: The routine use of positive end-expiratory pressure after open heart surgery. *Chest* 1979;76:397–400.
31. Marvel SL, Elliott G, Tocino I, et al: Positive end-expiratory pressure following coronary artery bypass grafting. *Chest* 1986;90:537–540.
32. Hertzberg LB, Glass DD: ?, in Kaplan JA (ed): *Management of ventilation, in Cardiac Anesthesia.* Orlando, Grune & Stratton, 1987, vol 2, pp 1041–1058.
33. Robotham JL, Lixfield W, Holland L, et al: The effects of positive end-expiratory pressure on right and left ventricular performance. *Am Rev Resp Dis* 1980;121:677–683.
34. Midell AI, Skinner DB, DeBoer A, Bermudez G: A review of pulmonary problems following valve replacement in 100 consecutive patients. The case against routine use of assisted ventilation. *Ann Thorac Surg* 1974;18:219–227.

35. Prakash O, Jonson B, Meiz S, et al: Criteria for early extubation after intracardiac surgery in adults. *Anesth Analg* 1977;56:703–708.

36. Quasha AL, Loeber N, Feeley TW, et al: Postoperative respiratory care: A controlled trial of early and late extubation following coronary artery bypass grafting. *Anesthesiology* 1980;52:135–141.

37. Gall SA, Olsen CO, Reves JG, et al: Beneficial effects of endotracheal extubation on ventricular performance. *J Thorac Cardiovasc Surg* 1988;95:819–827.

38. Kouchoukos NT, Korp RB: Functional disturbance following extracorporeal circulatory support in cardiac surgery, in Ionescu MI, Wooler GH (eds): *Current Techniques in Extracorporeal Circulation.* London, Butterworth, 1976, p 245.

39. Marsh HM, Abel MD: Postoperative management of the adult cardiac surgical patient, in Tarhan S (ed): *Cardiovascular Anesthesia and Post Operative Care.* Chicago, Year Book, 1989, pp 609–630.

40. Gillespie DJ, Marsh HM, Divertie MB, et al: Clinical outcome of respiratory failure in patients requiring prolonged (greater than 24 hours) mechanical ventilation. *Chest* 1986;90:364–369.

41. Matsumoto M, Oka Y, Strom J: Application transesophageal echocardiography to continuous intraoperative monitoring of left ventricular performance. *Am J Cardiol* 1980;46:95–105.

42. Terai C, Masaaki U, Sugimoto H: Transesophageal echocardiographic dimensional analysis of four cardiac chambers during positive end-expiratory pressure. *Anesthesiology* 1985;63:640–646.

43. Blanche C, Chaux A: Spasm in mammary artery grafts. *Ann Thorac Surg* 1988;45:586.

44. Sarabu MR, McClung JA, Fass A, Reed GE: Early postoperative spasm in left internal mammary artery bypass graft. *Ann Thorac Surg* 1987;44:199.

45. Jett GK, Arcidi JM, Dorsey LM, et al: Vasoactive drug effects on blood flow in the internal mammary artery and saphenous vein grafts. *J Thorac Cardiovasc Surg* 1987;94:2–8.

46. Estafanous FG, Tarazi RC, Viljoen JF, et al: Hypertension following myocardial revascularization. *Am Heart J* 1973;85:732–738.

47. Fremes SE, Weisel RD, Baird RJ, et al: The effects of post operative hypertension and its treatment. *J Thorac Cardiovasc Surg* 1983;86:47–56.

48. Patel CB, Laboy V, Venus B, et al: Use of sodium nitroprusside in post coronary bypass surgery: a plea for conservation. *Chest* 1986;89:663–667.

49. Selzer JL, Doto JB, Jacoby J: Decreased arterial oxygenation during sodium nitroprusside administration for intraoperative hypotension. *Anesth Analg* 1976;55:880–881.

50. Fremes SE, Weisel RD, Mickle DA, Teasdale SJ, et al: A comparison of nitroglycerin and nitroprusside: Treatment of postoperative hypertension. *Ann Thorac Surg* 1985;35:53–59.

51. Kaplan LA, Jones E: Vasodilator therapy during coronary artery surgery: comparison of nitroglycerin and nitroprusside. *J Thorac Cardiovasc Surg* 1979;77:301–309.

52. Mullen JC, Miller DR, Weisel RD, et al: Postoperative hypertension: A comparison of diltiazem, nifedepine, and nitroprusside. *J Thorac Cardiovasc Surg* 1988;96:122–131.

53. Chiariello M, Gold HK, Leinbach RC, et al: Comparison between the effects of nitroprusside and nitroglycerin on ischemic injury during acute myocardial infarction. *Circulation* 1976;54:766–773.

54. Donegani E, Costa P, De Paulis R, et al: Myocardial protection by perioperative diltiazem drip: a clinical evaluation. *J Thorac Cardiovasc Surg* 1986;34:168–171.

55. Floyd J, Komer CA, Frishman R, et al: The treatment of acute hypertension post coronary artery bypass grafting with intravenous nicardipine. *Crit Care Med* 1989;17:S11.

56. Slogoff S, Keats AS: Does chronic treatment with calcium entry blocking drugs reduce perioperative myocardial ischemia? *Anesthesiology* 1988;68:676–680.

57. Chung F, Houston PL, Cheng DCH, et al: Calcium channel blockade does not offer adequate protection from perioperative myocardial ischemia. *Anesthesiology* 1988;69:343–347.

58. Stone JG, Foex P, Sear JW, et al: Myocardial ischemia in untreated hypertensive patients: effect of a single small oral dose of a beta-adrenergic blocking agent. *Anesthesiology* 1988;68:495–500.

59. Gray RJ, Bateman M, Conklin C, Matloff JM: Comparison of esmolol and nitroprusside for acute post cardiac surgical hypertension. *Am J Cardiol* 1987;59:887–891.

60. Leslie JB, Kalavjian RW, Sergio MA, et al: Intravenous labetalol for treatment of postoperative hypertension. *Anesthesiology* 1987;67:413–416.

61. Weeks KR, Chatterjee K, Block S, et al: Bedside hemodynamic monitoring: Its value in the diagnosis of tamponade complicating cardiac surgery. *J Thorac Cardiovasc Surg* 1976;71:250–252.

62. Johnson LW, Dickstein RA, Fruehan CT, et al: Prophylactic digitalization for coronary artery bypass surgery. *Circulation* 1976;53:819–822.

63. Baerman JM, Kirsh MM, Buitlier M, et al: Natural history and determinants of conduction defects following coronary artery bypass surgery. *Ann Thorac Surg* 1987;44:150–153.

64. O'Connell JB, Wallis D, Johnson SA, et al: Transient bundle branch block following use of hypothermic cardioplegia in coronary artery bypass surgery: High incidence without perioperative myocardial infarction. *Am Heart J* 1982;103:85–91.

65. Williams JB, Stephenson LW, Holford FD, et al: Arhythmia prophylaxis using propanolol after coronary artery surgery. *Ann Thorac Surg* 1982;34:435–438.

66. Mohr R, Smolinsky A, Goor DA: Prevention of supraventricular tachyarrhythmia with low dose propanolol after coronary bypass. *J Thorac Cardiovasc Surg* 1981;81:840–845.

67. Daudon P, Corcos T, Gandjbakhch I, et al: Prevention of atrial fibrillation or flutter by acebutolol after coronary artery bypass grafting. *Am J Cardiol* 1986;58:933–936.

68. Bick R, Arbegast N, Crawford L, et al: Hemostatic de-

fects induced by cardiopulmonary bypass. *Vasc Surg* 1975;9:228–243.

69. Beall AC Jr, Yow EM, Bloodwell RD, et al: Open heart surgery without blood transfusion. *Arch Surg* 1967; 94:567–570.

70. Cohen JA, Frederickson EL, Kaplan JA: Plasma heparin activity and antagonism during cardiopulmonary bypass with hypothermia. *Anesth Analg* 1977;56:564–570.

71. Ellison N, Ominsky AJ, Wollman H: Is protamine a clinically important anticoagulant? *Anesthesiology* 1971; 35:621–629.

72. Bull BS, Huse WM, Brauer FS, Korpman RA: Heparin therapy during extracorporeal circulation, II. The use of dose–response curves to individualize the heparin and protamine dose. *J Thoracic Cardiovasc Surg* 1975; 69:685–689.

73. Berger RL: Reduced protamine dosage for heparin neutralization in open heart operations. *Circulation* 1967;suppl 2:154–157.

74. Esposito RA, Culliford AT, Colvin SB, et al: The role of activated clotting time in heparin administration and neutralization for cardiopulmonary bypass. *J Thorac Cardiov Surg* 1983;85:174–185.

75. Kolff WJ, Effler DB, Groves LK, et al: Disposable membrane oxygenator and its use in experimental surgery. *Cleve Clin Q* 1956;23:69–73.

76. Ellison NE, Beatty CP, Blake DR, et al: Heparin rebound in patients and volunteers. *J Thorac Cardiovasc Surg* 1974;67:723–729.

77. Estas JW: Kinetics of the anticoagulant effect of heparin. *JAMA* 1970;212:1492–1495.

78. Bernstein E, Indelglia R, Shea M, Varco R: Sublethal damage to the red blood cell from pumping. *Circulation* 1987;35:S:226.

79. Eika C: On the mechanism of platelet aggregation induced by heparin, protamine and polybrene. *Scand J Haematol* 1972;9:247.

80. Thompson C, Forbes C, Martin E, Prentice C: Potentiation of the platelet aggregation and adhesion of heparin both in vivo and in vitro. *Clin Sci* 1973;44:21.

81. O'Brien JR, Etherington M, Jamieson S: Refractory state of platelet aggregation with major operations. *Lancet* 1971;2:741–743.

82. Hershgold EJ, Pasquini R, Christensen D: Effect of heparin–protamine complexes on in vitro platelet aggregation. Third congress of the International Society on Thrombosis and Haemostasis, Washington, DC, Aug 22–26, 1972, p 204.

83. Schmidt P, Peden J, Brecher G, Baranovsky A: Thrombocytopenia and bleeding tendency after extracorporeal circulation. *N Engl J Med* 1961;265:1181–1185.

84. Karpatkin S: Heterogenicity of human platelets. II. Functional evidence suggestive of young and old platelets. *J Clin Invest* 1969;47:1083–1087.

85. Laufer N, Merin NB, Grover B, et al: The influence of cardiopulmonary bypass on the size of human platelets. *J Thorac Cardiovasc Surg* 1975;70:728–731.

86. Parker-Williams EJ: Platelets in prosthesis and pumps. *Clin Haematol* 1972;1:413.

87. McKenna R, Bachman F, Whittaker B, et al: The hemo-

static mechanism after open heart surgery, II. Frequency of abnormal platelet functions during and after extracorporeal circulation. *J Thorac Cardiovasc Surg* 1975;70:298–308.

88. Teoh K, Van Christaris MD, Weisel RD, et al: Dipyridamole preserved platelets and reduced blood loss after cardiopulmonary bypass. *J Thorac Cardiovasc Surg* 1988;96:332–341.

89. Becker RM, Smils ML, Dobell AR: Effects of platelet inhibition phenomena in cardiopulmonary bypass in pigs. *Ann Surg* 1974;179:52–57.

90. Addonizio VP Jr, Fisher CA, Jenkin BK, et al: Iloprost, a stable analogue of prostacyclin, preserved platelets during stimulated extracorporeal circulation. *J Thorac Cardiovasc Surg* 1985;89:926–933.

91. Bachman F, McKenna R, Cole E, Hassan N: The hemostatic mechanism after open-heart surgery. *J Thorac Cardiovasc Surg* 1975;70:76–85.

92. Jobes DR, Ellison N: Effective hemostasis in the cardiac surgical patient: Current status, in Ellison N, Jobes D (eds): *Effective Hemostasis in Cardiac Surgery.* Philadelphia, Saunders, 1988, pp 195–201.

93. Bowie EJW, Owen CA: The clinical and laboratory diagnosis of hemorrhagic disorders, in Miescher PA, et al (eds): *Disorders of Hemostasis.* Orlando, Grune & Stratton, 1984, pp 73–78.

94. Consensus Conference: Platelet transfusion therapy. *JAMA* 1987;257:1777–1780.

95. Salzman EW, Weinstein MJ, Weintraub RM, et al: Treatment with desmopressin acetate to reduce blood loss after cardiac surgery. *N Engl J Med* 1986;314:1402–1406.

96. Gravlee GP, Hopkins MB: Blood plasma products, in Ellison N, Jobes D (eds): *Effective Hemostasis in Cardiac Surgery.* Philadelphia, Saunders, 1988, pp 69–83.

97. Ware AI: Desmopressin acetate in hemorrhegic conditions, with emphasis on use after cardiopulmonary bypass, in Ellison N, Jobes D (eds): *Effective Hemostasis in Cardiac Surgery.* Philadelphia, Saunders, 1988, pp 137–153.

98. Ware JA, Reaves WH, Horak JK, Solis RT: Defective platelet aggregation in patients undergoing surgical repair of cyanotic congenital heart disease. *Ann Thorac Surg* 1983;36:289–294.

99. Mannucci PM: Desmopressin (DDAVP) for treatment of disorders of hemostasis, in Coller BS (ed): *Progress in Hemostasis and Thrombosis.* Orlando, Grune & Stratton, 1986, pp 19–45.

100. Spiess BD, Ivankovich AD: Thromboelastography: A coagulation-monitoring technique applied to cardiopulmonary bypass, in Ellison N, Jobes D (eds): *Effective Hemostasis in Cardiac Surgery.* Philadelphia, Saunders, 1988, pp 163–182.

101. Spiess B, Tuman K, McCarthy R, et al: Thrombo-elastography (TEG) as an indication of post cardiopulmonary bypass coagulopathies. *J Clin Monitor* 1987;3:25–30.

102. Sladen RN: Temperature and ventilation after hypothermic cardiopulmonary bypass. *Anesth Analg* 1985; 64:816–820.

103. Michenfelder JD, Uihlein A, Daw EF, et al: Moderate

hypothermia in man: Haemodynamic and metabolic effects. *Br J Anaesth* 1965;37:738–745.

104. Rodriguez JL, Weissman C, Damask MC, et al: Physiologic requirements during rewarming: Suppression of the shivering response. *Crit Care Med* 1983;11:490–497.

105. DeBakey ME, Cooley DA, Creech O Jr: Surgical considerations of dissecting aneurysm of the aorta. *Ann Surg* 1955;142:586–612.

106. DeBakey ME, McCollum CH, Grahm GM: Surgical treatment of aneurysms of the descending thoracic aorta: Long term results in over 500 patients. *J Cardiovasc Surg* 1978;19:571–576.

107. Vasco JS, Raess DH, Williams TE, et al: Nonpenetrating trauma to the thoracic aorta. *Surgery* 1977;82:400–406.

108. Symbas PN, Pfarnder LM, Drucker MH, et al: Crossclamping of the descending aorta, hemodynamic and neurohumoral effects. *J Thorac Cardiovasc Surg* 1983;85:300–305.

109. Rosenberg JN, Shine T, Nugent M: Thoracic aortic disease, in Kaplan JA (ed): *Cardiac Anesthesia.* Orlando, Grune & Stratton, 1987, pp 725–749.

110. Shenaq SA, Chelly JE, Karlberg H, et al: Use of nitroprusside during surgery for thoracoabdominal aortic aneurysm. *Circulation* 1984;70:10–17.

111. Crawford ES, Fenstermacher JM, Richardson W, et al: Reappraisal of adjuncts to avoid ischemia in the treatment of thoracic aortic aneursyms. *Surgery* 1970;67:182–196.

112. Katz NW, Blackstone EH, Kirklin JW, et al: Incremental risk factors for spinal cord injury following operation for acute traumatic aortic transection. *J Thorac Cardiovasc Surg* 1981;81:669–674.

113. Cunningham JN, Laschinger JC, Spencer FC: Monitoring of somatosensory evoked potentials during surgical procedures on the thoracoabdominal aorta. *J Thorac Cardiovasc Surg* 1987;94:275–285.

114. Whittemore AD, Clowes AW, Hechtman HB, et al: Aortic aneurysm repair: reduced operative mortality associated with maintenance of optimal cardiac performance. *Ann Surg* 1980;192:414–421.

115. Diehl JT, Cali RF, Hertzer NR, et al: Complications of abdominal aortic reconstruction—An analysis of perioperative risk factors in 557 patients. *Ann Surg* 1983;197:49–56.

116. Young AE, Sandberg GW, Couch NP: The reduction of mortality of abdominal aortic aneurysm resection. *Am J Surg* 1977;134:585–590.

117. Meloche R, Pottecher T, Audit, et al: Hemodynamic changes due to clamping of the abdominal aorta. *Can Anaesth Soc J* 1977;24:20–34.

118. Attia RR, Murphy JD, Snider M, et al: Myocardial ischemia due to infrarenal aortic crossclamping during aortic surgery in patients with severe coronary artery disease. *Circulation* 1976;53:961–965.

119. Gamulin Z, Forster A, Morel D, et al: Effects of infrarenal aortic crossclamping on renal hemodynamics in humans. *Anesthesiology* 1984;61:394–399.

120. Bush HL Jr. Renal failure following abdominal aortic reconstruction. *Surgery* 1983;93:107–111.

121. Starm JT, Billiar TR, Luxenberg MG, Perry JF: Risk factors for the development of renal failure following the surgical treatment of traumatic aortic rupture. *Ann Thorac Surg* 1987;43:425–427.

122. Ostri P, Mouritsen L, Jorgensen B, et al: Renal function following aneurysmectomy of the abdominal aorta. *J Cardiovasc Surg* 1986;27:714–718.

123. Paul MD, Mazer CD, Byrick RJ, et al: Influence of mannitol and dopamine on renal failure during elective infrarenal aortic clamping in man. *Am J Nephrol* 1986;6:422–434.

124. Mault JR, Dechert RE, Lees P, et al: Continuous arteriovenous filtration: An effective treatment for surgical acute renal failure. *Surgery* 1987;101:470–484.

125. Gornick CC, Kjellstrand CM: Acute renal failure complicating aortic aneurysm surgery. *Nephron* 1985;35:145–157.

126. Grace RR, Mattax KL: Anterior spinal artery syndrome following abdominal aortic aneurysmectomy. *Arch Surg* 1987;112:813–817.

127. Weissman C: Postoperative care after major vascular surgery. *Anesth Rep* 1989;1:304–315.

128. Sheng FC, Burns R, Baker JD, et al: Determinants of gastrointestinal complications in aortic surgery. *Vasc Surg* 1987;6:257–267.

129. Campbell WB, Collin J, Morris PJ: The mortality of abdominal aortic aneurysm. *Ann R Coll Surg Engl* 1986;68:275–278.

130. Smead WL, Vascaro PS: Infrarenal aortic aneurysmectomy. *Surg Clin North Am* 1983;63:1269–1292.

131. Kaiser AB, Clayson KR, Mulkerin JL Jr. et al: Antibiotic prophylaxis in vascular surgery. *Ann Surg* 1978;188:283–294.

132. Alexander JI, Spence AA, Pavkl RK, et al: The role of airway closure in postoperative hypoxemia. *Br J Anaesth* 1973;45:34–40.

133. Davis FG, Jackson JM: Postoperative care, in Thomas SJ (ed): *Manual of Cardiac Anesthesia.* New York, Churchill Livingstone, 1984, pp 419–456.

134. Bromage PR, Camperesi E, Chestnut D: Epidural narcotics for postoperative analgesia. *Anesth Analg* 1980;59:473–480.

135. Ali J, Yaffe CS, Serrette C. The effect of transcutaneous electric nerve stimulation on postoperative pain and pulmonary function. *Surgery* 1981;89:507–512.

136. Schemin B, Lindgen L, Rosenberg PH: Treatment of post thoracotomy pain with intermittent instillations of intrapleural bupivicaine. *Acta Anaesth Scand* 1989;33:156–159.

12 | The Neurosurgical Patient

Griselda A. Jones

Meticulous postanesthetic care is essential for good outcome in the neuroanesthetic patient because of the critical relationships between the cardiorespiratory system and intracranial contents.

Continued monitoring by the anesthesiologist must extend during transport into the postanesthetic care unit (PACU), as changes in vital signs may signal the development of an untoward neurological event. A team approach including cooperation between the anesthesiologist, neurosurgeon, and PACU staff, is necessary to ensure success of the neurosurgical procedure.

PATHOPHYSIOLOGY OF INTRACRANIAL PRESSURE

Maintaining adequate cerebral perfusion is of paramount concern. The brain depends almost exclusively on its energy from glycolysis, with minimal glucose and glycogen and low concentrations of high-energy phosphate compounds available for utilization. Thus, cerebral hypoxia usually results from decreased oxygen delivery rather than increased oxygen consumption.[1] Oxygen delivery is decreased due either to hypoxemia, from decreased arterial oxygen content with an adequate cerebral blood flow; or to ischemia, from a pathologic decrease in cerebral blood flow with little or no reduction in arterial oxygen content.[1]

Cerebral Blood Flow

Ischemia results when blood flow is inadequate for the metabolic demands of the tissue. It is caused by inadequate delivery of oxygen and other substrates, inadequate removal of carbon dioxide, and increased production of lactic acid secondary to a shift from aerobic to anaerobic metabolism.[2] The cerebral blood flow (CBF) at which cerebral ischemia occurs has been termed the critical cerebral blood flow. Normal CBF is 45 to 60 mL(100 g)/min. The critical cerebral blood flow is 16 to 17 mL(100 g)/min.[3] However, this figure may be modified by several factors, including certain anesthetic agents and hypothermia. CBF is directly proportional to cerebral perfusion pressure

(CPP). The CPP is defined according to the equation CPP = MABP − ICP, where MABP is the mean systemic arterial blood pressure and ICP is the intracranial pressure. The normal range of CPP is 70 to 100 mm Hg. Any factors that decrease the MABP and increase the ICP, decrease CPP. CPP is more important than ICP or MABP alone in determining brain ischemia.

Intracranial components include brain tissue (84%), cerebrospinal fluid (12%), and blood (4%). The intracranial compartment communicates with the spinal column via the spinal canal and with the thorax via the venous system.[4] The relationship between the three components is described in the Monro-Kellie doctrine developed in the 18th and 19th centuries, modified later by Cushing.[5] The total volume of these factors in the physiological state is constant, and an increase in one is compensated by a decrease in another. The relationship is best demonstrated by the pressure–volume diagram (Fig. 12–1). The horizontal portion of the curve, referred to as the initial phase of compensation, is accounted for by the displacement from the cranial cavity of a volume of cerebrospinal fluid (CSF) sufficient to offset the increase in volume from the mass effect (eg, tumor, hematoma). As the added volume is increased, the compensatory mechanisms are exhausted, and a further increase results

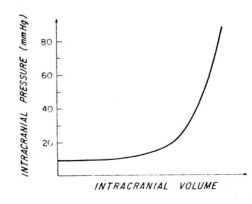

Figure 12-1. Intracranial compliance curve–ICP measurements may be within normal limits although the limits of compliance may have been reached and small increases in value can cause large increases in pressure.

in a rapid rise in ICP. This portion of the curve is known as the phase of decompensation, which represents relatively incompressible brain tissue. The pressure developed by additional volume is a measure of stiffness, or elastance, of the brain. The elastance depends on the physical state of the brain and may be increased by arterial hypertension and decreased by osmotic diuretics.[6]

Autoregulation and Cerebral Blood Flow

The ability of the cerebral vasculature to alter resistance and maintain CBF constant over a wide range in CPP is termed *autoregulation*. Although average CBF is approximately 50 mL/100 g/min, flow is not uniform, being four times greater in gray than in white matter. The limits of autoregulation in normal humans are at a MABP of approximately 50 to 160 mm Hg. Beyond the limits of autoregulation, CBF depends on CPP, which increases the risks of cerebral edema and spontaneous hemorrhage (Fig. 12–2).

Loss or impairment of autoregulation is associated with many of the causes of increased ICP, such as hypercapnia, high concentrations of inhaled anesthetics, hypoxia, trauma, and focal ischemia. Chronic hypertension shifts the autoregulatory curve to the right. When the phenomenon of autoregulation is lost, the CBF becomes passively dependent on systemic pressure.

The arterial carbon dioxide level (Pa_{CO_2}) influences blood flow and ICP. The primary mechanism involved in cerebrovascular response to change in Pa_{CO_2} or localized cerebral metabolic rate is believed to be a change in hydrogen ion concentration (H+) in the extracellular fluid (ECF) of the smooth muscle cells in the arteriolar walls.[7] Carbon dioxide (CO_2) is the most readily available clinical means of altering

ECF (H+) and ultimately cerebrovascular resistance, because CO_2 is an un-ionized gas and can readily diffuse into and out of the ECF. CBF changes by 2 to 3% for each change of 1 mm Hg in Pa_{CO_2} from the normal level of 40 mm Hg. Other determinants of the ECF (H+) include CO_2 produced by local cerebral mechanisms, CSF bicarbonate ion concentration (HCO_3^-), and lactic acidosis. In chronic hypercapnia, CBF tends to return toward normal as adjustment in CSF (HCO_3^-) equilibrates. CBF normalizes in four to six hours from initial hypocapnia with complete adaptation within 24 to 36 hours.[7]

Thus, an increase in blood volume has little effect on ICP if the ICP is low; if the ICP is already elevated, the increase in volume due to hypercarbia can bring about a major rise in pressure.

TRANSFER TO THE PACU

Following uneventful elective procedures, a patient who was conscious preoperatively should be responsive and breathing adequately with intact upper airway reflexes. Effects of the inhalational and intravenous anesthetics should be dissipated or pharmacologically reversed at the end of the surgical procedure. Ideally, the trachea should be extubated prior to leaving the operating room suite. Anesthesiologists and surgeons, especially, find this practice most appealing. Immediate realization of a satisfactory outcome and the ease of detecting any subsequent deterioration in neurological status allows careful monitoring of neurological function.

Several factors may preclude early extubation including intraoperative trauma to the respiratory centers of cranial nerves impairing ventilation postoperatively; drug-induced respiratory depression; inadequate reversal of muscle relaxation; and patients in whom airway or pulmonary decompensation existed preoperatively.

To prevent excessive reaction to the endotracheal tube, intravenous lidocaine (0.5 to 1.5 mg/kg) may be used to diminish laryngeal responses. However, lidocaine can depress the central nervous system (CNS) and decrease protective upper airway reflexes. Ensuring adequate ventilation is of the utmost importance because any rise of Pa_{CO_2} increases cerebral blood flow, which increases ICP. If ventilation with positive end-expiratory pressure (PEEP) is indicated, patients should be nursed in the head-up 30-degree position to avoid an increase in ICP.

Transport of the patient to the PACU requires careful observation. Patients should be kept at a 30-degree head-up position unless contraindicated, as in shunt procedures. Supplemental oxygen should be given. Monitoring devices for transport should in-

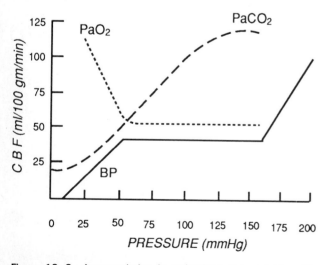

Figure 12–2. Autoregulation is maintained over a fairly wide range of systemic arterial blood pressure under normal conditions.

clude ECG, arterial blood pressure trace, and pulse oximetry. If the endotracheal tube is still present, care should be taken to ensure its stability without any compromise to venous drainage (avoid constrictive circumferential securing of the endotracheal tube).

INITIAL EVALUATION IN THE PACU

On arrival in the PACU, vital signs and neurological assessment are immediately measured and charted. Serum electrolytes, hemoglobin, hematocrit, arterial blood gas values, and skull and chest films are obtained and evaluated. A basic neurological assessment consists of determination of the level of consciousness, the degree of motor activity, and the size, quality, and reaction to light of the pupils. Since early evaluation of mental status and response is often subjective and inconsistent between members of the team, assessment by the Glasgow Coma Scale[8] is appropriate (Table 12–1). Although the scale was originally devised as a prognostic indicator after head injuries, it has been shown to be useful in the standardization of the neurological examination.

Pupillary size and light responses are useful signs of intracranial integrity, especially in the unconscious patient. Regional increases in ICP and herniation of the uncus around the tentorium cerebelli cause the pupil on the same side to dilate. In cases of midbrain lesions, the pupil on the same side constricts.[9] When evaluating pupillary size and response, it is important to note that certain drugs such as atropine, epinephrine, and trimethaphan camsylate all cause dilatation. Opiates and fentanyl constrict the pupil, an effect reversed by naloxone hydrochloride. Also, dur-

ing emergence after inhalation anesthesia, a divergent effect on the pupils (or even nystagmus) may be seen.

A head-up 30-degree position should be maintained throughout the PACU stay. This position promotes venous drainage from the brain and improves oxygenation by increasing the functional residual capacity. Notable exceptions to remaining in the head-up position are patients following lumbar laminectomy, ventriculo-peritoneal shunting, and carotid endarterectomy, and in those patients with absent pharyngeal reflexes. In these cases, there are risks of aspiration and arterial hypotension (which may promote cerebral infarction, arterial spasm, and, in the failing heart, myocardial infarction).

MONITORING

Conventional monitors in the PACU include electrocardiogram, sphygmomanometer, direct intraarterial pressure measurements, and pulse oximetry. Baseline neurological status should be immediately assessed and charted every 15 minutes as noted in a standard PACU neurological protocol. The Glasgow Coma Scale along with neurological function, level of consciousness, motor activity, and pupillary size and reaction to light, should be included in these assessments. A discharge summary or postanesthetic score that describes an awake and alert patient provides a baseline evaluation should any changes in mental status occur.[10]

Intracranial Pressure Monitoring

Invasive measurement of intracranial pressure is an acceptable and commonly used modality for both diagnostic and therapeutic assessment of the neurosurgical patient in the PACU. Direct monitoring of ICP in the immediate postoperative period enables early detection of neurological complications before changes in pupillary responses, mental status, or other vital signs are evident.

Most intracranial pressure monitors are hydrostatic pressure devices. One end is attached to the pia arachnoid and placed in the ventricle and the other end is attached to a Luer lock stopcock/syringe connector, attached to pressure tubing and a transducer.[11] Three types of intracranial monitors exist: intraventricular catheters, subarachnoid bolts, and epidural transducers.

Intraventricular Catheters

ADVANTAGE. These catheters provide therapeutic drainage of CSF, sampling of CSF, the most reliable measurement of ICP, easily analyzed waveform, sim-

TABLE 12–1. THE GLASGOW COMA SCALE

Eyes		
Open	Spontaneously	4
	To command	3
	To pain	2
	No response	1
Best motor response		
To command	Obeys	6
To pain	Localizes	5
	Flexion withdrawal	4
	Decorticate response (abnormal flexion)	3
	Decerebrate rigidity	2
	No response	1
Best verbal response	Oriented	5
	Disoriented	4
	Inappropriate words	3
	Incomprehensible sounds	2
	No response	1

Allowance should be made if the eyes are swollen shut or the trachea is intubated.

ple calibration, and accurate calculation of compliance.

DISADVANTAGES. Drawbacks include the potential for high infection rates, difficulty in cannulating ventricles due to small size or dislocation by mass effect, intracranial hematoma, inaccurate measurements due to progressive brain swelling that may compress the ventricles, and clogging of the catheter after intermittent drainage of ventricular fluid.

Subarachnoid Bolts

ADVANTAGES. Subarachnoid bolts *(most popular: Richmond bolt)* offer ease of positioning, decreased risk of infection, no penetration of the brain, and are useful if ventricles are small or displaced.

DISADVANTAGES. Drawbacks are an inability to drain CSF, unreliable pressures if the brain herniates into the bolt due to intracranial hypertension, and difficulty in measuring intracranial compliance.

Epidural Transducer

ADVANTAGES. Epidural transducers provide ease of insertion, no dural penetration, and a low risk of infection, and no adjustment of the transducer is needed.

DISADVANTAGES. This type of catheter is unable to drain CSF, cannot be recalibrated or rezeroed after placement, and provides questionable accuracy of ICP measurement through dura.[12-15]

All fluid-filled systems must be closed and strict aseptic conditions maintained. No heparin or external pressure from pressure bag systems should be used. No more than 0.1 mL of physiologic fluid should be used to clear any obstruction or flush the system. For the reference point, the base of the skull or the external auditory meatus should be used. Measurements should be made at the end of expiration. Because of the narrow range of normal values, careful calibration is important.[16]

Recently, a new disposable 4 French fiber-optic transducer-tipped catheter (FTC) has been described.[17] The system depends on a miniature transducer at the tip of the catheter. Inside the transducer, the movement of a mirrored diaphragm in response to pressure is sensed by the light fibers. This information is converted into an analog signal and displayed on a portable pressure monitor. The digital mean pressure is continuously displayed and interfaces with conventional monitoring systems for oscilloscopic hardcopy. The catheter is calibrated by the manufacturer and requires no further manipulation. If faulty calibration is suspected, the unit must be re-

placed. The zero or atmospheric balance is done once, prior to insertion of the catheter.

The FTC can be inserted in the same manner as the hydrostatic systems—intraventricularly through a ventriculostomy or by subarachnoid, or subdural placement. Advantages of this new system include elimination of problems of most fluid-filled systems such as dampening, kinked tubing, loose connectors, air bubbles, air entrapment in tubing, and movement artifact associated with fluid column pressure transmission. The ability to continuously monitor ICP during drainage of CSF is especially appealing. During patient transfer, the system uses a battery-powered portable monitor and can be displayed on the monitor as a mean digital value. Disadvantages include inaccurate pressures both when the catheter is "wedged" between the dura and the table of the skull and when the catheter records through tough, fibrous dura. The need for separate equipment for oscilloscopic and hard copy is a further disadvantage. Due to the fragility of the catheter, careful handling to avoid damage is essential.

The normal ICP tracing shows a pulsation with each heartbeat and with respiration. Lundberg classified ICP values into four groups:

Normal	0–10 mm Hg
Slight increase	11–20 mm Hg
Moderate increase	21–40 mm Hg
Severe increase	more than 40 mm Hg

Three types of waves—designated A, B, and C waves—are differentiated. A-waves (plateau waves) are associated with ICP up to 80 mm Hg and may persist for 15 to 20 minutes. These waves indicate that the patient is nearing the limits of the compensatory mechanism on the compliance curve. They may be associated with clinical signs of an acute increase in ICP and may be precipitated by several factors such as pain, surgical stimulation, tracheal intubation, positive-pressure ventilation, or laryngoscopic examination. B-waves are smaller, 20 to 25 mm Hg, occur once per minute, and are thought to be precursors of A-waves. The less-sustained C-waves occur at a rate of six per minute. Their significance presently is not known, although they seem to be benign.[18]

Once an increase in ICP is suspected, diagnostic testing includes skull roentgenograms, arterial blood gas analyses, and computed tomography scans. Hematomas require immediate surgical evacuation. Coagulation profiles should be recorded. Pneumocephalus can be released through a twist drill hole. Cerebral edema is treated with hyperventilation (PaCO$_2$ 25 to 30 mm Hg); diuretics (mainly furosemide 0.5 to 1.0 mg/kg); steroids (dexamethasone 4 mg every six hours, although they are of questionable therapeutic value); and barbiturates. Mannitol is administered in doses of 0.5 to 1.0 g/kg infused over 30 minutes. The onset of action is within 20 minutes and the maximum effect is seen in one to two hours.

Electroencephalographic (EEG) monitoring in the PACU may provide feedback concerning cerebral cortical function when clinical examination is limited or impossible (eg, general anesthesia, altered states of consciousness, barbiturate coma, or paralysis). EEG data may identify seizure activity not associated with clinical phenomena. EEG findings offer a reliable indicator of cerebral ischemia. There is a close correlation between EEG findings and cerebral blood flow and persistent EEG changes during clamping and development of a postoperative neurological defect. EEG data are now conveniently displayed as a three-dimensional display showing amplitude versus frequency versus time; and in a power spectral array (PSA), where the computer performs a Fourier analysis to convert the EEG signal to equivalent sine waves of known frequencies and amplitudes. Monitoring the PSA, the anesthesiologist can assist the neurosurgeon in rapid analysis of cortical function.[19,20]

DELAY IN REGAINING CONSCIOUSNESS

Many factors can combine to delay return to consciousness (Table 12-2). Intracranial surgery is usually not conducted on a "normal" brain. There are some obvious exceptions to this, such as procedures involving cranial nerves and their central pathways for control of pain; removal of small tumors of these nerves; excision of predominantly intrasellar tumors; and clipping of small and medium-sized aneurysms. Reactive swelling and consequent raised ICP are not infrequent accompaniments of neoplasms and ab-

TABLE 12-2. DELAY IN REGAINING CONSCIOUSNESS

Preoperative condition	Depressed sensorium
Intraoperative manifestation	Cerebral edema
Surgical catastrophe	Hematoma, stroke, pneumocephalus, air embolism
Prolonged anesthetic effect	Narcotics, barbiturates, tranquilizers, muscle relaxants
Respiratory depression	Drug effect, central damage
Temperature alteration	Hypothermia, hyperthermia
Cardiac instability	Hypertension, hypotension, arrythmias
Electrolyte imbalance	Hyperglycemia, hypoglycemia, hypernatremia, hyponatremia

Several factors may combine to delay return to consciousness in the neurosurgical patient.

scesses. If ischemia from increased pressure or reactive swelling occurs pre- or intraoperatively, recovery may be delayed or even limited. The brain is less tolerant of traction, manipulation, or rapid alterations of pressure. Preoperative status of the patient is an important determinent of postoperative function. Premedication, especially in elderly, hypovolemic (uncorrected), and other debilitated patients may contribute to delay in regaining consciousness. Patients who were intoxicated with alcohol or other "street drugs" may show a delay in awakening.

Intraoperative events must be considered. If narcotics were used for maintenance of anesthesia, the patient may still be narcotized. Naloxone hydrochloride should be avoided whenever possible, to prevent vomiting and untoward hemodynamic changes that occur with increased levels of pain. Small incremental doses, such as 0.05 to 0.1 mg, can be given intravenously until the desired response is attained. Temperature abnormalities, both hypothermia and hyperthermia, can delay recovery and must be corrected. The blood–brain barrier protects the CNS against excesses or deficits of sodium and water in isotonic proportions. This mechanism may fail if there is a major shift in osmolality of body fluids or after surgical intervention. Derangements of water, electrolytes, and acid–base homeostasis are manifest frequently as altered sensorium, disorientation, or focal or generalized manifestations. Fluid shifts intraoperatively or in the immediate postoperative period, caused by hypovolemia or as a result of diuretic administration, as well as hypervolemia, due to subsequent fluid overload, diabetes insipidus, or the syndrome of inappropriate antidiuretic release, may further complicate postoperative neurologic assessment.

An intraoperative catastrophe such as a paradoxical air embolism may cause prolonged unconsciousness. Air is entrained into the venous system of a patient with a right-to-left shunt, either an atrial or ventricular septal defect on a probe-patent foramen ovale. Although the valve is normally closed, should the pressure on the right side of the heart exceed that of the left side, it may open. Such a pressure change can be caused by the presence of air in the right heart or, in rare instances, by the sitting position. As only very small amounts of air (insufficient enough to be detected clinically) in the arteries of the brainstem can have devastating effects, the event might have passed unnoticed intraoperatively. Significant venous air embolism occurs in approximately 30% of patients in the sitting position. The complication may manifest as hypoxia postoperatively.

Other intraoperative occurrences that delay recovery include cerebral infarction, intracranial hematoma, and cerebral edema. After any intracranial pro-

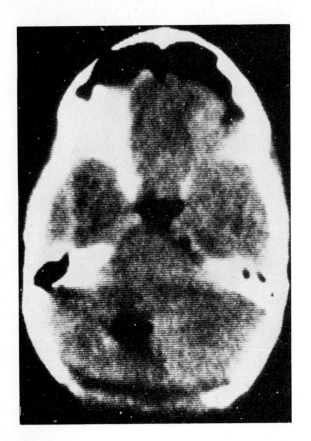

Figure 12–3. Tension pneumocephalus depicted in skull radiograms and by computerized tomography. Two to three weeks may be required for absorption of entrapped air. (Courtesy of Daniel Spitzer, Department of Neurosurgery, Montefiore Hospital, Bronx, New York.)

cedure, a small amount of air remains under the dura. This volume depends on the extent of decrease of cerebral volume caused by hyperventilation, diuretic administration, and mass removal. After closure of the dura, the brain size increases as brain fluid reaccumulates, normocarbia returns, hypothermia is corrected, and the pressure within the air pocket increases. Tension pneumocephalus can cause a profound decrease in level of consciousness. Diagnosis is made by skull radiographs or computerized tomography (Fig. 12–3).

THE RESPIRATORY SYSTEM

Respiratory inadequacy of any degree is undesirable in neurosurgical patients because of the deleterious effects of raised intracranial pressure and possible edema formation from both hypoxia and hypercarbia. Systemic hypoxia causes tissue lactic acidosis with a decrease in cerebral vascular resistance and a vasodilatory effect contributing both to an increase in cerebral blood flow and intracranial pressure.

The preoperative respiratory status of the patient impacts on the postoperative management. The safety of early extubation is decreased by chronic lung disease such as smoking, gross obesity, or other prexisting lung pathology; and by acute disease such as in aspiration from alcohol intoxication, cervical cord injuries, drowning, or smoke inhalation.

Surgical dissection in areas near the respiratory center, or increased pressure on the brainstem from edema or hemorrhage, can lead to respiratory irregularity. The earliest sign of bleeding in the posterior fossa can be hyperventilation. Carotid endarterectomy may damage the carotid body, which is the chemoreceptor responsible for the reflex increase in ventilation in response to arterial hypoxemia or acidosis. If the patient was breathing spontaneously prior to surgery, the goal of postoperative management is to return the patient to the same preoperative state. Neuromuscular blockade must be adequately reversed and those factors that may prolong blockade—such as hypothermia, hypokalemia, previous muscular weakness, and antibiotic administration—should be closely identified. If the sitting position is utilized, careful evaluation of the airway must be made prior to extubation. Edema of the airway with subsequent obstruction is not uncommon. Prolonged hyperventilation intraoperatively depletes CO_2 stores. These stores are reaccumulated by hypoventilation and as there are no oxygen stores, hypoxia may develop. Prolonged procedures with mechanical ventilation may predispose the patient to a degree of atelectasis. Diffusion hypoxia must be considered if nitrous oxide has been employed as an anesthetic. Tracheobronchial toilet, including suctioning of the endotracheal tube, must be accomplished with the minimal amount of trauma to prevent increasing intracranial pressure and hypoxia.[21] Postoperative shivering, which may increase oxygen requirements up to 400%, should be avoided if at all possible. Neurogenic pulmonary edema is a rare cause of hypoxia and is associated with severe intracranial damage.

Upon admission to the PACU, basic measurements include recording of respiratory rate, tidal volume, inspiratory force, and arterial blood gas analyses. Postoperative chest films should be obtained and evaluated. If one or more of the criteria listed in Table 12–3 exists, continued tracheal intubation with respiratory support should be considered.

If endotracheal intubation must be extended into the postanesthetic period, the criteria listed in Table 12–4 may help in determining an appropriate time for extubation.

Hypercoagulability

Intracranial malignancies and surgical procedures predispose to pulmonary embolism. Other factors

TABLE 12–3. CRITERIA FOR THE DIAGNOSIS OF RESPIRATORY INSUFFICIENCY

Rate of respiration	> 40/min, < 8/min
Tidal volume	< 3.5 mL/kg
Vital capacity	< 15 mL/kg
Vd/Vt	> 0.5
Maximal inspiratory force	< −25 cm H_2O
% pulmonary shunt	> 15%
$Paco_2$	> 45 mm Hg
Respiratory pattern	Irregular

If one or more of these criteria exist, reintubation and continued ventilatory support should be considered.

that increase the risk of thrombosis include previous venous thrombosis, varicose veins, obesity, and increased age.

Antithrombotic therapy includes placement of antiembolic stockings. Anticoagulant therapy including heparin or warfarin sodium is rarely justified immediately after intracranial surgery because of the dangers of cerebral hemorrhage.

THE CARDIOVASCULAR SYSTEM

Cardiovascular instability in the postoperative period can have disastrous CNS effects. Hypertension is one of the most frequently encountered problems in neurosurgical patients. Besides the added stress placed on the myocardium, hypertension can raise the intracranial pressure if autoregulation is impaired. The tendency to bleed at the operative site and edema formation may be increased.

The causes of hypertension are varied. Intraoperative fluid overload (which becomes more apparent during emergence as vascular tone returns); shivering; hypercarbia; preoperative hypertension (especially uncontrolled); rapid rewarming; vasoconstriction from hypothermia; hypoxemia; and pharmacologic intervention; all must be considered as possible etiologies. Rebound hypertension due to interference with the renin–angiotensin system may oc-

cur following the use of sodium nitroprusside. Resetting of the carotid baroreceptors and alterations of cerebral flow have been implicated as causes of hypertension following carotid endarterectomy. Tissue hypoxia in ischemic areas may cause the release of vasopressor substances triggering a hypertensive response.

Treatment of hypertension should be aimed at identifying the cause and treating appropriately. Labetalol, in intermittent boluses or by infusion, has been used with good results. Esmolol, with its rapid onset and short half-life, is also a good choice when beta-blockade is desired. While monitoring intravascular volume, diuretics have been used to control blood pressure postoperatively. Vasodilator drugs such as sodium nitroprusside may be used, although the increase obtained in cerebral venous pressure (CVP) may critically decrease CPP. Trimethaphan camsylate causes tachyphylaxis, tachycardia, and prolonged muscle weakness. It should be avoided although it has little effect on cerebral dynamics. Although hydralazine may cause cerebral vasodilation, increases in ICP, and decreases in CPP, it has been used to control blood pressure throughout the PACU stay.

Hypotension postoperatively is usually due to hypovolemia, especially secondary to diuretic administration. Measurement of CVP guides appropriate volume replacement. Other causes of hypotension are chronic hypovolemia from long-term diuretic therapy; adrenal insufficiency in the patient on steroid administration; anaphylactic reaction to antibiotics or blood products; a late response to sodium nitroprusside administration; catastrophic brainstem injury; persistent anesthetic effect; a late effect of beta-blockade; myocardial damage; hypothermia; and electrolyte imbalance.

Electrocardiographic abnormalities postoperatively may be related to intracranial injury or a result of therapy. T-wave inversion or ST depression can occur after ruptured cerebral aneurysm.[22] Bradycardia or supraventricular arrhythmias may be related to intracranial pathology or hypokalemia caused by diuretic therapy aggravated by respiratory alkalosis from hyperventilation. Tachycardia can be a result of vasodilator therapy or even associated with hypertension and elevated ICP.

TABLE 12–4. CRITERIA FOR EXTUBATION

History	Awake preoperatively; smooth intraoperative course
Respiratory rate	12–35/min
Respiratory pattern	Regular
Vital capacity	> −30 cm H_2O
Maximal inspiratory force	> −20 cm H_2O
Vd/Vt	< 0.5
Pulmonary Shunt	< 12%
$Paco_2$	30–45 mm Hg
Pao_2	> 75 mm Hg (FIO_2 = 0.3)

If these conditions are realized, extubation can usually be safely accomplished.

POSTOPERATIVE SEIZURES

Seizures occur in about 20% of neurosurgical patients postoperatively. A higher incidence occurs in patients with brain abscess or subdural empyema (up to 72%), and in those patients who had uncontrolled epilepsy preoperatively.[23] Seizures are also more likely to occur if the surgery involved a vascular lesion (intracranial aneurysm, arteriovenous malformation, hematoma) or if the surgical approach was transfrontal or required marked retraction of neural tissue.[24,25]

The dangers of seizures include the risk of aspiration, an increased incidence of focal and generalized neurological deficits possibly as a result of increased cerebral edema, and increased oxygen consumption during a period when ventilation may be suboptimal.

Phenytoin is used both for the treatment and prevention of postcraniotomy seizures. Preoperative administration of phenytoin has now become standard therapy. Dosages of 7 to 15 mg/kg given slowly (no more than 50 mg/min) achieve therapeutic blood levels.[26] Careful monitoring of the electrocardiogram and arterial blood pressure is necessary as arrhythmias and hypotension may occur. Decreased sensorium may occur with more rapid administration.

NERVE PALSIES

Effects of malpositioning during surgery may manifest as nerve palsies postoperatively. Brachial plexus and peroneal nerve palsies have been described in patients after craniotomy in the sitting position. The prone position in a circular face-piece has led to monocular blindness due to reduction in retinal artery flow secondary to compression of the globe. Hypoglossal nerve palsy following carotid endarterectomy may be associated with airway obstruction due to weakness of the tongue. Also, carotid endarterectomy may cause dysfunction of cranial nerves VII, IX, X, and XII, causing interference with vocal cord function, and gag reflexes, and ablating the ability to manage secretions necessitating prolonged intubation or even reintubation. Removal of cerebellopontine angle tumors may be associated with lower cranial nerve paresis (IX, X, XI, XII). Cranial nerve dysfunction may also occur after surgery in the fourth ventricle or for syringomyelia.

Damage to the cranial nerves can pose a diagnostic and patient care problem in the PACU. Temporary or permanent diplopia may result from direct injury. Keratitis may develop if corneal protection is inadequate both intraoperatively and during the PACU stay. Immediate prophylactic tarsorrhaphy is indicated. Diplopia on lateral gaze to the ipsilateral side may occur as a result of direct injury to the sixth nerve or brainstem dysfunction. With the use of the microscope, fewer facial nerve palsies occur.

GASTROINTESTINAL SYSTEM

Gastrointestinal bleeding occurs in about 2% of neurosurgical patients.[27] The etiology of this complication is associated with damage to the orbital surface of the frontal lobe, hypothalamus, or the tegmental area of the pons, rather than with the routine administration of steroids. Damage from surgery around the fourth ventricle, in close proximity to the vagal nuclei and parasympathetic pathways, has been associated with gastrointestinal bleeding. Decreased gastric motility is associated with increased ICP. Efforts made to evacuate the stomach contents prior to extubation are important.[28] Perioperative use of H_2-blockers (cimetidine 300 mg every 12 hours or ranitidine 150 mg every 12 hours beginning preferably 8 hours prior to surgery) and antacids (nonparticulate, such as sodium citrate 15 to 30 mL 15 to 30 minutes prior to surgery) is indicated.

THERMOREGULATORY SYSTEM

During prolonged surgical procedures, hypothermia is caused by heat loss convection, conduction, and radiation. The result may be (1) prolonged neuromuscular block, aggravating hypoventilation and hypercarbia; (2) shivering and rewarming, increasing oxygen consumption and hypoxemia; (3) a shift to the left of the oxygen dissociation curve; (4) vasoconstriction contributing to hypertension; (5) prolongation of recovery from general anesthesia; and (6) increase in pressure in a pneumocephalus.[29] Lesions of the brainstem or hypothalamus that cause hypothermia are rare. More common causes are severe injury, removal of a pituitary tumor or craniopharyngioma, or after spinal cord transection.

Immediate postoperative therapy includes warming of intravenous fluids and blood products, elevation of ambient temperature (if at all possible), use of radiant warmers, and humidification of inspired gases.

Hyperthermia can be caused by autonomic disturbances such as injury to the floor of the fourth ventricle, or the thalamus; and blood in the ventricular system. This may be accompanied by deep unconsciousness, shallow respirations, hypotension, and tachycardia. Although malignant hyperthermia usually occurs intraoperatively, it can manifest itself during the immediate postoperative period. Detection and treatment must begin immediately. An approach through infected surgical cavities, such as the sphenoid sinus or mastoid, increases the risk of postoperative meningitis.

SPECIAL CONSIDERATIONS

Several specific procedures require special considerations.

Spinal Column Surgery

The level of the spinal column at which the surgical intervention occurred determines the care necessary and the complications that may be seen in the PACU. Pain is usually related to muscle spasm in the immediate postoperative period, necessitating the use of narcotics for analgesia. The consequence of respiratory depression is not as severe as after craniotomy. Postoperatively the patient is nursed in a supine position to improve venous drainage. This position decreases functional residual capacity. Pulse oximetry is indicated.

Lumbar and Thoracic Laminectomy

Frequent neurovascular checks of the lower extremities are necessary to detect early hematoma formation that may cause cord compression. Therapy requires immediate reexploration.

Arteriovenous malformations of the cord may be extensive and require prolonged microsurgical dissection. Postoperative requirements include monitoring of cardiovascular stability due to the large blood loss and replacement. Hypothermia may be problematic. Frequent neurological examinations are necessary.

Patients who undergo Harrington-rod instrumentation for idiopathic scoliosis may have respiratory impairment preoperatively. Severe postoperative pain and administration of narcotics may further impair respiratory efforts. The major neurologic complication is damage to the spinal cord causing paresis or paralysis. Eliciting ankle clonus bilaterally is a satisfactory method of ensuring intact lower motor neuron function.

Cervical Spine Fusion

Cervical cord trauma may require emergency surgery for decompression and stabilization. Intercostal muscle function is lost with injury above T1, and therefore the incidence of respiratory embarrassment increases. Spasm and edema of the auxiliary musculature, especially if anterior stabilization has been done, can further contribute to ventilatory failure.[30] Careful assessment of the airway must be undertaken before extubation.

Hypoxemia secondary to neuromuscular deficit is found in approximately 50% of patients with a high spinal cord injury. Tracheal suctioning or intermittent ventilatory assistance may result in reflex bradycardia or even cardiac arrest due to vasovagal reflex in sympathectomized patients. This reflex can be blocked by administering atropine 0.4 mg intravenously. Cardiovascular instability after a high cord injury caused by poor sympathetic tone can result in hypotension and bradycardia. Pulmonary artery pressure monitoring may be essential to guide the resuscitation and prevent pulmonary edema formation. Atropine 0.4 mg intravenously, and even vasopressors, may be necessary to maintain cardiac stability.

Absence of neural drive to ventilation when voluntary control of breathing is diminished by sleep (Ondine's syndrome) is a rare but very serious postoperative respiratory complication. After severe high spinal cord injury or following bilateral percutaneous cervical cordotomy performed to relieve pain, there is interruption of ascending spinothalamic pathways transmitting pain sensation and also a block of involuntary respiratory tracts in the ventral quadrant of the cord. An apnea alarm or pulse oximeter must be utilized. Prophylactic intubation or tracheostomy may be performed. The disease is self-limiting over several days.[28]

Aneurysm Clipping

One of the more common causes of deterioration after apparently successful aneurysm surgery is arterial vasospasm. Cerebral vasospasm as a complication of subarachnoid hemorrhage has been well documented.[31] Neurological deficit may occur if the CBF level falls below 15 to 20 mL (100 g)/min.[32] Immediate correction of the flow insufficiency and avoidance of its direct consequences of capillary sludging and postischemic edema may allow improvement of the neurological deficit. Impairment of the ionic pump function results in a large extracellular efflux of potassium and leads to cell death, an effect that occurs at CBF levels of 7 to 11 mL (100 g)/min. Reversal of this decrease of CBF by increasing systemic blood pressure without further compromising ICP has proved useful. Volume expansion with whole blood does not cause vasodilation and does not increase collateral perfusion to ischemic areas of the blood because of the increased delivery of oxygen causing vasoconstriction. However, crystalloid-induced hypervolemia does result in vasodilation, which may be a response to decreased hemoglobin concentration and oxygen delivery.[33]

Induced hypotension intraoperatively is usually achieved by sodium nitroprusside infusion. Complications that may be seen in the immediate postoperative period include metabolic acidosis, tachycardia, hypotension, ventricular arrhythmias, and cardiac arrest. The treatment of cyanide toxicity requires sodium nitrite 300 mg intravenously, or sodium thiosulfate 150 mg/kg. Both therapies are aimed at increasing elimination through nontoxic breakdown.

Stereotactic Surgery

Stereotactic procedures are usually performed under local anesthesia with minimal sedation, unless the patient is too young, confused, or agitated to lie quietly, or has such severe involuntary movements that general anesthesia is essential. The patient is able to cooperate with simple commands, which allows accurate assessment of mental status. The most common complications are intracranial bleeding and edema. Performing these procedures under local anesthesia affords an additional degree of safety since neurologic deterioration can be quickly evaluated. Although the procedure appears relatively benign, frequent neurological examinations in the PACU are still essential.

Hypophysectomy

A major complication after hypophysectomy is the development of diabetes insipidus (DI). DI, a dysfunction of the neurohypophyseal tract, may occur following subarachnoid hemorrhage, aneurysmal surgery, craniofacial trauma, or surgery involving the pituitary and hypothalamic areas. Patients develop massive polyuria (16 to 24 L/day); excessive thirst; polydypsia; dilute urine (< 290 mOsmol/kg), specific gravity under 1.010; and serum sodium levels above 155 mg/dL. ''Essential hypernatremia'' has also been shown to present as intermittent hypernatremia and represent a variant of postoperative or posttraumatic diabetes insipidus, especially when there is an associated impairment in thirst mechanisms.[34]

The diagnosis of DI is made by either dehydration test or infusion of hypertonic saline.[35] The dehydration test is positive for DI after fluids are held long enough to show an hourly rise in urinary osmolality. Plasma osmolality is measured and five units of aqueous pitressin are administered subcutaneously and urine osmolality is measured. An increase in urine osmolality of greater than 9% indicates DI. Infusion of hypertonic saline can establish DI after a patient is given a water load of 20 mL/kg, which is followed by slow infusion of 5% saline to replace the water and solute lost in urine volume measured every 15 minutes. Following this a 5% saline infusion (0.05 mL/kg/min) is given. Osmolality of urine and plasma is measured every 15 minutes and the free water clearance is calculated. In patients with DI, both urine volume and free water clearance are unchanged.

Therapy consists of replacement of antidiuretic hormone. Nasal preparations are available, but due to the likely presence of nasal packing postoperatively, an intramuscular or intravenous preparation must be used. Desmopressin acetate injection,

(DDAVP) is a synthetic analogue of 8-arginine vasopressin indicated for antidiuretic replacement therapy in central DI. Dosages of 0.3 to 0.4 μg/kg have been recommended. Steroid replacement should be continued. Fluid replacement should avoid glucose-containing solutions.

Other causes of polyuria include solute diuresis caused by diuretics, hyperglycemia, and mineralocorticoid deficiency. Fluid and electrolytes should be closely monitored because of large fluid shifts that occurred intraoperatively.

Posterior Cranial Fossa Surgery

Intraoperatively, much effort has been expended to decrease brain size. The patient is predisposed to the development of a tension pneumocephalus. Airtight closure of the dura over a contracted brain may create a closed air space.[36] Craniotomies performed in the sitting position have been shown to create a siphon-like effect for air flow into the cranium,[37] as may the use of ventricular or lumbar subarachnoid drains.[38,39] Nitrous oxide expansion of all closed intracranial spaces is well documented.[40,41]

Controversy concerning the use of the sitting position in neurosurgery continues. The advantages and disadvantages intraoperatively are currently reviewed in the literature.[42] Complications of arterial and venous air embolism may include hypoxia; cor pulmonale; pulmonary edema[43]; cervical cord ischemia; midcervical quadriplegia[44]; postural hypotension; injury to the brachial plexus, sciatic, and peroneal nerves; obstruction of the internal jugular veins[45]; and increased incidence of myocardial infarction, especially in those patients with preexisting hypertensive disease.[46]

In the PACU, caution must be exercised in evaluating respiratory function. Lower cranial nerve dysfunction may cause vocal cord paralysis, swallowing difficulty, and airway obstruction, resulting in respiratory stridor, retained secretions, and the risk of aspiration. Blood from vigorous suctioning may accumulate in the posterior pharynx causing laryngospasm and respiratory arrest. Pharyngeal and tracheal edema may develop during prolonged intubation in a flexed position.

Because of the manipulation of the brain stem in posterior cranial fossa surgery, prolonged ventilatory disturbances may occur. In these situations evaluation of the respiratory pattern through pneumotachography, monitoring of ventilatory CO_2 response through capnography, and evaluation of intraairway pressure at occlusion before and during CO_2 challenge, have been used to evaluate adequacy of ventilation before extubation.[47] If there is still doubt, extubation should be delayed pending complete return to consciousness. Prior to extubation, laryngoscopy will help to confirm the presence of adequate protective laryngeal function.

Carotid Endarterectomy

Postoperatively, careful monitoring is essential for at least 24 hours, beginning in the PACU and continuing into an intensive care setting. Hypertension following carotid endarterectomy occurs with relative frequency.[48] New neurologic deficits have correlated positively with postoperative hypertension. Intracranial hemorrhage is a risk of cerebral revascularization that is markedly increased by hypertension.[49] Hypertension may also increase capillary hydrostatic pressure, especially in ischemic areas of the brain, leading to protein leak, edema, or hemorrhagic infarction. Ideally, arterial blood pressure should be stabilized prior to transport to the PACU. Close monitoring of arterial pressure during transport is essential. Hypotension may be seen as another alteration of the baroreceptor function postoperatively. Treatment consists of fluid replacement and infusion of phenylephrine hydrochloride if indicated.

Perioperative myocardial infarction is the leading cause of morbidity and mortality in these patients. A preoperative history of cardiac disease must be aggressively assessed and managed prior to surgery. Alterations in systemic blood pressure must be managed promptly to decrease the likelihood of an ischemic event. Cardiac medications should be continued up until the surgical procedure and restarted as soon as possible. Intraoperative and continued postoperative monitoring by a pulmonary catheter should be considered. Useful therapeutic modalities include intravenous infusions of labetalol (2 mg/kg/h), esmolol (50 to 100 μg/kg/min), infusions of sodium nitroprusside, and hydralazine (5 to 20 mg) to control hypertension.

Neurologic deficits caused by thrombosis require immediate reexploration. Postoperative bleeding can cause progressive impingement on the airway, causing respiratory difficulty and nearly impossible endotracheal intubation. The wound may need surgical evacuation prior to intubation.

Trauma to the carotid body may cause a decreased ventilatory response to increasing $PaCO_2$ and hypoxia, especially in patients who have undergone a staged bilateral procedure. Narcotics and other drugs that depress respiration should be administered cautiously or not at all. Patients should receive a high inspired oxygen concentration and an apnea monitor should be used.

Macroglossia and Facial Edema

Massive macroglossia and facial edema (Fig. 12–4) can be a postoperative complication related to positioning intraoperatively. Extreme flexion of the head

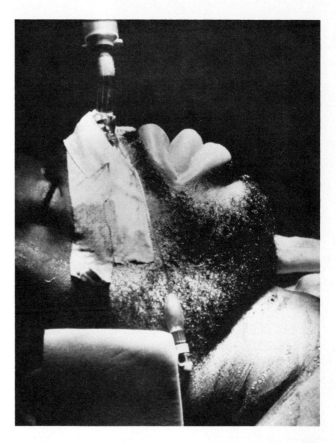

Figure 12–4. Massive facial edema prohibiting immediate postoperative extubation. The patient had been maintained in a flexed prone position for about five hours. (Courtesy of Daniel Spitzer, Department of Neurosugery, Montefiore Hospital, Bronx, New York.)

and neck may lead to venous thrombosis and swelling of the face and tongue. Bilateral occlusion of the internal jugular veins occur when the neck is flexed. Reintubation and even tracheostomy has been necessary in several cases.[50,51]

Neurogenic Pulmonary Edema

Acute neurogenic pulmonary edema (NPE) has been associated with several neurological states including severe head injury, multiple seizures, meningitis, subarachnoid hemorrhage, thrombosis, and intracranial tumors. The edema is fulminant and responds poorly to traditional treatment modalities such as digitalis and diuretics. It appears that NPE is initiated by a predominant alpha-receptor stimulation resulting from excessive increase in intracranial pressure. Left ventricular failure, as a result of increased preload and afterload due to intense systemic vasoconstriction with central pooling of blood, precedes NPE. As hypotension can further damage the already compromised cerebral circulation and autoregulation, a short-acting alpha-blocking agent such as phentolamine is indicated. The mainstay of therapy is directed toward the underlying brain injury or disease. Intubation and mechanical ventilation have proven to be beneficial.[52]

Postsurgical Testing

If a patient's neurological status is deteriorating, it may be necessary to transport the patient to the computerized tomography (CT) or magnetic resonance imaging (MRI) suite and continue monitoring and care in that environment. Ventilator support for controlled ventilation, intraarterial blood pressure monitoring, intracranial pressure monitoring, pharmacological paralysis, capnography, and pulse oximetry have been described and used successfully.[53]

Some studies[54] after carotid endarterectomy have shown that postoperative thrombosis occurred in the transition period between the end of the operation and shortly after the arrival of the patient in the PACU. The use of the ocular pneumoplethysmography in the PACU can determine the necessity of immediate reoperation for documented thrombosis of the carotid endarterectomy site. Conjunctival edema occurring intraoperatively can cause false positive tests, resulting in unnecessary reoperation.[54]

NEW ANESTHETICS AND THEIR IMPACT ON NEUROANESTHESIA

Propofol

Propofol (Diprivan, 2,6-diisopropylphenol) was first studied in Europe as an intravenous anesthetic agent, administered by either single injection for induction of anesthesia or by continuous infusion for maintenance of anesthesia. Now available as an aqueous emulsion, to avoid anaphylactic reactions, propofol has the advantage of a rapid recovery described as a "clear-headedness," with the alertness to accomplish minor tasks.[55] Clinical trials are still ongoing, but to date patterns are emerging. Encouraging results of earlier studies from Europe and later studies from the United States have shown that propofol decreases CBF (30%), cerebral vascular resistance (50%), and cerebral oxygen consumption (20%).[56] CPP remains unchanged during induction with propofol but CSF and mean arterial pressures decrease significantly.[57] As is the case with barbiturates and etomidate, propofol decreases ICP, presumably related to a decrease in cerebral blood volume.[58] The ventilatory effects of thiopental, etomidate, and propofol are comparable.[59] In comparison with thiopental, propofol shows more cardiovascular depressant effects such as a decrease in systemic arterial pressure, decrease in systemic vascular resistance, and a decrease in cardiac output.[55] Lower dosage administration (2 mg/kg) can maintain better cardiac stability.[55]

The rapid onset of action and short duration with remarkable recovery attributes may allow for even better neurological evaluation of a patient postoperatively. An uneventful PACU recovery that may be possible with this nearly "perfect" intravenous anesthetic agent would be a welcomed addition to the anesthesiologist's armamentarium. More study is needed.

Flumazenil

Flumazenil (Anexate) is an imidazobenzodiazepine that acts as a potent benzodiazepine antagonist, and blocks the central effects of the benzodiazepines at the receptor level.[60] Studies [61-63] have shown that patients intoxicated with benzodiazepines were fully awake within two to five minutes after careful titration of flumazenil. No significant changes in heart rate, blood pressure, or respiratory rate were observed. While monitoring EEG through PSA, patients sedated with benzodiazepines awakened smoothly with an abrupt change in the median EEG frequency from less than 3 to more than 6 Hz.[64] Some investigators have noted a slight drowsiness about one hour after reversal of sedation, which coincides with flumazenil's short elimination half-life of 50 minutes. Further studies are needed to determine the efficacy of this antagonism and to verify the lack of a stress response. The ability to safely "reverse" the effects of the benzodiazepines will provide another intravenous technique to the neuroanesthesiologist that allows early neurological assessment.

REFERENCES

1. Michenfelder JD: Brain hypoxia: Current status of experimental and clinical therapy. *Semin Anesth* 1983; 2:81–90.
2. Messick JM: Principles of neuroanesthesia for the non-neurosurgical patient with CNS pathophysiology. *Anesth Analg* 1985;64:143–174.
3. Astrup J, Siesjo BK, Symon L: Thresholds in cerebral ischemia—the ischemic penumbra. *Stroke* 1985;12: 723–725.
4. Frost EAM: *Recovery Room Practice.* Boston, Blackwell, 1985, p 151.
5. Miller JD, Sullivan HG: Severe intracranial hypertension. *Int Anesthesiol Clin* 1979;17:19–75.
6. McGillicuddy JE: Cerebral protection: Pathophysiology and treatment of increased intracranial pressure. *Chest* 1985;87:85–93.
7. Michenfelder JD: The cerebral circulation, in Prys-Roberts C (ed): *The Circulation in Anaesthesia: Applied Physiology and Pharmacology.* Oxford, Blackwell, 1980, pp 209–225.
8. Teasdale G, Jennett BB: Assessment of coma and impaired consciousness. A practical scale. *Lancet* 1974; 2:81.

9. Thiagarajah S: Postoperative care of neurosurgical patients. *Int Anesthesiol Clin* 1983;21:139–156.

10. Cramer C: Lumbar laminectomy: PACU standard or malpractice? *J Postanesth Nurs* 1987;11:149–158.

11. Aucoin PJ, Kotilainen HR, Gantz NM, et al: Intracranial pressure monitors and infection risks. *Am J Med* 1986;80:369–376.

12. North B, Reilly P: Comparison among three methods of intracranial pressure recording. *Neurosurgery* 1986;18:730–732.

13. Ostrup RC, Luerssen TG, Marshall LF, et al: Continuous monitoring of intracranial pressure with a miniaturized fiberoptic device. *J Neurosurg* 1987;67:206–209.

14. Sundbarg G, Nordstrom C, Messeter K, et al: Intraparenchymatous and intraventricular pressure recording. *J Neurosurg* 1987;67:841–845.

15. Mollman HD, Rockswold GL, Ford SE: Comparative methods of intracranial pressure monitorings. *J Neurosurg* 1988;68:737–741.

16. Thiagarajah S: Postoperative care of neurosurgical patients. *Int Anesthesiol Clin* 1983;21:139–154.

17. Hollingsworth-Fridlund P, Vos H, Daily EK: Use of fiber-optic pressure transducer for intracranial pressure measurements: A preliminary report. *Heart Lung* 1988;17:111–120.

18. Thiagarajah S: Postoperative care of neurosurgical patients, in *Recovery Room Practice*. Boston, Blackwell, 1985, pp 150–167.

19. Cascino GD: Neurophysiological monitoring in the intensive care unit. *J Intensive Care Med* 1988;3:215–223.

20. Hug CC: Monitoring, in Miller RD (ed): *Anesthesia*. New York, Churchill Livingstone, 1986, pp 420–422.

21. Rudy EB, Baun M, Stone K, et al: The relationship between endotracheal suctioning and changes in intracranial pressure: A review of the literature. *Heart Lung* 1986;15:488–493.

22. Drummond JC, Todd MM: Acute sinus arrhythmia during surgery in the fourth ventricle: An indicator of brain-stem irritation. *Anesthesiology* 1984;6:232.

23. Calliauw L, de Praetere P, Verbeke L: Postoperative epilepsy in subdural suppurations. *Acta Neurochir* 1984;71:217–223.

24. Deutschman CS, Haines SJ: Anticonvulsant prophylaxis in neurological surgery. *Neurosurgery* 1985;17:510–515.

25. Shaw MDM, Foy P, Chadwick D: The effectiveness of prophylactic anticonvulsants following neurosurgery. *Acta Neurochir* 1983;69:253–258.

26. Tsolaki M, Yannacou-Peftoulidou M, Grammaticos P, et al: Phenytoin plasma levels after intraoperative administration for the prevention of post-craniotomy seizures. *Acta Neurochir* 1987;84:36–38.

27. Takaku A, Tanaka SM, Mori T, et al: Postoperative complications in 1000 cases of intracranial aneurysms. *Surg Neurol* 1979;12:137.

28. Frost EAM: Recovery room care, in Frost E (ed): *Clinical Anesthesia in Neurosurgery*. Boston, Butterworths, 1984, pp 399–415.

29. Rosenlund RC: Postanesthetic care of the neurosurgical patient. *Anes Clin North Am* 1987;5:646.

30. Rosenlund RC: Postanesthetic care of the neurosurgical patient. *Anes Clin North Am* 1987;5:646.

31. Spallone A: Cerebral vasospasm as a complication of aneurysmal subarachnoid hemorrhage: A brief review. *Ital J Neurol Sci* 1985;6:19–26.

32. Symon L: Disordered cerebro-vascular physiology in aneurysmal subarachnoid haemorrhage. *Acta Neurochir* 1978;41:7–22.

33. Wood JH, Snyder LL, Simeone FA: Failure of intravascular volume expansion without hemodilution to elevate cortical blood flow in regions of essential focal ischemia. *J Neurosurg* 1982;56:80–91.

34. Arem R, Rushford FE, Segal J, et al: Selective osmoreceptor dysfunction presenting as intermittent hypernatremia following surgery for a pituitary chromophobe adenoma. *Am J Med* 1986;80:1217–1223.

35. Malhotra N, Roizen MF: Patients with abnormalities of vasopressin secretion and responsiveness. *Anes Clin North Am* 1987;5:395–409.

36. Raggio JF, Fleischer AS, Sung UF, Hoffman JC: Expanding pneumocephalus due to nitrous oxide anesthesia: Case report. *Neurosurgery* 1979;4:261–263.

37. Kitahata LM, Katz JD: Tension pneumocephalus after posterior-fossa craniotomy, a complication of the sitting position. *Anesthesiology* 1976;44:448–450.

38. Steinberfer A, Antunes JL, Michelsen WJ: Pneumocephalus after ventriculoatrial shunt. *Neurosurgery* 1979;5:708–710.

39. Grundy BL, Spetzler RF: Subdural pneumocephalus resulting from drainage of cerebrospinal fluid during craniotomy. *Anesthesiology* 1980;52:269–271.

40. Saidman LJ, Eger EI: Change in cerebrospinal fluid pressure during pneumoencephalography under nitrous oxide anesthesia. *Anesthesiology* 1965;26:67–72.

41. Miller CF, Furman WR: Symptomatic pneumocephalus after translabrynthine acoustic neuroma excision and nitrous oxide anesthesia. *Anesthesiology* 1983;58:281–283.

42. Nelson RJ, Lovick AHJ, Pickard JD, et al: Changes in cerebral blood flow during anaesthesia and surgery in the sitting position. *J Neuro Neurosurg Psych* 1987;50:971–975.

43. Gottdiener JS, Papademetriou V, Notargiacomo A, et al: Incidence and cardiac effects of systemic venous air embolism. *Arch Intern Med* 1988;148:795–800.

44. Hitselberger WE, House WF: A warning regarding the sitting position for acoustic tumor surgery. *Arch Otolaryngol* 1980;106:69.

45. Matjasko J, Petrozza P, Cohen M, et al: Anesthesia and surgery in the seated position: Analysis of 554 cases. *Neurosurgery* 1985;17:695–701.

46. Young ML, et al: Comparison of surgical and anesthetic complications in neurosurgical patients experiencing venous air embolism in the sitting position. *Neurosurgery* 1986;18:157–161.

47. Yates AP, Sumner E, Lindahl GE: Respiratory disturbance and posterior fossa surgery. *Anaesthesia* 1986;41:1214–1218.

48. Skydell JL, Machleder HI, Baker JD, et al: Incidence and mechanism of post-carotid endarterectomy hypertension. *Arch Surg* 1987;122:1153–1155.

49. Theisen GJ, Grundy BL: Anesthesia and monitoring for carotid endarterectomy. *Bull NY Acad Med* 1987;63:803–819.

50. Tattersall MP: Massive swelling of the face and tongue. *Anaesthesia* 1986;39:1015–1017.

51. Ellis SC, Bryan-Brown CW, Hyderally H: Massive swelling of the head and neck. *Anesthesiology* 1975;42:102–103.

52. Lagerkranser M, Pehrsson K, Sylven C: Neurogenic pulmonary oedema. *Acta Med Scand* 1982;212:267–271.

53. Barnett GH, Ropper AH, Johnson KA: Physiological support and monitoring of critically ill patients during magnetic resonance imaging. *J Neurosurg* 1988;68:246–250.

54. Gee W, Lucke JF, Madden AE: Reappraisal of ocular pneumoplethysmography after carotid endarterectomy. *J Vascular Surg* 1986;4:517–521.

55. Coates DP, Monk CR, Prys-Roberts C, et al: Hemodynamic effects of infusions of the emulsion formulation of propofol during nitrous oxide anesthesia in humans. *Anesth Analg* 1987;66:64–70.

56. Lippmann M, Paicius RM, Gingerich S, et al: A controlled study of the hemodynamic effects of propofol versus thiopental during anesthesia induction. *Semin Anesth* 1988;7(suppl):116–122.

57. Ravussin P, Guinard JP, Ralley F, et al: Effect of propofol on cerebrospinal fluid pressure and cerebral perfusion pressure in patients undergoing craniotomy. *Anaesthesia* 1988;43(suppl):37–41.

58. Vandesteene A, Trempont V, Engelman E, et al: Effect of propofol on cerebral blood flow and metabolism in man. *Anaesthesia* 1988;43(suppl):42–43.

59. Streisand JB, Stanley TH: The respiratory effects of Diprivan (propofol) with and without fentanyl. *Semin Anesth* 1988;7(suppl 1):123–126.

60. Darragh A, Lambre R, Scully M, et al: Investigation in man of the efficacy of a benzodiazepine antagonist Ro 15-1788. *Lancet* 1981;2:8–10.

61. Geller E, Niv D, Rudick V, et al: The use of RO 15-1788: A benzodiazepine antagonist, in the diagnosis and treatment of benzodiazepine overdose. *Anesthesiology* 1984;61:A135.

62. Geller E, Niv D, Rudick V, et al: RO 15-1788: A benzodiazepine antagonist, in the treatment of 34 intoxicated patients. *Anesthesiology* 1985;63:A157.

63. Geller E, Niv D, Rudick V, et al: The antagonism of Midazolam sedation by RO15-1788 in 50 postoperative patients. *Anesthesiology* 1985;63:A369.

64. Lauven PM, Ebeling B, Stoeckel H, et al: The efficacy of the benzodiazepine antagonist flumazenil (RO 15-1788) on unconscious intubated intensive care patients. Abstracts, Ninth world congress of anaesthesiologists, Washington, D.C., 1988, vol 2, p A0655.

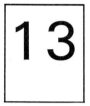

13 | The Obstetric Suite

Steven S. Schwalbe, Gertie F. Marx

The modern gravida considers pregnancy to be a natural process, not a disease, and does not want to be called a "patient." We have therefore elected to refer, whenever possible, to gravida, pregnant woman, puerpera, postpartum woman, or mother, rather than patient.

The puerperal woman's postsurgical recovery period differs markedly from that of the surgical patient's, both psychologically and physiologically. Whereas the surgical patient is nursed in a room without visitors, the postpartum woman is attended by a member of her family and may, after a suitable interval, be reunited with her baby. And while the surgical patient's physiologic adjustments result from the underlying pathologic condition, those of the puerpera are due to the natural sequelae of the loss of the products of conception. Since the postpartum physiological changes may initiate certain postoperative complications, a brief review of the major components is indicated.

PHYSIOLOGIC ADJUSTMENTS

Physiologic adjustments toward the nonpregant state begin immediately after delivery of the products of conception. Although the complete return to basal levels is not achieved until 6 weeks postpartum, circulatory, respiratory, and hepatic parameters change rapidly, and these developments may be of clinical importance to the care of the puerperal woman (Table 13–1).

Circulatory Changes

The augmented venous return from the emptying uterine blood pool leads to an increase in cardiac output over and beyond that accumulated during labor contractions. In 10 healthy multiparae treated with paracervical and pudendal blocks during labor (some pain experienced), cardiac output after vaginal delivery was 80% higher than prelabor (from a mean of 5.1 to 9.3 L/min), while in 13 comparable parturients given continuous caudal analgesia (no pain experi-

enced), the rise amounted to 58% (from a mean of 5.2 to 8.3 L/min).[1] These increases compare well with a 52% rise in cardiac output following delivery by elective cesarean section under spinal block in 12 normal women (from a mean of 5.5 to 8.4 L/min) and a 34% increase after scheduled section under general anesthesia in 17 gravidae (from a mean of 5.0 to 6.7 L/min).[2,3] During the first hour postpartum, cardiac output declines moderately independent of the method of delivery or anesthesia—despite average blood losses of 500 to 600 mL in vaginal deliveries and 900 to 1000 mL in abdominal deliveries—but is still 25 to 40% above predelivery values at 60 minutes after delivery,[4] and remains elevated for at least 48 hours after normal delivery.[5] The increase in cardiac output is due solely to a rise in stroke volume, while the heart rate, following closure of the arteriovenous shunt across the placenta, slows by approximately 10 to 14%.[5] As a consequence, left ventricular work is markedly elevated during the early puerperium at an average value of 11 kg m/min as compared with an average of 8 kg m/min during the early first stage of labor.[6]

These increases in stroke volume and left ventricular work, added to the strain placed on the heart by labor and parturition, favor the development of congestive heart failure in women with a predisposing medical condition such as rheumatic heart disease. Failure is more frequent in older parturients and occurs more often with mitral stenosis than with any other valvular lesion. Other common etiologies of heart failure in postpartum women are peripartum cardiomyopathy and certain congenital diseases, primarily stenotic lesions (pressure overload) and left-to-right shunts (volume overload).[7] Szekely and Snaith[8] differentiated three types of cardiac failure in obstetric patients and proposed the following diagnostic criteria.

- Right heart failure: abnormal jugular venous distension and extensive peripheral edema.
- Pulmonary congestion: exertional dyspnea, pulmonary rales, and/or radiologic evidence of interstitial edema.

TABLE 13-1. IMMEDIATE POSTPARTUM CHANGES

Cardiovascular	Cardiac output
	Heart rate
Respiratory	Functional residual capacity
	Alveolar ventilation
Hepatic	Plasma cholinesterase

- Pulmonary edema: dyspnea with cough, frothy sputum, pulmonary congestion, and intraalveolar edema.

Other common causes of postpartum pulmonary edema include:

- Recently discontinued beta-adrenergic tocolytic therapy.
- Pregnancy-induced hypertension.
- Aspiration pneumonitis.
- Water intoxication (prolonged oxytocin administration combined with either infusion of dextrose/water or large volumes of electrolyte solution).

The treatment of postpartum cardiac failure is the same as that in surgical patients, but prevention is feasible and therapy is facilitated in many puerperae by the sympathetic blockade accompanying regional analgesia. A catheter block initiated during labor or for cesarean section can be extended with dispatch to reduce venous return and decrease afterload should signs of impending failure occur. The block may be continued for 12 to 24 hours to reduce cardiac work, and then be allowed to dissipate slowly.

The heart rate, as mentioned earlier, does not normally rise after delivery. Tachycardia, therefore, is a sign of a complication the etiology of which must be elucidated. Common causes of postpartum tachycardia include pain; hypoventilation; bleeding; fever; drugs (hydralazine, diazoxide, etc); urinary bladder overdistension; pulmonary aspiration of gastric contents; pulmonary embolism; hyperthyroidism; and opiate withdrawal.

Respiratory Changes

The most impressive respiratory alteration produced by pregnancy is a progressive augmentation in resting ventilation, which is achieved primarily by an increase in tidal volume (40% at term) and only slightly by a rise in respiratory rate (average of two breaths/min). Since dead space remains unchanged, alveolar ventilation increases to an even greater degree, on the order of 60%.[9] Oxygen consumption also rises throughout gestation to a maximal increase of 20% (50 to 60 mL/min) at term.[10] During labor, there is further hyperventilation initiated unconsciously or advocated by prenatal childbirth education. Bonica[9]

studied four primigravidae who had no antenatal psychologic preparation and no sedation or analgesia during the first stage of labor; their ventilation increased from a mean of 10.5 L/min between contractions to a mean of 22.4 L/min at the peak of a contraction. Sedation and particularly extradural block significantly attenuate this added overbreathing. Yet, at delivery, most parturients show high PA_{O_2} and Pa_{O_2} values, low Pa_{CO_2} values, and somewhat elevated pH levels.[11] Hyperventilation ends shortly after parturition, and the respiratory values start to return to normal ranges. In an analysis of 23 healthy women delivering spontaneously without analgesia, both minute and tidal volume had decreased significantly (p < 0.01) one hour after delivery, alveolar ventilation was reduced from a mean of 11.5 to 6.8 L/min, Pa_{O_2} from a mean of 108 to 94 mm Hg (p < 0.0025), Pa_{CO_2} had risen from 25.5 to 29.4 mm Hg (p < 0.0025), and pH had changed from a mean of 7.48 to 7.43 (p < 0.0025).[11]

The increased alveolar ventilation affects the course of inhalation anesthesia. Since the alveolar concentration of the anesthetic is the primary determinant of the tension in the brain, induction of anesthesia with soluble agents (ether, halogenated agents) is enhanced. Similarly, emergence may be hastened. However, the rapid postdelivery reexpansion of the functional residual capacity which, at term, is reduced approximately 20% due primarily to the elevation of the diaphragm,[9] may tend to slow exhalation of the agents. Thus, awakening of postpartum women from general anesthesia should not differ markedly from that of nongravid patients, and their postanesthetic care should be the same. A patent airway must be maintained by appropriate positioning (tonsilar posture), vital signs must be monitored at regular short intervals, and supplemental oxygen must be administered by face mask for at least one hour, since metabolic rate and oxygen uptake remain elevated (although not at peak level) in the early postpartum period.[10]

Aspiration pneumonitis is the second leading cause of anesthesia-induced maternal morbidity and mortality, with failed intubation being the first.[12] Pulmonary inhalation of gastric contents may follow vomiting or regurgitation during induction of as well as during emergence from general anesthesia, and may involve solid food particles, liquid gastric juice, or a mixture of both. Aspiration of solid material produces mechanical obstruction of the trachea or smaller airways; aspiration of gastric juice with a pH of 2.5 or less causes a chemical bronchopneumonitis (Mendelson's syndrome); associated with both is reflex bronchospasm.

Aspiration may be "silent" and unsuspected until the characteristic triad of dyspnea, tachycardia, and cyanosis suddenly develops. Immediate action is necessary. The treatment of particulate aspiration is directed toward removal of the foreign material, by bronchoscopy if necessary. The therapy of acid aspiration begins with thorough suctioning of the upper airway followed by insertion of a cuffed endotracheal tube, endotracheal suctioning, and mechanical ventilation with 100% oxygen. Positive end-expiratory pressure is often necessary to permit adequate oxygenation. Despite their frequent use, parenteral corticosteroids have not been found to be helpful, but bronchodilators such as terbutaline improve oxygenation. Extended treatment includes continuous respiratory assistance, humidification and chest physiotherapy, antibiotics if appropriate, and continued bronchodilators. Progress of the disease process should be followed by chest radiograms and arterial oxygenation should be monitored by pulse oximetry and arterial blood gas determinations.

Hepatic Changes

Pregnancy induces many changes in liver function. Lipid metabolism is increased, that of cholesterol as much 150 to 200%. Total protein concentration is decreased primarily due to a reduction in albumin concentration and alphaglobulin levels. Fibrinogen, ceruloplasmin, and transferrin, in contrast, are elevated. Hepatic sulfobromophthalein (BSP) storage is increased but its retention in serum may remain normal because of rapid removal in hypoalbuminemic states.[13]

The changes in BSP metabolism revert to normal soon after delivery and the concentration of cholesterol, triglycerides, and lipoproteins decrease significantly within the first 24 hours postpartum.[14,15] These alterations may be important for the evaluation of laboratory results. All other hepatic parameters return to nonpregnant levels within 3 weeks of parturition.

Total alkaline phosphatase rises two- to four-fold during gestation, partly due to hepatic production of the enzyme and partly derived from the placenta. Levels return to the normal range by 20 days postpartum.[15] SGOT and SGPT, however, remain unchanged during uncomplicated pregnancy.

Plasma cholinesterase activity decreases markedly during pregnancy with a further reduction in the early puerperium. Blitt and coworkers[16] demonstrated a decline in activity of 21% on the second and 18% on the fourth postpartum day as compared with the values at the time of cesarean section. Although succinylcholine recovery is not normally prolonged in term-pregnant patients, two investigations have demonstrated longer action of the relaxant in postpartum women.[17,18] A comparison of the response to succinylcholine in women undergoing tubal ligation on the first or second postpartum day, and women

undergoing interval tubal ligation, showed that the dose that produced 80% of control twitch was significantly (p < 0.01) lower in the puerperal patients (3.1 ± 0.2 vs 5.5 ± 0.5 mg/m² BSA). Similarly, recovery times following injection of a 20-mg bolus of the drug were significantly longer (p < 0.01) in the postpartum than the nonobstetric group (625 ± 37 vs 434 ± 24 sec). Cholinesterase activity in the puerperae was inversely related to the time to maximal recovery.[17] Thus, when clinically relevant doses of succinylcholine are administered, paralysis lasts three to four minutes longer in postpartum than in either nonpregnant or term-pregnant women. This may become significant when a succinylcholine infusion has been continued to the end of cesarean section, particularly if airway difficulty occurs[18] or if magnesium sulfate or another drug degraded by cholinesterase, such as trimethaphan, has been administered.

REGIONAL ANALGESIA

Regional anesthetic techniques are in frequent use in the delivery suite. Epidural analgesia is commonly administered to women in the first stage of labor. Epidural and spinal blockade are both routine methods of anesthesia for operative procedures such as cesarean section and postpartum tubal ligation. The most important physiologic effect of these techniques is blockade of the sympathetic nervous system. Such a blockade may extend for varying distances above the level of the sensory block and may last well into the recovery period.[19,20]

When the level of sympathetic blockade is below T4, the predominant effect is loss of vasomotor tone and relaxation of both arterioles and capacitance vessels.[21] The resulting decrease in cardiac preload as venous capacitance increases leads to a diminished cardiac output and a fall in blood pressure. It is routine clinical practice to guard against such hypotension by proper preparation, monitoring, and treatment when regional anesthesia is instituted. However, it must be remembered that residual sympathetic blockade is often present well after the surgical procedure has finished.[20] Sudden changes in the puerpera's position, such as occurs when she is transferred to the postanesthetic care unit (PACU), may result in hypotension due to lack of compensatory sympathetic response. The treatment for this hypotension is the same as that for hypotension that occurs at the onset of anesthesia, namely, intravenous hydration and the judicious use of vasopressors such as ephedrine.

If the sympathetic block has extended into the region of T1 to T4, the paralysis of cardiac sympathetic fibers can result in bradycardia and diminished inotropic force.[22,23] Such a situation may yield a dangerously low cardiac output, particularly if hypotension already exists as a result of diminished venous return. Once again, venous return should be increased through rapid hydration and the use of vasopressors, while the bradycardia may be corrected with the use of atropine.

This situation is made even more severe if the parturient has received sedation in addition to the regional anesthetic. A recent analysis of cases of cardiac arrest during spinal anesthesia[24] has suggested that intravenous sedation and a high sympathetic blockade can act synergistically to create a sequence of respiratory insufficiency leading to hypoxia and hypercarbia, which in turn causes further vasodilatation and loss of venous return. The bradycardia and hypotension that ensue may be severe enough to lead to circulatory failure and arrest. In this extreme situation, ephedrine will no longer be effective in restoring adequate cardiac output and an alpha-adrenergic agent, such as phenylephrine or norepinephrine, must be used.

Even in a less extreme situation, sedation combined with paralysis of the intercostal muscles from a high regional blockade may lead to profound hypoventilation. Clearly, women who have received sedation with their conduction blockade must be monitored frequently during the recovery period not only for adequate blood pressure and heart rate, but also for adequacy of ventilation. Supplemental oxygen is indicated for all women during the recovery period.

When assessing a puerpera who has had a regional blockade for discharge from the PACU, the practice in most institutions is to check for return of motor function in the legs. While movement of the lower extremities may indicate that normal resolution of the block is taking place, such return of motor control does not insure the return of sympathetic control, since the latter may last for a significantly longer period. The puerpera may still experience signs and symptoms of hypotension with sudden postural changes. In addition, some degree of residual motor weakness may be present. Therefore, the first time the mother is allowed to ambulate, assistance should be provided.

Postdural Puncture Headache

The occurrence of a headache during the postpartum period is a frequent event independent of the use of regional anesthesia.[25] Common etiologies for headaches during this period include hypertensive disorders (chronic hypertension or pregnancy-induced hypertension); drug effects (ergotamine, ephedrine, and so on); hormonal effects from progesterone–estrogen imbalance; migraine headaches; postpartum depression; cortical vein thrombosis; and cerebral hemorrhage from arteriovenous malformation or a berry aneurysm.[26]

Postdural puncture headache (PDPH) is not usually seen in the PACU. Although it can occur only a few hours following the procedure, it will generally not appear until the following day. The incidence of PDPH following spinal anesthesia varies widely (0.33 to 22%)[27,28] depending on technique, hydration status of the parturient, experience of the anesthesiologist, and so on, but appears to correlate best with the size of the needle used. Following an accidental dural puncture with a 16-gauge epidural needle, the reported incidence of headache is close to 80%.[29] The headache itself is caused by a persistent leak of cerebrospinal fluid (CSF) through the hole that remains in the dura. This loss of CSF can cause movement of the brain within the cranial vault when the mother assumes an upright position. The resulting tension on meningeal structures causes pain referred to the frontal or occipital regions of the head, the posterior cervical region, or even the shoulders. This condition, when it appears, is usually self-limiting, resolving in a few days with no permanent neurologic sequelae. It can, however, be very distressing for the mother, and may delay her discharge from the hospital if not treated.

Following a spinal anesthetic, it has become common practice in some institutions to restrict a woman to prolonged bedrest, in some cases up to 12 or 24 hours postprocedure, in order to avoid a PDPH. This is probably counterproductive, since studies by Jones[30] and by Carbaat and van Crevel[31] indicate that early ambulation has no effect on the incidence of postdural puncture headache. In addition, the maintenance of a supine position for this long a period of time may aggravate backache and muscle spasm, and precipitate a headache from nonanesthetic causes. A woman who has received a spinal block should be restricted to bed only as long as the blockade lasts. Lying supine should be avoided, as this position tends to favor continued leakage of CSF.[32] The puerpera should instead be encouraged to lie on her side, with a pillow under her head and with her back slightly flexed.

If a PDPH develops and the pain is of mild to moderate severity, conservative treatment includes bedrest, intravenous hydration, analgesics, and an abdominal binder to increase intraabdominal pressure. Some success has also been reported with the use of intravenous caffeine sodium benzoate,[33,34] administering 500 mg in 1L of intravenous fluid. If conservative treatment should prove ineffective, a saline or blood patch may be considered.

The administration of an autologous epidural blood patch during the first 24 hours after dural puncture has often been eschewed because of evidence of lesser efficacy and a greater incidence of recurrence if administered during this period.[35,36] Recent work has challenged this assumption, and suggested that early placement of an epidural blood patch may be just as effective as later placement.[37] However, controversy still remains over the use of a so-called "prophylactic" blood patch, placed in a woman who has not yet developed any symptoms. This course of action subjects a woman who may never develop a headache to an invasive procedure that may be unnecessary.

Shivering

Shivering is a well-recognized complication in labor and delivery that can occur even in the absence of anesthesia. The reported incidence in parturients who receive epidural analgesia varies between 20 and 61%.[38-40] When shivering becomes severe it is not only distressing to the puerpera, but can interfere with proper monitoring of blood pressure and ECG, increase oxygen consumption as much as 400% above normal,[41] and increase myocardial work.

Various mechanisms have been proposed to explain this phenomenon. A decrease in core temperature may result from cold intravenous fluids, a cold operating room, or both. This may be augmented by heat loss due to cutaneous vasodilation. There may be a differential inhibition of afferent CNS pathways carrying warm and cold sensations, or some other modification of afferent impulses by the local anesthetic.[42]

Mild degrees of shivering usually resolve within 5 to 15 minutes and require only supplemental oxygen and reassurance. More severe shivering has been treated in a variety of ways with varying degrees of success. Warm blankets, warmed air, radiant heat, warmed IV fluids, phenothiazines, and diazepam have all been used; however, the most effective means appears to be the use of meperidine.[40,43] Intravenous injection of 12.5 to 50 mg, or epidural administration of 25 mg in 5 mL of saline, will resolve most cases of shivering within 5 minutes. The mechanism of action is unclear, but is probably a centrally mediated effect.

Backache

The incidence of backache following delivery is high (40%) even in the absence of any regional anesthetic.[25] This may be due to ligamentous strain from the lordosis of pregnancy or improper patient positioning. There is a small incidence (2.7%)[44] of women who will develop backache from the epidural puncture itself, probably as a result of trauma to the ligaments from the needle puncture. Such pain is usually mild and self-limiting. Conservative treatment includes heat, reassurance, early ambulation, and analgesics. The rare occurance of more severe pain, or persistent pain in the area of the lumbar puncture, warrants further investigation for signs of injury to the disc or for an epidural hematoma.

EPIDURAL NARCOTICS

The use of epidural narcotics has become increasingly popular in the labor and delivery suite. This route of administration provides a safe and effective means of achieving postpartum or postoperative analgesia, and is often given in conjunction with local anesthetics for either labor analgesia or operative anesthesia. However, the use of any drug requires monitoring for the development of side effects, and this is certainly true when epidural or intrathecal narcotics are in use.

Certainly the most feared, albeit the rarest complication of epidural opiates, is that of respiratory depression. This tends to be more of a problem with the poorly lipid-soluble agents, such as morphine. Following diffusion across the dural membranes into the cerebrospinal fluid, morphine is carried by diffusion and circulation of the CSF, to reach medullary centers 6 to 16 hours later. High concentrations of the free drug may persist in the CSF for 16 to 24 hours.[45] Fentanyl, on the other hand, a much more lipid-soluble narcotic than morphine, has a correspondingly shorter duration of action, and carries less danger of delayed respiratory depression.[46]

Women who have received epidural or intrathecal narcotics should have vital signs with respiratory rate taken at least every 15 minutes, to check for respiratory depression. In the case of fentanyl, it is probably necessary to do this for only three to four hours following injection. However, in the case of morphine, the respiratory rate should be checked for 16 to 24 hours following injection. If respiratory depression does develop, it can be treated with small doses of intravenous naloxone or by an intravenous naloxone infusion of 5 $\mu g/kg/hr$, while still retaining analgesia.[47]

If parenteral narcotics are going to be administered to a woman who has received epidural or intrathecal narcotics, the first injection should be half the dose that is normally used. After waiting the proper amount of time for peak onset of the parenterally administered narcotic, the puerpera's need for further analgesia can then be reevaluated. Needless to say, monitoring of respiratory rate should continue, as outlined earlier.

Nausea and vomiting have been reported as common side effects with morphine,[48] but less so with the more lipid-soluble agents such as fentanyl, sufentanil, and meperidine.[49] With these latter agents, the incidence of nausea and vomiting is not much different than the incidence that normally follows labor or surgery. This complication is usually self-limiting. If treatment is desired, low-dose droperidol or naloxone is effective.

Pruritus occurs frequently (70 to 100%)[50] following epidural or intrathecal morphine, but only requires treatment in a small number of cases (1 to 5%).[51] Again, the lipid-soluble agents have a much lower incidence of this side effect, which can be treated with either small doses of intravenous naloxone (0.1 to 0.3 mg) or diphenhydramine.

Urinary retention occurs more frequently in patients who have received morphine as opposed to the more lipid-soluble agents. This is not usually a problem in women who have undergone cesarean section, since a bladder catheter will be in place. A small number of women who have received fentanyl for labor may require either catheterization or intravenous naloxone (0.4 to 0.8 mg).[52,53]

There is evidence to suggest a relationship between epidural morphine administration and the occurrence or reactivation of herpes simplex type I (HSV-I) in the face.[54,55] The involved mechanism remains unclear. The morphine may cause a change in the woman's immunologic status. Alternatively, the drug may act as a ''triggering factor'' for the latent virus. More likely, the virus may be reactivated indirectly by irritation of the sensory nerves when patients who develop pruritus scratch or rub their faces. At the present time, there is no evidence to suggest a relationship between HSV-I and the use of other narcotics epidurally.

As a final consideration, if epidural narcotics are used in a parturient who has a narcotic addiction, it should be kept in mind that the doses used for analgesia will not be enough to prevent a withdrawal syndrome. Parenteral or oral narcotics will be required at some point for that purpose.

POSTPARTUM HEMORRHAGE

Postpartum hemorrhage occurs in about 3 to 5%[56] of all deliveries, and is a major cause of maternal mortality.[57] It can be defined as an abnormal blood loss during the first 24 hours following delivery.

The normal blood loss with vaginal delivery is approximately 500 mL, and 900 mL with cesarean section.[58] The average healthy puerpera is well equipped to handle these losses, since she has had increases in plasma volume and red cell mass during gestation and because she can increase her stroke volume and cardiac output to meet metabolic demands. Postpartum blood loss, however, can be severe enough to compromise this situation, leading to hypovolemic shock. Such blood loss, although severe, may not always be obvious in the delivery room. A slow, continuous ooze can occur throughout the early postpartum period, resulting in an underestimation of the degree of blood loss.

The most common causes of postpartum hemorrhage are uterine atony, retained placenta or remnants of the placenta, and trauma and lacerations to the birth canal. Other causes include coagulation defects, uterine rupture, uterine inversion, and placenta accreta. Twenty percent of all parturients who experience antepartum bleeding will develop a postpartum hemorrhage.[56] Proper treatment rests on the establishment of the correct diagnosis and the initiation of specific corrective measures.

Uterine atony is responsible for about 80% of the cases of postpartum hemorrhage.[59] This may occur immediately following delivery of the infant or develop several hours later. The degree of atony can be quite variable, but a completely atonic uterus can loose 2 L of blood in less than 5 minutes.[56]

There are a number of factors that interfere with the normal ability of the uterus to contract adequately following delivery. These include prolonged labor; uterine overdistention (as with multiple gestations, a large fetus, or hydramnios); uterorelaxant drugs (ritodrine, magnesium sulfate, halogenated anesthetic agents, etc); multiparity; uterine myomas; and severe hypotension with resulting hypoxia of the myometrium.

Immediate treatment of uterine atony involves gentle massage of the uterus through the abdominal wall, expression of blood clots, fluid replacement, and intravenous oxytocin (50 to 100 mU/min). Care should be taken not to give oxytocin in a rapid intravenous bolus, which can create hypotension through vasodilation.[60] Oxygen may be administered by face mask and vital signs should be watched closely, including urine output and central venous pressure if necessary. Prostaglandin $F_2\alpha$ may be given intramuscularly or by injection into the uterus. If this is used in an asthmatic puerpera, she must be monitored for the development of bronchospasm. Ergotamine (0.2 mg) can also be given intramuscularly or by slow intravenous injection, but this should be used cautiously, if at all, in a woman who has received ephedrine or other pressor agents to support her blood pressure, lest a hypertensive crisis develop. Likewise, the presence of hypertension or preeclampsia should also be considered a contraindication to the use of methylergonovine.[61,62] If pharmacologic measures fail to control the hemorrhage of atony, surgical intervention may be required.

Retained placenta occurs in approximately 1% of all births and is defined as a failure to deliver the placenta within 30 minutes after delivery of the infant. Treatment will require manual removal of the placenta or the remnants of the placenta, and occasionally curettage of the uterus.[63]

Lacerations of the birth canal may follow a tumultuous labor, a traumatic forceps delivery, or a breech extraction, and sometimes occur during an otherwise normal delivery. The vagina and cervix should be visually inspected and any lacerations repaired. If bleeding continues, the uterus should be explored for the possibilities of uterine rupture or retained placental fragments.

CLINICAL IMPLICATIONS

Following an uncomplicated vaginal delivery, a healthy postpartum woman requires minimal monitoring in the PACU. Blood loss from an atonic uterus or a birth canal laceration are the most frequent complications; therefore, uterine tone and vaginal bleeding should be checked every 15 minutes for 1½ to 2 hours together with vital signs (systolic and diastolic pressure, heart rate, and respiratory rate). When regional analgesia is administered for labor or delivery, recovery from both motor and sympathetic block must be ascertained before discharge from the PACU to prevent a fall from weakness of the legs or from postural hypotension. In this regard, it must be kept in mind that the duration of sensory, motor, and sympathetic blockade is significantly (2 to 3½ times) longer in the obstetric population than in nongravid patients of similar age and habitus.[64]

In contrast, the postcesarean puerpera needs the same care as a surgical patient following laparotomy. Vital signs and vaginal bleeding should be monitored every 15 minutes for the first 1½ to 2 hours, every 30 minutes for the next 1 to 2 hours, and hourly thereafter. Continuous pulse oximetry is recommended. When vaginal bleeding is excessive, a physician should be summoned to check uterine tone. Again, recovery from regional analgesia is retarded. When opioids have been used extradurally or intrathecally for postoperative pain relief, the hazard of sudden respiratory depression for up to 24 hours must be recognized and appropriate monitoring instituted as discussed earlier. Following general anesthesia, positioning and supplemental oxygen inhalation are the same as advocated for the surgical patient. However, the effect of muscle relaxants may be prolonged as reported for succinylcholine (vide supra) and suggested for vecuronium.[65]

There are, however, "high-risk" puerperae in whom additional prophylactic or therapeutic mea-sures are indicated. In most cases, such measures do not differ from those employed in the nongravid surgical patient. The rare disorders in which the pregnant or postpartum state necessitates special consideration will be briefly discussed.

Pregnancy-Induced Hypertension

Although delivery of the products of conception is the definitive treatment of pregnancy-induced hypertension, the clinical onset of both the nonconvulsive and the convulsive form may occur following parturition. Postpartum preeclampsia manifests as hypertensive crisis accompanied by hyperreflexia, oliguria, rapidly increasing facial edema, and complaints of headache, nausea, and visual disturbances. Immediate antihypertensive therapy is required because of the danger of primary cerebral hemorrhage, and should be combined with intravenous magnesium sulfate, preferably by continuous infusion. Chlorpromazine (thorazine) is not the drug of choice as it may enhance potential hepatic impairment.[66]

Postpartum eclampsia—convulsions with loss of consciousness—usually appears during the first 12 hours of the puerperium but has been reported as late as 11 days after delivery.[67] The differential diagnosis includes epilepsy and water intoxication, the latter generally due to intravenous administration of hypotonic solutions in combination with oxytocin, which has an antidiuretic effect. Eclamptic convulsions are treated according to the same principles as convulsions from other causes.

Asthma

Stimuli inducing acute asthmatic attacks include emotional stress (anxiety, fear, pain) and physical exertion (hyperventilation, bearing-down)—common developments during labor and delivery.[68] Thus, the risk of postpartum bronchospasm cannot be underestimated. Emotional support, mild sedation, and inhalation of humidifed oxygen may be preventive. If an attack occurs, previously proven drug therapy should immediately be restarted with one important caveat: terbutaline, a beta-2 agonist which is very effective during pregnancy, may produce undesirable postpartum depression of uterine contractility.[69]

Diabetes Mellitus

Following delivery, insulin requirements fall precipitously but to varying degrees.[70] In the gestational diabetic, we discontinue insulin administration at this time. In the overt diabetic, we monitor blood glucose concentration at regular three-hour intervals for two days and maintain the level around 100 mg/dL (5.6 mmol/L)[71] by use of regular insulin. Women who were delivered under regional block fare better than those who received general anesthesia, due to a smaller metabolic expenditure and lower incidence of vomiting, as well as earlier ability to return to oral food intake, which facilitates glucose control.

Sickle Cell Disease

The postpartum period is a difficult time for women with sickle cell anemia, particularly when delivery was by cesarean section. Pain, the parenteral use of analgesics, and anticipated reduction in arterial oxygen partial pressure, will all predispose to the formation of sickle cells. Supplemental oxygen and maintenance of intravascular fluid volume, prepregnancy hematocrit level, and body temperature, are important considerations.[72] Extradural analgesia, used for labor or parturition, should be maintained for pain relief in the postpartum period, but position should be changed frequently to prevent stasis.

Myasthenia Gravis

A myasthenic crisis may be precipitated by emotional stress (labor, delivery) as well as by infection (chorioamnionitis, pulmonary complication consequent to respiratory muscle weakness). However, the obligatory anticholinesterases potentiate the effects of narcotics while most antibiotics possess muscle-relaxing properties. Thus, opioids and tranquilizers must be used cautiously to avoid respiratory depression, and antibiotics devoid of neuromuscular blocking action should be preferred. The first ten postpartum days appear to be particularly hazardous. A review of 128 cases revealed that exacerbation of symptoms was common during the puerperium while remission was most unusual.[73] The patient's normal oral medications should be resumed as soon as possible, making regional block the preferred method of analgesia/anesthesia. If oral drugs cannot be tolerated, intravenous or intramuscular equivalents must be substituted (neostigmine, oral 10 to 20 mg, IM 0.5 to 1.5 mg, IV 0.25 to 0.75 mg; pyridostigmine, oral 50 to 70 mg, IM 3 to 5 mg, IV 1 to 3 mg).[74]

Cerebral Vascular Anomaly

In contrast to cerebral aneurysms, which tend to bleed during the period of parturition, hemorrhage from arteriovenous anomaly occurs more frequently during the early puerperium, possibly related to the maximum increase in cardiac output. The clinical picture of sudden severe headache followed by semistupor (without convulsion) is suggestive of this complication, and warrants immediate specific neurologic workup.[66]

Addiction

The incidence of pregnant women addicted to narcotics or cocaine has been rising steadily in urban centers. Two complications may arise in the postpartum period, abstinence and acute overdose.

Narcotic abstinence may not become evident until some hours after delivery since the addiction drug is usually taken just prior to hospital admission. The severity of withdrawal increases with the addictive dose and the duration of dependence. Methadone abstinence develops gradually and the onset of the syndrome is delayed. Withdrawal manifestations include anxiety, jitteriness, yawning, sweating, rhinorrhea, hypotension, and hypoglycemia. Although the treatment recommended for withdrawal, in general, is oral methadone substitution (in the smallest effective dose), the postpartum patient requires initial therapy with intramuscular methadone (10-mg increments) or intravenous opiate injection(s). Of the latter, fentanyl has the advantage of short action, while meperidine is pharmacologically more closely related to the addicted drug (meperidine or heroin).

Overdose leading to respiratory depression or even apnea has been observed after an opiate—hidden in the mother's handbag or smuggled in by the father—is injected by either into the intravenous line or into a peripheral vein. Known addicted women should therefore be assigned a bed close to the nurses' station, an intravenous tubing without injection ports should be substituted, and the infusion should be discontinued at the earliest possible time. Naloxone (0.4 to 0.8 mg IV) is the treatment for narcotic overdose. Pulmonary edema caused by heroin requires intensive care management.[75]

Cocaine, whether injected or inhaled, produces hypertension, tachycardia, nervousness, and lack of cooperation. In overdose, convulsions may develop. In most cases, treatment is unnecessary because of the short duration of the drug. If intervention is necessary, neurolept agents are used to treat delusions, benzodiazepines for anxiety states. Beta blockers are no longer recommended because they increase the risk of cardiovascular toxicity.[76] In contrast, calcium channel blockers appear to be beneficial. Well-controlled rat studies led to the conclusion that nitrendipine (a clinically used antiarrhythmic and coronary vasodilator) "might be considered in clinical trials in the treatment of acute toxicity of cocaine in man."[77]

AMNIOTIC FLUID EMBOLISM SYNDROME

Amniotic fluid embolism is a rare obstetric complication associated with a high maternal mortality rate (approximately 80%). The disorder is neither predicatable nor preventable. It is triggered by the sudden entry of amniotic fluid and/or debris of fetal origin into the maternal venous circulation. This may occur during labor and vaginal delivery, cesarean section, or postpartum (due to trapping of the noxious material in venous sinuses with later release). Rupture of the membranes is a prerequisite.[78-80]

The chronology of events is usually triphasic. The initial phase is mostly respiratory; mechanical and anaphylactic reactions to the foreign substances produce pulmonary arterial spasm, ventilation/perfusion aberrations, and bronchospasm, leading to severe hypoxia and right heart strain. A secondary phase, consequent to left ventricular and pulmonary capillary injury, is evidenced by left heart failure and ARDS. Pulmonary edema may be of cardiac or noncardiac origin. In the third phase, uncontrollable hemorrhage due to coagulation activation, and uterine atony, supervene. However, in 10 to 15% of patients, bleeding diathesis is the initial presenting manifestation.[78,79]

The classical clinical picture is that of sudden respiratory distress (without chest pain), hypotension, and pulmonary edema often leading to cardiorespiratory distress.[78,79] A fall in oxygen saturation occurs immediately.[4] If the patient survives this episode, disseminated intravascular coagulopathy and uterine atony almost always follow.[78,79]

The definitive diagnosis is based on the detection of substantial amounts of fetal squamous cells, vernix, hair and/or meconium in maternal blood obtained from a central venous or pulmonary artery catheter or, in survivors, on evidence of perfusion defects on pulmonary scanning in conjunction with coagulation profile abnormalities.[78–80] The new term *amniotic fluid embolism syndrome* has been coined because fetal squamous cells have been detected in the pulmonary artery circulation in normal, uncomplicated cases.[78]

Therapy must have three objectives: (1) support of the cardiopulmonary system; (2) control of the coagulopathy; and (3) reestablishment of uterine tone. The following measures have been advocated: 100% O_2 with positive pressure ventilation via endotracheal tube; optimization of cardiac preload by intravenous infusion of an electrolyte solution with subsequent dopamine infusion if necessary; rapid digitalization, hydrocortisone (2 to 4 g IV), terbutaline, isoproterenol; replacement of blood and clotting factors and, if the response is not adequate, uterine packing followed by maintained manual uterine massage together with judiciously administered oxytocics including prostaglandin $F_2\alpha$. An avenue for the measurement of pulmonary and central venous pressure is recommended for continued hemodynamic assessment.[78–81]

CARDIOPULMONARY RESUSCITATION IN THE PREGNANT PATIENT

Although most patients in the PACU or intensive care unit have already delivered their fetuses, occasionally a pregnancy may still be ongoing (for example, fol-

lowing head injury). Although cardiac arrest is very rare in pregnant patients, resuscitative (CPR) effects must be adapted because of altered physiologic responses.

Aspiration is an ever-present danger in the unconscious parturient. Mechanical and hormonal factors retard gastric emptying and food may be retained for more than 24 hours.[82] Therefore, even if ventilation is believed to be adequate by bag-valve-mark technique, endotracheal intubation should be secured as soon as possible.

Because of the changes in hemodynamics in the gravid patient even minor degrees of aortocaval compression imposed by the gravid uterus may have a profound effect on the success or failure of resuscitative efforts. Any compression of the inferior vena cava seriously impedes venous return. In addition, obstruction of the lower aorta represents a significant obstacle to flow, hindering the development of an appropriate arteriovenous pressure gradient during chest compressions.

It is therefore imperative that uterine displacement be maintained during CPR. A wedge or sandbag should be placed under the right hip to provide a left lateral tilt to the pelvis of approximately 30 degrees. The position of the torso is not greatly affected and chest compressions should still be possible without difficulty. If circumstances make this approach cumbersome or impractical, the uterus can be deviated manually by displacing the patient's abdomen to the left and slightly cephalad.

If hemodynamic stability still cannot be achieved despite uterine displacement, then abdominal delivery of the baby must be immediately performed. Stabilization of the mother may never occur without delivery and relief of the aortocaval compression.[83] Several cases have occurred in which prompt delivery allowed adequate maternal resuscitation and recovery.[84,85]

A review of agonal and postmortem cesarean section has demonstrated the vitality of this procedure to the infant.[86] Approximately 70% of babies survive if delivery is within five minutes of arrest as compared to a 13% survival rate in those delivered after 6 to 15 minutes.

In the first and second trimesters the degree of aortocaval compression exerted by the uterus may be minimal, and an emergency abdominal delivery may offer little in terms of effective resuscitation.

If CPR fails to maintain peripheral circulation, emergency thoracotomy with open chest cardiac massage should be considered as a last resort.[83]

Selection of vasopressors is very important. The uterine vascular supply appears to lack autoregulation and flow depends on mean perfusion pressure.[87] Therefore, hypotension has severe consequences for the fetus. Although the uterine vascular bed is almost maximally dilated under normal conditions, it can respond with marked vasoconstriction to any exogenous or endogenous alpha-adrenergic stimulation. Uterine blood flow is well maintained by administration of ephedrine, but agents with alpha-adrenergic activity reduce uterine blood flow as maternal blood pressure increases. Ephedrine, through its predominant beta-adrenergic effects, increases cardiac output, blood pressure, and uterine blood flow without deleterious effects on the fetus, making it the agent of choice for maternal hypotension.

During cardiac arrest, ephedrine may not be a sufficient myocardial stimulant. Epinephrine has been used in these situations primarily for its alpha-adrenergic properties,[88,89] and the value of its beta-adrenergic effects in these situations is controversial.[90] The recommended intravenous dose of epinephrine (0.5 to 1.0 mg every five minutes during resuscitation) is more than enough to reduce uterine blood flow and adversely affect an already compromised fetus.[91] Early delivery of the infant gives the child the best chance of survival.

CONCLUSION

The puerperal woman without medical or obstetric complications is managed satisfactorily in an obstetric PACU—that is, a PACU lacking equipment and staff for intensive monitoring of circulatory, respiratory, or metabolic parameters. However, whenever intensive monitoring is desirable or the necessity for rapid intervention is possible, postpartum care should be provided in the surgical PACU or an intensive care unit.

REFERENCES

1. Ueland K, Hansen JM: Maternal cardiovascular dynamics. III. Labor and delivery under local and caudal analgesia. *Am J Obstet Gynecol* 1968;103:8–18.
2. Ueland K, Gills RE, Hansen JM: Maternal cardiovascular dynamics. I. Cesarean section under subarachnoid block anesthesia. *Am J Obstet Gynecol* 1968;100:45–54.
3. Ueland K, Hansen JM, Eng M, et al: Maternal cardiovascular dynamics. V. Cesarean section under thiopental-nitrous oxide-succinylcholine anesthesia. *Am J Obstet Gynecol* 1970;108:615–622.
4. Hansen JM, Ueland K: Maternal cardiovascular dynamics during pregnancy and parturition, in Marx GF (ed): *Parturition and Perinatology.* Philadelphia, Davis, 1973, pp 21–36.
5. Robson SC, Dunlop W: Haemodynamic changes during the early puerperium. *Br Med J* 1987;294:1065.
6. Adams JQ, Alexander AM: Alteration in cardiovascular physiology during labor. *Obstet Gynecol* 1958;12:542–549.
7. Mason SJ: Cardiac failure and arrhythmias during pregnancy, in Berkowitz RL (ed): *Critical Care of the Obstetric Patient.* New York, Churchill Livingstone, 1983, pp 481–504.
8. Szekely P, Snaith L: *Heart Disease and Pregnancy.* Edinburgh, Churchill Livingstone, 1974.
9. Bonica JJ: Maternal respiratory changes during pregnancy and parturition, in Marx GF (ed): *Parturition and Perinatology.* Philadelphia, Davis, 1973, pp 1–19.
10. Pernoll ML, Metcalf J, Schlenker TL, et al: Oxygen consumption at rest and during exercise in pregnancy. *Respir Physiol* 1975;25:285–293.
11. Fisher A, Prys-Roberts C: Maternal pulmonary gas exchange. A study during normal labour and extradural blockade. *Anaesthesia* 1968;23:350–356.
12. Marx GF, Berman JA: Anesthesia-related maternal mortality. *Bull NY Acad Med* 1985;61:323–330.
13. Monheit AG, Cousins L, Resnik R: The puerpium: Anatomic and physiologic readjustments. *Clin Obstet Gynecol* 1980;23:973–984.
14. Fallon HG: Liver diseases, in Burrow GN, Ferris TF (eds): *Medical Complications During Pregnancy.* Philadelphia, Saunders, 1975, pp 318–344.
15. Potter JM, Nestel PJ: The hyperlipidemia of pregnancy in normal and complicated pregnancies. *Am J Obstet Gynecol* 1979;133:165–170.
16. Blitt CD, Petty WC, Alberternst EE, Wright BJ: Correlation of plasma cholinesterase activity and duration of action of succinylcholine during pregnancy. *Anesth Analg* 1977;56:78–83.
17. Ganga CC, Heyduk JV, Marx GF, Sklar GS: A comparison of the response to suxamethonium in post-partum and gynaecological patients. *Anaesthesia* 1982;37:903–906.
18. Leighton BL, Cheek TG, Gross JB, et al: Succinylcholine pharmacodynamics in peripartum patients. *Anesthesiology* 1986;64:202–205.
19. Marx GF, Orkin LR: *Physiology of Obstetric Anesthesia.* Springfield, IL, Chas. C Thomas, 1969, pp 96–100.
20. Chamberlain DP, Chamberlain BDL: Changes in the skin temperature of the trunk and their relationship to sympathetic blockade during spinal anesthesia. *Anesthesiology* 1986;65:139–143.
21. Shimosato S, Etsten BE: The role of the venous system in cardiocirculatory dynamics during spinal and epidural anesthesia in man. *Anesthesiology* 1964;30:619–628.
22. Malliani A, Peterson DF, Bishop VS, Brown AM: Spinal sympathetic cardiocardiac reflexes. *Circ Res* 1972;30:158–166.
23. Otton PE, Wilson EJ: The cardiocirculatory effects of upper thoracic epidural analgesia. *Canad Anaesth Soc J* 1966;13:541–549.
24. Caplan RA, Ward RJ, Posner K, Cheney FW: Unexpected cardiac arrest during spinal anesthesia: A closed claims analysis of predisposing factors. *Anesthesiology* 1988;68:5–11.
25. Grove LH: Backache, headache and bladder dysfunction after delivery. *Br J Anaesth* 1973;45:1147–1149.

26. Ostheimer GW: Headache in the postpartum period, in Marx GF (ed): *Clinical Management of Mother and Newborn*. New York, Springer-Verlag, 1979, pp 27–41.

27. Myers L, Rosenberg M: The use of the 26-gauge spinal needle: A survey. *Anesth Analg* 1962;41:509–515.

28. Krueger JE: Etiology and treatment of postspinal headaches. *Anesth Analg* 1953;32:190–198.

29. Craft JB, Epstein BS, Coakley CS: Prophylaxis of dural-puncture headache with epidural saline. *Anesth Analg* 1973;52:228–231.

30. Jones RL: The role of recumbency in the prevention and treatment of postspinal headache. *Anesth Analg* 1974;53:788–796.

31. Carbaat PAT, van Crevel H: Lumbar puncture headache: Controlled study on the preventive effect of 24 hours' bed rest. *Lancet* 1981;2:1133–1135.

32. Jawalekar SR, Marx GF: Cutaneous cerebrospinal fluid leakage following attempted extradural block. *Anesthesiology* 1981;54:348–349.

33. Sechzer PH, Abel L: Post spinal anesthesia headache treated with caffeine I. Evaluation with demand method. *Curr Ther Res* 1978;24:307–312.

34. Jarvis AP, Greenawalt JW, Fagraeus L: Intravenous caffeine for postdural puncture headache. *Anesth Analg* 1986;65:313–321.

35. Palahniuk RJ, Cumming M: Prophylactic blood patch does not prevent post lumbar puncture headache. *Canad Anaesth Soc J* 1979;26:132–133.

36. Loeser EA, Hill GE, Bennett GM, Sederberg JH: Time vs success rate for epidural blood patch. *Anesthesiology* 1978;49:147–148.

37. Cheek TG, Banner R, Sauter J, Gutsche BB: Prophylactic extradural blood patch is effective—A preliminary communication. *Br J Anaesth* 1988;61:340–342.

38. Downing JW: Bupivacaine: A clinical assessment in lumbar extradural block. *Brit J Anaesth* 1969;41:427–432.

39. Waters HR, Rosen N, Perkins DH: Extradural blockade with bupivacaine: A double blind trial of bupivacaine with adrenaline 1/200,000 and bupivacaine plain. *Anaesthesia* 1970;25:184–190.

40. Brownridge P: Shivering related to epidural blockade with bupivacaine in labour and the influence of epidural pethidine. *Anaesth Intens Care* 1986;14:412–417.

41. Bay J, Nunn JF, Prys-Roberts C: Factors influencing arterial PO_2 during recovery from anaesthesia. *Brit J Anaesth* 1968;40:398–407.

42. Nathan PW: Observations on sensory and sympathetic function during intrathecal analgesia. *J Neurol Neurosurg Psychiatry* 1976;39:114–121.

43. Claybon LE, Hirsh RA: Meperidine arrests postanesthesia shivering. *Anesthesiology* 1980;53:S180.

44. Phillips OC: Neurologic complications following spinal anesthesia with lidocaine: A prospective review of 10,440 cases. *Anesthesiology* 1969;30:284–289.

45. Naulty JS: Intraspinal narcotics. *Clin Anaesth* 1986;4:145–156.

46. Negre I, Gueneron JP, Ecoffey C, et al: Ventilatory response to carbon dioxide after intramuscular and epidural fentanyl. *Anesth Analg* 1987;66:707–710.

47. Rawal N, Schott U, Tandon B, et al: Influence of intravenous naloxone infusion on analgesia and un-

48. Stenseth R, Sellevold O, Breivik H: Epidural morphine for postoperative pain: Experience with 1095 patients. *Acta Anaesth Scand* 1985;29:148–156.

49. Brownridge P: Epidural and intrathecal opiates for postoperative pain relief. *Anaesthesia* 1983;38:74–75.

50. Martin R, Salbaing J, Blaise G, et al: Epidural morphine for post-operative pain relief. A dose–response curve. *Anesthesiology* 1982;56:423–426.

51. Bromage PR, Camporesi E, Chestnut D: Epidural narcotics for postoperative analgesia. *Anesth Analg* 1980;59:473–480.

52. Rawal N, Mollefors K, Axelsson K, et al: Naloxone reversal of urinary retention after epidural morphine. *Lancet* 1981;2:1411.

53. Rawal N, Mollefors K, Axelsson K, et al: An experimental study of urodynamic effects of epidural morphine and of naloxone reversal. *Anesth Analg* 1983;62:641–647.

54. Crone LL, Conly JM, Clark KM, et al: Recurrent herpes simplex virus labialis and the use of epidural morphine in obstetric patients. *Anesth Analg* 1988;67:318–323.

55. Gieraerts R, Navalgund A, Vaes L, et al: Increased incidence of itching and herpes simplex in patients given epidural morphine after cesarean section. *Anesth Analg* 1987;66:1321–1324.

56. Biehl DR: Antepartum and postpartum hemorrhage, in Shnider S, Levinson G (eds): *Anesthesia for Obstetrics*, ed 2. Baltimore, Williams & Wilkins, 1987, pp 281–292.

57. Gibbs CE, Locke WE: Maternal deaths in Texas, 1969 to 1973. *Am J Obstet Gynecol* 1976;126:687–692.

58. Pritchard JA, Baldwin RM, Dickey JC, et al: Blood volume changes in pregnancy and the puerperium. II. Red blood cell loss and changes in apparent blood volume during and following vaginal delivery, cesarean section and cesarean section plus total hysterectomy. *Am J Obstet Gynecol* 1962;84:1271–1282.

59. Marx GF: Shock in the obstetric patient. *Anesthesiology* 1965;26:423–434.

60. Rall TW, Schleifer LS: Oxytocin, prostaglandins, ergot alkaloids and other drugs; tocolytic agents, in Gilman AG, Goodman LS, Rall TW, Murad F (eds): *The Pharmacological Basis of Therapeutics*, ed 7. New York, Macmillan, 1985, pp 926–945.

61. Abouleish E: Postpartum hypertension and convulsion after oxytocic drugs. *Anesth Analg* 1976;55:813–815.

62. Munson WM: The pressor effect of various vasopressor–oxytocic combinations: A laboratory study and a review. *Anesth Analg* 1965;44:114–119.

63. Ferguson JE II, Joyce TH III, Pearl RG, Rahlfs T: Obstetric shock, pulmonary disorders, hemorrhage and postpartum intensive care, in Albright GA, Ferguson JE II, Joyce TH III, Stevenson DK (eds): *Anesthesia in Obstetrics: Maternal, Fetal and Neonatal Aspects*. Boston, Butterworths, 1986, pp 458–489.

64. Marx GF, Orkin LR: *Physiology of Obstetric Anesthesia*. Springfield, IL, Chas. C Thomas, 1969, pp 96–100.

65. Camp CE, Tessem J, Adenwala J, Joyce TH: Vecuronium and prolonged neuromuscular blockade in postpartum patients. *Anesthesiology* 1987;67:1006–1008.

66. Marx GF: Pathophysiology and therapy of postpartum complications, in Marx GF (ed): *Clinical Management of Mother and Newborn.* New York, Springer-Verlag, 1979, pp 13–25.

67. Sibai BM, Abdella TN, Spinnato JA, Anderson GA: Eclampsia V. The incidence of nonpreventable eclampsia. *Am J Obstet Gynecol* 1986;154:581–586.

68. Niederman MS, Matthay RA: Asthma and other severe respiratory diseases during pregnancy, in Berkowitz (ed): *Critical Care of the Obstetric Patient.* New York, Churchill Livingstone, 1983, pp 335–366.

69. Cohen WR: Personal Communication

70. Singer F, Horlick M, Poretsky L: Recovery of beta-cell function postpartum in a patient with insulin-dependent diabetes mellitus. *NY J Med* 198;88:496–498.

71. Gabbe SG: Management of diabetes mellitus in pregnancy. ACOG Technical Bulletin No. 92, 1986.

72. Stoelting RK, Dierdorf SF, McCammon RL: Anemia, in *Anesthesia and Co-Existing Disease,* ed 2. New York, Churchill Livingstone, 1988, pp 557–573.

73. Plauche WC: Myasthenia gravis in pregnancy. *Am J Obstet Gynecol* 1964;88:404–409.

74. Aboulesh E: Neurologic diseases, in James FM, Wheeler AS (eds): *Obstetric Anesthesia: The Complicated Patient.* Philadelphia, Davis, 1982, pp 57–86.

75. Rolbin SH, Rolbin SB: Drug addiction: Anesthetic considerations for the mother, fetus and newborn, in James FN, Wheeler AS (eds): *Obstetric Anesthesia: The Complicated Patient.* Philadelphia, Davis, 1982, pp 317–331.

76. Gawin FH, Ellinwood EH: Cocaine and other stimulants. Actions, abuse, and treatment. *New Engl J Med* 1988; 118:173–182.

77. Nahas G, Trouve R, Demus JF, von Sitbon M: A calcium-channel blocker as antidote to the cardiac effects of cocaine intoxication. *New Engl J Med* 1985;313:519–520.

78. Clark SL: Amniotic fluid embolism, in Clark SL, Phelan JP, Cotton DB (eds): *Critical Care Obstetrics.* Oradell, NJ, Medical Economics Books, 1987, pp 315–331.

79. Mulder JI: Amniotic fluid embolism: An overview and case report. *Am J Obstet Gynecol* 1985;152:430–435.

80. Duff P, Engelsgjerd B, Zingery LW, et al: Hemodynamic observations in a patient with intrapartum amniotic fluid embolism. *Am J Obstet Gynecol* 1983;146:112–115.

81. Quance D: Amniotic fluid embolism detected by pulse oximetry. *Anesthesiology* 1988;68:951–952.

82. Crawford JS: Some aspects of obstetric anesthesia. *Br J Anaesth* 1956;28:201–208.

83. Lee RV, Rodgers BD, White LM, et al: Cardiopulmonary resuscitation of pregnant women. *Am J Med* 1986;81:311–18.

84. Depace NL, Betesh JS, Kotle MN: "Postmortem" cesarean section with recovery of both mother and offspring. *JAMA* 1982;248:971–975.

85. Marx GF: Cardiopulmonary resuscitation of late-pregnant women. *Anesthesiology* 1986;65:116.

86. Katz VL, Dotters DJ, Droegmueller W: Perimortem cesarean delivery. *Obstet Gynecol* 1986;68:571–576.

87. Ralston DH, Shnider SM, deLorimier AA: Effects of equipotent ephedrine, metaraminol, mephentermine, and methoxamine on uterine blood flow in the pregnant ewe. *Anesthesiology* 1974;40:354–370.

88. Redding JS, Pearson JW: Evaluation of drugs for cardiac resuscitation. *Anesthesiology* 1963;24:203–207.

89. Yakatis RW, Otto CW, Blitt CD: Relative importance of alpha and beta adrenergic receptors during resuscitation. *Crit Care Med* 1979;7:293–296.

90. Standards and guidelines for cardiopulmonary resuscitation (CPR) and emergency cardiac care (ECC). *JAMA* 1986;255:2905–2984.

91. Rosenfield CR, Barton MD, Meschia G: Effects of epinephrine on distribution of blood flow in the pregnant ewe. *Am J Obstet Gynecol* 1976;124:156–163.

Ingrid B. Hollinger

The postanesthesia care of the pediatric patient covers the transition from general or regional anesthesia with central nervous system depression and respiratory and cardiovascular instability to full alertness with recovery of all protective reflexes. In some patients, this includes various periods of intensive respiratory management, cardiovascular management, or both, due to preexisting medical conditions or as a result of surgery (eg, a neonate with cardiac abnormalities). Although the majority of patients requiring prolonged intensive care are transferred to an intensive care unit, they frequently spend many hours in the postanesthetic care unit (PACU), either until they are sufficiently stable to be transported to a distant unit or until an intensive care unit bed becomes available.

This chapter reviews the general principles of postanesthetic care of infants and children and some of the problems encountered clinically in certain patient groups or after specific procedures.

Those involved in the postanesthetic care of infants and children should be familiar with the anatomical and physiological differences of these patients compared to adults and understand the emotional needs and psychological problems of these patients and their parents.

ANATOMY AND PHYSIOLOGY

The differences in size between adults and infants is obvious. However, the proportion of various body areas to each other and the body surface area to weight is different and changes with age (Table 14–1).[1,2]

Respiratory System

The upper airway is characterized by the following major differences.[3,4]

- The tongue is large relative to the size of the oral cavity and located closer to the roof of the mouth.
- The larynx is positioned approximately one interspace higher (C3–C4) in the neck when compared to the adult (C4–C5). The more immature the infant, the higher the position of the larynx.
- The epiglottis is narrow and omega-shaped; it is tilted posterior to the axis of the trachea.
- The vocal cords are slanted upwards and posteriorly. The loose alveolar tissue of the glottis is prone to edematous swelling with minor trauma or overhydration.
- The narrowest portion of the infant larynx is the nondistensible cricoid ring, the only circumferential cartilaginous structure. This feature persists until puberty when cricoid and thyrocartilage grow. Thereafter the rima glottidis becomes the narrowest part of the larynx.
- The ribs of the infant are cartilaginous and the configuration of the rib cage tends to be circular rather than ellipsoid as in the adult.[5] The horizontal position of the ribs prevents the "bucket handle" effect of intercostal muscle contraction.
- The angle of insertion of the diaphragm is almost horizontal instead of oblique as in the adult, which results in decreased efficiency of contraction.[6] In addition, the diaphragm contains less type I (slow twitch, high oxidative) fatigue-resistant muscle fiber in the newborn and young infant.[7] The diaphragm of the premature infant contains only about 10% high oxidative fibers; in the newborn approximately 25% type I fibers are present. The proportion of high oxidative fibers progressively increases until the adult composition of 50 to 55% type I fibers is reached towards the end of the first year.[6,7]

Development of the conducting airways down to the terminal bronchioli is completed at the end of the 16th week of gestation. Until birth only primitive terminal saccules have developed with sufficient capillary network to allow gas exchange.[8] The major portion of alveolar development occurs postnatally within the first decade of life.[9] Absolute lung compliance, expressed as mL/cm H_2O, is directly related to lung size, and the newborn has only 3 to 5% of adult

TABLE 14–1. RELATIONSHIP OF WEIGHT, BODY SURFACE, AND DISTRIBUTION OF BODY SURFACE AREA THROUGH INFANCY AND CHILDHOOD

Group	Wt. (kg)	BSA (mL)	%BSA Head	%BSA Trunk	%BSA Upper Extremity	%BSA Lower Extremity	BSA/wt
Neonate (0–1 mo)	3	0.2	21	30	19	28	0.066
Infant (6 wk–2					19	30	
yr)	3–15	0.45	19	32			0.045
Child (2–10 yr)	15–30	1.05	15	32	19	34	0.035
(10–14					19	36	
yr)	30–50	1.25	13	32			0.025
Adult (> 17 yr)	50–70	1.75	10	32	19	36	0.025

values (Table 14–2).[10] However, since the lungs of the newborn and infant contains less elastic elements, the result is a higher specific compliance, which is compliance standardized to lung volume (functional residual capacity, vital capacity, or total lung capacity) or greater distensibility of the infant lung.[11] The extremely compliant rib cage contributes little to maintenance of negative intrathoracic pressure and lung volumes. Together with the lack of elastic recoil in the lung tissue, this leads to collapse of small airways and increased closing capacity.[12]

While the abdominal contents in the upright position act as a pull on the diaphragm, increasing lung volumes, they tend to push the diaphragm cephalad in the supine position in a nonuniform pattern, resulting in a loss of functional residual capacity.[11,13]

Most of the work of breathing in the infant is expended to overcome flow resistance. While in the adult 60% of total airway resistance is contributed by the nose and 80% rests in the upper airway, in infants bronchioles and small airways contribute the majority of resistance to airflow; the nasal passages account for only about 25%.[14,15] This is due to the small airway diameter and the lack of supporting structures.[16,17] According to Poiseuille's law for flow through hollow tubes, resistance (R) is proportional to length and radius[18] for laminar flow:

$$R \alpha \frac{L}{r^4}$$

and for turbulent flow:

$$R \alpha \frac{L}{r^5}$$

where L = length of tube, r = radius.

Flow is laminar in the trachea and distal airways but turbulent in the central airways below the ca-

TABLE 14–2. NORMAL PULMONARY FUNCTION VALUES

	Infant	Adult	Denominator
Respiratory frequency	34–45	13	BPM
Tidal volume	6–8	7	mL/kg
Alveolar ventilation	100–150	60	mL/kg/min
Minute ventilation	200–260	90	mL/kg/min
Dead space to tidal volume ratio	0.3–0.4	0.3	mL/kg/min
Functional residual capacity	30	34	mL/kg
Pulmonary compliance	4–6	130–160	mL/cm H_2O
Specific compliance (CL/FRC)	0.04–0.05	0.05–0.06	mL/cm H_2O/L
Airway resistance	18–29	2–3	cm H_2O/L/
Oxygen consumption	6–8	3–4	sec
Arterial blood gases			mL/kg/min
Pad_2	55–85	85–100	
Paco_2	30–35	37–44	tore
pH	7.32–7.38	7.35–7.45	

rina.[19] The most important factor determining flow resistance is obviously the radius of the airflow passages, which explains the higher absolute airway resistance of infants. Because of the small absolute diameter of the airway even minor degrees of swelling markedly elevate airway resistance and the work of breathing (Fig. 14–1).

The signs and symptoms of small airway disease (eg, bronchiolitis) are more marked in infants and children and relatively small amounts of mucosal swelling may lead to symptomatic airway obstruction (eg, croup).

A major determinant of minute ventilation is oxygen requirement. Infants have an oxygen consumption of 6 to 8 mL/kg/min, twice that of the adult (2 to 3 mL/kg).[10,21] They adapt to this metabolic demand by increasing minute ventilation. Alveolar ventilation based on weight is twice that of an adult—100 to 150 mL/kg/min compared to 60 mL/kg/min.[20,21] The increased ventilatory requirement explains the higher ventilatory frequency seen in infancy and childhood since tidal volume remains constant on a weight basis at 5 to 7 mL/kg. The proportion of wasted ventilation (dead space) is 0.4 during the first month and then attains adult levels 0.3.[10,21,22] Table 14–2 lists normal values for lung function in infants and adults. Although in general alveolar ventilation is more effi-

ciently increased by higher tidal volume than faster respiratory rates,[22] the relationship between elastic and flow resistive forces in the infant lung is such that the minimum work of breathing is achieved with respiratory rates around 37 breaths per minute.[17] The metabolic cost of breathing in adults is approximately 2% of oxygen consumption. In premature infants this value increases to 6%.[23] Because of the small absolute size of the infant airways and the high resistive work required under basal conditions, any degree of narrowing of even an inappropriately small, long endotracheal tube may result in such an increase in work of breathing that exhaustion and ventilatory failure ensue.[24,25]

In infants, as in adults, ventilation is controlled by peripheral and central chemoreceptors. The ventilatory response to CO_2 is mediated through H^+ receptors located in the medulla oblongata. The slope of the CO_2 response curve of the newborn is equal to that of the adult. It is, however, shifted to the left, possibly due to the high minute ventilation or residual progesterone effect.[22] CO_2 responsivity is easily depressed by hypoxemia, sedatives, and anesthetics.[26,27] In addition, it is influenced by the sleep state of the infant. During rapid eye movement (REM) sleep, motor tone of skeletal muscles is depressed, resulting in loss of tone of the chest wall and pharyn-

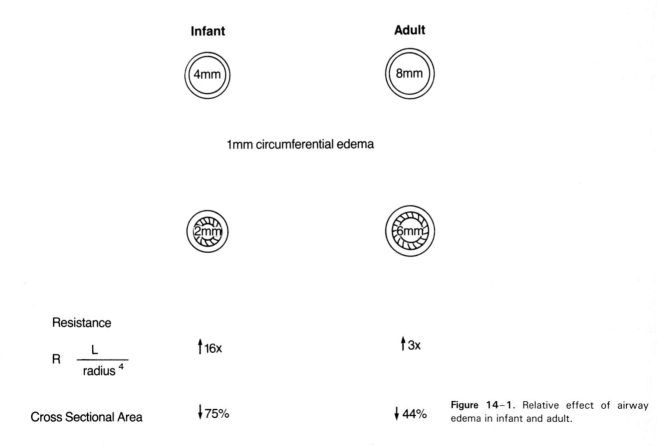

Figure 14–1. Relative effect of airway edema in infant and adult.

geal muscles. Functional residual capacity is reduced by approximately 30%, resulting in intrapulmonary shunting.[27,28] Loss of tone of upper airway muscles results in various forms of upper airway obstruction.[29] The response to CO_2 is irregular or depressed.[27] Normal newborns may sleep up to 20 hours a day while the normal adult sleeps only an average of 8 hours a day. In addition, adult sleep consists of only 20% REM sleep while newborns spend more than 40% and prematures up to 80% of their sleep time in REM sleep. The adult relationship of REM and non-REM sleep of 1:4 is not reached until the second half of the first year.[27,28] Prematures have a CO_2 response curve shifted towards adult values, particularly if they exhibit periodic breathing,[30] probably due to immaturity of chemoreceptor centers. The ventilatory response to changes in oxygenation is mediated via the carotid chemoreceptors. Inhalation of 100% oxygen will result in an immediate (30 sec) decrease in ventilation. This response is unchanged in prematures, normal newborns, infants, and adults.[26] The response to hypoxia, however, is different in the premature and newborn when compared to adults. While adult subjects exhibit sustained hyperventilation with hypoxia, preterm and newborn infants exhibit only a brief period of hyperventilation (if at all), followed by progressive hypoventilation.[26,31] In preterm babies periodic breathing or apnea may occur. In addition, these infants fail to arouse in response to hypoxia.[26,27] The abnormal response to hypoxia is independent of gestational age but changes with postnatal age. After about the third postnatal week, infants demonstrate appropriate hyperventilation and arousal when exposed to hypoxia.[26,27,31] Hypoxia significantly flattens the slope of the CO_2 response curve in newborns and prematures.[26,27]

Chemoreceptor responses are depressed by anesthetics and sedatives. While inhalational anesthetics flatten CO_2 response and increase apneic threshold, narcotics and ketamine are followed by hypoventilation largely due to a reduction in respiratory rate and a parallel shift to the right of the CO_2 response curve, although some flattening of the response to CO_2 also occurs.[32]

In addition to chemoreceptor influences, ventilation in the premature and newborn is influenced by a number of peripheral receptors that are mostly vagally mediated. Slow lung inflation leads to inhibition of inspiration (Hering-Breuer); rapid lung inflation to inspiratory gasp followed by apnea (Head's paradoxical reflex).[21] Stimulation of the superior laryngeal nerve leads to glottic closure and prolonged apnea.[33] Muscle spindles in the intercostal muscles are responsive to changes in inspiratory or expiratory load.[27] They are not fully active, similar to the muscles of respiration in the premature, resulting in

hypoventilation in the presence of increased respiratory load.[27] Of interest is the fact that temperature-sensitive receptors located in the nose or face, when exposed to warmth, may trigger apnea, while colder ambient temperature stimulates respiration.[21]

Cardiovascular System

At birth, half of the myocardium consists of connective tissue, with fewer sarcomers per gram of tissue.[37] Myocardial function is characterized by poor compliance, increased resting tension, and the development of less active tension when stimulated.[37]

Augmenting preload does little to increase cardiac output and heart rate becomes the major determinant of cardiac performance.[38] Since the right ventricle carries a higher workload during fetal life, right ventricular mass is increased and at birth the right ventricle is larger. Distensibility of both ventricles is equal (contrary to adults) but reduced. With the changes in pulmonary and systemic vascular resistances with birth, stress on the right ventricle is reduced postnatally by 47%, while the workload for the left ventricle increases 116%.[21] As a result, right ventricular muscle mass decreases and left ventricular muscle mass increases until the adult ratio is achieved at about 3 to 4 months of age. Despite the relative underdevelopment of the myocardium, infants have a cardiac output, based on weight, of three to four times adult values at the end of the first year.[21] Output ranges from 130 to 240 mL/kg/min (adult value is 70 mL/kg/min).

Heart rate is controlled by sympathetic and parasympathetic innervation. While parasympathetic innervation develops early in fetal life, sympathetic innervation of the myocardium is incomplete at birth and consists mostly of beta receptors. Because alpha-adrenergic receptor development is lagging centrally as well as peripherally, vasoconstrictor response to sympathetic stimulation is limited. Direct stimulation through infusion of catecholamines, however, results in prolonged effect. Cardiac output increases with application of catecholamines, mostly through increase in cardiac rate.[21,39] As a result of the immaturity of the sympathetic nervous system the newborn and infant display exaggerated responses to vagal stimulation (eg, bradycardia and apnea with nasopharyngeal stimulation such as suctioning).[40] Episodic bradycardia, sinus bradycardia with nodal escape, and varying degrees of atrioventricular block, as well as atrial and ventricular extrasystoles, can be observed in normal newborns and particular prematures as a result of autonomic imbalance and developmental changes in the conduction system.[21]

While the newborn heart is sensitive to vagal stimulation it is relatively insensitive to the direct effects of hypoxemia. In adults, cardiac output and myocardial contractility are decreased by hypoxemia, while in the newborn under similar conditions high energy phosphate levels and myocardial function are maintained, presumably due to the newborn's ability to use anaerobic metabolic pathways more efficiently.[41] However, if hypoxemia is combined with acidosis, myocardial function declines.[42]

As a result of the immaturity of the sympathetic nervous system, cardiovascular reflexes that maintain perfusion under conditions of hypovolemia are not fully functional. The infant is unable to mount massive vasoconstriction to maintain cardiac output. Maintenance of an adequate blood volume and central venous pressure is therefore essential for maintenance of blood pressure and organ perfusion. Inhalational anesthetics depress myocardial function to various degrees[43,44] and suppress baroreceptor response,[43] an effect that may persist into the postanesthetic period.

During the first weeks of life the infant's circulation remains in a transitional state. The two main fetal channels diverting blood flow from the lungs in utero, the ductus arteriosus and the foramen ovale, are only functionally closed. The main stimulus to ductal closure is the postnatal increase in arterial oxygenation, which causes constriction of the ductal musculature.[21] The foramen ovale closes as left atrial pressure exceeds right atrial pressure following the increase in pulmonary blood flow and systemic vascular resistance after birth. Conditions that increase pulmonary vascular resistance, particularly hypoxia and acidosis, may lead to reopening of these fetal channels, bypassing the lung and leading to severe cyanosis and rapid cardiovascular deterioration.[45,46] Shunting across the ductus arteriosus normally persists in the first few days of life.[47] Anatomic closure is not complete until 2 to 3 months of age.[48] In premature infants, ductal closure may be delayed and the ductus may reopen particularly under conditions of hypoxia or hypervolemia.[49,50] Pulmonary artery pressure, which is suprasystemic in the fetus at birth, declines rapidly with expansion of the lung postnatally but does not reach adult levels until the end of the first year. This is accompanied by a decrease in the muscle thickness of the pulmonary arteries.[51,52]

As pointed out earlier, the immaturity of vascular reflexes requires maintenance of an adequate filling pressure to maintain cardiac output, blood pressure, and organ perfusion. Blood pressure in the absence of compensatory vasoconstriction becomes an indicator for adequacy of blood volume and can be used as a guide for volume replacement.[21] Table 14–3 lists normal values for heart rate and blood pressure for various ages. Blood pressure should be measured with a cuff the width of which is equivalent to 40 to 50% of the circumference of the extremity.[55,56]

Blood volume in the newborn and infant is larger on a weight basis than later in life. In the newborn, blood volume is 9 to 10% of body weight and declines to adult values (7% of body weight) by 2 years of age.[21,57] In the newborn, the expanded blood volume consists mostly of red cell volume. The more immature the infant the larger the red cell volume per unit body weight.[21] The neonatal red cells contain nearly exclusively fetal hemoglobin, which has an increased affinity for oxygen due to reduced levels of 2,3 disphosphoglycerate (2-3 DPG). P_{50} of the neonate is 19 mm Hg and gradually increases to adult levels (P_{50} - 27 mm Hg) by 4 to 6 months. P_{50} increases to 30 mm Hg by the end of the first year and remains high through childhood, compensating for the reduced levels of hemoglobin seen during this period.[2,58] Hemoglobin levels decline after birth due to a decrease in erythropoesis and a shorter life span of the fetal red blood cell. In prematures, the fall in hemoglobin is greater and occurs earlier. The lowest hemoglobin concentration is seen between the 9th and 12th week postnatally and then gradually rises (physiologic anemia).[59] White cell count may reach 21,000/mm³ in the first 24 hours of life and may still be normal at 12,000/mm³ by the end of the first week. Adult levels are reached at puberty. Throughout the first few years of

TABLE 14–3. NORMAL VALUES FOR BLOOD PRESSURE AND HEART RATE

| | Heart Rate | | Blood Pressure | |
	Mean	Range	Mean Systolic (± 2 sd)	Mean Diastolic (± 2 sd)
Newborn	145	70–190	65 ± 18	40 ± 16
1–11 mo	120	80–160	96 ± 27	65 ± 27
2 years	110	80–130	95 ± 25	61 ± 24
4 years	100	80–120	99 ± 20	65 ± 20
6 years	100	75–115	95 ± 15	55 ± 9
8 years	90	70–110	100 ± 16	55 ± 9
10 years	90	70–110	110 ± 17	58 ± 10
12 years	88	70–110	115 ± 19±	59 ± 10
14 years	83	60–105	118 ± 19±	60 ± 10

life relative lymphocytosis is present.[60] Normal hematologic values during infancy and childhood are listed in Table 14–4.

Temperature Regulation

Maintenance of normal body temperature is of major importance in caring for pediatric surgical patients. Body temperature is the result of a balance between heat production from metabolism and heat loss due to environmental factors. Heat is produced by activity; metabolism of food, particularly proteins (specific dynamic action); and in response to lower environmental temperatures.[61] In newborn infants, a major source of metabolic heat production rests in brown fat located between the scapula, the vessels of the neck, in the axilla and the mediastinum, and around the kidneys and adrenals. This tissue is particularly rich in mitochondria. Cold exposure or norepinephrine infusion will result in large increases in fat metabolism in these tissues with concomitant heat production, the so-called nonshivering thermogenesis. The maximal metabolic rate of brown fat is approximately 40 times the whole body metabolic rate, with an oxygen consumption of 600 mL/kg/min.[61-63] Hypoxia prevents heat production in brown fat. The sedated infant is unable to increase heat production by activity. Involuntary muscle activity (shivering) is practically absent under 3 to 6 months of age (Fig. 14–2).[64,65]

Heat is distributed predominantly by convection through the circulation. Thermal insulation is minimal in the small infant with poorly developed subcutaneous fat and high skin blood flow. The disproportional large head surface area combined with a high cerebral blood flow contribute to the major influence of this area on temperature maintenance and whole body metabolic rate.[61] Heat loss from the organism occurs predominantly through radiation and convection. Radiation of heat occurs to the nearest surface, irrespective of the temperature of the surrounding air, and is proportional to the temperature difference between the radiating body and the surface. Convective heat loss is due to air movement around the organism. Radiation and convective heat loss are most efficiently reduced by reduction of exposed body surface area (blankets, caps, wrapping in plastic foil). Conductive heat loss occurs to air and is negligible due to the low thermal conductivity of air. Considerable amounts of heat, however, can be lost to cold mattresses or blankets. Heat loss due to evaporation occurs from the skin and respiratory tract. This heat loss varies with ambient humidity, and, for example, the presence of wet skin. The increased alveolar ventilation, the large body surface area relative to weight, and the more water-permeable skin of the neonate, lead to higher evaporation water losses in this age group. In the term baby, 20 to 30% of metabolic heat is lost in this manner.[61]

Temperature sensitive receptors are located in the skin, particularly in the trigeminal area and in the central nervous system in the hypothalamus.[61,66] Central integration of various thermal stimuli adjust the balance between heat loss and heat gain.[67] This central integrating system is depressed by general anesthesia and not fully active in the premature and newborn.[61,68] A thermoneutral state is achieved when vasomotor adjustments alone without changes in metabolic rate are sufficient to maintain normothermia.[61] The set point for temperature in a neutral thermal environment is a rectal or core temperature of 36.5 to 37°C. In small babies, however, a lower core temperature between 36.0 and 36.5°C may be found without signs of thermal stress (increased oxygen consumption).[61,68] The sensors for thermoregulation are predominantly located in the skin, particularly of the face and abdomen, and their sensitivity changes with age and weight of the infant. In small young infants a gradient of only 1.5°C between skin and environment or rectal and environmental temperature may be permissible for minimal O_2 consumption. In older infants a gradient of 2.5 to 5°C is generally acceptable. A skin temperature of the ab-

TABLE 14–4. NORMAL HEMATOLOGIC VALUES

	Hemoglobin (g/dL)	HCT	Leukocytes (wbc/mm³)	Neutrophil (%)	Lymphocytes (%)
Cord blood	16.8 (13.7–20.1)	55 (45–65)	18,000 (9–30,000)	61	31
2 wk	16.5 (13.0–20.0)	50 (42–66)	12,000 (5–21,000)	40	48
3 mo	12.0 (9.5–14.5)	36 (31–41)	12,000 (6–18,000)	30	63
6 mo–6 yr	12.0 (10.5–14.0)	37 (33–42)	10,000 (6–15,000)	45	48
7–12 yr	13.0 (11.0–16.0)	38 (34–40)	8000 (4500–13,500)	55	38
Adult					
Female	14 (12.0–16.0)	42 (37–47)	7500 (5–10,000)	55	35
Male	16 (14.0–18.0)	47 (42–52)	7500 (5–10,000)		

Adapted from Pearson HA: Diseases of the blood, in Behrman RE, Vaughan VC (eds): Nelson's Textbook of Pediatrics, ed 13. Philadelphia, Saunders, 1987, pp 1035–1078.

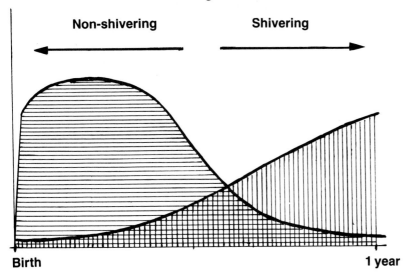

Thermogenesis

Non-shivering   Shivering

Birth   1 year

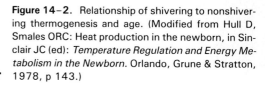

Figure 14–2. Relationship of shivering to nonshivering thermogenesis and age. (Modified from Hull D, Smales ORC: Heat production in the newborn, in Sinclair JC (ed): *Temperature Regulation and Energy Metabolism in the Newborn.* Orlando, Grune & Stratton, 1978, p 143.)

dominal wall of 36.5°C corresponding to an average skin temperature of 35 to 36°C is usually optimal.

As pointed out previously, reduction of exposed body surface area significantly reduces cold stress. Exposure to lower-than-thermoneutral environmental temperatures has multiple deleterious consequences. Nonprotein energy stores are depleted, and release of catecholamines with increase in pulmonary vascular resistance occurs, followed by metabolic acidosis, lethargy, and in extreme cases, pulmonary hemorrhage and death.[61] To avoid the metabolic stress of temperature maintenance, not only core but also skin temperature has to be maintained. Stimulation of temperature-sensitive receptors located particularly in the face by, for example, cold drafts (high-flow oxygen) will result in a noticeable rise in metabolism.[69,70] Recommended environmental temepratures for various ages are listed in Table 14–5. The use of overhead infrared lamps can mitigate the effects of a cool environment to a large extent.

Intensive efforts at prevention of heat loss will occasionally result in iatrogenic increases in temperature. Infants lose heat through peripheral vasodilatation and increase in evaporative heat loss (sweating). Prematures are unable to sweat and the ability to sweat is not fully matured at birth. Dehydration and infection as well as excessive atropinization may cause elevation in body temperature. Metabolic rate is increased by 12% for each degree C above 37[71] and fluid therapy has to be adjusted accordingly. Physical measures to reduce elevated body temperature include uncovering of the patient, increasing evaporative and convective heat loss with wet sponging and increased air circulation (fan), and the application of cold packs.[61] An unusual cause for severe elevation in body temperature in the postanesthetic period with a concomitant maximal increase in metabolic rate is the development of the malignant hyperthermia syndrome (discussed in a later section).

Renal Physiology and Fluid Electrolyte Metabolism

Water is the main constituent of body mass, the remainder consisting of fat and skeletal mineral and cell solids. Fat contains only about 10% water and contributes therefore mostly to weight, not body water content.[72] The younger the individual the higher the proportion of water in total body weight. While the 3-month-old fetus consists of 95% water, total body water declines to 78% of weight at birth, 65% of weight at 12 months, and continues to decline until it reaches adult values of 55 to 60% of total weight at approximately 2 years of age. The changes in body composition with age are illustrated in Figure 14–3. Total body water can be divided into two compartments separated by the cell membrane and intra- and extra cellular fluid space. The extracellular compartment is further divided by the capillary membrane into intravascular and interstitial fluid space (Fig. 14–4).[73] Intracellular water comprises about 33% of body weight at birth and rapidly rises to adult levels of 44% within the first 3 months.[74] Extracellular water

TABLE 14–5. RECOMMENDED ENVIRONMENTAL TEMPERATURES FOR VARIOUS AGES

Premature or neonate	27°C
Infant 1–6 months	26°C
6 months–2 years	25°C

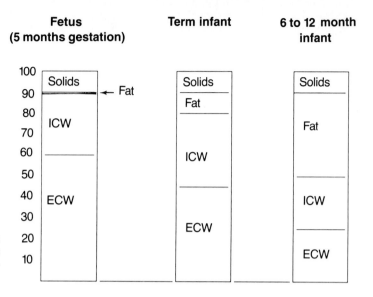

Figure 14-3. Changes in body composition with age. (From Driscoll JM, Heird WL: Maintenance fluid therapy during the neonatal period, in Winters RW (ed): *The Body Fluids in Pediatrics.* Boston, Little, Brown, 1973, p 266.)

makes up a much larger proportion of total body water in the infant. A small premature may have an extracellular fluid space of 60% of total body water. At birth, extracellular water constitutes 45% of total body weight, which rapidly declines in the first few months. It reaches 25 to 30% by 1 year and adult levels of 20% at puberty (Fig. 14–5).[74] Much of the reduction in extracellular fluid and total body water occurs immediately postnatally.[73] Excessive parental fluid therapy in the premature and neonate interferes with this physiologic process and may result in undesirable consequences. Patent ductus arteriosus, respiratory distress syndrome, and necrotizing enterocolitis have been linked to high fluid intake.[75-77] Plasma and interstitial fluid contain large amounts of sodium and chloride as predominant cation and anion, while intracellular fluid contains potassium, magnesium, and phosphate. The electrolye content of extracellular water is 150 mEq/L, that of intracellular water 200 mEq/L (Table 14–6).[72,78]

Renal function at birth is immature. Glomerular filtration rate (GFR) is only 25% of adult values.[78,79]

GFR increases rapidly within the first 2 weeks of life but does not reach adult values until after the end of the first year.[78] Prematures have an even lower GFR, which increases slower than in term babies.[80] The low GFR results in an inability to excrete large fluid loads rapidly. The concentrating capacity of the preterm and full-term kidney is also poorly developed. Maximal concentration capacity is between 500 to 600 mOsm/L compared to the adult value of 1200 mOsm/L.[81] Tubular capacity for secretion or reabsorption is disproportionately limited compared to glomerular filtration. This is particularly important for the regulation of serum sodium content, the major cation of the extracellular space. The infant, and particularly the premature, is unable to excrete excess sodium efficiently but is also unable to conserve sodium[82] (obligatory sodium loss). Prematures are "salt-wasters" and need excess sodium adminstration to prevent hyponatremia. Plasma osmolality is principally regulated by antidiuretic hormone and serum sodium concentration by aldosterone. The tubular system of the small infant is unresponsive to both

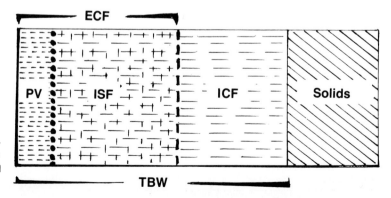

Figure 14-4. Subdivision of total body mass in the newborn. PV = plasma volume; ISF = interstitial fluid; ICF = intracellular fluid; ECF = extracellular fluid; TBW = total body water.

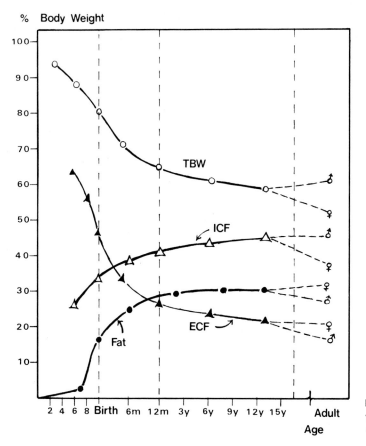

Figure 14-5. Extracellular water as a percentage of total body weight. TBW = total body water; ICF = intracellular fluid; ECF = extracellular fluid.

these hormones.[83-85] Renal function matures rapidly after birth and reaches 80 to 90% of adult function by 4 to 6 weeks of age. Full maturation is achieved towards the end of the first year of life. Because of the inability of the immature kidney to conserve either water or salt, fluid deprivation, abnormal losses, or hydration with non-sodium-containing fluids can lead rapidly to severe dehydration and electrolyte imbalance, particularly hyponatremia.[81]

Obligatory water losses occur as insensible loss through the skin and respiratory tract and in the urine volume necessary to excrete the solute load of metabolism. Insensible water loss depends on the temperature and humidity of the environment. Cutaneous losses are higher in the low-birth-weight infant. Under conditions of thermoneutrality and 50% relative humidity, cutaneous losses are approximately 30 mL/100 cal and respiratory losses 15 mL/100 cal.[86] Insensible water loss may be increased up to 300% in premature infants and is increased between 50 and 115% by phototherapy or a radiant warmer. The latter two modalities lead to additive water losses.[87] Under baseline conditions normal adults have an oral water requirement of approximately 35 mL/kg/day, and normal infants, 130 to 150 mL/kg/day. This explains their greater propensity for dehydration. Besides water, electrolytes and calories have to be provided to maintain a patient in zero balance.[71,87,88]

In the perioperative period, maintenance fluid therapy generally only addresses water and electrolyte balance and caloric requirements only insofar as to prevent ketosis and gluconeogenesis. The latter can be provided by infusion of 5% dextrose solution. Fluid and electrolyte requirements are conveniently based on caloric need and body weight.[71,88]

TABLE 14-6. CONCENTRATION OF ELECTROLYTES IN PLASMA AND INTRACELLULAR FLUID

	Newborn	Plasma Infant	Intracellular All Ages
Cations			
Na^+	145	140	10
K^+	6.3	4	150
Ca^{++}	4	5	—
Mg^{++}	2	2	40
Anions			
Cl^-	103	103	—
HCO_3^-	20	27	10
Protein	15	16	40
Organic			
Phosphates	5.5	16	150
Undetermined	3.0	6.0	—

Usual requirements for water, electrolytes, and glucose are sumarized in Table 14–7. These requirements are met by 5% dextrose with 0.25% NaCl and 20 mEq/L K$^+$ in infants. Newborns and prematures require glucose concentration to be increased to 10% to prevent hypoglycemia. Sodium concentration of maintenance solutions need to be increased to 40 mEq/L in prematures to prevent hyponatremia. The amount of fluids required based on caloric need varies with weight[71] and is outlined in Table 14–8.

During the first day of life maintenance requirements are decreased to approximately 75 mL/kg/24 hours. Glucose-containing solutions should not be given to replace abnormal losses and should not exceed 15 to 20 mL/kg/h to avoid hyperglycemia and hyperosmolarity, resulting in cellular dehydration and increased renal water losses.[87] In premature infants hyperglycemia may cause intracerebral hemorrhage.[89]

Maintenance fluid requirements are increased by fever (12% for each degree above 37°C).[71] They are also increased by hyperventilation and hypermetabolic states (eg, thyrotoxicosis) and decreased during hypothermia without compensatory increase in metabolic rate (12% for each degree below 37°C).[71]

Central Nervous System

The basic tubular and multiventricular form of the brain is established in the first trimester. However, neuronal connection and support structures and myelinization develop only during the last trimester and in infancy. This development coincides with the period of most rapid brain growth. Brain weight doubles in the first 6 months and by 2 years reaches approximately 80% of its final weight.[90] Although cerebral blood flow and oxygen consumption are relatively low at birth (40 mL/100 g/min or 2.3 mL O$_2$/100 g/min, respectively) they rise with the rapid brain growth to as high as 90 to 100 mL/100 g/min and oxygen consumptions of 4.5 to 4 mL/100 g/min in older infants and children.[91] During its rapid growth phase the brain is particularly sensitive to hypoxic ischemic injury leading to microcephaly and major neurologic deficit.[92]

Since myelinization of the nervous system continues throughout childhood[93] inadequate neurologic function results, causing instability of respiration and

TABLE 14–7. MAINTENANCE REQUIREMENTS FOR WATER, ELECTROLYTES, AND GLUCOSE

Water	100 mL	per 100 cal
Sodium	2.5 mEq	" " "
Potassium	2.5 mEq	" " "
Chloride	5.0 mEq	" " "
Glucose	5 g	" " "

TABLE 14–8. MAINTENANCE FLUID REQUIREMENTS[71]

0–10 kg	100 mL/kg/24 h
11–20 kg	50 mL/kg/24 h for each kg over 10
Over 20 kg	20 mL/kg/24 h for each kg over 20

From Winters RW: Maintenance fluid therapy, in Winters RW (ed): The Body Fluids in Pediatrics. *Boston, Little, Brown, 1973, p 117 & 124.*

muscular activity. The increased permeability of the blood–brain barrier and the lack of myelinization lead to accumulation of drugs such as barbiturates and narcotics in the CNS,[94] particularly in the neonate and premature. This may lead to prolonged action and depression in the postanesthesia period. In older infants and children less effect of these drugs is seen when compared to the adult, probably due to distribution in a large extracellular fluid space.[94] Because of the immaturity of the newborn, brain anesthetic requirements are reduced during the neonatal period.[95] Anesthetic requirements rise rapidly during the first few months of life and are highest between 3 months and 3 years. Because of the high fraction of minute ventilation to FRC seen in infants and children, emergence from inhalation anesthetics is rapid.[95] Similar to the central nervous system, development of the neuromuscular junction is immature.[96] This results in increased sensitivity and prolongation of action of nondepolarizing muscle relaxants. After 6 months of age, infants and children require larger and more frequent doses of nondepolarizing relaxants.[97,98] As mentioned earlier, the diaphragm consists of less fatigue-resistant muscle in the newborn and infant. Residual neuromuscular block combined with the prolonged effects of intravenous anesthetic agents can lead to respiratory muscle fatigue, respiratory depression, and apnea in the postanesthetic period, particularly in the young infant.

The developmental changes in the autonomic system have been outlined previously. In summary: parasympathetic innervation is more complete than sympathetic innervation in the young infant, resulting in a propensity to exaggerated vagal reflexes such as bradycardia.

Psychological Differences

The child characteristically has a lack of self-control, and it is usually difficult to persuade children in the preschool age to act against their will. Hospitalization may lead to lasting psychological disturbance.[99] Induction of anesthesia and the waking-up process in the PACU are critical times.[100] While the infant less than 1 year old recovering from surgery is often satisfied with a loving hug to make him or her comfortable, the toddler waking up in strange surroundings requires comforting and compassionate care by the PACU care team to avoid lasting psychological sequelae. Causes of hypoxia of hypoventilation should be excluded before sedating an agitated child. Protection from self-inflicted injury during a period of disorientation is important. Presence of a parent may be the best sedative for the child, although this is less often required than perceived.[101]

SPECIAL CONSIDERATIONS

The recovery process begins in the operating room when surgery and anesthesia are terminated. Unless postoperative mechanical ventilation is planned, transfer to the PACU is carried out after the child is awake and has regained protective airway reflexes and is breathing spontaneously. During transfer to the PACU, as many as 50% of pediatric patients may become mildly hypoxic when breathing room air.[102-105] The reason for this may lay in the altered pulmonary physiology. General anesthesia causes a reduction in functional residual capacity[106,107] and increases closing capacity.[108] These effects are exaggerated in infants and children[109] due to the lack of elastic recoil and increased closing capacity.[12,102] In addition, respiratory depression due to the residual effects of inhalation anesthesia agents, narcotics, or sedatives may contribute to the development of hypoxemia.[110,111] The use of pulse oximetry in transport will alert the anesthesiologist to the development of hypoxemia since clinical signs of hypoxemia (cyanosis and bradycardia) are either absent or occur much later.[112] Patients who are not fully awake should be positioned on their side during transport to prevent airway obstruction from the tongue and reduce the chances of aspiration of secretions. Heart and breath sounds should be monitored continuously, if possible, with a precordial stethoscope. The anesthesiologist should stay with the patient until the PACU team has assessed the patient, a report about the patient's condition has been given, basic monitoring has been established, and care of the patient has been transferred to the PACU team.

The process of awakening begun in the operating room continues in the PACU, where the patient regains full consciousness and cardiopulmonary stability. In the majority of cases, the patients are retained in the PACU for a minimum of 1 hour following any general anesthetic. During this period, close observation includes monitoring of heart rate, respiration, oxygenation, blood pressure, core temperature, skin color and temperature, and delayed awakening.

Heart Rate
All patients should be connected to a cardiac monitor with display of an ECG trace. A three-lead monitor is sufficient, although due to the variability of lead placement, changes like hyperkalemia or bundle branch block should not be made without formal 12-lead EKG tracing. However, most cardiac dysrhythmias and presence of sinus rhythm can be recognized from these tracings.[113] Since atrial contraction is a significant contribution to cardiac output, particularly in the failing heart (up to 30%),[114,115] maintenance of sinus rhythm is important. Bradycardia should be assumed to be a sign of hypoxia unless this has been ruled out.

Respiration
Respiration should be monitored for rate and depth and the presence of upper airway obstruction. Auscultation should be done for presence of adequate breath sounds bilaterally and presence of abnormal sounds like wheezing and rales. Small infants, particularly prematures and former prematures up to 50 weeks postconceptual age, require monitoring with an apnea monitor (described later).

Oxygenation
The ability to assess oxygenation by judging skin color is fraught with errors.[36] In unconscious or deeply sedated patients, pulse oximetry should be used to assess adequacy of oxygenation.[112] In the neonate, oxygenation and ventilation may be assessed noninvasively with the use of transcutaneous O_2 and CO_2 monitoring. Changes in skin blood flow interfere with these measurements, particularly transcutaneous CO_2 ($P_{tc} CO_2$). While transcutaneous measurement of O_2 and CO_2 change in the same direction with ventilatory changes, they increasingly diverge during hypovolemia and low-flow states. Reversal of this divergence may be used to assess adequacy of resuscitation.[116]

Blood Pressure
Proper width of the cuff should equal two-thirds the length of the upper arm. A narrow cuff will give an erroneously high reading.[55,56] In older children who have undergone relatively simple procedures, systolic blood pressure alone may be measured by the palpatory method or by watching the bounce of the needle on the pressure gauge as the cuff is deflated. In infants, blood pressure can be measured accurately by either Doppler or electronic ausculatory or oscillometric methods.[53,55,56]

Core Temperature
In general, measurement of rectal temperature is adequate. Tympanic membrane or bladder temperature may be substituted.

Skin Color and Temperature
Warm pink toes are a sign of adequate cardiac output.[113] Normal toe temperature ranges from 32 to 34°C. A rectal skin temperature gradient of less than

4°C has been shown to correlate with normal cardiac performance.[117] After major surgery, perfusion of the skin varies widely with volume states and cardiac output. If toe temperature approaches environmental temperature the prognosis of the patient is poor.[118] Improvement in skin temperature of the extremities can be used to gauge therapy.[119].

Level of Consciousness; Delayed Awakening

Delayed awakening (discussed in Chapter 2) may have multiple etiologies. The patient may have received large amounts of barbiturates or other sedatives and narcotics, inhalational anesthetics may have been discontinued late, and with the patient still hypoventilating, removal of these agents from the CNS will be delayed. Hypoxia and hypercarbia need to be excluded. Hypovolemia and hypotension with poor cerebral perfusion may result in drowsiness. Parenteral fluid therapy with solutions containing insufficient amounts of sodium may cause hyponatremia with CNS depression. In the small infant hypoglycemia may be present, resulting in obtundedness. Residual neuromuscular block may lead to hypoventilation with hypercarbia. Hypothermia results in delayed awakening. Rare causes of delayed awakening include CNS pathology like intracranial hemorrhage, or the child may have sustained an intraoperative hypoxic–ischemic insult to the brain. Awakening with agitation and confusion is not infrequently seen in young children, particularly after inhalation anesthetics.[120] It is more common after the use of large doses of belladonna alkaloids, particularly scopolamine,[121] and may be reversed under these circumstances with intravenous physostigmine at a dose twice that of the initial belladonna dose.[1] Hypoxia may lead to confusion and should be excluded before treating restlessness. The use of ketamine (particularly large doses) leads to delayed awakening with hallucinations. This is more common in older children.[122] However, one of the most common reasons for agitation is postoperative pain. Relief of postoperative pain can be achieved by titrated doses of narcotics or prevented by judicious use of local and regional blocks (discussed later in the chapter).

Fluid intake should include maintenance and replacement for ongoing third-space losses plus replacement for measured losses as from drains and suction devices.

REPLACEMENT FLUID THERAPY

The purpose of replacement fluids as opposed to maintenance fluids is to correct body fluid deficits caused by external losses (vomiting, nasogastric suc-

tion) or internal sequestration (burns, loss into the bowel wall and lumen in intestinal obstruction, or due to surgery). Surgery results in less sodium and water retention and less catabolic response in the infant when compared to the adult.[123] However, there appears to be increased renal potassium loss. Translocation of isotonic fluid into a nonfunctional interstitial compartment is related to the degree of surgical trauma.[124] It is highest with intraabdominal procedures.[125] Unreplaced translocation—third-space losses—result in clinical signs of dehydration.

Third-space fluid is derived initially from the plasma volume, which in turn is replenished from the interstitial fluid. Thus this fluid loss is nearly isotonic and suitable replacement fluids include lactated Ringer's solution, normal saline, and Normosol. Large amounts of normal saline may cause hyperchloremic acidosis due to the inappropriate high chloride content (150 mEq/L versus 103 mEq/L in serum).

The amount of third-space loss and, therefore, the amount of replacement required depends upon the severity of trauma. For example,

- Minimal surgical trauma (hernia repair) = 1 to 2 mL/kg/h.
- Moderate surgical trauma (pyloromyotomy) = 2 to 4 mL/kg/h.
- Major surgical trauma (bowel resection) = 4 to 6 mL/kg/h.

Much larger amounts may be required to achieve the endpoint of adequate replacement therapy—a stable blood pressure and adequate urine output.[87] A minimal urine output of 0.5 to 1 mL/kg/h should be maintained under any circumstances.[79,123]

In prematures and small infants requiring large amounts of replacement fluids, one fourth to one third should be replaced with 5% albumin to effect a more equal distribution between extra- and intracellular fluid and plasma volume.[125,126] Ongoing abnormal losses due to drains should be measured and replaced with appropriate solutions.[123,127] Clinical signs of dehydration are illustrated in Table 14–9. Hypotonic dehydration generally results in more severe signs of dehydration; hypertonic dehydration in less.[128] Table 14–10 lists composition of replacement fluid for specific gastrointestinal losses.[83]

BLOOD REPLACEMENT

The allowable whole blood loss in pediatric surgical patients is calculated to attain a final postoperative hematocrit of not less than 30% for infants and children and 40% for prematures and newborns.[129]

TABLE 14–9. CLINICAL SIGNS OF DEHYDRATION

	Mild	Moderate	Severe
Body weight	−5%	−10%	−15%
Skin turgor			
Mucous membranes	Dry	Very dry	Parched
Skin color	Pale	Grey	Mottled
Urine	Mild oliguria	Oliguria	Severe oliguria and acotemia
Blood pressure	Normal	±normal	Reduced
Pulse	±	↑	↑↑

From Dell RB: Pathophysiology of dehydration, in Winters RW (ed): The Body Fluids in Pediatrics. Boston, Little, Brown, 1973, p 142.

EBV = wt in kg × y mL/kg, where y = 90 for newborn, 80 up to 1 year, 70 up to 12 years, 65 for adolescents.

$$ERCM = EBV \times \frac{Hct}{100} \quad (A)$$

$$ECRM_{30} = EBV \times \frac{30}{100} \quad (B)$$

$$ARCL = A - B$$

$$AWBL = (A - B) \times 3$$

where:

EBV = estimated blood volume
ERCM = estimated red cell mass (depends on patient's preoperative hematocrit)
$ERCM_{30}$ = estimated red cell mass at a hematocrit of 30%
ARCL = Allowable red cell loss
AWBL = Allowable whole blood loss

The assumption made is that blood loss is occurring at a hematocrit of 30%. For practical purposes the following management protocol may be used:

Amount of Blood Loss	Therapy
Blood loss is less than one third of AWBL	Ringer's lactated solution
Blood loss is more than one third but less than total AWBL	Colloid, preferably 5% albumin
Blood loss is equal to or more than AWBL	Blood

When replacing blood loss with isotonic electrolyte solution, each mL of blood has to be replaced with 3 mL of crystalloid since the latter is also redistributed to the interstitial fluid volume.[127] Postoperative anemia can be treated with a transfusion of packed red cells, which have an average hematocrit of 75. 1 mL/kg of packed cells increases the hematocrit by 1 to 1.5%.[127,130]

Persistent surgical bleeding in the postanesthetic period may indicate presence of a coagulopathy, particularly after massive intraoperative blood transfusion. In newborns, and particularly prematures, sepsis may cause depression in platelet count.[129] Clinical bleeding may be apparent with counts below 50,000. Production of various coagulation factors is reduced in the neonate and infant. Factors II, X, VII, IX, and XII are affected and adult levels are sometimes not reached until 12 months of age. For this reason, prothrombin (PT) and partial thromboplastin (PTT) times vary widely in this age group. PT may range from 13 to 20 sec and PTT from 45 to 70 sec.[129] Treatment with specific blood components or factors may be indicated.[130,131] Transfusion of 0.3 units of platelets/kg will usually result in a platelet count above 65,000/mm[3].[132]

Replacement of coagulation factors in the form of fresh frozen plasma may be required in patients after the loss of one blood volume, particularly if blood replacement is carried out with packed or frozen red cells. Replacement is calculated as 20 to 30% of blood volume lost as volume of fresh frozen plasma (FFP).[133] Our practice is to tranfuse equal volumes of packed red cells and fresh frozen plasma after one blood volume loss. Since fresh frozen plasma has the highest citrate content of any blood product, rapid

TABLE 14–10. REPLACEMENT SOLUTIONS FOR GASTROINTESTINAL LOSSES

	Na+ (mEq/L)	K+ (mEq/L)	Cl+ (mEq/L)	H3 (mEq/L)	Destrose (g)
To replace gastric drainage	140	15	155	0	0
To replace small intestine losses	140	15	115	40	0
To replace diarrheal losses	40	40	40	40	50.0

From Winters RW: Maintenance fluid therapy, in Winters RW (ed): The Body Fluids in Pediatrics, Boston, Little, Brown, 1973, p 129.

administration of this component may result in a significant fall of ionized calcium, particularly in the small infant or newborn with reduced calcium stores. If the rate of administration of FFP exceeds 1 mL/kg/min, clinical signs of hypocalcemia may occur, particularly cardiovascular depression.[133] Therapy with intravenous calcium during rapid infusion of FFP is required to avoid this complication. Calcium chloride 2.5 mg/kg or calcium gluconate 7.5 mg/kg are equally efficacious.[134]

INVASIVE MONITORING

In critically ill children and after major surgery, invasive monitoring of cardiovascular and respiratory function is indicated. Percutaneous cannulation of the radial, dorsalis pedis, or posterior tibialis arteries is possible even in small premature infants and carries a minimal risk of complications.[135,136] Use of transillumination or Doppler location of the vessel may help in location of the vessel. In newborns, the umbilical artery may be utilized for arterial access, but in the presence of intermittent right-to-left shunting in the perinatal period, oxygen tensions in the distal aorta, which are postductal, may not adequately reflect *retinal* oxygenation. Complications, including ischemia of the lower extremities and renal or mesenteric artery occlusion, occur in 2 to 5% of patients.[137]

The femoral and axillary artery may be used if other vessels cannot be cannulated.[138,139] Although easy to cannulate the temporal artery should be avoided since it has been associated with cerebral infarction due to retrograde flushing.[140] Brachial artery cannulation may result in increased incidence of ischemic complications since this vessel has no collateral circulation.[141] An intraarterial cannula allows direct continuous blood pressure measurement and intermittent sampling for blood gas analysis and blood chemistry. Continuous monitoring of blood gases will eventually be possible in clinical practice with the use of an intraarterial fluorescent optode system.[142] Normal values for arterial blood gases in pediatrics are listed in Table 14–2.

Central venous access may be required to judge adequacy of preload, for establishment of a major access for fluid administration, and as a means of infusion for *sclerosing* solution (eg, vasopressors, hyperalimentation, cetain antibiotics, and K⁺ supplements). Acid–base status and oxygen extraction in situations with reduced cardiac output may be judged by the difference in arterial and central venous blood gas values and oxygen content.[143] The most popular route in pediatric patients is the right internal jugular vein using the ''Seldinger'' technique.[144,145] Cannulation of the external jugular vein results in failure to reach in-

trathoracic location in at least 25% of cases.[146] Cannulation of the subclavian vein is more difficult than cannulation of the internal jugular vein in infants and can cause life-threatening complications like pneumo- and/or hemothorax.[147] Cannulation of the femoral vein requires the use of a long catheter to pass into the thorax for adequate pressure measurement. It is more difficult to prevent dislodgement of these cannulae and to keep the site sterile.[148] Use of the umbilical vein in newborns has been associated with hemorrhagic necrosis of the liver when hyperosmolar solutions (eg, 25 or 50% dextrose, full-strength $NaHCO_3$, or THAM) have been infused through this line. Correct positioning above the hepatic vein is of utmost importance and should be verified radiographically and by displaying of the normal central venous wave form.[148,149] Pulmonary artery catheters are not commonly used in pediatric patients since their size makes them difficult to place and isolated left heart failure is uncommon in the pediatric age group. Their use may be associated with a higher risk of pulmonary embolization, infarction, dysrhythmias, and valvular damage because of their relatively large diameter compared to the infant's or child's vascular structures.[150] Besides measurement of right- and left-sided filling pressures they allow measurement of thermodilution cardiac output and treatment of pulmonary hypertension by direct infusion of vasodilators into the pulmonary circulation.[151]

RESPIRATORY COMPLICATIONS

Respiratory complications cause most of the postanesthetic problems seen within the first hour following the end of anesthesia. In one study[152] published in 1975, 26% of all anesthesia-related cardiac arrests occurred in the PACU, with a mortality rate of 38%. Overall anesthesia-related mortality was 1 in 10,000 anesthetics. In a later study,[153] anesthesia-related problems occurred in 22 to 33% of all patients in the PACU. The mortality rate for this study was very low, 1:40,000, but the only mortality observed in 40,240 anesthetics occurred in the postanesthesia period due to unrecognized respiratory depression.

In children, the major respiratory complications encountered in the postanesthetic period include airway obstruction; postextubation croup; respiratory depression; aspiration; apnea; and acute respiratory failure.

Airway Obstruction
In the early postoperative period, the most frequent and serious complication is airway obstruction.[154] Soft tissue obstruction of the upper airway occurs during general anesthesia, in deep sleep stages, in patients

with apnea–hypersomnia, and in sleeping infants whose necks are slightly flexed.[155] Due to relaxation of the pharyngeal musculature the tongue is displaced posteriorly and the negative pressure of inspiration results in airway collapse.[156] Extension of the neck decreases the tendency to airway closure; however, positive pressure is required to reopen the collapsed airway.[155] Repeated upper airway collapse may be treated with low-level continuous positive airway pressure (CPAP).[155] Insertion of an oropharyngeal airway may alleviate the problem until the patient is fully awake.

Obstructive sleep apnea may be present in as many as 10% of patients after cleft palate surgery immediately postoperatively.[157] The incidence of airway obstruction is particularly high in patients with Treacher Collins syndrome, hemifacial microsomia, and Stickler syndrome.[157]

Other common causes for postanesthetic upper airway obstruction in the pediatric age group include enlarged tonsils and adenoids, laryngeal spasm, laryngeal edema, and swelling due to surgery of the airway and surrounding tissues.

The hallmarks of airway obstruction are retractions (suprasternal, subcostal, intercostal), nasal flaring, inspiratory stridor or crowing, and decreased or absent air entry.[158]

As already mentioned, obstruction of the upper airway may follow surgery for cleft palate repair. The pharyngeal flap may cause complete nasal airway obstruction, resulting in airway obstruction when the mouth closes[159] or in the development of obstructive sleep apnea.[160] Swelling of the tongue as a result of excessive pressure from the mouth gag may result in increasing upper airway obstruction as the tongue progressively increases in size over one to two hours following the end of the procedure.[161,162] If at the conclusion of the surgical procedure some lingual edema is noticed, the endotracheal tube should not be removed until sufficient time has elapsed for further swelling of the tongue to occur.[162] Airway obstruction may follow tongue resection, resection of a cystic hygroma, and tonsillectomy and adenoidectomy.[163,164] Clot formation due to ongoing bleeding from the surgical site may result in complete airway obstruction. Positioning of the patient in a lateral decubitus or prone position with the head turned to the side assists in maintenance of upper airway patency and facilitates drainage of blood and secretions from the mouth.[165] A rare cause of upper airway obstruction is uvular edema following even atraumatic endotracheal intubation, where the enlarged uvula occludes the glottic opening when the patient assumes an upright position.[166]

Airway obstruction should be relieved promptly. With complete cessation of gas exchange, arterial carbon dioxide tension rises 6 mm Hg during the first minute and then 3 to 4 mm Hg per minute while alveolar P_{O_2} and arterial P_{O_2} decline.[167,168] These figures apply to adult patients. From a recent study[169] it appears that the rise in arterial P_{CO_2} and fall in arterial P_{O_2} are much more rapid in children. The P_{CO_2} increased between 10 and 12 mm Hg in the first minute, between 7 and 10 mm Hg in the second minute, and between 3 and 6 mm Hg during the third minute. Oxygenation rapidly declined from an average of 480 mm Hg to as low as 80 mm Hg after 3 minutes. Airway obstruction due to pharyngeal obstruction by the tongue can be effectively overcome by hyperextension of the head with anterior displacement of the mandible.[170] If obstruction is still not relieved, a nasal or oral airway can be inserted. The nasal airway is preferred because it is better tolerated. The oral airway may stimulate gagging, vomiting, and laryngospasm. One-hundred percent oxygen should be administered by face mask until the obstruction is relieved.

Laryngeal spasm is defined as laryngeal obstruction due to partial or complete spasm of the intrinsic or extrinsic muscles of the larynx.[171] Two mechanisms are in effect, reflex closure of the glottis and reflex closure of the larynx. Reflex closure of the glottis is due to a shutter-like adduction of the vocal cords— that is, it involves the intrinsic laryngeal muscles. The resulting airway obstruction is incomplete, intermittent, and occurs during inspiration or expiration. It usually occurs in response to somatic sensory stimulation, such as suctioning, or the presence of an airway during light planes of anesthesia and during recovery. Treatment includes discontinuation of the stimulus, application of positive pressure with bag and mask, and administration of 100% oxygen.

Reflex closure of the larynx is due to a ball valve mechanism involving the extrinsic muscles, particularly the thyrohyoid muscle,[171] and occurs in response to visceral sensory stimulation and as an exaggerated response to stimulation of the superior laryngeal nerve.[172] It results in complete laryngeal obstruction. To treat the laryngeal spasm, the stimulus should be stopped or any irritant removed from the larynx, such as secretions, blood, or a long airway. One hundred percent oxygen should be administered. This spasm cannot be broken by positive pressure but may be terminated by severe hypoxia, hypercarbia, or deep anesthesia.[173] The incidence of laryngospasm is higher below the age of 9 years and even higher between 1 to 3 months of age.[174] It is commonest following extubation, in the presence of a nasogastric tube, and after oral endoscopies. The highest incidence was found in children with respiratory tract infections—95.8/1000.[174] Forcing the chin forward by strong pressure applied behind the angles of the jaw is often an effective maneuver to relieve the problem.[171] Attempts to force air into the pharynx under positive pressure will worsen the obstruction when the larynx is completely closed, since it leads to distension of the pyriform fossa, pressing the aryepiglottic folds more firmly against each other.[171] If forward movement in the temperomandibular joint does not relieve the airway obstruction, a small dose of succinylcholine 0.5 to 1 mg/kg together with atropine should be administered.[173] Respiration must then be supported by positive pressure ventilation (eg, Ambu bag) until full muscle function has recovered.

In the absence of intravenous access, succinylcholine 4 mg/kg can be given intramuscularly to relieve the laryngospasm.[173] This has, however, been associated with the development of acute pulmonary edema.[175,176] If hypoxia and bradycardia are developing, intubation without relaxation should be performed to prevent further deterioration. Direct spraying of the cords with lidocaine 1 mg/kg will facilitate intubation by relaxing the larynx.[177] If the airway cannot be established, cricothyrotomy may be lifesaving.[173] Laryngospasm following extubation may be prevented by injection of lidocaine 2 mg/kg intravenously one minute before extubation,[178] and delaying extubation until the child is completely awake and resumes a normal breathing pattern after a cough.[176] Laryngospasm should be considered a serious complication, necessitating aggressive therapy. In a study by Olsson and Hallen,[174] 5 out of every 1000 patients who developed laryngospasm sustained a cardiac arrest.

Relief of acute upper airway obstruction of various etiologies may result in development of negative pressure pulmonary edema.[176-181] The pathophysiologic basis for the development of this noncardiac form of pulmonary edema includes creation of large negative intrathoracic pressure gradients across the alveolar–capillary membrane, hypoxic pulmonary vasoconstriction, and increased transmural pressure in the heart and great vessels with increased left-ventricular afterload.[176,181] Therapy includes positive pressure ventilation with positive end expiratory pressure and forced diuresis with furosemide, if necessary.[176-181]

Postextubation Croup
Laryngeal or better subglottic edema leads to the clinical picture of postintubation croup.[182] Infants are more prone to postintubation complications for the following reasons (in order of decreasing importance):

1. Small size of the larynx. In the adult, 1 mm of edema produces only slight hoarseness. In the infant the same amount of edema reduces the lumen by 75% and produces serious airway obstruction (see Fig. 14–1).[3]
2. Loose areolar tissue present in the submucosa of the subglottic area, where edema fluid easily accumulates.
3. Cricoid cartilage forming a complete ring.

The incidence of postextubation croup varies between 1 to 4% of intubated patients. It is most common in children 1 to 3 years of age.[182] Contributory factors include tight-fitting endotracheal tube; trauma during intubation; long duration of intubation (more than 48 hours); movement of the head and, therefore, of the endotracheal tube during positive pressure ventilation; surgery of the head, neck, or bronchoscopy; and hypotension.[182]

The incidence of postextubation croup is markedly diminished by use of an endotracheal tube that allows an initial audible leak at 25 to 35 cm H_2O.[183,184]

Symptoms of postextubation croup usually occur within 30 to 60 minutes following extubation.[185] The diagnosis is made on the basis of stridor, thoracic retraction, hoarseness, croup-like cough, and varying degrees of respiratory obstruction.[186] Treatment includes positioning the patient upright; administering cool, humidifed oxygen; and giving inhaled racemic epinephrine. The 2.25% solution is diluted with sterile water to a total volume of 2 mL in the following proportion: 1:8 for less than 5 kg; 1:6 for 5 to 10 kg; 1:4 for 10 to 15 kg; and 1:3 for 10 to 20 kg.[187] It may be delivered by face mask with nebulization or IPPB.[187-189]

If symptoms cannot be controlled with inhalation every 30 minutes, if hypoventilation with rising arterial carbon dioxide tension occurs, or if the patient appears obtunded, reintubation is necessary to stabilize the airway.[185,189] Reintubation should be performed with an endotracheal tube at least one size smaller than the original endotracheal tube, and an auscultatory air leak should be detectable over the larynx at 25 to 30 mm water airway pressure to avoid long-term sequelae.[183,184] The use of steroids for the treatment of postextubation croup remains controversial.[190] The drug and dosage most commonly recommended is dexamethasone 0.5 to 1.0 mg/kg.[185,189] Reintubation in croup is not associated with significant subglottic stenosis.[191]

Respiratory Depression
Respiratory depression in the PACU may occur for a variety of reasons. Ventilatory reflexes are depressed by anesthetics in a dose-dependent fashion. While the response to CO_2 is significantly depressed above 1 MAC for halothane, enflurane, and isoflurane, with flattening of the CO_2 response curve,[192] the response to hypoxemia is already severely depressed at

subanesthetic concentrations.[111] Patients who rely on their chemoreceptor drive for ventilatory control (eg, Pickwickian syndrome) may develop severe hypoventilation following anesthesia with potent inhalational anesthetics. Narcotics and ketamine produce depression of respiration with right shift of the CO_2 response curve.[193] Rate is primarily affected. Bolus doses of ketamine flatten the CO_2 response curve.[194] The newer synthetic opiates like fentanyl can cause chest wall rigidity and cause more marked ventilatory depression in the newborn and young infant compared to the older child.[195-197] Morphine sulfate causes more profound respiratory depression in newborns in equianalgesic doses when compared to meperidine, presumably due to higher blood–brain permeability.[198] Barbiturates depress rate and depth of respiration, which may be mitigated by noxious stimuli.

After arrival in the PACU, following large doses of barbiturates, severe respiratory depression may occur, since the patient is now undisturbed.[199] Sedatives of the benzodiazepine group cause only mild respiratory depression due to a reduction in tidal volume.[199] However, in combination with narcotics, they may lead to severe depression of respiration and apnea.[200]

Due to the high minute ventilation to functional residual capacity ratio of infants and children, recovery from inhalational anesthetics is rapid. Although on a theoretical basis, recovery from the less soluble agents isoflurane and enflurane should be more rapid, clinically no difference is seen[201] and airway irritability and stormy emergence is more common, particularly with enflurane.[202]

Residual neuromuscular block, due to inadequate reversal, may lead to muscle fatigue (particularly of the diaphragm) and respiratory failure. This is of particular importance during the first months of life when the neuromuscular function is still immature and the diaphragm has a high proportion of type-II (nonfatigue-resistant) muscle fibers (see the earlier section on ventilatory physiology p. 187).

Reversal of neuromuscular blockade cannot be ascertained by voluntary clinical signs like head lift and grip strength in the infant. However, reflex leg lift appears to be an adequate substitute since it is associated with a maximal negative inspiratory force of at least -32 cm H_2O.[203] This and a crying vital capacity of greater than 15 mL/kg have been shown to demonstrate adequate ventilatory reserve.[204] Use of a nerve stimulator to measure the response to supramaximal stimulation of, usually, the ulnar nerve, and using the train-of-four ratio of the force of contraction as assessment of degree of neuromuscular blockade,[205] gives an objective measurement of reversal of neuromuscular block. A train-of-four ratio higher than 0.8 indicates adequate reversal.[206]

Preexisting pulmonary disease and decrease ventilatory function as a result of surgery (eg, cardiothoracic) may result in respiratory failure.[207]

Treatment of respiratory depression involves the following:

1. Stir-up regimen by PACU personnel stimulates spontaneous respiration and is often sufficient. This involves verbal and tactile stimulation.
2. Naloxone (Narcan) may be used to reverse narcotic-induced respiratory depression. It is a pure narcotic antagonist, and acts by competitive inhibition. Its duration of action is short-lived (30 to 60 minutes), and hence respiratory depression may recur. Thus, patients must be observed closely, or an intravenous dose of naloxone must be followed by an intramuscular dose to provide a longer-lasting effect.[208]
3. Residual muscle relaxant may be reversed with an anticholinesterase and anticholinergic combination.
4. Controlled ventilation may be indicated to maintain a normal Pa_{CO_2} and to enhance the excretion of inhalational anesthetics by increasing alveolar ventilation.

Pulmonary Aspiration

Factors that make the infant more vulnerable than adults to regurgitation and aspiration of gastric contents include the following:[209]

1. Higher resting intragastric pressure due to the relatively small size of the stomach, excessive air swallowing during crying, encroachment of other abdominal organs, and strenuous diaphragmatic breathing.
2. Short esophagus.
3. Relaxation of the gastroesophageal junction. Regurgitation following feeding has been observed in normal infants up to 12 months of age. Gastroesophageal reflux has been well documented as a cause of apnea, wheezing, and pneumonia in small infants[210-211] and laryngeal competence is decreased for 6 to 8 hours following extubation.[212]
4. Cough reflex that may not be well developed.
5. Discordance of breathing and swallowing mechanisms, which may occur in premature and dyspneic infants.[209]
6. Atropine-relaxed tone of the esophageal–gastric junction.[213]

Aspiration continues to present a significant problem in pediatric anesthesia. Fifty percent of aspirations occur in the postanesthetic period.[153,214] Aspiration constituted 25% of all postanesthetic problems seen in the most recent series.[151] However, while aspiration caused 25% of anesthesia-related mortality in the 1960s,[214] perianesthetic mortality related to pulmonary aspiration has not been noted in recent reviews.[152,153]

Apnea and the Former Premature

Apnea in the newborn and premature is defined as a respiratory pause of 20 seconds or longer, or a briefer episode of apnea associated with bradycardia, cyanosis, or pallor.[215,216] Apnea of 5 to 10 seconds alternating with breathing is defined as periodic breathing.[215] Both are commonly seen in premature infants (25 to 60%).[217,218] Etiology includes immaturity of respiratory control, episodic airway obstruction, alteration in sleep state, and diaphragmatic fatigue.[28,29,215] The incidence of apnea episodes is increased with hypoxemia, sepsis, intracranial hemorrhage, patent ductus arteriosus, hyper- and hypothermia, hypoglycemia, and hypocalcemia.[215] Treatment of idiopathic apnea consists of therapy with theophylline. Theophylline improves apnea by increasing alveolar ventilation through central stimulation.[219] Low level CPAP also reduces the frequency of apneic episodes.[220] Apnea is rarely seen in normal term infants.[221] Apnea with bradycardia causes reduction in cerebral blood flow and may result in hypoxic–ischemic injury to the developing central nervous system.[222]

Since 1982,[223] it has been recognized that following minor operations (most commonly inguinal herniorrhaphy), infants who were born prematurely developed apnea episodes following an uneventful general anesthetic. Apnea occurred whether or not a previous history of apnea was present,[224,225] but occurred more frequently and at higher postconceptual age if a history of apnea or bronchopulmonary dysplasia was present.[224-228] The majority of infants developing apnea or periodic breathing were less than 44 weeks postconceptual age and less than 3000 g body weight.[223-228] However, in Kurth's series,[225] prolonged apnea was observed as late as 60 weeks postconceptual age. Apneic episodes in all series occurred within 12 hours of surgery and were common if neuromuscular blocking agents had been used intraoperatively.[224,228] Intraoperative therapy with caffeine 8 to 10 mg/kg prevented episodes of prolonged apnea in infants less than 44 weeks postconceptual age and with a history of apnea.[229,230] No general consensus has been reached about the postconceptual age up to which in-hospital monitoring is required in former premature infants following minor surgery.[231-233] Below 44 weeks postconceptual age, incidence of postoperative apnea is highest. Since apnea has been observed even in a term infant, below this age[234] monitoring for apnea following anesthesia for several hours is certainly indicated, and these patients may not be candidates for outpatient surgery. Infants with a history of apnea who are less than 48 weeks postconceptual age are also at significant risk and require monitoring for at least 12 hours.[224,225,228] Our policy at present is to admit all former prematures less than 48 weeks postconceptual age and to monitor them with an apnea monitor overnight; and to admit all term infants less than 1 month of age.

Acute Respiratory Failure

Acute respiratory failure is defined as an impairment of alveolar ventilation and pulmonary gas exchange resulting in failure to deliver sufficient oxygen to meet the demands of the body and/or inability to eliminate carbon dioxide adequately.[232] The impairment in gas exchange poses an immediate threat to life.[233]

Causes for acute respiratory failure vary with the age of the patient. Outside the newborn period, respiratory failure is most commonly due to bronchopneumonia, upper airway obstruction, congenital heart disease, and asthma.[232,233] Postoperatively, respiratory failure can occur due to preexisting lung disease (eg, asthma, cystic fibrosis, upper respiratory tract infection),[234-236], as a complication of surgery (particularly thoracic or cardiac; or as a result of anesthetic overdose (respiratory depression from anesthetic agents, persistent neuromuscular blockade).

Clinical criteria for the diagnosis of respiratory failure in infants and children include:[232,233,236,237]

- Severe inspiratory retractions and use of accessory muscles of respiration; flaring of alae nasi.
- Irregular respirations, tachybradypnea, prolonged apnea.
- Diminished or absent breath sounds.
- Cyanosis in 60% oxygen.[237]
- Decreased level of consciousness.
- Poor skeletal muscle tone.
- Signs of cardiovascular collapse: absent or diminished pulse and blood pressure, excessive tachycardia, pulsus paradoxus > 12 mm Hg.

Physiologic criteria include the following:[232,233,237,238]

- Hypercarbia with $PaCO_2 \geq 65$ mm Hg.
- Hypoxemia with $PaO_2 \leq 70$ mm Hg in FIO_2 0.6.
- For newborn, hypoxemia with $PaO_2 \leq 55$ mm Hg in FIO_2 0.6.

Three clinical and any one physiologic criteria confirm diagnosis of acute respiratory failure.[233]

Changes in pulmonary mechanics requiring mechanical ventilation include[233] vital capacity under 15 mL/kg; forced expiratory volume at 1 second (FEV_1) under 10 mL/kg; or negative inspiratory force under 20 cm H_2O.

Treatment aims at improvement of pulmonary

gas exchange. Since loss of lung volume occurs with anesthesia resulting in increased shunting, a trial of constant positive airway pressure (CPAP) may be used to improve oxygenation.[239,240] CPAP may be applied by nasal prongs in the newborn and via face mask in the infant and child. Face mask CPAP is generally poorly tolerated and leads to gastric distention.[237] CPAP is therefore best applied via endotracheal airway. CPAP results in increase in functional residual capacity and alveolar and airway dimensions.[240] The increased lung volume increases compliance and reduces the work of breathing.[237] The optimal level of CPAP is defined as that level at which maximal oxygen transport is achieved (oxygen content × cardiac output).[241] Excessive levels of CPAP increase dead-space ventilation, which may lead to hypercarbia, reduction in venous return and cardiac output, and barotrauma of the lung.[242]

If oxygenation cannot be improved or if hypoventilation and hypercarbia are present, mechanical ventilation via an artificial airway must be instituted. Mechnical ventilators in use in pediatric intensive care can be classified into four categories: volume-preset, pressure-preset, time-flow-preset, and negative-pressure ventilators.[243] While negative-pressure ventilators provide the most physiological approach to artificial ventilation, they severely restrict access to the patient. Infants less than 10 kg are usually easily ventilated with time-flow or pressure-preset ventilators. These ventilators readily compensate for a variable leak around the endotracheal tube and allow for rapid ventilatory rates and continuous-flow intermittent mandatory ventilation. With rapid changes in pulmonary compliance, pressure-preset ventilators may lead to over- or underventilation of the lung.[237] Volume-preset ventilators will deliver the set tidal volume at whatever pressure is required, and are therefore less influenced by changes in compliance. With large internal compliance volume, measurement of delivered volume becomes difficult for small tidal volumes. All modern ventilators have the capability to provide positive end-expiratory pressure (PEEP). Methods of achieving PEEP that allow unimpeded exhalation to the desired pressure are preferable, since they increase mean intrathoracic pressure less and do not lead to overinflation as easily as breathing through an expiratory resistance. The latter method has theoretical advantages in small airway disease, since it tends to stabilize the airways better and, by slowing respiration, improves compliance, which is frequency-dependent under these circumstances.[244]

All ventilators require humidification of respiratory gases with a heated humidifier, preferably with heated tubing, to minimize water condensation within the system.[245] Optimal humidification provides 33 g H_2O/L of gas which corresponds to 75%

relative humidity at body temperature.[246] All ventilators need to be equipped with alarms for excessive airway pressure (obstruction) and for sudden loss of airway pressure (disconnect). When heated humidifiers are used, temperature of the inspired air should be measured close to the airway to detect accidental overheating, which may result in tracheal damage.[247]

Intermittent mandatory ventilation (IMV) allows the patient to breathe spontaneously between ventilator cycles from a fresh gas source with low resistance.[248,249] PEEP is maintained throughout. Continuous-flow systems for provision of IMV are generally better tolerated since demand valves impose additional work to overcome valve resistance.[237]

Ventilatory patterns vary from patient to patient and depend on inspiratory and expiratory flow rates, tidal volume, ratio of inspiration to expiration (I:E ratio), and respiratory rate. With interstitial or alveolar disorders, commonly seen in the postanesthetic period, ventilation with large tidal volumes at relatively low ventilatory frequencies, with longer inspiratory times, low inspiratory flow, and end-expiratory plateau, maximizes the distribution of gases with minimal peak airway pressure.[250,251] Patients with obstructive airway disease (asthma, bronchiolitis) are better ventilated with higher inspiratory flow rates, shorter inspiratory times, and longer expiratory pauses to allow for exhalation from obstructed portions of the lung, thus minimizing the problem of air trapping and alveolar rupture.[237]

Assisted ventilation is started with tidal volumes of 10 to 15 mL/kg and respiratory rates of 25 to 30 for the infant and 16 to 20 for the child. With pressure- and time-flow-preset ventilators, adequacy of chest expansion and breath sounds will guide initial setup and analysis of arterial blood gases will determine final adjustment for each mode of ventilation. PEEP is added in increments of 2 to 3 mm H_2O to improve oxygenation. Since the resistance of the upper airway is bypassed by endotracheal intubation, a physiological PEEP of 2 to 3 mm H_2O should be provided for all intubated children to minimize loss of FRC.[252] If PEEP of higher than 10 cm H_2O is required to achieve adequate oxygenation, measurement of cardiac filling pressures should be instituted (central venous or pulmonary arterial pressure) to judge adequacy of cardiovascular performance. Ventilation with high mean intrathoracic pressures usually requires augmentation of cardiac filling.[253]

Provision of mechanical ventilation by positive pressure requires an artificial airway. Endotracheal intubation is presently preferred for management of ventilatory failure in infants and children even for prolonged periods of time, and is associated with minimal morbidity.[254] Tracheostomy is reserved for patients with upper airway anomalies or chronic lung disease requiring prolonged ventilatory assistance and for the provision of home ventilator care.[255,256]

ENDOTRACHEAL INTUBATION IN CHILDREN

Size

The optimal tube size is one that passes easily through the glottic and subglottic regions and produces a small leak of gas around the tube at 25 to 30 cm of water peak inspiratory pressure.[254] One formula for calculation of endotracheal tube size that we use is:

$$\text{diameter (mm)} = \frac{\text{age (years)}}{4} + 4$$

This formula is for uncuffed endotracheal tubes and is applicable for children over 2 years of age. Table 14–11 lists endotracheal tube sites for patients younger than 2 years. A few patients will require an endotracheal tube that is smaller or larger.

Cuffed endotracheal tubes should not be used in children less than 7 to 8 years of age, since they reduce the size of the lumen, thereby increasing airway resistance and putting pressure on the delicate tracheal mucosa, thus increasing the incidence of subglottic damage. The correct size of a cuffed endotracheal tube is 0.5 mm internal diameter less than that calculated by the above formula.

The composition of endotracheal tubes is important. Toxic substances form on gamma-ray-sterilized polyvinyl chloride (PVC) tubes after resterilization with ethylene oxide. The clear, polyvinyl, disposable tubes that have been tissue-implant-tested (Z 79) are the most satisfactory ones for general use. Because they are easier to stabilize, nasotracheal tubes are preferred for long-term ventilatory management. Endotracheal tubes move with movement of the neck. Flexion moves the tip caudal, extension cephalad.[257,258] A chest x-ray should be obtained after each endotracheal intubation to ascertain tube position and to be correlated with neck position.[258]

Complications of prolonged nasotracheal intubation include colonization with gram-negative organisms,[259] cosmetic nasal deformity,[260] chronic ear infection,[260] silent aspiration,[261] obstruction due to blockage or kinking, and accidental dislodgment. Partial obstruction results in significant increase in airway resistance.[262] Prevention of partial or complete obstruction requires adequate humidification of the inspired air and frequent suctioning, particulary in the presence of increased secretions. Since effective coughing is not possible with an artificial airway in place, chest physiotherapy should be utilized to propel mucous secretions centrally where they can be removed by suctioning. Suctioning should be performed with sterile technique using sterile gloves and catheters after preoxygenation with 100% oxygen. The suction catheter should not completely occlude the lumen, since excessive subatmospheric pressure may result in pulmonary collapse. Endotracheal suctioning always results in loss of FRC and may cause hypoxemia.[259] Suctioning should be limited to 10 seconds and be followed by manual hyperinflation with prolonged inspiratory time to reconstitute FRC.[259] Suction should only be applied on removal of the catheter. Sidehole catheters may result in suction damage to the walls of the trachea.[263] Trauma from suction catheters may result in ulceration and stenosis of the distal trachea and mainstem bronchi.[260]

Weaning from ventilatory support can be attempted in the presence of a stable cardiovascular system and with the child awake and alert. The infant and child should be able to generate at least −20 mm H_2O negative inspiratory pressure and a vital capacity of 10 mL/kg. Blood gases should be stable with an FIO_2 of less than 0.5 and arterial PO_2 of more than 60 mm Hg. $PaCO_2$ should be less than 60 mm Hg and PEEP less than 10 cm H_2O.[237,252] Peak inspiratory pressure is decreased as compliance improves and IMV rate is slowly decreased until the patient is weaned to a CPAP of 2 to 3 mm H_2O. After a period of spontaneous ventilation on a CPAP of 2 to 3 cm H_2O without deterioration of blood gases or signs of respiratory fatigue or stress, extubation is carried out.[264]

In the presence of unilateral lung disease the good lung should be positioned *uppermost* to optimize gas exchange.[265]

NAUSEA AND VOMITING

Vomiting is a frequent and unpleasant sequel of general anesthetics in children. It is more common after certain procedures, particularly strabismus repair,[266-269] where it occurs in 41 to 85% of patients. Vomiting is more common in the presence of surgical pain. Severe vomiting may preclude patient dis-

TABLE 14–11. ENDOTRACHEAL TUBE SIZES BELOW 2 YEARS OF AGE

Age	Size (ID) (mm)	Length (cm)
Premature		
<1000 g	2.5	8–10
1000 g	3.0	10
2500 g		
Newborn to 6 months	3.0–3.5	10–11
6 months to 1 year	3.5–4.0	12
1–2 years	4.5	13

charge after a planned outpatient surgery; result in dehydration; or, in the early stages of recovery, may lead to aspiration and development of aspiration pneumonitis. Unconscious patients should be positioned on their sides to prevent aspiration if vomiting should occur. Intraoperative pretreatment with droperidol 0.075 mg/kg intravenously, significantly lowers the incidence of postoperative vomiting. For greatest effectiveness it should be given 10 minutes before manipulation of the eye.[268] Droperidol may be given in the PACU in case of vomiting but is less effective under these circumstances. Treatment with doperidol does not cause delay in discharge but appears to provide a smooth recovery without restlessness or agitation.[268] Oral pretreatment with an equal dose of droperidol is less effective in prevention of vomiting.[269]

POSTOPERATIVE PAIN RELIEF

Postoperative pain is a common problem in pediatric postanesthesia care; however, it has only recently been addressed.[270,271] It appears that children frequently are provided with insufficient pain relief following surgery, partially because they may be unable to communicate. Signs of pain in infants and children include agitation, hypertension, hypoventilation with hypercarbia due to splinting,[272] and hypoxemia due to atelectasis.

In preterm babies and small infants, reaction to pain causes release of stress hormones and results in a variety of cardiorespiratory problems. Bradycardia, poor circulation, metabolic acidosis, and increased ventilatory requirements have been described.[273]

Pain varies with anxiety and apprehension and can be reduced by adequate preoperative preparation.[274,275] It is influenced by the site of surgery, with perineal and orthopedic procedures being more painful than abdominal or thoracic ones.[276]

Anesthetic technique influences the severity of postoperative pain. Inhalation anesthetics have no analgesic properties. If no narcotics have been administered pre- or intraoperatively, early use of narcotics in the postanesthesia period may be required for pain relief and reduction of agitation. Pain is easier prevented than treated. Small intravenous doses of morphine 0.05 to 0.1 mg/kg or fentanyl 5 to 10 μg/kg during emergence from inhalation anesthesia reduce pain and agitation on awakening. Continuous infusion with morphine 0.02 mg/kg/h can be used in children over 6 months of age to provide postoperative analgesia.[277] The analgesic effect of morphine appears shorter in younger infants.[278] Below 6 months of age, respiratory depression may occur more readily following intravenous morphine.[277] Patient-controlled analgesia (PCA) can be used for postoperative pain

relief in children over 6 years of age.[279-281] Doses of morphine vary between 0.015 and 0.03 mg/kg/h, after a loading dose of 0.05 mg/kg titrated with further doses to pain relief with a four-hour limit set at 0.25 mg/kg. Low-dose ketamine 1 mg/kg following an inhalational anesthetic also provides excellent pain relief without cardiorespiratory depression or psychological side effects.[282]

Regional Anesthesia for Postoperative Pain Relief

Use of regional anesthesia or nerve blocks of the surgical area prior to emergence from general anesthesia provides excellent pain relief with minimal physiological alterations. If the block has been established after induction but prior to the surgical procedure, lighter levels of general anesthesia are frequently tolerated and recovery is therefore more rapid. In addition, due to the lack of surgical pain, recovery tends to be smoother.[283,284] Patients require less narcotic and nonnarcotic analgesics postoperatively and are able to ambulate easier, resulting in earlier discharge from an ambulatory setting.[285]

Distribution and metabolism of local anesthetics varies in the pediatric age group. Neonates and small infants have low concentrations of plasma proteins, particularly alpha-glycoprotein, which is responsible for plasma binding of lidocaine. Plasma concentrations of 2.5 μg/L are toxic in the neonate while adults rarely show signs of neurotoxicity below levels of 5 μg/L.[286] Plasma protein binding does not reach adult levels until after the first year of life. The low plasma cholinesterase levels seen in the newborn can result in delayed metabolism of ester-type local anesthetics like procaine if given in large doses. This may be of particular importance if red-cell cholinesterase is also low, as is seen during physiologic anemia at 2 to 3 months of age.[287] Amide-type local anesthetics cannot be metabolized well since microsomal enzyme systems of the liver are immature in the neonate and as much as 90% of the drug may be excreted unchanged in the urine.[288] After the first few months of life children eliminate drugs at a greater rate than adults, possibly due to the fact that the liver mass constitutes a greater percentage of body weight and has relatively more metabolic sites for breakdown of local anesthetic drugs.[286] This accounts for the low blood concentrations seen after relatively large doses of local anesthetics in the older child.[288-292] Plasma concentrations rise more rapidly to peak blood concentrations in children,[288-292] which may be related to their greater cardiac output. Elimination half-life is, however, prolonged; which is thought to be due to the larger volume of distribution in children, which is related to the differences in body composition in the child.[286,291]

After 1 year of age children are quite tolerant to

high doses of local anesthetics and rarely exhibit signs of toxicity.[286] Dosage for local anesthetics is generally the maximum allowable dose. Addition of epinephrine retards absorption and permits use of larger doses of local anesthetics. Intravascular injection or injection into a very vascular area can lead to signs of toxicity with very small doses.[293,294] Table 14–12 lists anatomical sites and rapidity of absorption of local anesthetics in declining order. Table 14–13 lists maximum allowable amounts of local anesthetics at various sites.[293,294]

Contraindications to the use of local anesthetic techniques are the same as in adults: infection at the site of injection or a systemic coagulopathy. Relative contraindications are presence of anatomic abnormalities or degenerative nerve disease. Since most techniques are performed with the patient asleep or heavily sedated, a nerve stimulator should be used for localization in peripheral nerve blocks.

The most frequently performed blocks in pediatric patients are dorsal penile block for relief of circumcision pain, inguinal-ilio hypogastric nerve block for inguinal herniorrhaphy, and caudal epidural for relief of pain associated with major genitourinary and lower extremity orthopedic procedures.[293,294] The simplest method for relief of postcircumcision pain is application of topical lidocaine to the incision.[295] Block of the femoral nerve relieves the pain of fractures of the femoral shaft.[296] Thoracotomy pain is relieved by blocking the first six intercostal nerves, while blocking of the six lower intercostals provides analgesia of the abdominal wall.[297] For long-lasting postoperative pain relief, local anesthetics may be injected repeatedly or by continuous infusions through the catheter placed epidurally by the sacral or epidural route[298,299] or an interpleurally placed catheter positioned either by the surgeon or percutaneously.[300,301] For caudal and epidural blockade in children, various dosage schedules have been proposed. Dosage of 0.1 mL per segment per year of age of 0.25% bupivacaine or 1% lidocaine appears effective in prepubertal children.[302] Another formula to calculate dose is mL/segment = 0.056 × weight (kg).[303] The simplest method is to use 0.5 mL/kg of the desired local anesthetic solution for lumbar block; 1 mL/kg to achieve a lower thoracic

TABLE 14–13. LOCAL ANESTHETIC AGENTS AND MAXIMAL DOSAGE IN CHILDREN

Drug	Maximal Dosate (mg/kg)		
	Spinal	Epidural Caudal	Peripheral
Tetracaine	0.2–0.6 (minimal effective dose 1.5 mg)	2	2
Lidocaine	1–2.5 with 1:200,000 epinephrine	5 7–10	5 7–10
Bupivacaine	0.3–0.4 with 1:200,000 epinephrine	3 3–5	3 3–5
2-Chloroprocaine		15	15

level; and 1.25 mL/kg for a midthoracic level of analgesia.[304] The total mg/kg dose should be checked to be within the acceptable safe range of the drug.[286,293,294,298,305]

For continuous epidural infusion, bupivacaine 0.25% without epinephrine should be used. After a loading dose of 0.5 mL/kg an epidural infusion of 0.25% bupivacaine is started 30 minutes later at the rate of 0.08 mL/kg/h.[299] This corresponds to 0.2 mg/kg/h of bupivacaine. For continuous intrapleural block, 0.5% bupivacaine has been used. After a loading dose of 0.5 mL/kg given slowly at the rate of 1 mL/min, the catheter is infused with 0.5% bupivacaine at 0.1 to 0.5 mL/kg/h. Because of the prolonged elimination half-life of bupivacaine in children, the latter doses may lead to accumulation and patients must be observed closely for signs of central nervous system toxicity.[292]

The use of local anesthetics for pain control generally results in sympathetic blockade and motor weakness. Intrathecal or epidural narcotics result in similar pain relief and generally fewer side effects. Their use has not been widespread in pediatric anesthesia mostly due to the fact that patients require close observation for late respiratory depression for at least 12 hours following the injection of morphine.[306] Even in the absence of clinical signs of respiratory depression (decreased rate, increased end-tidal CO_2), ventilatory response to CO_2 is depressed for up to 22 hours.[307] Preservative-free morphine sulfate may be injected epidurally or caudally at a dose of 0.1 mg/kg for postoperative pain relief for surgical procedures involving the legs, abdomen, and chest. Caudal epidural morphine has been used for pain control in children following open heart surgery[308]; however, pain relief was not complete and had to be enforced with small doses of parenteral narcotics. Side effects in children as well as in adults include pruritus, nausea and vomiting, urinary retention, and (rarely) re-

TABLE 14–12. SPEED OF ABSORPTION FROM VARIOUS ANATOMIC SITES (IN DECLINING ORDER)

Fastest	Intratracheal
	Intercostal
	Caudal epidural
	Brachial plexus
	Distal peripheral nerves
Slowest	Subcutaneous infiltration

From Yaster M, Wetzel RC: Pediatric regional anesthesia. Anesth Rep 1988; 1:123

spiratory depression.[309] Pain relief following thoracotomies is of particular importance in pediatric patients with their limited ventilatory reserve. Pain may lead to instability of the chest wall, which must be stabilized by active muscle contraction; this, combined with diaphragmatic dysfunction, results in breathing at low tidal volumes, worsening airway closure, and can lead to atelectasis. Pain relief allows the patient to cough and reexpand the lung, reestablishing adequate functional residual capacity.[272] The undesirable side effects of epidural morphinelike nausea and pruritus and particular respiratory depression may be reversed with small doses of naloxon intravenously without reserving analgesia.[306]

THE PATIENT WITH SLEEP APNEA

Airway problems during sleep are often difficult to document and may not be recognized on routine examination of the child. The combination of obesity and hypersomnolence in a young boy was first described in 1837 by Charles Dickens in his *Pickwick Papers*.[310] More than 50 years elapsed before further studies showed that these patients suffered periodic states of airway obstruction and suffocation during sleep.[311] Not until 1937 was the association recognized of these clinical symptoms with significant cardiovascular problems, cor pulmonale, and congestive heart failure.[312] Systematic research undertaken in recent years has been able to elucidate the underlying physiologic and anatomic features of this and other syndromes associated with apnea during sleep. Apnea or an apneic period is defined as cessation of airflow for more than 10 seconds. A sleep apnea syndrome is characterized by 30 or more such episodes during a seven-hour sleep period.[313]

The most common significant airway problem associated with sleep in children is obstructive sleep apnea (OSAS).[314] Sleep apnea occurs more commonly in males than in females (2:1) and in children less than 6 years of age due to the lymphoid tissue hyperplasia common in this age group. Excessive daytime sleepiness, although common in adults and teenagers with sleep apnea, is not often recognized in small children. Principal clinical features in this group are restless sleep, sleepwalking, enuresis, and abnormal, particularly aggressive, behavior patterns. Withdrawal and even bizarre behavior may be present. Small children may show failure to thrive while older children tend to be obese. Children with obstructive sleep apnea frequently suffer recurrent otitis media.[314] The diagnosis is established objectively through monitoring during sleep in a controlled environment by polysomnography. Physiologic parameters monitored during sleep include EEG, ECG, respiratory effort (by chest and/or abdominal strain gauges or esophageal pressure transducer), airflow at the nostrils, extraocular eye movement, chin muscle tone, and arterial oxygen saturation.[315]

As already discussed in the section on respiratory control, normal sleep consists of a cyclic alteration between REM and non-REM sleep stages, with non-REM sleep as the predominant sleep pattern after the first year of life and during the first half of night sleep. During non-REM sleep, heart and respiratory rate are slower and more regular, and muscles are relaxed, but muscle tone is preserved. REM sleep, in contrast, is associated with profound physiologic changes. Muscle tone reaches its lowest level during REM sleep, most pronounced in the neck muscles. Extraocular muscles, however, are not paralyzed, and rapid conjugated eye movements together with muscle twitching occur. Phasic episodes of autonomic variability occur, including elevated and irregular heart rate, respiratory rate, and blood pressure. Cerebral blood flow is increased, as is cerebral oxygen consumption. Temperature regulation is suspended. Because of the profound muscle relaxation during REM sleep, airway obstruction tends to occur more readily and since arousal thresholds are increased, severe levels of oxygen desaturation may develop before the patient awakens.[316,317]

Sleep Apnea Syndromes

Sleep apnea syndromes are commonly classified into central sleep apnea, obstructive sleep apnea, and mixed apnea.[318]

Central Sleep Apnea. Central sleep apnea is characterized by repeated apneic periods without respiratory effort caused by a lack of neuronal output to the respiratory muscles. The underlying cause appears to be reduced or absent chemoreceptor sensitivity, particularly to CO_2. It is relatively uncommon (10% or less of all sleep apneas), but associated with various neurological disorders, particularly familial dysautonomia; Shy-Drager syndrome; central alveolar hypoventilation (Ondine's curse); diabetic neuropathy; brain stem lesions; encephalitis; bilateral cervical cordotomies; and bilateral carotid body resection. Congestive heart failure and nasal obstruction due to various causes including the common cold may be associated with central apnea.[319,320] Therapy is difficult. Acetazolamide has been used successfully in some cases. Inspiring low-flow oxygen-enriched air during sleep reduces the frequency of apneas. Severe cases of central sleep apnea require mechanical ventilation during sleep.[320]

Obstructive Sleep Apnea. More than 85% of patients with sleep apneas have the obstructive type and over two thirds of patients are overweight. Again the syndrome is more common in males and in the elderly.[321] Tiredness, fatigue, and daytime sleepiness are common complaints. Deterioration of memory and judgement with attacks of morning confusion occur. Patients snore loudly at night, with periods of snorting or silence during an apneic episode. This is followed by gasping and choking as respiration resumes. Sleep is restless with frequent movements.[314,322] Sleepwalking and, particularly in children, enuresis are common. The underlying cause is obstruction of the upper airway during sleep, resulting in cessation of airflow despite continuing respiratory efforts. Progressively asphyxia develops, which leads to arousal from sleep and restoration of upper airway patency. The primary site of obstruction appears to be the pharynx. Normally the pressure in the pharynx during inspiration is slightly subatmospheric. Collapse of the airway is prevented by the activity of the dilator and abductor muscles of the upper airway, which generally results in an actual dilatation of the upper airway. During REM sleep, muscle activity in the upper airway is reduced. With the onset of diaphragmatic contraction, negative airway pressure is generated that may lead to collapse of the hypotonic pharyngeal walls and in a small pharyngeal cavity cause complete airway obstruction. Continuing diaphragmatic activity increases negative airway pressure and increases the obstruction. Progressive asphyxia with hypoxemia and respiratory acidosis develops, resulting in arousal from sleep, which is accompanied by activation of the upper airway muscles. Stimulation by these muscles is greater than diaphragmatic activity, resulting in dilatation of the upper airway and resumption of airflow.[322]

Patients are usually unaware of the arousal that results in reduction of deep non-REM sleep and some REM sleep, sleep fragmentation, and persistent sleepiness. The latter causes the common clinical features of obstructive sleep apnea—drowsiness and intellectual, personal, and behavioral deterioration. Obstructive sleep apnea is associated with a variety of anatomic abnormalities of the upper airway, particularly in children. These include facial dysmorphism with micrognathia or retrognathia or relative or absolute macroglossia. Obstructive sleep apnea is found in Pierre Robin and Treacher Collins syndrome, hemifacial microsomia, craniosynostosis (Aperts or Crouzons disease), frontometaphyseal dysplasia, and trisomy 21, and may occur following the repair of a cleft palate particularly after a pharyngeal flap reconstruction.[160] Achondroplasia, Prader Willi syndrome, congenital myxedema, and also various hemoglobinopathies are associated with obstructive sleep apnea.

Several neuromuscular disorders may present with obstructive sleep apnea. These include various forms of Arnold-Chiari malformation with or without Klippel-Feil syndrome, syringobulbia, cerebral palsy, and myotonic dystrophy.[319,323,326] The majority of children who present with signs of obstructive sleep apnea have adenotonsillar hypertrophy that has resulted in narrowing of the airway and increased airway resistance. As the negative intraluminal pressure during inspiration increases, the velocity of airflow rises. The decrease in muscle tone during sleep facilitates the development of pharyngeal wall collapse and airway obstruction.[324] The repeated episodes of nocturnal asphyxiation have several cardiovascular consequences. Arterial hypoxemia increases systemic and pulmonary arterial pressures. Negative intrathoracic pressure exerted against an upper airway obstruction increases left-ventricular transmural pressure and increases left-ventricular and left-atrial volumes and pressures. The increase in left-atrial pressure may precipitate pulmonary edema.

While systemic arterial pressures usually return to normal with relief of the obstruction, pulmonary pressures remain elevated. Persistent pulmonary hypertension and cor pulmonale usually develop only in the presence of either lung disease or persistent hypoventilation during daytime as well as sleep. The amount of arterial desaturation is determined in part by preapnea oxygen saturation and lung volumes. If lung volumes are reduced, as in obesity, significant desaturation occurs much more rapidly. Although systemic blood pressure tends to normalize with resumption of ventilation, systemic hypertension may persist during wakefulness even in the absence of daytime hypoventilation. Patients with obstructive sleep apnea have a high incidence of systemic hypertension.

Second-degree heart block is a further complication of low arterial oxygen saturation below 60%. Of greatest clinical significance are changes in heart rate and rhythm. During non-REM sleep heart rate decreases by 5 and 8% and returns to normal during REM sleep. Ventricular ectopy is decreased during sleep. All forms of sleep apnea causing arterial hypoxemia result in vagally mediated bradycardia. Sinus arrhythmia with variability exceeding 30 beats/min is present in nearly all patients. Severe sinus bradycardia (less than 30 beats/min), or sinus arrest with pauses in excess of 10 seconds, may be present in more than 10% of patients. Desaturation below 60% commonly results in second-degree heart block and ventricular ectopy. Malignant ventricular arrhythmias (multifocal, bigeminy, ventricular tachycardia) are observed. Increased sympathetic neural activity may play an important role in generating these arrhythmias. Sudden death during sleep in patients with obstructive sleep apnea is probably due to fatal cardiac arrhythmias (ventricular fibrillation or complete heart block without ventricular escape.[321,327,328]

Mixed Apnea. A mixed sleep apnea with both central and obstructive apnea has been observed. Central apnea usually preceeds an obstructive episode. Dickens' fat boy Joe exhibited this syndrome, characterized by marked obesity, somnolence, periodic breathing, hypoventilation and hypercarbia, hypoxia, polycythemia, and cor pulmonale.[329] The syndrome is rare and present in only about 5% of patients with sleep apnea. The degree of obesity, magnitude of hypoventilation, and severity of apnea do not necessarily correlate. Obesity imposes an increased load on the respiratory muscles. Ventilation perfusion relationships are abnormal. Lung volumes are diminished. Closing capacity increases, resulting in airway closure and intrapulmonary shunting. Central blood volume is increased, resulting in a decrease in lung compliance. Chest wall compliance is markedly diminished due to obesity. Hypoxemia and sleep fragmentation result in somnolence. Central control of ventilation is abnormal and in conjunction with the increased work of breathing leads to chronic hypercarbia and loss of hypoxic drive. Excess fat tissue leads to narrowing of the pharyngeal dimension and predisposes to the development of obstruction during sleep. The abnormal control of ventilation results in more severe hypoxia before arousal, and in slowly increasing hypercarbia even during waking hours.[329]

Therapy

Obstructive and mixed sleep apneas usually respond dramatically to therapy aimed at preventing upper airway closure during sleep. Positive nasal airway pressure via a mask or prongs acting as a pneumatic splint to hold the upper airway open may be sufficient.[330] Uvulopalato pharyngoplasty involving resection of tonsils, uvula, the nonmuscular portion of the soft palate, and redundant pharyngeal mucosa enlarges pharyngeal dimensions and is frequently curative, as is tonsillectomy with adenoidectomy in children with OSAS due to lymphoid hyperplasia.[331-333] With skeletal abnormalities, mandibular osteotomy with or without maxillary advancement and hyoid suspension may be necessary to enlarge the upper airway and prevent obstruction.[331] If obstruction cannot be relieved, tracheoplasty is performed, which bypasses the obstruction during sleep and allows the patient to function normally during the day with the tracheoplasty closed.[331-333]

In the immediate postoperative period patients are still at risk for development of airway obstruction and apnea.[334,335] We routinely place nasopharyngeal airways for 24 hours following surgery to maintain upper airway patency.[328] They require monitoring in an intensive care unit setting with apnea monitoring and pulse oximetry. Apnea monitors relying on thoracic or diaphragmatic motion will not detect airway obstruction.[336] Since obstructive episodes result in hypoxemia, pulse oximetry will detect the episode. Obstructive episodes result in addition in vagally mediated bradycardia, and patients may still exhibit cardiac dysrhythmias. Continuous electrocardiographic monitoring is therefore essential. Administration of supplemental oxygen should be tailored to acceptable arterial oxygenation. Patients with mixed forms of apnea may rely on peripheral chemoreceptor stimulation for control of ventilation, and elimination of hypoxic drive will result in central apnea.[337] The sensitivity to sedatives and narcotics remains for weeks following relief of chronic airway obstruction. Use of these drugs intraoperatively resuts in prolonged postoperative hypoventilation and apnea requiring mechanical ventilation.[338] Although inhalational anesthetics also cause significant respiratory depression, their effects are not prolonged and a normal ventilatory pattern is established quickly. Postoperative use of narcotics and sedatives must be controlled carefully with small titrated doses to avoid development of apnea.[335] Following removal of the nasopharyngeal airways the day after surgery, patients should remain in a monitored setting until a sleep period has been observed without recurrence of obstructive apnea.[328]

MALIGNANT HYPERTHERMIA

Malignant hyperthermia is an inherited metabolic disease of muscle. It is inherited as an autosomal dominant with reduced penetrance and variable expressivity.[339] In children the incidence of the disorder is quoted as 1:3000 to 1:15,000.[339] The pathophysiologic defect lies in the inabiliy of the sarcoplasmic reticulum of skeletal muscle to store calcium after triggering of the syndrome. This results in a tremendous increase in hydrolysis of high-energy phosphates with a large increase in oxygen consumption and carbon dioxide and heat production, outstripping the individual's ability to eliminate or dissipate the end products of metabolism. As oxygen demand outstrips oxygen supply, anaerobic pathways are utilized, resulting in metabolic acidosis. The marked increase in oxygen uptake results in very low venous oxygen content; and the equally increased CO_2 production in respiratory acidosis with high venous, and later arterial, CO_2. The high myoplasmic calcium levels lead to inability of the muscle to relax and clinical signs of rigidity. As the muscle disintegrates, swelling and rhabdomyolysis occurs with breakdown of cell mem-

TABLE 14-14. SIGNS AND SYMPTOMS OF MALIGNANT HYPERTHERMIA

Tachycardia (sudden, unexplained)
Tachypnea
Skeletal muscle rigidity
Rapid rise in temperature
Cyanotic mottling of skin
Cyanosis
Unstable blood pressure
Arrhythmia
Profuse sweating
Discolored urine
Hyperkalemia
Central venous desaturation and hypercarbia
Respiratory and metabolic acidosis
Elevated creatinephosphokinase
Coagulopathy

brane stability. Potassium, calcium, and myoglobin will leak from the cell. Hyperkalemia is a major cause of mortality. Myoglobinuria may lead to renal failure. Cardiac dysrhythmias are frequently seen due to sympathetic stimulation from the increased metabolism, hypoxia, acidosis, hyperkalemia, and hyperthermia. The syndrome occurs nearly exclusively during or following anesthesia with potent inhalational agents and/or the use of succinylcholine.[339,340] It can be triggered by stress in susceptible individuals and can occur in patients with muscle disease (eg, muscular dystrophy). There is a very close association with central core disease.[341] A similar syndrome with common pathways has been described following high doses of neuroleptic drugs, neuroleptic malignant syndrome.[342,343]

Since increased metabolism is the hallmark of the

TABLE 14-15. TREATMENT PLAN FOR MALIGNANT HYPERTHERMIA EPISODE

100% oxygen
Hyperventilation
Dantrolene sodium (2.5-3 mg/kg IV)
Surface cooling
Internal cooling (cold gastric lavage)
Correct acidosis with sodium bicarbonate
Forced diuresis (Mannitol, Lasix)
Give large amounts cold intravenous fluids (non-calcium-containing)
Establish monitoring
  ECG, temperature, indwelling urinary catheter, arterial and central venous lines
Monitor arterial and venous gases and electrolytes
Hyperkalemia can be treated with glucose and insulin (1mL/kg 50% dextrose and 0.2 units/kg of regular insulin).
Cardiac arrhythmias should be treated with procainamide 15 mg/kg slowly IV.

From Ryan JF: Malignant hyperthermia, in Ryan JF, Todres ID, Cote CJ, Goudsouzian N (eds): A Practice of Anesthesia for Infants and Children. Orlando, Grune & Stratton, 1986, p 247.

syndrome, signs of cardiorespiratory stimulation—*tachycardia and tachypnea*—are the initial symptoms. Table 14-14 lists signs and symptoms of malignant hyperthermia.

Treatment centers on therapy with dantrolene sodium.[344] The effective dose is 2.5 mg/kg intravenously. If this does not result in complete resolution of the symptoms, a bolus dose of 10 mg/kg should be given 45 minutes later.[339] Besides treatment with dantrolene, ancillary measures to correct the physiologic sequelae of hypermetabolism should be instituted (Table 14-15). Successful therapy is indicated by resolution of all symptoms within 30 minutes. Until this has been achieved, supplemental doses of dantrolene should be given.[339] Patients require monitoring for 24 hours, while they are maintained on intravenous dantrolene 1 mg/kg every 8 hours.

REFERENCES

1. Pang LM: Special pediatric problems, in Israel JS, DeKornfeld TJ (eds): *Recovery Room Care.* Chicago, Year Book, 1987, pp 237-260.
2. Smith RM: Fundamental differences, in Smith RM (ed): *Anesthesia for Infants and Children.* St. Louis, Mosby, 1980, pp 5-37.
3. Eckenhoff J: Some anatomic considerations of the infant larynx influencing endotracheal anesthesia. *Anesthesiology* 1951; 12:401-410.
4. Coté J, Todres ID: The pediatric airway, in Ryan JF, Todres ID, Cote CJ, Goudsouzian N (eds): *A Practice of Anesthesia in Infants and Children.* New York, Grune & Stratton, 1986, pp 35-54.
5. Krahl VE: Anatomy of the mammalian lung, in Fenn WO, Rahn H (eds): *Handbook of Physiology.* Baltimore, Williams & Wilkins, 1965, vol 1, pp 213-284.
6. Muller NL, Bryan AC: Chest wall mechanics and respiratory muscles in infants. *Ped Clin N Am* 1979; 26:503-516.
7. Keen TG, Ianuzzo CD: Development of fatigue resistant muscle fibers in human ventilatory muscle. *Am Rev Resp Dis* 1979; 119:139-141.
8. Hislop A, Reid L: Development of the acinus in the human lung. *Thorax* 1974; 29:90-94.
9. Thurlbeck WM: Postnatal growth and development of the lung, *Am Rev Resp Dis* 1975; 111:803-844.
10. Motoyama EK: Pulmonary mechanics during early postnatal years. *Pediatri Res* 1977; 11:220-223.
11. Agostoni E, Mead J: Statics of the respiratory system, in Feen WO, Rahn H (eds): *Handbook of Physiology.* Baltimore, Williams & Wilkins, 1965, vol 1, pp 387-409.
12. Mansell A, Bryan AC, Levison H: Airway closure in children. *J Appl Physiol* 1972; 33:711-714.
13. Agostoni E, Mognoni P, Torri G, et al: Relation between changes of rib cage circumference and lung volume. *J Appl Physiol* 1965; 20:1179-1186.

14. Polgar G, Kong GP: Nasal resistance of the newborn infant. *J Pediatr* 1965; 67:557–567.

15. Briscoe WA, DuBois AB: The relationship between airway resistance, airway conductance and lung volume in subjects of different age and body size. *J Clin Invest* 1958; 37:1279–1285.

16. Polgar G: Airway resistance in the newborn infant. *J Pediatr* 1961; 59:915–921.

17. Cook CD, Sutherland JM, Segal S, et al: Studies of respiratory physiology in the newborn infant. *J Clin Invest* 1957; 36:440–448.

18. Hill DW: *Physics Applied to Anesthesia*, ed 4. London, Butterworths, 1980, pp 170–179.

19. Motoyama EK: Airway function tests in infants and children. *Int Anesthesiol Clin* 1988; 26:6–13.

20. Cross KW, Tizard LPM, Trythall DAH: The gaseous metabolism of the newborn infant. *Acta Paediatr* 1957; 46:265–285.

21. Nelson NM: Respiration and circulation after birth, in Smith CA, Nelson NM (eds): *Physiology of the Newborn Infant*. Springfield, IL, Chas. C Thomas, 1976, pp 117–262.

22. Motoyama EK, Cook CD: Respiratory physiology, in Smith RM (ed): *Anesthesia for Infants and Children*. St. Louis, Mosby, 1980, pp 38–86.

23. Thibeault DW, Clutario B, Auld PAM: The oxygen cost of breathing in the premature infant. *Pediatrics* 1966; 37:954–959.

24. Cave P, Fletcher G: Resistance of nasotracheal tubes used in infants. *Anesthesiology* 1968; 29:588–590.

25. LeSouef PN, England SJ, Bryan CA: Total resistance of the respiratory system in preterm infants with and without an endotrachael tube. *J Pediatr* 1984; 104:108–111.

26. Rigatto H: Respiratory control and apnea in the newborn infant. *Critical Care Med* 1972; 5:2–9.

27. Bryan AC, Bryan MH: Control of respiration in the newborn, in Thibeault DW, Gregory GA (eds): *Neonatal Pulmonary Care*, ed 2. Norwalk CT, Appleton-Century-Crofts, 1986, pp 33–48.

28. Parmelee AH Jr, Wenner WH, Akiyama Y, et al: Sleep states in premature infants. *Dev Med Child Neurol* 1967; 9:70–77.

29. Dransfield DA, Spitzer AA, Fox WW: Episodic airway obstruction in premature infants. *Am J Dis Child* 1983; 137:441–443.

30. Rigatto H, Brady JP, de la Torre Verduzco R: The effect of gestational age on the ventilatory response to inhaled carbon dioxide. *Pediatrics* 1975; 55:614–620.

31. Rigatto H, Brady JP, de la Torre Verduzco R: The effect of gestational age on the ventilatory response to inhalation of 100% and 15% oxygen. *Pediatrics* 1975; 55:604–613.

32. Kafer ER, Marsh HM: The effect of anesthetic drugs and disease on the clinical regulation of ventilation. *Int Anesthes Clin* 1977; 45:1–38.

33. Lawson EE: Prolonged central respiratory inhibition following reflex induced apnea. *J Appl Physiol* 1981; 50:874–879.

34. Doeshuk CF, Fisher BJ, Matthews LW, et al: Pulmo-

nary physiology of the young child, in Scarpelli E, Auld P (eds): *Pulmonary Physiology of the Fetus, Newborn and Child*. Philadelaphia, Lea & Febiger, 1975, pp 166–182.

35. Polgar G, Weng TR: Functional development of the respiratory system. *Am Rev Resp Dis* 1979; 120:625–695.

36. Crone RK: The respiratory system, in Gregory GA (ed): *Pediatric Anesthesia*. New York, Churchill Livingstone, 1983, pp 54–62.

37. Friedman WF: The intrinsic properties of the developing heart. *Progr CV Dis* 1972; 15:87–111.

38. Rudolph AM: *Congenital Diseases of the Heart*. Chicago, Year Book, 1974, pp 11–12.

39. Nelson NM: Respiration and circulation before birth, in Smith CA, Nelson NM (eds): *The Physiology of the Newborn Infant*. Springfield, IL, Chas. C Thomas, 1976, pp 15–116.

40. Cordero L Jr, Hon EH: Neonatal bradycardia following pharyngeal stimulation. *J Pediatr* 1971; 78:441–447.

41. Robinson S: Cardiovascular physiology in pediatrics, in Gregory GA (ed): *Pediatric Anesthesia*. New York, Churchill Livingstone, 1983, vol 1, pp 9–33.

42. Downing SE, Talner NS, Gardner TH: Influences of arterial oxygen tension and pH on cardiac function in the newborn lamb. *Am J Physiol* 1966; 211:1203–1208.

43. Hickey RF, Eger EI: Circulatory effects of inhaled anesthetic agents, in Prys-Roberts C (ed): *The Circulation in Anesthesia*. Oxford, Blackwell, 1980, pp 441–457.

44. Hug CC Jr: Anesthetic agents and the patient with cardiovascular disease, in Ream AK, Fogdall RP (eds): *Acute Cardiovascular Management*. Philadelphia, Lippincott, 1982, pp 247–291.

45. Rudolph Am, Yuan S: Response of the pulmonary vascular circulation to hypoxia and H^+ ion concentration changes. *J Clin Invest* 1966; 45:399–411.

46. Pang LM, Mellins RB: Neonatal cardiorespiratory physiology. *Anesthesiology* 1975; 43:171–196.

47. Mahoney LT, Coryell KG, Lauer RM: The newborn transitional circulation: An echocardiographic study. *J Am Coll Cardiol* 1985; 6:623–629.

48. Heyman MA, Rudolph AM: Control of the ductus arteriosus. *Physiol Rev* 1975; 55:62–78.

49. Baylen BG, Emmanouilides GC: Patent ductus arteriosus in the newborn, in Thiebeault DW, Gregory GA (eds): *Neonatal Pulmonary Care*, ed 2. Norwalk, CT, Appleton-Century-Crofts, 1986, pp 519–550.

50. Bell EF, Warburton D, Stonestreet BS, et al: Effect of fluid administration on the development of symptomatic patent ductus arteriosus and congestive heart failure in premature infants. *N Engl J Med* 1980; 302:598–604.

51. Rudolph AM: The changes in the circulation after birth. *Circulation* 1970; 41:343–359.

52. Rowe RD, James LS: The normal pulmonary arterial pressure during the first year of life. *J Pediatr* 1957; 51:1–4.

53. Park MK, Lee DH: Normative arm and calf pressure values in the newborn. *Pediatrics* 1989; 83:240–243.

54. Gersony WM: The cardiovascular system, in Behrman

RE, Vaughan VC (eds): *Nelsons Textbook of Pediatrics,* ed 13. Philadelphia, Saunders, 1987, pp 943–944.

55. Kirkendall WM, Feinleib M, Freis M: Recommendation for blood pressure determination by sphygmomanometers. *Circulation* 1980; 62:1145A–1155A.

56. Lum LG, Jones MD: The effect of cuff width on systolic blood pressure measurement in the neonate. *Pediatrics* 1974; 91:963–966.

57. Smith RM: Fluid therapy and blood replacement, in Smith RM (ed). *Anesthesia for Infants and Children,* ed 4. St. Louis, Mosby, 1980, pp 547–586.

58. Delivoria-Papadopoulos M, Roncevic N, Oshi FA: Postnatal changes in oxygen transport of term, premature and sick infants: The role of 2,3 disphosphoglycerate and adult hemoglobin. *Ped Res* 1971; 5:235–245.

59. O'Brien RT, Pearson HA: Physiologic anemia of the newborn infant. *J Pediatr* 1971; 70:132–138.

60. Pearson HA: Diseases of the blood, in Behrman RE, Vaughan VC (eds): *Nelson's Textbook of Pediatrics,* ed 13. Philadelphia, Saunders, 1987, pp 1033–1078.

61. Sinclair JC: Metabolic rate and temperature control, in Smith CA, Nelson NM (eds): *Physiology of the Newborn Infant.* Springfield, IL, Chas. C Thomas, 1976, pp 354–415.

62. Schiff D, Stern L, Leduc J: Chemical thermogenesis in newborn infants. *Pediatrics* 1966; 37:577–582.

63. Smith RE, Horwitz BA: Brown fat and thermogenesis. *Physiol Rev* 1969; 49:330–425.

64. Hull D, Smales ORC: Heat production in the newborn, in Sinclair JC (ed): *Temperature Regulation and Energy Metabolism in the Newborn.* Orlando, Grune & Stratton, 1978, pp 129–156.

65. Brueck K, Wuennenberg B: The influence of ambient temperature in the process of replacement of nonshivering by shivering thermogenesis during postnatal development. *Fed Proc* 1965; 25:1332–1336.

66. Hellon RF: Neurophysiology of temperature regulation, problems and perspectives. *Fed Proc* 1981; 40:2804–2807.

67. Hensel H: Neural processes in long term thermal adaptation. *Fed Proc* 1981; 40:2830–2834.

68. Davis PJ: Thermoregulation of the newborn, in Cook OR, Marcy JH (eds): *Neonatal Anesthesia.* Pasadena, Appleton Davies, 1988, pp 63–70.

69. Mestyan J, Jarai I, Bata B, et al: The significance of facial skin temperture in the chemical heat regulation of premature infants. *Biol Neonat* 1964; 7:243–254.

70. Brueck K: Temperature regulation in the newborn infant. *Biol Neonat* 1961; 3:65–119.

71. Winters RW: Maintenance fluid therapy, in Winters RW (ed): *The Body Fluids in Pediatrics.* Boston, Little, Brown, 1973, pp 113–133.

72. Winters RW: Regulation of normal water and electrolyte metabolism, in Winters RW (ed): *The Body Fluids in Pediatrics.* Boston, Little, Brown, 1973, pp 95–112.

73. Driscoll JM, Heird WL: Maintenance fluid therapy during the neonatal period, in Winters RW (ed): *The Body Fluids in Pediatrics.* Boston, Little, Brown, 1973, pp 265–278.

74. Friis-Hansen B: Body water compartments in children: Changes during growth and related changes in body composition. *Pediatrics* 1981; 28:169–181.

75. Bell EF, Warburton D, Stonestreet BS, et al: Effect of fluid administration on the development of symptomatic patent ductus arteriosus and congestive heart failure in the premature infant. *N Engl J Med* 1980; 302:598–604.

76. Stevenson JG: Fluid administration in the association of patent ductus arteriosus complicating respiratory distress syndrome. *J Pediatr* 1977; 90:257–261.

77. Bell EF, Warburton D, Stonestreet BS: High volume fluid intake predisposes premature infants to necrotizing enterocolitis. *Lancet* 1979; 90:7–14.

78. Edelman CM, Spitzer A: The kidney, in Smith CA, Nelson NM (ed): *The Physiology of the Newborn Infant.* Springfield, IL, Chas. C Thomas, 1976, pp 416–458.

79. Graves S: Fluid and electrolyte therapy in children. *ASA Refresher Courses* 1981; 114.

80. Aperia A, Broberger O, Herlin P, et al: Postnatal control of water and electrolyte homeostasis in premature and full term infants. *Acta Paediatr Scand* 1982; 305(suppl):61–65.

81. Edelman CM, Barnett HL: Role of the kidney in water metabolism in young infants. *J Pediatr* 1960; 56:154–179.

82. Aperia A, Broberger O, Thodenius D, et al: Renal control of sodium and fluid balance in newborn infants during intravenous maintenance therapy. *Acta Paediatr Scand* 1978; 64:725–731.

83. Siegel SR: Hormonal and renal interaction in body fluid regulation in the newborn infant. *Clin Perinatol* 1982; 9:535–557.

84. Aperia A, Broberger O, Herin P, et al: A comparative study of the response to an oral NaCl and NaHCO$_3$ load in newborn preterm and full term infants. *Ped Res* 1977; 11:1109–1111.

85. Sulyok E, Nemeth M, Tenyl I, et al: Postnatal development of the renin-angiotension aldosterone system RAAs in relation to electrolyte balance in premature infants. *Pediatr Res* 1979; 13:817–820.

86. Sosulski R, Polin RA, Baumgart S: Respiratory water loss and heat balance in intubated infants receiving humidified air. *J Pediatr* 1983; 103:307–310.

87. Cook DR, Row MI: Parenteral fluid therapy, in Cook DR, Marcy JH (eds): *Neonatal Anesthesia.* Pasadena, Appleton Davies, 1988, pp 71–85.

88. Holliday MA, Segar WE: The maintenance need for water in parenteral fluid therapy. *Pediatrics* 1975; 19:823–832.

89. Kliegman RM, Wald MK: Problems in metabolic adaptation: Glucose, calcium and magnesium, in Klaus MH, Faranoff AA (eds): *Care of the High Risk Neonate,* ed 3. Philadelphia, Saunders, 1986, pp 220–238.

90. Coppoletta JM: Wolbach SB: Body length and organ weights of infants and children. *Am J Pathol* 1933; 9:55–70.

91. Donnegan J: Anesthesia for pediatric neurosurgery, in Cottrell TE, Turndorf H (eds): *Anesthesia and Neurosurgery,* ed 2. St. Louis, Mosby, 1986, pp 173–187.

92. Kandt RS, Johnston MV, Goldstein GW: The central

nervous system: Basic concepts, in Gregory GA (ed): *Pediatric Anesthesia*. New York, Churchill Livingstone, 1983, pp 129–167.

93. Freeman JM, Braun AW: Central nervous system disturbances, in Behrmann RE (ed): *Neonatal-Perinatal Medicine*, ed 2. St. Louis, Mosby, 1977, pp 787–836.

94. Gregory GA: Pharmacology, in Gregory GA (ed): *Pediatric Anesthesia*. New York, Churchill Livingstone, 1983, pp 315–339.

95. Cook DR, Marcy JH: Pediatric anesthetic pharmacology, in Cook DR, Marcy JH (eds): *Neonatal Anesthesia*. Pasadena, Appleton Davies, 1988, pp 87–125.

96. Crumrine RS, Yodlowski EH: Assessment of neuromuscular function in infants. *Anesthesiology* 1981; 54:29–32.

97. Cook DR: Muscle relaxants in infants and children. *Anesthesiology* 1981; 60:335–343.

98. Goudsouzian N: Muscle relaxants in children, in Ryan JF, Todres ID, Cote CJ, Goudsouzian N (eds): *A Practice of Anesthesia for Infants and Children*. Orlando, Grune & Stratton, 1986, pp 105–114.

99. Chapman AH, Loeb DG, Gibbons MJ: Psychiatric aspects of hospitalization of children. *Arch Paed* 1956; 73:77–88.

100. Davenport HT, Wessy JS: The effect of general anesthesia, surgery and hospitalization on the behavior of children. *Am J Orthopsychiatry* 1970; 40:806–824.

101. Smith RM: Normal recovery, in Smith RM (ed): *Anesthesia for Infants and Children*, ed 4. St. Louis, Mosby, 1980, pp 216–228.

102. Motoyama E, Glazener CH: Hypoxemia after general anesthesia. *Anesth Analg* 1986; 65:267–272.

103. Pullerits J, Burrows FA, Roy WL: Arterial desaturation in healthy children during transfer to the recovery room. *Can J Anaesth* 1987; 34:470–473.

104. Kataria BK, Haznik EV, Mitchard R, et al: Postoperative aterial oxygen saturation in the pediatric population during transport. *Anesth Analg* 1988; 67:280–282.

105. Chripko DL, Bevan JC, Archer DP, et al: Decreases in arterial oxygen saturation in paediatric outpatients during transfer to the postanesthetic recovery room. *Can J Anaesth* 1989; 36:128–132.

106. Westbrook PR, Stubbs SE, Sessler AD, et al: Effects of anaesthesia and muscular paralysis on respiratory mechanics in man. *J Appl Physiol* 1973; 34:81–86.

107. Don HF, Wahba M, Cuadrado L, et al: The effects of anesthesia and 100% oxygen on the functional residual capacity of the lungs. *Anesthesiology* 1970; 32:521–529.

108. Alexander JI, Spence AA, Parish RK, et al: The role of airway closure in postoperative hypoxaemia. *Br J Anaesth* 1973; 45:34–40.

109. Dobbinson TL, Nisbett HLA, Pelton DA, et al: Functional residual capacity and compliance in anaesthetized paralyzed children. II: Clinical results. *Can Anaesth Soc J* 1973; 20:322–323.

110. Hickey RF, Severinghaus DW: Regulation of breathing: Drug effects, in Hornbein TF (ed): *Regulation of Breathing*. New York, Marcel Dekker, 1981, pp 1251–1312.

111. Knill RL, Gelb AW: Ventilatory response to hypoxia and hypercapnia during halothane sedation and anesthesia in man. *Anesthesiology* 1978; 49:244–251.

112. Cote CJ, Goldstein EA, Cote MA, et al: A single blinded study of pulse oximetry in children. *Anesthesiology* 1988; 68:184–188.

113. Edmonds JF, Barker GA, Conn AW: Current concepts in cardiovascular monitoring in children. *Crit Care Med* 1980; 8:548–553.

114. Ruskin J, Harley A, Rembert J, et al: Contribution of atrial systole to ventricular stroke volume in man. *Circulation* 1968; 38(suppl 6):168.

115. Hartzer GO, Maloney JD, Curtis JJ, et al: Hemodynamic benefits of atrioventricular sequential pacing after cardiac surgery. *Am J Cardiol* 1977; 40:232–236.

116. Shoemaker WC, Vidyasagar D: Physiological and clinical significance of $P_{tc}O_2$ and $P_{tc}CO_2$ measurements. Guest editorial. *Crit Care Med* 1981; 9:689–690.

117. Alexi-Meskhishvili V, Popov SA, Nikoljuk AP: Evaluation of hemodynamics in infants and babies after open-heart surgery. *Thorac Cardiovasc Surg* 1984; 32:4–9.

118. Joly HR, Weil MH: Temperature of the great toe as an indication of the severity of shock. *Circulation* 1969; 39:131–138.

119. Ibsen B: Treatment of shock with vasodilators measuring skin temperature on the big toe. *Dis Chest* 1967; 52:425–429.

120. Downes JJ, Nicodemus H: Preparation for and recovery from anesthesia. *Ped Clin North Am* 1969; 16:601–611.

121. Eckenhoff JE, Kneale DH, Dripps RD: The incidence and etiology of postanesthetic excitement. *Anesthesiology* 1961; 22:667–673.

122. Hollister GR, Burn JMB: Side effects of ketamine in pediatric anesthesia. *Anesth Analg* 1974; 53:264–267.

123. Liu LMP: Perioperative fluid management, in Ryan JF, Todres ID, Cote CJ, Goudsouzian N (eds): *A Practice of Anesthesia for Infants and Children*. Orlando, Grune & Stratton, 1986, pp 115–121.

124. Heird WC, Winters RW: Fluid therapy for the pediatric surgical patient, in Winters RW (ed): *The Body Fluids in Pediatrics*. Boston, Little, Brown, 1973, pp 595–611.

125. Shires T, Williams J, Brown F: Acute changes in extracellular fluids associated with major surgical procedures. *Ann Surg* 1961; 154:803–810.

126. Mollit DL, Ballantine TVN, Gosfeld JL, et al: A critical assessment of fluid requirements in gastroschisis. *J Pediatr Surg* 1978; 13:217–219.

127. Furman EB, Roman DG, Lemmer LAS, et al: Specific therapy in water, electrolyte and blood volume replacement during pediatric surgery. *Anesthesiology* 1975; 42:187–193.

128. Dell RB: Pathophysiology of dehydration, in Winters RW (ed): *The Body Fluids in Pediatrics*. Boston, Little, Brown, 1973, pp 134–154.

129. Honig GR, Hruby MA: Disorders of the blood and hematopoetic system, in Behrman RE (ed): *Neonatal-Perinatal Medicine*. St. Louis, Mosby, 1977, pp 345–393.

130. Buchholz DH: Blood transfusion: Merits of component therapy: I. *J Pediatr* 1974; 84:1–15.

131. Buchholz DH: Blood transfusion: Merits of component therapy: II. *J Pediatr* 1974; 84:165–172.

132. Cote CJ, Liu LM, Szyfelbein SK, et al: Changes in serial platelet counts following massive transfusion in pediatric patients. *Anesthesiology* 1985; 62:197–201.

133. Cote CJ, Drop LJ, Daniels AL: Ionized hypocalcemia following fresh frozen plasma adminstration to thermally injured children. *Anesthesiology* 1984; 61:A421.

134. Cote CJ, Drop LJ, Daniels AL: Calcium chloride versus calciumgluconate: Comparison of ionization and cardiovascular effects in children and dogs. *Anesthesiology* 1987; 66:465–470.

135. Miyasaka K, Edmonds JF, Conn AW: Complications of radial artery lines in paediatric patients. *Can Anaesth Soc J* 1976; 23:9–14.

136. Todres ID, Coté CJ: Procedures, in Ryan RF, Todres ID, Cote CJ, Goudsouzian N (eds): *A Practice of Anesthesia for Infants and Children.* Orlando, Grune & Stratton, 1986, pp 289–304.

137. Goetzman BW, Stadalnik RC, Bogren HG, et al: Thrombotic complications of umbilical artery catheters: A clinical and radiographic study. *Pediatrics* 1975; 56:374–379.

138. Glenski TP, Beynen FM, Brady T: A prospective evaluation of femoral artery monitoring in pediatric patients. *Anesthesiology* 1987; 66:227–229.

139. Adler DC, Bryan-Brown CW: Use of the axillary artery for intravascular monitoring. *Crit Care Med* 1973; 1:148–150.

140. Prian AW, Wright GB, Rumack CM, et al: Apparent cerebral embolization after temporal artery cannulation. *J Pediatr* 1978; 93:115–118.

141. Hug CC: Monitoring, in Miller E (ed): *Anesthesia,* ed 2. New York, Churchill Livingstone, 1986, pp 411–463.

142. Shapiro BA, Cane RD, Chomka CM, et al: Preliminary evaluation of an intra-arterial blood gas system in dogs and humans. *Crit Care Med* 1989; 17:455–460.

143. Adrogué HJ, Rashad NM, Gorin AB, et al: Assessing acid–base status in circulatory failurre. *N Engl J Med* 1989; 320:1312–1316.

144. Prince SR, Sullivan RL, Hackel A: Percutaneous catheterization of the internal jugular vein in infants and children. *Anesthesiology* 1976; 44:170–174.

145. Coté CJ, Jobes DR, Schwartz AJ, et al: Two approaches to cannulation of the child's internal jugular vein. *Anesthesiology* 1979; 50:371–373.

146. Belanin KG, Buckley JJ, Gordon JR, et al: Percutaneous cervical central venous line placement: A comparison of the internal and external jugular vein routes. *Anesth Analg* 1980; 59:40–44.

147. Groff DB, Ahmed N: Subclavian vein catherization in the infant. *J Pediatr Surg* 1974; 9:171–174.

148. Bausmer G, Keith D, Tesluk H: Complications following use of indwelling catheters of the inferior vena cava. *JAMA* 1958; 167:1606–1611.

149. James LS: Emergencies in the delivery room, in Behrmann RE (ed): *Neonatal-Perinatal Medicine.* St. Louis, Mosby, 1977, pp 128–145.

150. Loomis JC: Care of the pediatric patient following cardiovascular surgery, in Ream AK, Fogdall RP (eds): *Acute Cardiovascular Management.* Philadelphia, Lippincott, 1982, pp 635–700.

151. Ein SH, Barker G, Olley P, et al: The pharmacologic treatment of newborn diaphragmatic hernia—A 2 year evaluation. *J Pediatr Surg* 1980; 15:384–394.

152. Salem MR, Bennett EJ, Schweiss JF, et al: Cardiac arrest related to anesthesia: Contributing factors in infants and children. *JAMA* 1975; 233:238–241.

153. Tiret L, Nivoche Y, Hatton F, et al: Complications related to anaesthesia in infants and children. *Br J Anaesth* 1988; 61:263–269.

154. Berry FA: The child in the recovery room, in Berry FA (ed): *Anesthetic Management of Difficult and Routine Pediatric Patients.* New York, Churchill Livingstone, 1986, pp 425–440.

155. Wilson SL, Thach BT, Brouillette RT, et al: Upper airway patency in human infant: Influence of airway pressure and posture. *J Appl Physiol* 1980; 48:500–504.

156. Remmers JE, DeGroot WT, Sauerland EK, et al: Pathogenesis of upper airway occlusion during sleep. *J Appl Physiol* 1978; 44:931–938.

157. Shprintzen RJ: Pharyngeal flap surgery and the pediatric airway. *Int Anesthesiol Clin* 1988; 26:79–88.

158. Badgwell JM, McLeod ME, Friedberg J: Airway obstruction in infants and children. *Can J Anaesth* 1987; 34:90–98.

159. Jackson P, Whitaker LA, Randall P: Airway hazards associated with pharyngeal flaps in patients who have the Pierre Robin syndrome. *Plast Reconstr Surg* 1976; 58:184–186.

160. Kravath RE, Pollak CP, Borowiecki B: Obstructive sleep apnea and death associated with surgical correction in velopharyngeal incompetence. *J Pediatr* 1980; 86:645–648.

161. Lee JTR, Kingston HGG: Airway obstruction due to massive lingual edema following cleft palate surgery. *Can Anaesth Soc J* 1985; 32:265–267.

162. Bell C, Oh TH, Loeffler J: Massive macroglossia and airway obstruction after cleft palate repair. *Anesth Analg* 1988; 67:71–74.

163. Tate N: Deaths from tonsillectomy. *Lancet* 1963; 2:1090–1091.

164. Alexander DW, Graft TD, Kelley E: Factors in tonsillectomy mortality. *Arch Otolaryngol* 1965; 82:409–411.

165. Smith RM: Anesthesia for plastic surgery, in Smith RM (ed): *Anesthesia for Infants and Children,* ed 4. St. Louis, Mosby, 1980, pp 408–421.

166. Haselby KA, McNiece WL: Respiratory obstruction from uvular edema in a pediatric patient. *Anesth Analg* 1983; 62:1127–1128.

167. Eger EI, Severinghaus JW: The rate of rise of $PaCO_2$ in the apneic anesthetized patient. *Anesthesiology* 1961; 22:419–425.

168. Frumin MJ, Epstein RM, Cohen G: Apneic oxygenation in man. *Anesthesiology* 1959; 20:789–798.

169. Emhardt JD, Weisberger EC, Dierdorf SF, et al: The rise of arterial carbondioxide during apnea in children. *Anesthesiology* 1988; 69:A779.

170. Morikawa S, Safar P, DeCarlo J: Influence of head-jaw

position on upper airway patency. *Anesthesiology* 1961; 22:265–270.

171. Fink BR: The etiology and treatment of laryngeal spasm. *Anesthesiology* 1956; 17:569–577.

172. Suruki M, Sasaki CT: Laryngeal spasm: A neurophysiologic redifinition. *Ann Otol* 1977; 86:150–157.

173. Roy WL, Lerman J: Laryngospasm in paediatric anaesthesia. *Can J Anaesth* 1988; 35:93–98.

174. Olsson GL, Hallen B: Laryngospasm during anesthesia. A computer aided incidence study in 136,929 patients. *Acta Anaesthesiol Scand* 1984; 28:2567–575.

175. Cook DR, Westman H, Rosenfeld L, et al: Pulmonary edema in infants: Possible association with intramuscular succinylcholine. *Anesth Analg* 1981; 60:220–223.

176. Lee KWT, Downes JJ: Pulmonary edema secondary to laryngospasm in children. *Anesthesiology* 1983; 59:347–349.

177. Baraka A: Intravenous lidocaine controls extubation laryngospasm in children. *Anesth Analg* 1978; 57:506–507.

178. Barin ES, Stevenson IF, Donnelly GL: Pulmonary edema following acute upper airway obstruction. *Anaesth Intens Care* 1986; 14:54–57.

179. Kanter RK, Watchko JF: Pulmonary edema associated with upper airway obstruction. *Am J Dis Child* 1984; 138:356–358.

180. Sofer S, Bar-Ziv J, Scharf SM: Pulmonary edema following relief of upper airway obstruction. *Chest* 1984; 86:401–403.

181. Warner LO, Beach TP, Martino JD: Negative pressure pulmonary oedema secondary to airway obstruction in an intubated infant. *Can J Anaesth* 1988; 35:507–510.

182. Koka BV, Jeon IS, Andre JM, et al: Postintubation croup in children. *Anesth Analg* 1977; 56:501–505.

183. Finholt DA, Henry DB, Raphaely RC: Factors affecting leak around tracheal tubes in children. *Can Anaesth Soc J* 1985; 32:326–329.

184. DiCarlo JV, Sanders AI, Sweeney MF: Airway complications of endotracheal intubation in pediatric patients: Effect of endotracheal tube fit. *Anesthesiology* 1988; 69:A775.

185. Berry FA: Clinical course of traumatic croup, in Berry FA (ed): *Anesthetic Management of Difficult and Routine Pediatric Patients.* New York, Churchill Livingstone, 1986, pp 437–438.

186. Maze A, Block E: Stridor in pediatric patients: A Review. *Anesthesiology* 1979; 50:132–145.

187. Adair JC, Ring WH, Jordan WS, et al: Ten year experience with IPPB in the treatment of acute laryngo tracheobronchitis. *Anesth Analg* 1971; 50:649–655.

188. Westley CR, Brooks JG, Cotton EK: Nebulized racemic epinephrine by IPPB for the treatment of croup. *Am J Dis Child* 1978; 132:484–487.

189. Loomis JC: Pediatric intensive care, in Gregory GA (ed): *Pediatric Anesthesia.* New York, Churchill Livingstone, 1983, pp 915–1020.

190. Tunnessen WW, Feinstein AR: The steroid croup controversy: An analytical review of methodologic problems. *J Pediatr* 1980; 96:751–756.

191. Cantrell RW, Bell RA, Morioka WT: Acute epiglottitis:

Intubation versus tracheostomy. *Laryngoscope* 1978; 88:994–1005.

192. Pavlin EG: Respiratory pharmacology of inhaled anesthetic agents, in Miller RD (ed): *Anesthesia,* ed 2. New York, Churchill Livingstone, 1986, pp 667–699.

193. Bailey PL, Stanley TH: Pharmacology of intravenous narcotic anesthetics, in Miller RD (ed): *Anesthesia,* ed 2. New York, Churchill Livingstone, 1986, pp 745–797.

194. Hamza J, Ecoffey C, Gross JB: Ventilatory response to CO_2 following intravenous ketamine in children. *Anesthesiology* 1989; 70:422–425.

195. Koehntop DE, Rodman JH, Brundage DM, et al: Pharmacokinetics of fentanyl in neonates. *Anesth Analg* 1986; 65:227–233.

196. Hertzka RE, Gauntlett IS, Fisher DM, et al: Fentanyl induced ventilatory depression: Effects of age. *Anesthesiology* 1989; 70:213–218.

197. Yaster M, Koehler RC, Traystman RJ: Effects of fentanyl on peripheral and cerebral hemodynamics in neonatal lambs. *Anesthesiology* 1987; 66:524–530.

198. Way WL, Costley EC, Way EL: Respiratory sensitivity of newborn infants to meperidine and morphine. *Clin Pharmacol Ther* 1965; 6:454–461.

199. Way WL, Trevor AJ: Pharmacology of intravenous nonnarcotic anaesthetics, in Miller RD (ed): *Anesthesia,* ed 2. New York, Churchill Livingstone, 1986, pp 799–833.

200. Stanley TH, Webster LR: Anesthetic requirements and cardiovascular effects of fentanyl-oxygen and fentanyl-diazepam-oxygen anesthesia in man. *Anesth Analg* 1978; 57:411–416.

201. Chinyanga HM, Vandenberghe H, MacLeod S, et al: Assessment of immediate postanesthetic recovery in young children following intravenous morphine infusions, halothane and isoflurane. *Can Anaesth Soc J* 1984; 31:28–35.

202. Steward DJ: A trial of enflurane for paediatric outpatient anaesthesia. *Can Anaesth Soc J* 1977; 24:603–608.

203. Mason LJ, Betts EK: Leg lift and maximum inspiratory force, clinical signs of neuromuscular blockade reversal in neonates and infants. *Anesthesiology* 1980; 52:441–442.

204. Shimada Y, Yoshiya I, Tanaka K, et al: Crying vital capacity and maximal inspiratory pressure as clinical indicators of readiness for weaning of infants less than one year of age. *Anesthesiology* 1979; 51:456–459.

205. Ali HH, Savavese JJ: Monitoring of neuromuscular function. *Anesthesiology* 1976; 45:216–249.

206. Ali HH, Uhing JE, Gray TC: Quantative assessment of residual antidepolarizing block. Part II. *Br J Anaesth* 1971; 43:478–485.

207. Edmonds JF: Postoperative cardiorespiratory care, in Steward DJ (ed): Some aspects of paediatric anaesthesia. New York, Elsevier, 1982, pp 355–369.

208. Ngai SH, Berkowitz BA, Yan JC, et al: Pharmacokinetics of naloxone in rats and in man. *Anesthesiology* 1976; 44:398–401.

209. Salem MR, Wong AY, Collins VJ: The pediatric patient with a full stomach. *Anesthesiology* 1973; 39:435–440.

210. Berquist WE, Rachelefsky GS, et al: Gastroesophageal

reflux associated recurrent pneumonia and chronic asthma in children. *Pediatrics* 1981; 68:29–35.

211. Johnson DG, Jolley SG: Gastroesophageal reflux in infants and children: *Surg Clin North Am* 1981; 61:1101–1115.

212. Burgess GE, Cooper JR, Marino RJ, et al: Laryngeal compliance after tracheal extubation. *Anesthesiology* 1979; 51:73–77.

213. Opie JC, Chayne H, Steward DJ: Intravenous atropine rapidly reduces lower esophageal sphincter pressure in infants and children. *Anesthesiology* 1987; 67:899–900.

214. Graff TD, Phillips OC, Benson BW, et al: Baltimore anesthesia study committee: Factors in pediatric anesthesia mortality. *Anesth Analg* 1964; 43:407–414.

215. Rigatto H: Apnea. *Ped Clin North Am* 1982; 29:1105–1116.

216. American Academy of Pediatrics task force on prolonged infantile apnea: Prolonged infantile apnea, 1985. *Pediatrics* 1985; 76:129–131.

217. Daily WJR, Klaus M, Meyer HBP: Apnea in premature infants: Monitoring, incidence, heart rate changes and an effect of environmental temperature. *Pediatrics* 1969; 43:510–518.

218. Fenner A, Schalk U, Hoenicke JE, et al: Periodic breathing in prematures and neonatal babies. *Pediatr Res* 1973; 7:174–183.

219. Davi M, Sankaran K, Simons K, et al: Physiological changes induced by theophylline in the treatment of apnea of preterm infants. *J Pediatr* 1978; 92:91–95.

220. Kattwinkel J: Neonatal apnea: Pathogenesis and therapy. *J Pediatr* 1977; 90:342–347.

221. Hoppenbrouwers T, Hodgman JE, Harper RN, et al: Polygraphic studies of normal infants during the first six months of life: Incidence of apnea and periodic breathing. *Pediatrics* 1977; 60:418–425.

222. Perlman JM, Volpe JJ: Episodes of apnea and bradycardia in the preterm newborn: Impact on cerebral circulation. *Pediatrics* 1985; 76:333–338.

223. Steward DJ: Preterm infants are more prone to complications following minor surgery than are term infants. *Anesthesiology* 1982; 56:304–306.

224. Liu LMP, Cote CJ, Goudsouzian NG, et al: Life-threatening apnea in infants recovering from anesthesia. *Anesthesiology* 1983; 59:506–510.

225. Kurth CD, Spitzer AR, Broennle AM, et al: Postoperative apnea in preterm infants. *Anesthesiology* 1987; 66:483–488.

226. Welborn LG, Ramirez N, Oh TH, et al: Postanesthetic apnea and periodic breathing in infants. *Anesthesiology* 1986; 65:658–661.

227. Gregory GA, Steward DJ: Life-threatening perioperative apnea in the ex "preemie." *Anesthesiology* 1983; 59:495–498.

228. Mayhew JF, Bourke DJ, Guinee WS: Evaluation of the premature infant at risk for postoperative complications. *Can J Anaesth* 1987; 34:627–631.

229. Welborn LG, DeSoto H, Hannallah RS, et al: The use of caffeine in the control of post-anesthetic apnea in former premature infants. *Anesthesiology* 1988; 68:796–798.

230. Welborn LG, Hannallah RS, Fink K, et al: The role of caffeine in the prevention of postoperative apnea in former premature infants. *Anesthesiology* 1988; 69: A753.

231. Tetzlaff JE, Anand DW, Pudimat MA, et al: Postoperative apnea in a full term infant. *Anesthesiology* 1988; 69:426–428.

232. Vidyasagar D: Clinical diagnosis of respiratory failure in infants and children, in Gregory GA (ed): Respiratory failure in the child. *Clin Crit Care Med* 1981; 3:1–10.

233. Downes JJ, Fulgencio T, Raphael RC: Acute respiratory failure in infants and children. *Ped Clin North Am* 1972; 19:423–445.

234. McGill WA, Coveler LA, Epstein BS: Subacute upper respiratory tract infection in small children. *Anesth Analg* 1979; 58:331–333.

235. Rockoff MA: Pre-existing medical conditions in pediatric anesthesia. *ASA Refresher Course* 1983; 236.

236. Downes JJ, Nicodemus HF, Pierce WS, et al: Acute respiratory failure in infants following cardiovascular surgery. *J Thorac Cardiovasc Surg* 1970; 59:21–37.

237. Crone RK: Assisted ventilation in children, in Gregory GA (ed): Respiratory failure in the child. *Clin Crit Care Med* 1981; 3:17–29.

238. Yeh TS, Holbrook PR: Monitoring during assisted ventilation of children, in Gregory GA (ed): Respiratory failure in the child. *Clin Crit Care Med* 1981; 3:31–51.

239. Daly BDT, Hughes DA, Norman JC: Alveolar masophometrics: Effects of positive endexpiratory pressure. *Surgery* 1974; 76:624–629.

240. Johnson B, Ahlstrom H, Lindroth M, et al: Continuous positive airway pressure: Modes in relation to clinical application. *Ped Clin North Am* 1980; 27:687–699.

241. Suter PM, Fairley HB, Isenberg M: Optimum end expiratory airway pressure in patients with acute pulmonary failure. *N Engl J Med* 1975; 292:284–289.

242. Perkins RM, Levin DL: Adverse effects of positive pressure ventilation in children, in Gregory GA (ed): Respiratory failure in the child. *Clin Critic Care Med* 1981; 3:163–187.

243. Downes JJ, Goldberg AI: Airway management, mechanical ventilation, and cardiopulmonary resuscitation, in Scarpelli EM, Auld PAM, Goldman HS (eds): *Pulmonary Disease of the Fetus, Newborn and Child.* Philadelphia, Lea & Febiger, 1978, pp 99–131.

244. Woolcock AJ, Vincent NJ, Macklem PT: Frequency dependence of compliance as test for obstruction in the small airways. *J Clin Invest* 1969; 48:1097–1106.

245. Hayes B, Robinson JJ: An assessment of methods of humidification of inspired gas. *Br J Anaesth* 1970; 42:94–104.

246. Forbes AR: Temperature, humidity and mucous flow in the intubated trachea. *Br J Anaesth* 1974; 46:29–34.

247. Klein EF, Graves SA: "Hot pot" tracheitis. *Chest* 1974; 65:225–226.

248. Downs JB, Klein EF, Desautels D, et al: Intermittent mandatory ventilation: A new approach to weaning patients from mechanical ventilators. *Chest* 1973; 64:331–335.

249. Kirby RR, Robinson EJ, Shultz J: Continuous flow

ventilation as an alternative to assisted or controlled ventilation in infants. *Anesth Analg* 1972; 51:871–875.

250. Dammann JF, McAslan TC: Optimal flow pattern for mechanical ventilation of the lungs. *Crit Care Med* 1977; 5:129–136.

251. Fuleihan SF, Wilson RS, Pontoppidan H: Effect of mechanical ventilation with end-expiratory pause on blood–gas exchange. *Anesth Analg* 1976; 55:122–130.

252. McWilliams BC: Mechanical ventilation in pediatric patients. *Clin Chest Med* 1987; 8:597–609.

253. Crone RK: Acute circulatory failure in children. *Pediatr Clin North Am* 1980; 27:525–538.

254. Battersby EF, Hatch DJ, Towey RM: The effects of prolonged naso-endotracheal intubation in children. *Anaesthesia* 1977; 32:154–157.

255. Raphaely R: Pediatric intensive care. *ASA Refresher Course* 1981; 232A.

256. Othersen HB: Intubation injuries of the trachea in children. *Ann Surg* 1979; 189:601–606.

257. Donn SM, Kuhus LR: Mechanism of endotracheal tube movement with change of head position in the neonate. *Ped Radiol* 1980; 9:32–40.

258. Todres ID, Debros F, Kramer SS, et al: Endotracheal tube displacement in the newborn infant. *J Pediatr* 1976; 89:126–127.

259. Gregory GA: Respiratory care of the child. *Crit Care Med* 1980; 8:582–587.

260. Perkin RM, Levin DL: Adverse effects of positive pressure ventilation in children, in Gregory GA (ed): Respiratory failure in the child. *Clin Crit Care Med* 1981; 3:163–187.

261. Browning DH, Graves SA: Incidence of aspiration with endotracheal tubes in children. *J Pediatr* 1983; 102:582–584.

262. Redding GJ, Fan L, Cotton EK, et al: Partial obstruction of endotracheal tubes in children. *Crit Care Med* 1979; 7:227–231.

263. Todres ID, Hinkle AJ: Pulmonary care during endotracheal intubation. *Clin Crit Care Med* 1981; 3:11–16.

264. Berman LS, Fox WW, Raphaely RC: Optimum levels of CPAP for tracheal extubation of newborn infants. *J Pediatr* 1976; 89:109–112.

265. Davies H, Kichtmann R, Gordon I, et al: Regional ventilation in infancy. *N Engl J Med* 1985; 313:1626–1628.

266. Abramowitz MD, Oh TH, Epstein BS, et al: The antiemetic effect of droperidol following outpatient strabismus surgery in children. *Anesthesiology* 1983; 59:579–583.

267. Hardy JF, Charest J, Gironard G, et al: Nausea and vomiting after strabismus surgery in preschool children. *Can Anaesth Soc J* 1986; 33:57–62.

268. Lerman J, Eustis S, Smith DR: Effect of droperidol pretreatment on postanesthetic vomiting in children undergoing strabismus surgery. *Anesthesiology* 1986; 65:322–325.

269. Nicolson SC, Kaya KM, Betts EK: The effect of preoperative oral droperidol on the incidence of postoperative emesis after paediatric strabismus surgery. *Can J Anaesth* 1988; 35:364–367.

270. Mather L, Mackie J: The incidence of postoperative pain in children. *Pain* 1983; 15:271–282.

271. Beyer JE, DeGood DE, Ashley LC, et al: Patterns of

postoperative analgesic use with adults and children following cardiac surgery. *Pain* 1983; 17:71–81.

272. Tyler DC: Respiratory effects of pain in a child after thoracotomy. *Anesthesiology* 1989; 70:873–874.

273. Anand KJS, Hickey PR: Pain and its effect in the human neonate and fetus. *N Engl J Med* 1987; 317:1322–1329.

274. Steward DJ: Psychological preparation and premedication, in Gregory GA (ed): *Pediatric Anesthesia.* New York, Churchill Livingstone, 1983, pp 423–436.

275. Egbert LD, Battit GE, Welch CF, et al: Reduction of postoperative pain by encouragement and instruction of patients. *N Engl J Med* 1964; 270:825–927.

276. Smith RM, Steston J, Sanchez-Salazar A: Postoperative distress in children. *Anesthesiology* 1961; 22:145.

277. Bray RJ: Postoperative analgesia provided by morphine infusion in children. *Anaesthesia* 1983; 38:1075–1078.

278. Olkkola KT, Maunuksela EL, Korpela R, et al: Kinetics and dynamics of postoperative intravenous morphine in children. *Clin Pharm Therap* 1988; 44:128–136.

279. Dodd E, Wang JM, Rauck RL: Patient controlled analgesia for post surgical pediatric patients ages 6–16 years. *Anesthesiology* 1988; 69:A372.

280. Means LJ, Allen HM, Lockabill SJ, et al: Recovery room initiation of patient-controlled analgesia in pediatric patients. *Anesthesiology* 1988; 69:A772.

281. Rodgers BM, Webb CJ, Stergios D, et al: Patient-controlled analgesia in pediatric patients. *J Pediatr Surg* 1988; 23:259–262.

282. Forestner JD: Postoperative Ketamine analgesia in children. *South Med J* 1988; 81:1253–1257.

283. Shandling B, Steward DJ: Regional anesthesia for postoperative pain in pediatric outpatient surgery. *J Pediatr Surg* 1980; 15:477–480.

284. Blaise G, Roy WL: Postoperative pain relief after hypospadias repair in pediatric patients: Regional analgesia versus systemic analgesics. *Anesthesiology* 1986; 65:84–86.

285. Hannallah RS, Broadman LM, Belman AB, et al: Comparison of ilio inguinal/ilio hypogastric block for control of postorchiopexy pain in pediatric ambulatory surgery. *Anesthesiology* 1987; 66:832–834.

286. Arthur DS, McNicol LR: Local anesthetic techniques in paediatric surgery. *Br J Anaesth* 1986; 58:760–778.

287. Zsigmond EK, Downs JR: Plasma cholinesterase activity in newborns and infants. *Can Anaesth Soc J* 1971; 18:278–285.

288. Meffin P, Long GJ, Thomas J: Clearance and metabolism of mepivacaine in the human neonate. *Clin Pharmacol Ther* 1973; 14:218–225.

289. Rothstein P, Arthur GR, Feldman H, et al: Pharmacokinetics of bupivacaine in children following intercostal block. *Anesthesiology* 1982; 57:A426.

290. Eyres RL, Oppenheim RC, Brown TCK: Plasma bupivacaine concentration in children during caudal epidural analgesia. *Anaesth Intens Care* 1983; 11:20–22.

291. Ecoffey C, Desparmet J, Berdeaux A, et al: Pharmokinetics of lidocaine in children following caudal anesthesia. *Br J Anaesth* 1984; 56:1399–1402.

292. Ecoffey C, Desparmet J, Maury M, et al: Bupivacaine

in children Pharmokinetics following caudal anesthesia. *Anesthesiology* 1985; 63:447–448.

293. Rice LJ, Broadman LM, Hannallah RS: Regional anesthesia in pediatric patients. *Adv Anesthesia* 1989; 6:291–324.

294. Yaster M, Wetzel RC: Pediatric regional anesthesia. *Anesth Rep* 1988; 1:120–129.

295. Tree-Trakarn T, Pirayavaraporn S, Lerta-Kyamance J: Topical anesthesia for relief of post-circumcision pain. *Anesthesiology* 1987; 67:395–399.

296. Berry FR: Analgesia in patients with fractured shaft of the femur. *Anaesthesia* 1977; 32:576–577.

297. Shelly FR: Analgesia in patients with fractured shaft of the femur. *Anaesthesia* 1977; 32:576–577.

297. Shelley MP: Intercostal nerve blockade for children. *Anaesthesia* 1987; 41:541–544.

298. Ecoffey C, Dubousset AM, Samii K: Lumbar and thoracic epidural anesthesia for urologic and upper abdominal surgery in infants and children. *Anesthesiology* 1986; 65:87–90.

299. Desparmet J, Meistelmann C, Barre J, et al: Continuous epidural infusion of bupivacaine for postoperative pain relief in children. *Anesthesiology* 1987; 67:108–111.

300. McIlvaine WB, Knox RF, Jones MA, et al: Intrapleural bupivacaine for analgesia after subcostal incision in children. *Reg Anesth* 1988; 13:31.

301. McIlvaine WB, Knox RF, Jones MA, et al: Continuous infusion of bupivacaine via intrapleural catheter for analgesia after thoracotomy in children. *Anesthesiology* 1988; 69:261–264.

302. Schulte-Steinberg O, Rahlf VW: Spread of extradural analgesia following caudal injection in children. *Br J Anaesth* 1977; 49:1027–1034.

303. Takasaki M, Dohi S, Kawabata Y, et al: Dosage of lidocaine for caudal anesthesia in infants and children. *Anesthesiology* 1977; 47:527–529.

304. Armitage EN: Regional anesthesia in pediatrics. *Clin Anaesth* 1985; 3:553–568.

305. Rice LJ: Regional anesthesia in pediatrics. *ASA Refresher Course* 1988; 123.

306. Krane EJ: Delayed respiratory depression in a child after caudal epidural morphine. *Anesth Analg* 1988; 67:79–82.

307. Attia J, Ecoffey C, Saudouk P, et al: Epidural morphine in children: Pharmacokinetics and CO_2 sensitivity. *Anesthesiology* 1986; 65:590–594.

308. Rosen KR, Rosen DA: Caudal epidural morphine for control of pain followig open heart surgery in children. *Anesthesiology* 1989; 70:418–421.

309. Glenski JA, Warner MA, Dawson B, et al: Postoperative use of epidurally administered morphine in children and adolescents. *Mayo Clin Proc* 1984; 59:530–533.

310. Dickens C: *The Posthumous Papers of the Pickwick Club.* London, Chapman & Hall, 1837.

311. Caton R: A case of narcolepsy. *Br Med J* 1880; 358.

312. Kerr WJ, Lagen JB: Postural syndrome related to obesity leading to postural emphysema and cardiorespiratory failure. *Ann Intern Med* 1936; 10:569–595.

313. Guilleminault C, Tilkian A, Dement WC: The sleep apnea syndromes. *Annu Rev Med* 1976; 27:465–484.

314. Mandel EM, Reynolds CF: Sleep disorders associated with upper airway obstruction in children. *Ped Clin North Am* 1981; 28:897–903.

315. Orr WC: Utilization of polysomnography in the assessment of sleep disorders. *Med Clin North Am* 1985; 69:1153–1167.

316. Phillipson EA: Breathing disorders during sleep. *Basics of RD* 1979; 7:18–23.

317. Baker TL: Introduction to sleep and sleep disorders. *Med Clin North Am* 1985; 69:1123–1152.

318. Gastaut H, Tassinari CA, Duron B: Polygraphic study of the episodic diurnal and nocturnal manifestations of the Pickwickian syndrome 1966; *Brain Res* 2:167–186.

319. Chung F, Crago RR: Sleep apnea syndrome and anesthesia. *Can Anaesth Soc J* 1982; 29:439–445.

320. White DP: Central sleep apnea. *Med Clin North Am* 1985; 69:1205–1219.

321. Guilleminault C: Obstructive sleep apnea. The clinical syndrome and historical perspective. *Med Clin North Am* 1985; 69:1187–1203.

322. Brouillette RT, Fernback SK, Hunt CE: Obstructive sleep apnea in infants and children. *J Pediatr* 1982; 100:31–40.

323. Bradley TD, Phillipson EA: Pathogenesis and pathophysiology of the obstructive sleep apnea syndrome. *Med Clin North Am* 1985; 69:1169–1185.

324. Kuna ST, Remmers JE: Neural and anatomic factors related to upper airway occlusion during sleep. *Med Clin North Am* 1985; 69:1221–1242.

325. Schaefer M: Upper airway obstruction and sleep disorders in children with craniofacial anomalies. *Clin Plast Surg* 1982; 9:555–567.

326. Roa NL, Moss KS: Treacher Collins' syndrome with sleep apnea: Anesthetic considerations. *Anesthesiology* 1984; 60:71–73.

327. Shepard JW: Gas exchange and hemodynamics during sleep. *Med Clin North Am* 1985; 69:1243–1264.

328. Weinberg S, Kravath R, Phillips L, et al: Episodic complete airway obstruction in children with undiagnosed obstructive sleep apnea. *Anesthesiology* 1984; 60:356–358.

329. Wittels EH: Obesity and hormonal factors in sleep and sleep apnea. *Med Clin North Am* 1985; 69:1265–1280.

330. Lombard RM, Zwillich CN: Medical therapy of obstructive sleep apnea. *Med Clin North Am* 1985; 69:1317–1335.

331. Thawley SE: Surgical treatment of obstructive sleep apnea. *Med Clin North Am* 1985; 69:1337–1358.

332. Eliaschar I, Lavie P, Halpern E, et al: Sleep apneic episodes as indication for adeno-tonsillectomy. *Arch Otolaryngol* 1980; 106:492–496.

333. Frank Y, Kravath RE, Pollak CP, et al: Obstructive sleep apnea and its therapy: Clinical and polysomnographic manifestations. *Pediatrics* 1983; 71:737–742.

334. Gabrielczyk MR: Acute airway obstruction after palato pharnygoplasty for obstructive sleep apnea syndrome. *Anesthesiology* 1988; 69:941–943.

335. Tierney NM, Pollard BJ, Doran BRH: Obstructive sleep apnea. *Anesthesia* 1989; 44:235–237.

336. Warburton D, Stark AR, Taeusch HW: Apnea monitor

failure in infants with upper airway obstruction. *Pediatrics* 1977; 60:742–744.

337. Martin RJ, Sanders MH, Gray BA, et al: Acute and long term ventilatory effects of hyperoxia in the adult sleep apnea syndrome. *Am Rev Resp Dis* 1982; 125:175–180.

338. Rafferty TD, Ruskis A, Sasaki C, et al: Perioperative considerations in the management of tracheotomy for the obstructive sleep apnea patient. *Br J Anaesth* 1980; 52:619–622.

339. Ryan JF: Malignant hyperthermia, in Ryan JF, Todres ID, Cote CJ, Goudsouzian N (eds): *A Practice of Anesthesia for Infants and Children.* Orlando, Grune & Stratton, 1986, pp 243–251.

340. Gronert GA, Mott J, Lee J: Aetiology of malignant hyperthermia: Relationship to other diseases. *Br J Anaesth* 1988; 60:303–308.

341. Brownell AKW: Malignant hyperthermia: Relationship to other diseases. *Br J Anaesth* 1988; 60:303–308.

342. Dallman JH: Neuroleptic malignant syndrome: A review. *Milit Med* 1984; 149:471–473.

343. Caroff SN, Rosenberg H, Fletcher JE, et al: Malignant hyperthermia susceptibility in the neuroleptic malignant syndrome. *Anesthesiology* 1987; 67:20–25.

344. Kolb ME, Horne ML, Martz R: Dantrolene in human malignant hyperthermia: A multicenter study. *Anesthesiology* 1982; 56:254–262.

15 The Burned Patient

Steven A. Blau

Few patients require as much attention from the anesthesiologist at as many points in the course of their care as do the victims of thermal injury. The skills of the anesthesiologist are often required in the emergency room when the "acute" patient first presents and during the early days of his or her fluid resuscitation. The primary concerns at this time are respiratory and cardiovascular and include the "ABCs of trauma," namely the maintenance of airway, ventilation, and circulation. After the patient's cardiovascular status has stabilized, the patient will require the attention of the anesthesiologist during the repeated operative procedures that must be performed to "close" the burn wound. During this period of the hospital course, the *postanesthetic* care of the burn patient becomes merged with the *preanesthetic* care of the patient before the next operative procedure. In the surgical intensive care unit or the burn intensive care unit, the anesthesiologist will participate in the care of the patient between operative procedures especially in the areas of pulmonary management and pain control. The patient's course after the initial operative procedures to achieve wound coverage is marked by intensive rehabilitation and operative procedures aimed at reconstruction. At this point the anesthesiologist must deal with a "chronic" patient, possibly habituated to analgesics, and frequently presenting with anatomic and physiologic difficulties.

THE EARLY PERIOD: RESUSCITATION AND STABILIZATION

Respiratory Injuries
The major cause of death in childhood victims of fires in the United States today is smoke inhalation. Smoke inhalation in adults markedly affects the prognosis of patients in whom survival is likely based upon their age and the size of the burn. Few areas of the management of the burned patient, however, have caused as much confusion in those only casually associated with the care of these patients. Such terms as *respiratory burns, inhalation burns,* and the like are generally incorrect and should not be used. Rather, there are three distinct respiratory tract injuries in burn patients, which reflect different anatomic, physiologic, and pathologic processes; (1) upper airway injury; (2) smoke inhalation or lower tract injury; and (3) acute carbon monoxide poisoning. The patient may manifest any one or a combination of these complications early in his or her hospital course.

Upper Airway. Anatomically, an upper airway injury is an injury to the oropharynx, nasopharynx, or hypopharynx that leads to progressive edema with the risk of upper airway obstruction. The pathophysiologic process is heat injury with the consequent development of edema. The edema classically increases over the first 8 to 12 hours and usually resolves within 48 to 72 hours if no other injury is superimposed. The injury, with its concomitant risk of loss of airway, should be suspected in all patients who present with facial burns, especially those in which the patient has loss of mustache, nasal vibrissae, eyelashes, or eyebrows. Occasionally, patients will present with acute airway obstruction or frank stridor and no diagnostic efforts are required. Immediate intubation to protect the airway is indicated in these patients. Definitive diagnosis, however, usually requires upper endoscopy.

The standard endoscopic approach is usually direct laryngoscopy. The anesthesiologist examines the proximal airway down to the level of the vocal cords. Early evidence of erythema and edema is suggestive of burn injury and the trachea should be intubated to protect the airway. However, the signs of upper airway injury may not be visible at first and endoscopy should be repeated in a few hours.

In past years our own experience with laryngoscopy was generally unsatisfactory because less experienced staff members were unsure of the significance of the observations. Thus, almost all the patients with facial burns were intubated. This management is appropriate if the level of experience of the observer is inadequate. Several years ago, our primary diagnostic modality was changed to fiberoptic endoscopy with a flexible nasopharyngoscope, which is a more benign experience for the patient and allows reevaluation of the airway at frequent intervals. The incidence of intubation in our burn center fell consequent to the change without a significant increase in morbidity. The development of edema may be delayed by inadequate fluid resuscitation and therefore the significance of the absence of edema must be interpreted after considering other aspects of the patient's course.

In other centers where endoscopy of the lower tract is regularly performed (see below, "Smoke Inhalation & Lower Tract Injury"), the flexible fiberoptic bronchoscope provides the same view, and the endotracheal tube can easily be advanced over the bronchoscope if intubation is indicated. There is some question, however, whether this "violation" of the tracheobronchial tree does not by itself contribute to the morbidity of lower tract injuries.

Safety is a key issue when the decision is made *not* to intubate. Airway obstruction in these patients is a very acute event and the sudden obstruction of an already narrowed airway can result in death despite the prompt availability of medical assistance. Oxygen extraction may already be maximal and the tolerance of hypoxia is minimal. All patients in whom intubation has not been effected must be observed carefully with frequent assessment of the airway. The patients should be asked to phonate at regular intervals and their forced vital capacity assessed simply by asking them to exhale forcefully and rapidly. In the interests of patient safety, all patients with head and neck burns who are being transferred to another institution should be intubated prior to transfer.

Is nasotracheal intubation preferable to endotracheal intubation in these patients? Although the former probably reduces patient discomfort and is more commonly reported by burn centers,[1-3] the decision is usually made on the basis of the experience of the anesthesiologist. These patients will require extensive suctioning to maintain pulmonary toilet, especially if there is a lower tract injury, and some clinicians claim that the endotracheal route with the ability to place a larger-sized tube is therefore preferable.

Smoke Inhalation and Lower Tract Injury. Lower tract injuries, anatomically, are injuries to the tracheobronchial tree and the respiratory epithelium. The length of the airway proximal to the vocal cords and its structure make it generally difficult to transmit hot gases to the tracheobronchial tree. Thus the term "inhalation burn" is a physical misnomer. The only exception to this rule occurs with superheated steam, whose "particle" size is sufficiently small and hot microscopic droplets may actually reach the bronchi. Physiologically, this injury is not mediated by heat, but by chemicals, with various components of smoke producing atelectasis, the elaboration of fluid, an increase in vascular permeability, and pneumonitis.[4]

Patients presenting with isolated lower tract injuries and smoke inhalation are frequently asymptomatic on their presentation to the emergency room. Two important historical events should be sought in the patient with burn injury that are suggestive of increased risk of lower tract injuries: a history of a closed-space fire and a period of unconsciousness. The former suggests the physical confinement of smoke increasing the ambient concentration of toxic substances. The latter suggests that the patient experienced a period of hypoxemia or anoxemia.

If the patient has stridor and signs of upper airway injury, the initial management by intubation to protect the upper airway is initially sufficient for this injury. In the absence of obvious signs of upper airway injury, the physician must establish the diagnosis of a smoke inhalation. The most sensitive means of diagnosing these injuries is by demonstrating ventilation–perfusion mismatch using a xenon-133 scan.[5] Unfortunately, despite its sensitivity, financial and other considerations make use of this nuclear medicine study relatively uncommon. Bronchoscopy may establish the disease early by demonstrating erythema and edema of the tracheobronchial tree or blunting of the usually sharp bronchial septa or even frank ulceration of the respiratory mucosa.

Routine diagnostic techniques are generally unreliable. Few patients present in acute pulmonary edema and auscultation will often miss the diagnosis. Early chest radiographs usually demonstrate clear lung fields. Arterial blood gases may manifest hyperventilation with decreased P_{CO_2} and normal P_{O_2}, but these findings are only suggestive of smoke inhalation at best. Patients frequently have elevated carboxyhemoglobin levels, which should alert the staff to the *possibility* of smoke inhalation. The usual course of smoke inhalation injury is relatively insidious and severity of the injury increases over the first few days.

Management is expectant. With the development of pulmonary edema and the consequences of ventilation–perfusion (V/Q) mismatch, ventilatory support requires mechanical ventilation, enriched oxygen atmospheres, and the appropriate use of positive end-expiratory pressure (PEEP). Minimizing the volume of fluid infused, much as one would do for a patient with a pulmonary contusion, although theoretically beneficial, is not usually feasible in the burned patient. Few pharmacologic avenues of therapy are currently available.

Steroids are mentioned here to condemn their use. Although they may act to stabilize cell membranes and in animals the amount of fluid extravasated into the lungs is decreased,[6] their use is contraindicated by their concomitant immunosuppression. In other experimental studies, bacterial challenge increased the morbidity and mortality of animals receiving corticosteroids.[1] Moreover, in clinical studies,[7] steroids have not been shown to improve survival. The immunosuppression of the patient with extensive cutaneous injury and the increased portals of entry for bacteria in patients with large thermal burns contraindicates steroid use.

Prophylactic antibiotics are similarly condemned. The proteinaceous fluid that collects in the tracheobronchial tree, the loss of ciliary barrier function, and the diminished ability to the intubated patient to cough, all contribute to the incidence of postintubation pneumonia. Prophylactic antibiotics do not decrease the incidence, but rather increase the risk that the pathogens that are recovered will be more resistant to antibiotics.

The pharmacologic weapons of the future will probably take advantage of the role prostaglandins play in respiratory tract injury and the ability of specific drugs to interfere with and modify their metabolism. The adverse role of thromboxane is increasingly apparent.[8-11] Interventions with ibuprofen and indomethacin are today only at the level of laboratory animal studies, however.[12,13]

The role of oxygen-free radicals and other potent free radicals in potentiating damage is increasingly investigated.[14] Whereas some of the more benign antioxidant drugs such as vitamin C and vitamin A can be added to the patient's medical regimen with relatively little risk, their efficacy is unclear. Use of free radical scavengers will probably increase in the care of these patients either to interfere with the initial injury caused by smoke inhalation and its reperfusion component or as a means of dealing with the harmful effects of the enriched oxygen atmosphere that the patient must breathe.

Carbon Monoxide Poisoning. Although elevated levels of carbon monoxide may be *predictive* of the risk of smoke inhalation, there does not appear to be any evidence that carbon monoxide actually participates in the pathophysiology of that injury. Carbon monoxide affects all tissues, especially those of the brain and heart. Its mechanism of action stems from its increased affinity for hemoglobin (2000 times that of oxygen) and its consequent ability to displace oxygen from the hemoglobin moiety. The injury produced, however, is not exclusively one of anoxemia. There is a suggestion that carbon monoxide can be carried by hemoglobin and poison the cytochrome cascade in the mitochondria.[15-18] This latter mechanism has been suggested as an explanation for the incidence of cardiac damage,[16] neurologic impairment,[17] and fetal injury.[18]

The therapy for carbon monoxide poisoning is geared to the rapid elimination of the carbon monoxide by its competition with enriched oxygen environments. The half-life (T 1/2) of carboxyhemoglobin is almost four hours in room air at normal pressure ($FIO_2 = 0.21$, 1 atmosphere). By breathing 100% oxygen, the half-life falls to about an hour. In a hyperbaric pressure, breathing 100% oxygen (2.5 atmospheres), the T 1/2 falls to about 24 minutes.[19] Forced mechanical ventilation may also decrease the half-life of carboxyhemoglobin presumably by increasing the mass action of oxygen.[20] Few areas of respiratory management have provoked more controversy than the use of hyperbaric oxygen (HBO), which was generally discarded some years ago when the use of hyperbaric chambers for other conditions fell out of favor. This reaction may not have been warranted.

Published figures suggest a very high mortality in patients presenting with a carboxyhemoglobin level of 60% or greater. In our center, where hyperbaric oxygen is used extensively for this condition, many patients have survived these levels.[19] Additional support for HBO has been provided by other centers,[21,22] although many burn centers have found that the use of an out-of-hospital facility significantly compromises the management of the patient's thermal injury.[23]

There is very little experience with the use of free radical scavengers to combat the probably increased numbers of free radicals formed during treatment with these high concentrations of oxygen. Experiences with allopurinol, n-acetylcysteine (with its abundance of sulfhydryl bonds),[24] and vitamin E have been reported.

More important in the clinical management of patients after HBO therapy is a need to be aware of the problems associated with increased atmospheric pressure. The timing of the pressurization or ''dive,'' the recovery period, and the treatment interval are designed to avoid the problems of oxygen toxicity. Barotrauma is not uncommon, especially rupture of the tympanic membrane. Common problems that are experienced and recognized early in the course of caring for patients undergoing HBO therapy are consequent to the changing properties of gases at elevated pressures. Endotracheal tube balloons filled with air take up less volume at hyperbaric conditions and the ET tube can be dislodged. Consequently the balloon is inflated with water, which is less compressible under pressure. Similarly, a small pneumothorax resulting, for instance, from central venous cannulation and controlled during the pressurization, may develop into a bigger problem during decompression.

The neurologic recovery of our patients treated with HBO therapy for isolated carbon monoxide poisoning is generally good and appears to be better than for those patients treated by the more conventional means of forced mechanical ventilation at high oxygen concentrations but at atmospheric pressure. This observation, however, could reflect observer bias. There are no good prospective randomized trials of HBO therapy for carbon monoxide poisoning.

Tracheostomy. The role of tracheostomy in the management of the burned patient mirrors the enthusiasm for the technique in critically ill patients in general. The development of low pressure cuffs that allow longer periods of intubation without causing tracheal injury led to relatively long periods of naso- or orotracheal intubation prior to resorting to surgery. The burn patient was felt to be an especially poor candidate for tracheostomy because of the increased potential for mediastinitis. In recent years, however, the realization of the role of tracheostomy in helping to wean patients from mechanical ventilation has seen the return of this operation in burned patients.[25,26] Much like their critically ill surgical ''cousins,'' burn patients seem to be able to tolerate the procedure and to be removed more rapidly from mechanical ventilation.

FLUID RESUSCITATION

The second component of the resuscitative phase of burn injury is fluid resuscitation. The burn patient's intravascular volume decreases as a result of losses of fluid through the denuded burn wound, into non-burned tissues consequent to increases in vascular permeability, and evaporative losses into the circuit of the ventilator and into the room through the burn wound. The goal of restoration of the intravascular volume space is really the restoration of the cardiac output.

The ''normal'' relationship between preload (a function of intravascular volume) and cardiac output may not be maintained in patients with significant burn injuries. Ex vivo hearts of burned animals mirror the clinical picture seen in patients[27] and demonstrate fixed temporal defects in cardiac contractility.[28] The apparent defect in the Frank Starling relationship, which necessitates voluminous fluid expansion, was originally attributed to circulating burn toxins, a concept not universally accepted. Recent experience with free radical damage in other clinical situations has renewed interest in this cardiac defect and free radical scavengers have been applied in experimental animal models.[29] Despite the cardiac role in decreasing cardiac output seen in untreated burns, the principal clinical management continues to be fluid resuscitation. As in many other aspects of burn care, different centers—both in this country and abroad—have adopted specific resuscitation regimens[30] that provide satisfactory clinical results. Although the

most commonly used regimen is the Baxter or Parkland formula, it is far from a universally accepted therapy (Table 15–1).

Some general principles apply. The previous controversy about the role of colloid and crystalloid therapy in the first day of therapy has generally been resolved in favor of pure crystalloid expansion. The rationale for this lies in the increased capillary leak in the early burn period, which mitigates against any benefit from protein solutions. Extravascular protein exerts no beneficial oncotic pressure gradient.

The decision as to which crystalloid is usually between hypotonic or almost isotonic fluids (commonly Ringer's lactate) and hypertonic fluid regimens. Few clinical comparisons of these regimens have been reported.[31-35] Hypotonic regimens usually result in higher fluid volumes and patients tend to develop more peripheral edema. Some investigators have suggested that this increased fluid therapy adversely affects pulmonary management and the increased tissue edema increases the depth of the burn injury by increasing the distance between the burn wound and its blood supply.

Statistical analysis has demonstrated that patients resuscitated with the Baxter or Parkland formula receive an average of 4 cc per kilogram body weight per percentage burn surface area in the first 24 hours. This number thus became the ''formula'' for the resuscitation of the burn patient. The patient, however, is not treated by formula, but by the clinical response to fluid therapy, namely cardiac output. Although cardiac output is frequently assessed in the critically ill patient *invasively* by the use of pulmonary artery catheterizations, many burn centers tend to avoid this technique as a routine, employing it only in high-risk patients. The immunosuppression seen in the burn patient is so severe that invasive monitor-

TABLE 15–1. SEVERAL PROTOCOLS ARE USED IN THE FLUID RESUSCITATION OF THE BURN PATIENT

Name	Solution
Parkland	Ringer's lactated solution 4.0 mL/kg/% burn
Brooke	Ringer's lactated solution 1.5 mL/kg/% burn + colloid 0.5 mL/kg/% burn + 5% dextrose in water, 2000 mL
Modified Brooke	Ringer's lactated solution 2.0 mL/kg/% burn
Evans	Normal saline 0.1 mL/kg/% burn + colloid 1.0 mL/kg/% burn + 5% dextrose in water, 2000 mL
Hypertonic sodium chloride	Volume of fluid containing 250 mEq/L sodium to promote a urinary output of 30 mL/h

ing by placing a catheter in the heart and great vessels for two or three days seems physiologically expensive. Several centers have demonstrated that patients can be resuscitated without information from these catheters.

In the absence of hard data on cardiac output, most burn physicians rely on urine output as a guide to intravascular volume status, which is clinically practical for most patients without preexisting renal insufficiency. The goal in adults is to maintain an hourly urine output of 50 cc. In children, the goal is 1/2 to 1 cc per kilogram body weight per hour. The use of urine output is not as simple as it appears, however. Firstly, urine output often does not have the same association with cardiac output as it does in unburned patients. High levels of antidiuretic hormone (ADH) tend to cause oliguria. Secondly, the catecholamine response to injury increases circulating glucose levels and may lead to glycosuria. The osmotic effects tend to increase the urine output out of proportion to the cardiac output. Moreover, the therapy for hemoglobinemia or myoglobinemia requires the patient to have increased urine output to ''flush'' the kidneys. Finally, drugs such as dopamine result in increased diuresis and naturesis for the same volume of infused fluid and this increased urine output does not necessarily correlate with augmentation of cardiac output.

A 70-kilogram patient with burns over 50% of his or her body should require, according to the Parkland formula, $4 \times 70 \times 50$, or 14,000 cc in the first 24 hours, half of which is administered in the first 8 hours and half over the next 16. Patients with concomitant pulmonary injury have been shown to require more fluid. The peripheral edema produced by this prodigious volume of fluid infused prompted the development of hypertonic fluid regimens many years ago. The current interest in very hypertonic fluids (7.5% saline) in the management of hemorrhagic shock has led to an examination of the use of these fluids in burn patients.[36] The fluid infusion in burn patients, however, is continuous rather than bolus, perhaps minimizing the clinical value of these very hypertonic solutions.

Hypertonic fluid therapy in burn patients today usually means solutions whose sodium content ranges from 200 to 300 mEq/L. The anion composition used varies between centers. In general, the chloride content is less than 130 mEq/L because of the risk of development of hyperchloremic metabolic acidosis. Other ions used include lactate, bicarbonate, and acetate. Some studies in animals have suggested that there are differences in the physiologic and metabolic effects to these ions, but this area continues to remain controversial. What is generally accepted, though, is that patients resuscitated with hypertonic fluids require less total volume than do patients resuscitated with hypotonic fluid regimens. When the fluid therapy is described in terms of sodium infusion, however, the regimens are similar at 0.4 to 0.5 mEq sodium per kilogram body weight per percentage body surface area burned.

The sodium load, then, is not increased over that received in hypotonic fluid regimens. These solutions are well tolerated by all ages.[32–35,37] The regimens are not benign, however, and patients receiving therapy should be carefully monitored for electrolyte abnormalities, especially hypernatremia and hypokalemia.

The use of fluid resuscitation regimens in children is more complicated than that in adults. Formulas based upon weight are less reliable when they are applied to small children whose weight-to-volume ratio differs from that of adults. Blind application of the Parkland formula in a 15-kg child will result in the infusion of a volume of fluid that is actually less than maintenance. Modified volume schedules either add the extra volume to maintenance or calculate the fluid needs in terms of body surface area instead of weight. Other problems include the need for early glucose infusions, as children do not have adequate glycogen stores to maintain serum glucose; the need for supplemental calcium to maintain cardiac contractility; and inconsistencies in the ability of small children to metabolize lactate.

Somewhere between 16 and 24 hours after burn injury, the capillary leak that makes colloid therapy questionable decreases to the point that supplemental protein infusions are appropriate. These solutions include human serum albumin, fresh frozen plasma, and other oncotic products such as hydroxyethyl starch (HESPAN).[38] The rationale is obvious if one looks at the typical laboratory values of a patient resuscitated according to the Parkland formula, namely decreased serum sodium (133–135 mEq/L) and a markedly decreased serum albumin. The protein is infused largely to increase the colloid oncotic pressure and return fluid from the extravascular space into the intravascular space. There is some data that the protein infusion also increases cardiac output out of proportion to its ability to increase preload. This latter finding may not be completely valid as the temporal response of cardiac output must be considered. In experimental animals and in many patients, the cardiac output reaches a nadir some four to eight hours after burn injury and with program fluid resuscitation returns to normal about 24 hours after injury.[28,39,40] Experimental animals have been resuscitated more rapidly; however, the animals recieved four to five times the volumes usually administered early in comparable models of burn injury.[41]

After the first 24 hours, the goal has shifted somewhat mechanically from infusing fluids to retrieving fluids, and salt intake is restricted and colloid therapy predominates in most patients. Neurohumoral processes do not necessarily facilitate this task, however, and many patients will require some diuretic therapy during this phase of their resuscitation. Dopamine, as mentioned earlier, is especially useful at this point. The need to diurese the patient is predicated upon the desire to normalize the patient's cardiovascular status rapidly and bring the patient expeditiously to the operating room to begin excisional therapy.

THERMOREGULATION

One of the major problems with which the anesthesiologist must contend both during the operation and subsequently is altered thermoregulation. The burn patient has lost much of the normal ability to regulate his body temperature. A large portion of his vapor barrier has been lost with loss of the keratinized skin layer. The injured denuded skin weeps fluid into the dressing and water vapor into the air. The patient has also lost some of the ability to vasoconstrict unburned portions of the skin, thereby losing the ability to regulate evaporative losses of heat energy.

In the burn unit, the patient's environment is maintained at a high ambient temperature, usually on the order of 85 to 90°F., a point of thermoneutrality.[42] If the temperature is increased, the patient begins to perspire, and with the evaporation of that fluid continues to lose heat energy. Lowering the temperature increases the work that the patient must expend to maintain core temperature. This work of heating consumes calories that should support other vital activities.

In the operating room, the anesthesiologist must adequately warm the patient. Heating the room is relatively simple and effective although it tends to adversely affect the personnel caring for the patient. The expedient of leaving the room at frequent intervals or having a team of anesthesiologists, compromises the goal of decreasing traffic in the room to protect against infection.

A heating blanket under the patient is an acceptable alternative. In addition, inspired gases should be heated through the anesthetic apparatus using a heated nebulizer that results in a good heat exchange. It must be further remembered that in extensive excisions, a large surface is exposed during the procedure, further compromising the heating of the patient by increasing the surface area exposed to lose heat by radiation.

In the postanesthetic care unit (PACU) or in the burn unit, the methods to rewarm the patient are usually the use of a radiant heat shield or simply warming the room. The effect of this increased heat load on the patient and his or her fluid requirements is obvious.

The patient's own ability to rewarm after a surgical procedure can be directly compromised by the anesthesiologist. When placed in a cold environment, the patient responds by shivering, which is a manifestation of muscle contraction (with consumption of intracellular high energy phosphates and calories). This response can be blocked by prolonged anesthesia or by the use of neuromuscular blockers. Prolonged neuromuscular blockade has been shown to decrease the rate of return of core temperature in postoperative patients. Although no studies directly address this problem in thermally injured patients, they probably behave in a similar fashion.

All fluids administered during and immediately after the procedure should be heated, if possible. Blood products can be satisfactorily warmed through commercial blood warmers. Although these warmers *do* decrease the maximal flow rate of the intravenous line, the blood losses during burn excision are somewhat more predictable than those during operations performed in other types of trauma, and this diminution can be factored into the plan of fluid therapy.

FLUID MANAGEMENT DURING THE OPERATIVE PROCEDURE

The loss of vapor barrier obviously impacts upon fluid management intraoperatively. Although the patient is usually well hydrated prior to the operative procedure, as commonly evidenced by a good urine output or a satisfactory central venous pressure (CVP), a large amount of fluid will be lost during the procedure: both blood and proteinaceous fluid through wounds and salt and water. The patient should receive enough fluid to maintain a generous urine output during the procedure, but should not receive excessive amounts of salt, especially during the early days postburn. This is obvious as the patient generally has a positive sodium balance already and the anesthesiologist can only tip the balance further.

The most common procedure in the management of burn patients is excision and split-thickness skin grafting. Although in obvious third-degree burns, the tissue can be removed at the level of the superficial fascia, in deep second-degree burns and in burns where the depth is not readily apparent, the procedure of debridement is tangential excision or serial excision, increasing the depth of tissue exposed. The objective for the surgeon is to identify the most superficial tissue that can support a skin graft. This may be dermis in deep second-degree burns or fat, fascia, muscle, paratenon (but not tendon), or periosteum (but not bone). Serial excision is accompanied by major blood loss. Many, but not all, advocate the use of tourniquets when operating on extremities. The tourniquet definitely decreases the early blood loss but the avascular field sometimes makes it difficult to identify the end point of the excision. Moreover, the tourniquet is not suitable for the management of truncal or head and neck burns.

The amount of blood loss is prodigious and some centers have reported blood loss averaging from one-half to one unit of blood per percent burn excised. The anesthesiologist must be aware that the surgeon not only usually underestimates the amount of blood loss, but that he or she frequently unwittingly hides it in the sponges, sheets, and puddles on the floor. The anesthesiologist usually underestimates the blood loss as well, and patients require blood replacement in the postoperative period. Because of the significance of these fluid shifts, most surgeons restrict themselves to excision of 10 to 15% of the body surface area at one operation and try to contain their operation to about one and one-half hours.

Because patients are losing large amounts of colloid and protein along with blood, intraoperative colloid infusions are appropriate and indicated. The mild coagulopathy in these patients makes fresh frozen plasma (FFP) an especially useful colloid solution. This same thinking in terms of colloid replacement persists into the postoperative period with colloid playing an increasingly useful role in these patients.

The question of determining the end point of blood transfusion is more difficult to answer. The prevailing hematocrit in most critically ill patients in the ICU ranges from 25 to 30%, which represents a compromise between the rheologiocal properties of the blood (high hematocrits leading to increased microvascular viscosity) and the oxygen-carrying capacity of the blood. In the elderly patient and in the patient with preexisting cardiac disease, these numbers may be liberalized. Although the burn patient is frequently (especially after the fourth day of hospitalization) hypermetabolic and might be better served by a higher hematocrit, there is little data on the effect of higher hematocrits on the microvasculature flow of these patients.

Some concern has been raised over the effects of large-bolus infusions of albumin. It has been shown that aggressive exogenous albumin therapy results in higher serum albumins but lower nonalbumin proteins,[43,44] suggesting that the albumin in some way depressed the liver's synthesis of other proteins or caused redistribution of nonalbumin proteins. This problem has not been specifically addressed in burn patients.

A variety of pharmacologic techniques have been employed in decreasing the blood loss during excisional therapy. Topical thrombin solutions have been employed to decrease the blood loss during harvesting of split-thickness skin grafts and wound excision. Some anesthesiologists prefer this to the use of topical epinephrine solution because of the adverse effects of the latter as it is absorbed into the circulation. The risk of systemic effects from absorption may be overstated.[45] Other centers have demonstrated beneficial effects of vasopressin intravenously.[46]

Intraoperative maintenance of total parenteral nutrition (TPN) is probably still a necessity, although some recent studies have suggested that the cessation of a hyperglycemic solution does not always produce the rapid fall in serum glucose originally anticipated. The question is moot, however, as the anesthesiologist rarely has a need to decrease the rate of infusion of this solution. Moreover, the TPN line should never be interrupted for the infusion of other solutions. Not only might precipitation of the products in the line occur, but contamination may result.

Line contamination is a special problem in immunosuppressed patients. Peripheral intravenous sets should be changed at least every 72 hours, and preferably every 48 hours. Central venous cannulae are more difficult to change repeatedly, but a regimen wherein they are changed at three days over a guide wire and replaced completely into a new site at six days seems to be an acceptable compromise. The risks of multilumen CVP lines have not been addressed in burn patients specifically, but in general medical and surgical patients the data are somewhat conflicting. A recent series demonstrated that with sound technique and CVP "teams," the risks can be minimized. Arterial lines pose a greater problem because they are difficult to change frequently. Fortunately, documented arterial infection is uncommon and no maximal safe interval for maintenance of these in a single site is known. Pulmonary artery catheters when placed in burn patients are managed as they are in patients in the surgical ICU, namely they are removed at 72 hours and are not used for central parenteral alimentation.

MEDICATIONS

Drug therapy is complicated in burn patients by a series of complex physiological changes that affect many aspects of pharmacokinetics, including cardiovascular changes with diminished and then increased cardiac output and differences in regional blood flow; alterations in renal function; alterations in hepatic function; and shifts in concentrations of plasma protein and of specific component proteins. The clinical picture is further complicated by the temporal nature of disordered metabolism; the nonlinear metabolic changes that do not correlate absolutely with burn size;[47] differences between the drug responses of children and adults; and the lack of correlation between the limited animal data and clinical pharmacology.[47] A brief outline of the general changes in physiology follows.

Cardiovascular Changes

As described earlier, the ebb and flow of the metabolic response to injury is seen in the response of cardiac output in burn patients. The initial decreased cardiac output persists for about 8 to 12 hours on average and is replaced by a hyperdynamic cardiac response seen as early as 48 hours after burn and almost invariably presents by four days after burn injury. This response seems not to depend upon the etiology of the burn (scald, flame, etc), to occur in children as well as adults, and to be a common factor in burns over approximately 20% body surface area. The shift to hyperdynamic response may be slower in patients with inhalation injuries who tend to require more fluid for resuscitation. In very large burns, the hyperdynamic response may not be seen because many of these adult patients cannot be resuscitated. The elderly patient, even with a relatively small burn, may not manifest a hyperdynamic response because of fixed myocardial disease or concomitant administration of cardiac drugs such as beta blockers.

Muscle blood flow is diminished and cutaneous blood flow is further diminished as a consequence of the initial low cardiac output; hence the basis for the contraindication of intramuscular medications in the emergency room and during the first two days in the burn unit. Specifically, intramuscular analgesics must be avoided as they tend to remain in the periphery, offering no analgesia until the cardiac output recovers and they are rapidly absorbed into the central circulation. Analgesics, as discussed further in the section on pain, must be given intravenously in the early stages of burn care.

Renal Changes

The changes in renal blood flow generally mirror the changes in cardiac output, with relative hypoperfusion being replaced by hyperperfusion. Increased glomerular filtration can be seen by measurements of creatine clearance, which can exceed 200 mL per minute in previously healthy burn patients. Drugs whose metabolism depends upon tubular function, however, or on the metabolic functions of the kidney, exhibit a more complicated course in patients with burn injury.

Hepatic Changes

Like the kidney, part of the hepatic dysfunction in burn patients relates to the changes in hepatic blood flow consequent to alterations in cardiac output. Hepatic artery flow decreases in shock in step with changes in cardiac output; portal venous inflow is usually depressed to an even greater degree. Recovery of cardiac output directly increases hepatic artery blood flow, but factors that affect superior mesenteric artery (SMA) inflow into the gut must also be considered in the recovery of portal venous inflow. The liver's function in drug metabolism is more complicated. Microsomal enzyme levels are an important factor in the metabolism of many classes of drugs and these levels are changed as a consequence of the burn injury, possibly on the basis of the immune response to burn injury.

Changes in Protein Binding

Many classes of drugs are bound to protein in their transport through the plasma space. The protein-bound fraction of the drug is usually pharmacologically inactive. The two major proteins to which drugs are bound are albumin[48] and alpha-1-acid glycoprotein,[49] two acute-phase proteins (APP). Albumin is a negative APP in that its level falls after injury and trauma and in burn patients.[50] Part of its early fall is related to redistribution. Drugs that normally bind to circulating serum albumin are likely, then, to be pharmacologically more active. On the other hand, alpha-1-acid glycoprotein is a positive APP and increases after injury and trauma.[51] Thus drugs that are bound to this protein are likely to be less available to the tissues in patients with burn injuries and increased doses are needed to achieve the same physiologic effect.[52]

Specific Drugs

Muscle Relaxants

Succinylcholine Neuromuscular relaxants are divided into two groups: (1) depolarizing agents such as succinylcholine, which produce muscle fasciculation (depolarization) prior to producing paralysis; and (2) nondepolarizing agents such as d-tubucurarine, metacurine, pancuronium, atracurium, and vecuronium. The nondepolarizing agents compete with acetylcholine for receptors at the neuromuscular junction and are sometimes referred to as competitive blocking agents, succinylcholine being considered a ''noncompetitive'' blocking agent.

In normal, nonburned individuals, succinylcholine produces a rapid onset of paralysis and a rapid recovery of paralysis caused by the metabolism of the drug by circulating cholinesterase. The depolarization causes an efflux of potassium from the cell into the extracellular fluid and an influx of sodium. During repolarization, the direction of these ion shifts is reversed. The complications of the drug include muscle pain, myoglobinuria, and rarely, malignant hyperthermia. In burn patients, the principal complication of the drug is a profound hyperkalemia, which may be severe enough to cause a cardiac arrest.[53,54] The temporal response to this drug is important. There are no reported cases of cardiac arrest if the drug is administered during the few days after injury. Since abnormal elevations of plasma potassium have been recorded shortly after injury,[53,55,56] this may reflect the severity of the potassium increase. Most cases of cardiac arrest occurred from the third to the seventh week after injury; the peak response of plasma potassium occurs from three weeks to three months after injury.[53-56] The potassium response to succinylcholine administration decreases slowly[57] but may persist as long as 2 years after the burn injury.[58] In general, the more extensive the burn, the more likely the hyperkalemic response.[57] The response to succinylcholine is inconsistent. Some patients have sustained cardiac arrests after having received the drug earlier in their hospital course and have been resuscitated without untoward effects.[56,59,60] Patients with electrical burns with direct muscle injury may be more sensitive to the effects of the drug.[61] The hyperkalemic response may be dose related but can occur at relatively low doses.[57]

The rise in potassium in susceptible individuals occurs within the first minute, peaks at two to five minutes, and declines over the next ten to fifteen minutes.[53,56] The cardiac risk, in addition to the absolute level of the plasma potassium, is increased by beta-adrenergic blockade, alpha-adrenergic stimulation, verapamil, and dantrolene.[62-65]

Although several authors have suggested methods to ameliorate the response to succinylcholine such as pretreatment with diazepam, magnesium sulfate, or nondepolarizing drugs,[57,66-68] they do not seem to be universally successful and the complications of succinylcholine are best handled by avoiding the drug entirely. Avoidance should extend at least through the early period of reconstructive surgery.[57]

The suggested mechanism for the adverse effects of succinylcholine is based upon the similarity of the abnormal response to that seen in denervation injury, namely a "supersensitivity."[54,68] Soon after denervation, the entire muscle membrane surface, as opposed to just the motor end plate, develops acetylcholine receptors. In denervated patients and animals, a dose of succinylcholine or acetylcholine results in a greater efflux of potassium because the entire muscle membrane is "leaking," not just the motor end plate.[54,68] This model would explain the concomitant hyposensitivity to d-tubocurarine, whose action would be decreased by the increased number of receptors.[57] The data in humans that acetylcholine receptors increase are indirect, however.[69]

Nondepolarizing Drugs. In contrast to the experience in other critically ill patients, the intravenous dose and plasma concentrations of nondepolarizing drugs (NDMR) required for a given effect in burn patients are markedly increased. The shift in the dose–response curve for this class of drugs correlates both with time after burn injury and the burn surface area.[70,71] The hyposensitivity to NDMRs is usually not seen in patients whose burn surface area is less than 10%,[57] while in patients whose burn exceeds 40% of their body surface area, the effective dose must be increased 2.5 to 5-fold.[57] There is a temporal response pattern to these drugs as well, with a peak resistance about 2 weeks after injury that decreases but persists for as long as a year after injury.[72]

The mechanism of the hyposensitivity to these drugs seems to be associated with the increased plasma levels of the acute phase protein, alpha-1-acid glycoprotein. Further complications in ascribing etiology to this hyposensitivity stem from differences in renal excretion and hepatic metabolism among the various members of the class. Furthermore, the putative increase in acetylcholine receptors that is invoked to explain the increased sensitivity to succinylcholine also explains part of the increased hyposensitivity to the nondepolarizing agents, which must bond to more sites to compete against acetylcholine.

H-2 Blockers. H-2 blockers (cimetidine, ranitidine, famotidine) are used alone or in combination with antacids to decrease gastric pH and gastric volume to prevent stress ulceration and upper gastrointestinal bleeding. The relative value of antacid therapy versus H-2 blockers is still debated. Failures of H-2 blocker therapy in the critically ill are generally associated with the administration of inadequate drug to achieve an increase in gastric pH. In the early resuscitative period, the usual doses of cimetidine are effective to produce the desired change in gastric pH. During the hyperdynamic phase of increased glomerular filtration, the dose must be adjusted upwards to about twice the usual dose in adults and even higher in children.[73] As always, the clinical efficacy of the drug, as revealed by gastric pH, should guide subsequent therapy. The use of cimetidine by continuous infusion may be even more useful in burn patients. The pharmacokinetics of the other H-2 blockers have not been as well delineated.

Anxiolytics. Intravenous diazepam is rapidly cleared from the plasma pool and sequestered in adipose tissue, resulting in a long half-life but a brief hypnotic effect. The elimination of the drug from the body requires hepatic metabolism (oxidative metabolic reaction in the cytochrome p-450 system or phase I reaction). In burn patients, the accumulation of the drug in fat depots is worsened by the nonspecific decrease in the drug-metabolizing capacity of the liver[74] and the interactions of other drugs such as cimetidine.[75]

Lorazepam possesses a number of properties that make it preferable in burn patients. Its hepatic metabolism is a phase II reaction by conjugation and its metabolic products are pharmacologically inactive as opposed to the metabolic products of diazepam. Clearance is faster than that of diazepam and is unaffected by cimetidine.[75] The unbound volume of distribution is much less than that of diazepam, resulting in longer-acting sedation.[74]

Antibiotics. Our knowledge of the pharmacokinetics of antibiotics in burn patients is largely restricted to those drugs whose serum levels are monitored in clinical practice. The burn patient usually requires increased doses of aminoglycosides and vancomycin to achieve both satisfactory plasma drug levels and, probably, therapeutic effectiveness.[76–79] There are two possible mechanisms for the need for increased doses of medication: increased renal excretion of drug and losses of antibiotic into wound fluid. The first is probably the predominant mechanism, as each of these drugs is renally excreted and dose modifications based upon creatine clearance produce expected serum levels. In small children whose weight-to-surface-area relationship is altered, the amount of drug that enters the burn wound becomes more significant. Nevertheless, the clinical use of these potentially nephrotoxic drugs in burn patients requires frequent (as often as daily) monitoring of peak and trough serum levels. Both aminoglycosides and vancomycin are important drugs in burn patients and experience has demonstrated that appropriate dosing can produce clinical effectiveness without renal compromise. A further word of caution in the use of vancomycin: the dose should be infused over one hour because of the risk of hypotension in a hypovolemic patient.

Other classes of drugs that are renally excreted but whose dosage schedules are not ordinarily adjusted in cases of renal insufficiency are probably effective in burn patients at the usual dosages. Obviously, preexisting renal insufficiency, or secondary renal hypoperfusion during episodes of sepsis with inadequate maintenance of cardiac output, requires dose adjustments.

Topical Antimicrobials. Topical therapy is one of the mainstays of infection control in burn patients, but these agents applied to denuded skin are not without systemic side effects, both real and suspected. Plasma sulfadiazine has been recovered in patients treated with topical silver sulfadiazine (Silvadene). This could be of significance in patients with G-6-P-D deficiency. Acid–base problems can occur with topical

mafenide acetate, a potent carbonic anhydrase inhibitor.[80] Iodine ion accumulation can occur in patients treated with topical betadine or Helafoam,[81] but has never been proven to cause clinical problems. Silver nitrate applied topically is associated with significant electrolyte abnormalities—especially hyponatremia, hypokalemia, hypocalcemia, and hypochloremia—because of the leaching out of these minerals and the absorption of free water from the wet dressings.[82]

PAIN

Burn injuries are commonly thought of as being the most painful injuries experienced. In the context of the modern setting of burn care, this is largely true. The aggressive management of the burn wound prior to its closure (with passive and active exercise regimens and frequent dressing changes and bedside debridements), and the rehabilitation of the patient with closed wounds afterward, are also painful procedures. The goal of the physician must be one of minimizing pain without minimizing the active exercise that contributes to a reduction in the ultimate morbidity of the injury. Pain medication in this light is analogous to that seen in the patient with rib fractures; a condition of pain-free breathing without depression of the stimulus to breathing. Many of the principles outlined in Chapter 5 are applicable to burn patients.

In the early period of the patient's hospital course, analgesia is usually provided by potent narcotic agents such as morphine sulfate and meperidine given intravenously. Relatively long-acting narcotics may be safely administered as ventilation is usually supported in the severely burned patient and the danger of respiratory depression is largely obviated.

Some centers have reported the benefits of self-administered 50% nitrous oxide with oxygen during hydrotherapy and debridement. This preparation produces a prompt analgesia approximately 20 seconds after inhalation that lasts for about 40 seconds to two minutes. The bone marrow changes that can occur during long-term exposure have caused concern, however.

After the initial period of shock and resuscitation, the patient's pain begins to come under the more usual regimens of pain control. In the burn patient, as opposed to the patient after a cholecystectomy, for instance, there are two patterns of pain: (1) a continuous background pain that occurs when the patient moves in bed or takes a deep breath; and (2) the acute increased pain that comes from manipulation of the burn wound during burn care and active exercise. Narcotics continue to be the mainstay of analgesic therapy although some clinicians recommend the addition of tranquilizers and mood elevators.[83]

The patient whose pain is well controlled in the resting state requires increased pain medication during special procedures. Intramuscularly administered analgesics are satisfactory providing that the staff is aware of the time required before effective analgesia is achieved and the prolonged persistence of analgesia long after the source or cause of pain is removed. This latter effect is equivalent to the depressent effects of anesthesia without surgical stress. The regimen not infrequently leads to an inadequately anesthestized patient during the procedure who is obtunded several hours later.

Intravenous analgesia is preferable because the onset of action is obvious and the dose can be modified appropriately. The use of a morphine infusion for the background pain control allows a combination of the two techniques, the drip rate being increased during the procedure and reduced afterwards. This technique is obviously only applicable to the intensive care unit setting. The use of short-acting and very-short-acting analgesia would be beneficial in the acute-pain-provoking setting, but a continuous drip with a short-acting drug is economically and physiologically unwise. The use of patient-controlled pumps may improve upon the physician or nurse-controlled system.[84-86]

Some burn centers have used additional oral narcotic preparations such as hydromorphone hydrochloride and codeine or codeine and acetaminophen[87] for the acute pain or debridement procedures. In a few centers, the use of inhalation agents such as methoxyflurane (despite its renal problems) or a 50% nitrous oxide mixture[88-91] as an adjunct to the daily management of the burn wound has been described. In large series,[89] the incidence of complications has been minimal. Similarly, some burn centers[92-94] have used ketamine (1.5 to 2 mL/kg IM) as an adjunct to the burn care of their patients, especially in pediatric populations, but most physicians who employ this agent and technique do so in the operating room.

It is not clear how many burn patients become addicted or habituated to pain medications during their hospital stay. The best way of preventing this seems to be to separate the patient from the perception of pain and the alleviation of pain by medication. Preventing the acute pain by the timely use of analgesics will probably break this cycle.

Consideration must also be made to the relationship between analgesia and feeding and decreases in gastrointestinal motility. The metabolic needs of these patients require aggressive use of the gastrointestinal tract for nutrition. Analgesic techniques that require long periods where the patient is fasted beforehand and that cause the patient nausea and vom-iting intefere with caloric intake. Similarly, the physician must be aware of the constipating effects of many of these drugs and temper their use with stool softeners and laxatives.

NUTRITION

Current practices of hyperalimentation are discussed in Chapter 8, but like other aspects of their care, there are important modifications in burned patients because of their specifically altered physiology.

Burn patients differ from trauma or general surgery patients in that the gut is rarely compromised by the injury. These patients can and should be fed enterally, not parenterally, and feeding should commence with recovery of gastrointestinal function on about the second day after burn injury. Patients with large burns commonly develop an early acute gastric ileus, which requires that they be fasted and a nasogastric tube placed. Resuscitation can adversely affect the recovery of small bowel function by producing a fall of serum albumin and a consequent decrease in tissue oncotic pressure. At low levels of serum albumin, the gut becomes a secretory rather than an absorptive organ.[95] Studies have demonstrated that this dysfunction is rapidly reversed by the infusion of exogenous albumin in children[96] and less rapidly improved by these infusions in adults. In most patients, the enteral route is approached by a soft nasogastric or nasointestinal tube early in the patient's course when caloric needs are highest and subsequently by oral intake. Some patients have come to operation for the placement of feeding gastrostomies or feeding jejunostomies as adjuncts to their nutritional management.

There are specific contraindications to intravenous nutrition in burn patients apart from the availability of the simpler, safer enteral route. The immunological competence of these patients makes them poor candidates for maintenance of long-term intravenous lines. Moreover, a recent report suggests that TPN may actually be harmful in that the ratio of helper to suppressor T-lymphocytes is adversely effected.[97] Nevertheless, the patient with major burns may require parenteral nutritional support at some point during his or her hospitalization.

Common anesthesiologic practice makes enteral nutrition difficult. Fasting the patient for at least eight hours prior to general anesthesia is a sound rule but interrupts the nutrition important to these patients whose survival frequently correlates with the physician's ability to maintain lean body mass and immunocompetence. This interval is reduced to four hours in some centers that have found that aspirating the stomach prior to induction is an adequate safeguard against the risk of aspiration.

The burn patient is the paradigm of the stressed patient with increased caloric needs. The classic Harris-Benedict equation measuring energy expenditure is usually cited as a guide to the feeding of these patients. Recent evidence suggests that this formula errs in the seriously burned patient and patients whose nutrition is guided by it will be overfed. In adults the Curreri formula (25 kcal per kilogram body weight plus 40 kcal per percentage body surface area burned) has been generally successful in estimating the caloric demands of the patient. This is a "dynamic" formula in that the caloric intake is modified as the wound is increased by donor sites and decreased by closure of the burn wound. Similar formulas exist for burned children.

Unlike most general surgical patients, fat may not be as useful a substitute for glucose calories in the burn patient. This may reflect the demands of the burn wound for glucose or the neuroendocrine milieu of the burn patient, which is characterized by persistant elevated levels of circulating catecholamines. The burn patient requires a different protein intake than other surgical patients to compensate for the extensive protein losses through the wounded skin and for healing of extensive wounds. In our center, we supplement the patient with increased doses of vitamin C (a cofactor in collagen synthesis) and vitamin A (which also decreases the incidence of stress gastritis).

INFECTION

Infection is a major risk in the burn patient and the major cause of death in patients who survive their first days in the hospital. In addition to the loss of an effective skin barrier to invasion by microorganisms, the burn patient has decreased neutrophil function both endogenous to the neutrophils with documented defects in chemotaxis and cell killing and also secondary to the acute fall in plasma fibronectin, one of the body's principal opsonins. This lack is particularly important in the body's handling of encapsulated gram-positive microorganisms. There are also defects in T-cell function and number, with an adverse change in the ratio of helper to suppressor lymphocytes. Prolonged periods of hyponutrition or malnutrition further decrease the humoral immune system. Many of the important topics in infection control are discussed in Chapter 4, but some unique features of the burn patient require elaboration.

Because of the aforementioned defects in immunological function, the patient with significant surface area cutaneous burns should be approached as any other patient in protective isolation. This should include wearing of caps, gowns, gloves, and masks for all personnel having physical contact with the patient. It is as important during patient transport to the operating room as at any other time in the patient's course.

The burn patient's status can frequently be assessed by screening for infection with serial sputum gram stains and cultures, urine cultures for patients with indwelling catheters, and quantitative biopsies of skin for the detection of invading microorganisms. The need for frequent changes in intravenous line sites has already been discussed.

The well-described changes in the immune system secondary to the use of certain inhalation anesthetic agents is probably overstated clinically. The aseptic techniques of the anesthesiologist is more important. Intraoperatively the anesthesia staff must be as gowned and gloved as the surgical staff. Similarly, postoperative visits require the anesthesia staff to gown and glove before seeing the patient in all but the most acute emergencies.

REFERENCES

1. Herndon DN, Thompson PB, Traber DL: Pulmonary injury in burned patients. *Crit Care Clin* 1985;1:79–96.
2. Via-Reque E, Rattenborg CC; Prolonged oro- or nasotracheal intubation. *Crit Care Med* 1981;9:637–639.
3. Robinson L, Miller RH: Smoke inhalation injuries. *Am J Otolaryngol* 1986;7:375–380.
4. Traber DL, Linares HA, Herndon DN, Prien T: The pathophysiology of inhalation injury—A review. *Burns Therm Inj* 1988;14:357–364.
5. Moylan JA, Wilmore DW, Morton DE, Pruitt BA Jr.: Early diagnosis of inhalation injury using Xenon 133 lung scan. *Ann Surg* 1972;176:477–484.
6. Dressler DP, Skornik WA, Kupersmith S: Corticosteroid treatment of experimental smoke inhalation. *Ann Surg* 1976;183:46–52.
7. Robinson NB, Hudson LD, Riem M, et al: Steroid therapy following isolated smoke inhalation injury. *J Trauma* 1982;22:876–889.
8. Herndon DN, Traber DL, Linares H, et al: Etiology of the pulmonary pathophysiology associated with inhalation injury. *Resuscitation* 1986;14:43–59.
9. Traber DL, Herndon DN, Stein MD, et al: The pulmonary lesion of smoke inhalation in an ovine model. *Circ Shock* 1986;18:311–323.
10. Sharar SR, Heimbach DM, Howard M, et al: Cardiopulmonary response after spontaneous inhalation of Douglas fir smoke in goats. *J Trauma* 1988;28:164–170.
11. Demling R, Ryan P, Katz A, Lalonde C: Pulmonary dysfunction after burn wound excision: Role of thromboxane, chemotactic (factors and oxygen radicals) (abstract). Presented at the 18th annual meeting of the American Burn Association, Chicago, April 1986.
12. Shinozawa Y, Hales C, Jung W, Burke J: Ibuprofen pre-

vents synthetic smoke-induced pulmonary edema. *Am Rev Respir Dis* 1986;134:1145–1148.

13. Kimura R, Traber L, Heimbach D, et al: Ibuprofen reduces the lung lymph flow changes associated with inhalation injury. *Circ Shock* 1988;24:183–191.

14. Brown M, Desai M, Traber LD, et al: Dimethylsulfoxide with heparin in the treatment of smoke inhalation injury. *J Burn Care Rehabil* 1988;9:22–25.

15. Goldbaum LR, Orellano T, Dergal E: Joint Committee on Aviation Pathology: XVI. Studies on the relation between carboxyhemoglobin concentration and toxicity. *Aviat Space Environ Med* 1977;48:969–970.

16. Sotonyi P, Somogyi E, Balogh I, Nemes A: The evaluation of electron microscopic cytochrome-oxidase reaction in experimental heart muscle hypoxia. *Cell Mol Biol* 1980;26:9–15.

17. Somogyi E, Balogh I, Rubanyi G, et al: New findings concerning the pathogenesis of acute carbon monoxide (CO) poisoning. *Am J Forensic Med Pathol* 1981;2:31–39.

18. Penney DG, Baylerian MS, Thill JE, et al: Cardiac response of the fetal rat to carbon monoxide exposure. *Am J Physiol* 1983;244:H289–297.

19. Hyperbaric Center Advisory Committee Emergency Medical Service, City of New York: A registry for carbon monoxide poisoning in New York City. *J Toxicol Clin Toxicol* 1988;26:419–441.

20. Halebian P, Cabrales S, Barie P, et al: Carbon monoxide excretion by different modes of mechanical ventilation (abstract). Presented at the 18th annual meeting of the American Burn Association, Chicago, April 1986.

21. Van Hoeson KB, Camporesi EM, Moon RE, Hage ML: Should hyperbaric oxygen be used to treat the pregnant patient for acute carbon monoxide poisoning? A case report and literature review. *JAMA* 1989;261:1039–1043.

22. Meyers RA, Snyder SK, Lindberg S, Cowley RA: Value of hyperbaric oxygen in suspected carbon monoxide poisoning. *JAMA* 1981;246:2478–2480.

23. Grube BJ, Marvin JA, Heimbach DM: Therapeutic hyperbaric oxygen: Help or hindrance in burn patients with carbon monoxide poisoning (abstract)? Presented at the 19th annual meeting of the American Burn Association, Washington, DC April 1987.

24. Howard RJ, Blake DR, Pall H, et al: Allopurinol/N-acetylcysteine for carbon monoxide poisoning (letter). *Lancet* 1987;2:628–629.

25. Hunt JL, Purdue GF, Gunning T: Is tracheostomy warranted in the burn patient? Indications and complications (abstract). Presented at the 18th annual meeting of the American Burn Association, Chicago, April 1986.

26. Jones WG, Goodwin CW, Madden M, et al: Tracheostomies in burn patients (abstract). Presented at the 20th annual meeting of the American Burn Association, Seattle, March 1988.

27. Adams HR, Baxter CR, Parker JL, Senning R: Development of acute burn shock in unresuscitated guinea pigs. *Circ Shock* 1981;8:613–625.

28. Temples TE, Burns AH, Nance FC, Miller HI: Effect of burn shock on myocardial function in guinea pigs. *Circ Shock* 1984;14:81–92.

29. Horton JW, White J, Baxter CR: The role of oxygen-

30. Rubin WD, Mani MM, Hievert, JM: Fluid resuscitation of the thermally injured patient: Current concepts with definition of clinical subsets and their specialized treatment. *Clin Plastic Surg* 1986;13:9–20.

31. Jelenko C III, Williams JB, Wheeler ML, et al: Studies in shock and resuscitation, I: Use of a hypertonic, albumin-containing, fluid demand regimen (HALFD) in resuscitation. *Crit Care Med* 1979;7:157–167.

32. Caldwell FT Jr, Bowser BH: Critical evaluation of hypertonic and hypotonic solutions to resuscitate severely burned children: A propsective study. *Ann Surg* 1979;189:546–552.

33. Bowser BH, Caldwell FT Jr: The effects of resuscitation with hypertonic vs hypotonic vs coloid on wound and urine fluid and electrolyte losses in severely burned children. *J Trauma* 1983;23:916–923.

34. Bowser-Wallace BH, Caldwell FT Jr: A prospective analysis of hypertonic lactated saline v Ringer's lactate-colloid for the resuscitation of severely burned children. *Burns Therm Inj* 1986;12:402–409.

35. Bowser-Wallace BH, Caldwell FT Jr: Fluid requirements of severely burned children up to 3 years old: Hypertonic lactated saline vs Ringer's lactate-colloid. *Burns Therm Inj* 1986;12:549–555.

36. Horton JW, White DJ, Baxter CR: Small volume hypertonic saline dextran resuscitation from thermal injury (abstract). Presented at the 21st annual meeting of the American Burn Association, New Orleans, March 1989.

37. Bowser-Wallace BH, Cone JB, Caldwell FT Jr: Hypertonic lactated saline resuscitation of severely burned patients over 60 years of age. *J Trauma* 1985;25:22–26.

38. Waters LM, Christensen MA, Sato RM: HEtastarch: A new colloid for burn resuscitation (abstract). Presented at the 19th annual meeting of the American Burn Association, Washington DC April 1987.

39. Ferguson JL, Merrill GF, Miller HI, Spitzer JJ: Regional blood flow redistribution during early burn shock in the guinea pig. *Circ Shock* 1977;4:317–326.

40. Ferguson JL, Hikawyj-Yevich I, Miller HI: Body fluid compartment changes during burn shock in the guinea pig. *Circ Shock* 1980;7:457–466.

41. Moore DB, Rainey WC, Caldwell FT, et al: The effect of rapid resuscitation upon cardiac index following thermal trauma in a porcine model (abstract). Presented at the 18th annual meeting of the American Burn Association, Chicago, April 1986.

42. Roberts ML, Pruitt BA Jr: Nursing care and psychological considerations, in Moncrief JA, Pruitt BA Jr (eds): *Burns: A Team Approach.* Philadelphia, Saunders, 1979.

43. Lucas CE, Bouwman DL, Ledgerwood AM, Higgins R: Differential serum protein changes following supplemental albumin resuscitation for hypovolemic shock. *J Trauma* 1980;20:47–51.

44. Denis R, Smith RW, Grabow D, et al: Relocation of nonalbumin proteins after albumin resuscitation. *J Surg Res* 1987;43:413–419.

45. Brezel BS, McGeever KE, Stein JM: Topical epinephrine solutions vs thrombin solution for hemostasis on split thickness skin donor sites (abstract). Presented at

derived free radicals in burn-induced myocardial contractile depression. *J Burn Care Rehabil* 1988;9:589–598.

the 18th annual meeting of the American Burn Association, Chicago, April 1986.

46. Achauer BM, Hernandez J, Parker A: Minimimizing blood loss in primary excision with intraoperative vasopressin (abstract). Presented at the 18th annual meeting of the American Burn Association, Chicago, April 1986.

47. Martyn J: Clinical pharmacology and drug therapy in the burned patient. *Anesthesiology* 1986;65:67–75.

48. Koch-Weser J, Sellers EM: Binding of drugs to serum albumin. *N Engl J Med* 1976;311–316:294:526–531.

49. Piaksky KM, Borga O: Plasma protein binding of basic drugs. *Clin Pharmacol Ther* 1977;22:545–549.

50. Moncrief JA: The body's response to heat, in Artz CP, Moncrief JA, Pruitt BA Jr (eds): *Burns: A Team Approach.* Philadelphia, Saunders. 1979.

51. Piaksky KM: Disease-induced changes in the plasma binding of basic drugs. *Clin Pharmacokin* 1980;5:246–267.

52. Martyn JAJ, Abernathy DR, Greenblatt DJ: Plasma protein binding of drugs after severe burn injury. *Clin Pharmacol Ther* 1984;35:535–539.

53. Viby-Mogensen J, Hanet HK, Hansen E, et al: Serum cholinesterase activity in burned patients. *Acta Anaesthesiol Scand* 1975;19:159–179.

54. Gronert GA, Theye RA: Pathophysiology of hyperkalemia induced by succinylcholine. *Anesthesiology* 1975;43:89–99.

55. Gronert GA, Dotin LN, Richey CR, et al: Succinylcholine-induced hyperkalemia in burned patients, Part II. *Anesth Analg* 1969;48:958–962.

56. Shaner PJ, Brown RL, Kirksey TD, et al: Succinylcholine-induced hyperkalemia in burned patients, Part I. *Anesth Analg* 1969;48:764–770.

57. Martyn J, Goldhill DR, Goudsouzian NG: Clinical pharmacology of muscle relaxants in patients with burns. *Clin Pharmacol* 1986;26:680–685.

58. Elridge L, Liebhold M, Steinbach JH: Alterations in cat skeletal muscle neuromuscular junctions following prolonged inactivity. *J Physiol* 1981;313:529–545.

59. Allan CM, Cullen WG, Gillies DVM: Ventricular fibrillation in a burned boy. *Can Med Assoc J* 1961;85:432–434.

60. Tolmie JD, Joyce TH, Mitchell GD: Succinylcholine danger in the burned patient. *Anesthesiology* 1967;28:467–470.

61. Artz CP: Electrical injury simulates crush injury. *Surg Gynecol Obstet* 1967;125:1316–1321.

62. McCammon RL, Stoetling RK: Exaggerated increase in serum potassium following succinylcholine in dogs with beta blockage. *Anesthesiology* 1984;61:723–725.

63. Williams ME, Rosa RM, Silva P, et al: Impairment of extrarenal potassium disposal by alpha-adrenergic stimulation. *N Engl J Med* 1984;311:145–149.

64. Nugent M, Tinker JH, Moyer JP: Verapamil versus rate of development and hemodynamic effects of acute hyperkalemia in halothane-anesthetized dogs: Effect of calcium therapy. *Anesthesiology* 1984;60:435–439.

65. Nigrovic V: Succinylcholine, cholinoceptors and proposed mechanism of early adverse hemodynamic reaction. *Can Anesth Soc J* 1984;31:382–394.

66. Blitt CD, Carlson GL, Rollins GD, et al: A comparative evaluation of pretreatment with non-depolarizing neuromuscular blockers prior to administration of succinylcholine. *Anesthesiology* 1981;55:687–689.

67. Erkola O, Salmenpera M, Tammisto T: Does diazepam pretreatment prevent succinylcholine induced fasiculations? A double blind comparison of diazepam and d-tubocurarine pretreatment. *Anesth Analg* 1980;59:932–934.

68. Ali HH, Savarese JJ: Monitoring of neuromuscular function. *Anesthesiology* 1976;45:216–249.

69. Aulick LH, Wilmore DW, Mason AD, et al: Depressed reflex vasomotor control of the burn wound. *Cardiovasc Res* 1982;16:113–119.

70. Marathe PH, Dwersteg JF, Pavlin EG, et al: Effect of thermal injury on the pharmacokinetics and pharmacodynamics of atracurium in humans. *Anesthesiology* 1989;70:752–755.

71. Martyn JAJ, Liu LMP, Szyfelbein SK, et al: Neuromuscular effects of pancuronium in burned children. *Anesthesiology* 1983;59:561–564.

72. Martyn JAJ, Mateo RS, Szyfelbein SK, et al: Unprecedented resistance to neuromuscular blocking effect of metocurine with persistence after complete recovery in a burned patient. *Anesth Analg* 1982;61:614–617.

73. Martyn JAJ, Greenblatt DJ: Cimetidine pharmacokinetics and pharmacodynamics in pediatric burned patients (abstract). Presented at the 18th annual meeting of the American Burn Association, Chicago, April, 1986.

74. Klotz V, Reimann I: Delayed clearance of diazepam due to cimetidine. *N Engl J Med* 1980;302:1012–1014.

75. Ruffalo RL, Thompson JF: Effect of cimetidine on the clearance of benzodiazepines. *N Engl J Med* 1980;303:753–754.

76. Zaske DE, Dipolle RJ, Strate RJ: Gentamicin dosage requirements: Wide variation in 242 patients with normal renal function. *Surgery* 1980;87:164–169.

77. Zaske DE, Sawchuk RJ, Strate RG: The necessity for increased doses of amikacin in burn patients. *Surgery* 1978;84:603–608.

78. Loirat P, Rohan J, Bailet A, et al: Increased glomerular filtration rate in patients with major burns and its effect on pharmacokinetics of tobramycin. *N Engl J Med* 1978;299:915–919.

79. Glew RH, Moellering RC, Burke JF: Gentamicin dosage in children with extensive burns. *J Trauma* 1976;16:819–823.

80. Petroff PA, Handler EW, Mason AD: Ventilatory patterns following burn injury and effect of sulfamylon. *J Trauma* 1975;15:650–656.

81. Notea E, Hirshowitz B: Comparison of blood serum iodine levels with the use of Iodex and Povidone iodide ointment. *J Trauma* 1985;25:247–249.

82. Moncrief JA: Topical antibacterial therapy of the burn wound, in Moncrief JA, Pruitt BA Jr (eds): *Burns: A Team Approach.* Philadelphia, Saunders 1979.

83. Steiner H, Clark WR: Psychiatric complications of burned adults: A classification. *J Trauma* 1977;17:134–143.

84. Tamsen A, Hartvig P, Fagerlund C, et al: Patient-controlled analgesic therapy. Part I: Pharmacokinetics of

pethidine in the pre and postoperative periods. *Clin Pharmacokin* 1982;7:149–163.

85. Tamsen A, Hartvig P, Fagerlund C, et al: Patient-controlled analgesic therapy. Part II: Individual analgesic demand and analgesic plasma concentrations of pethidine in postoperative pain. *Clin Pharmacokin* 1982;7:164–175.

86. Tamsen A, Hartvig P, Fagerlund C, et al: Patient-controlled analgesic therapy. Part III: Pharmacokinetics and analgesic plasma concentrations of ketobemidone. *Clin Pharmacokin* 1982;7:252–265.

87. Marvin JA, Heimbach DM: Pain control during the intensive care phase of burn care. *Crit Care Clin* 1985;1:147–158.

88. Filkins SA, Cosgrav P, Marvin JA, et al: Self-administered anesthesia: A method of pain control. *J Burn Care Rehabil* 1981;2:33–34.

89. Marvin JA, Engrav LH, Heimbach, DNM: Self-administered nitrous oxide analgesia for debridement: A five-year experience (abstract). Presented at the American Burn Association meeting, San Francisco, April 1984.

90. Baskett PJF: Analgesia for the dressing of burns in children: A method using neuroleptanagesia and Entonox.

Postgrad Med J 1972;48:138–142.

91. Oduro KA: Experiences with the penthrane analgizer. *Ghana Med J* 1971;10:43–47.

92. Demling RH, Ellerbee S, Jarrett F: Ketamine anesthesia for tangential excision of burn eschar: A burn unit procedure. *J Trauma* 1978;18:269–270.

93. Ward CM, Diamond AW: An appraisal of ketamine in the dressing of burns. *Postgrad Med J* 1976;5:222–223.

94. Slogoff S, Allen GW, Wessels JV, et al: Clinical experience with subanesthetic ketamine. *Anesth Anal Curr Res* 1974;53:354–358.

95. Andrassy RJ, Durr ED: Albumin: Use in nutrition and support. *Nutr Clin Prac* 1988;3:226–229.

96. Ford EG, Jennings LM, Andrassy RJ: Serum albumin (oncotic pressure) correlates with enteral feeding tolerance in the pediatric surgical patient. *J Pediat Surg* 1987;22:597–599.

97. Stein MD, Herndon DN, Abston S, Rutan TC: Lack of beneficial effects of TPN administration on immunity and mortality in thermal injury patients (abstract). Presented at the 18th annual meeting of the American Burn Association, Chicago, April 1986.

16 The Trauma Victim

Werner K. Pfisterer

While heart disease and cancer often claim victims beyond the middle years, trauma is the leading cause of death for those aged 1 to 44 years. Thirty-three percent of Americans are involved in traumatic injuries each year, accounting for 100,000 deaths and 200,000 major disabilities. Over $100 billion is spent annually on trauma victims, prompting the National Academy of Science's reference to injury as "the principal public health problem in America today."[1]

Traumatic injuries, methods of treatment, and trauma-related surgical procedures appear in the oldest western medical texts, Edwin Smith's papyrus, and Hammurabi's Code. Cautery–thermal debridement (5th century BC boiling oil), ligature for bleeding control (300 BC), and suture closure (150 AD) as methods of traumatic wound treatment have their roots in antiquity.[2] Since then, much of what is medically offered the trauma victim today is based on lessons learned during combat. The modern concept of first aid was introduced during the Napoleonic wars, when casualties were immediately transported to medical stations instead of receiving attention only after the fighting had subsided. Organized mobile field hospitals and ambulance corps equipped for resuscitation enroute were introduced during the American Civil War. The surgical treatment of trauma-related injury was advanced further in 1846 when John C. Warren first used general anesthetics. Wilson first proposed the concept of triage in 1846 as a method to prioritize surgical treatment into three categories: surgery for those in most immediate need first; palliation to those already mortally wounded second; and treatment for those with only minor injuries deferred until last.[3]

Although injuries incurred during battle have been numerous, the most common causes of multiple trauma-related injuries in modern times are motor vehicle accidents, violence, and industrial accidents.[2] Since the first reported automobile-related death in 1898, motor vehicle trauma alone has claimed more American lives than those lost in all the American battles combined.[4] Major advancements made during World War I in the diagnosis, treatment, and management of the trauma victim are listed in Table 16–1. The increased incidence of trauma to civilians

in the post-World-War-I era resulted in the founding of the American Association for the Surgery of Trauma in 1937, which endeavored to curtail the rising morbidity and mortality.

Trauma care of civilians improved significantly as a result of the experience attained during the Korean and Vietnam wars. Important developments are listed in Table 16–2. Reduction between time of injury and definitive treatment is a critical element for higher survival rates in the multiple trauma victim.[5] Rapid transport using helicopters for quick evacuation of casualties during the Vietnam War without prior resuscitation has been applauded by some and criticized by others.[6] Military anti-shock trousers (MAST), introduced during the Korean War, remain a useful adjunct in the management of certain trauma victims. Advanced trauma life support, introduced into the Emergency Medical Services (EMS) system, is now a common part of the prehospital resuscitation process.

The organization and systemization of modern trauma care can be traced to a report published by the Committee on Trauma, Division of Medical Sciences, sponsored by the United States National Academy of Sciences. Entitled "Accidental Death and Disability: the Neglected Disease of Modern Society," it proposed a system of trauma care involving the regionalization and categorization of hospitals especially equipped to manage the multiply traumatized patient. In that same year (1966) Cook County Hospital opened the first civilian trauma unit. Since then, the management of the trauma victim has been organized into prehospital emergency services (immediate care involving resuscitation and evaluation during

TABLE 16–1. IMPORTANT DEVELOPMENTS IN TRAUMA CARE DURING WORLD WAR I

Recognition of hypovolemic shock
Pathophysiology of wounding recognized
Recognition of injury complications
Treatment of infection by antibiotics
Whole blood administration began
Establishment of field hospital shock units
Mass casualty situation plan established
Average injury to surgery time nine hours

TABLE 16–2. IMPORTANT DEVELOPMENTS IN TRAUMA CARE AFTER WORLD WAR II

Korean War

Refinement of echeloning medical care
Direct evacuation by helicopter
Introduction of regional medical service
Military antishock trousers
Average injury to surgery time three hours

Vietnam War

Scoop and run helicopter evacuation policy
Efficient and plentiful surgical units
Improved regional emergency medical services
Average injury to surgery time eighty minutes

---

evacuation by ground or air while in communication with the trauma center); and inhospital management (resuscitation, evaluation, definitive treatment, and follow-up care). Emergency Medical Services follows a system based on a suggestion by Boyd in 1971 in which trauma victims are transported only to the regionally designated trauma center.[7] Hospitals are permitted to engage in various levels of trauma care according to one of four categories listed in Table 16–3. The system of categorization and regionalization of hospitals for trauma care has apparently resulted in a significant reduction in mortality.[8]

ACUTE MANAGEMENT OF THE MULTIPLY INJURED PATIENT

Fifty percent of all major trauma fatalities succumb within minutes due to extreme injury to the central nervous or cardiovascular systems.[9] This is despite the best of care. Another 30% will die within 24 hours, usually from extensive injury with massive blood loss; some of these are considered salvagable. The remaining 20% survive several months or more, with most eventually yielding to infection and multiple organ failure (renal dysfunction is very common.)[10] The fate of patients surviving beyond the "trial of life" during the initial minutes after injury will depend on proper and efficient management during the "golden hour" after medical assistance has begun. The priorities in the multiple trauma patient are, in the following order: (1) rapid airway evaluation and management; (2) avoidance of prolonged shock with

TABLE 16–3. LEVEL TRAUMA CARE HOSPITAL CATEGORIES

Level 1—Fully equipped emergency facility with a full surgical service immediately available 24 hours every day
Level 2—Limited emergency treatment facility
Level 3—Restricted emergency treatment facility
Level 4—Resuscitation only; patients then transferred

TABLE 16–4. INDICATIONS FOR INTUBATION OF THE TRAUMA VICTIM

Arrest: cardiac or respiratory
Impending respiratory failure
Unresponsive patient posttrauma
Pulmonary toilet postaspiration
Obstructive airway not relieved by chin lift
Glasgow coma scale 8 or less

---

cardiovascular stabilization, fluid resuscitation, and control of external sources of hemorrhage; and (3) rapid diagnosis and treatment of potentially life-threatening injuries. Resuscitation of the trauma victim begins in the field and is continued in the emergency room, operating room, postanesthetic care unit (PACU), and intensive care unit as necessary. The anesthesiologist is critically involved in four of five areas. Patients may require several operative procedures or close observation in the intensive care unit following anesthetic interventions, making the "postanesthetic care period" less well defined. Thus, to better understand this dynamic process, discussion of the trauma patient in the PACU is expanded to include critical aspects of initial resuscitation, diagnosis, and management.

Airway Assessment and Management

The immediate concerns in airway evaluation are twofold: (1) maintenance of patency allowing for adequate gas exchange; and (2) protection against aspiration. Upper airway obstruction is commonly caused by the tongue, blood, vomitus, dentures, and edema. The airway can often be maintained by oral and/or nasal airway insertion in addition to a chin lift moving the mandible and tongue anteriorly, especially in those breathing spontaneously. The Resusitube, esophageal obturator airway, pharyngeal tracheal lumen airway, and the anti-vomiting anti-aspiration tube are other alternatives preceeding tracheal intubation in the field, but are not without complication of misplacement and/or mucosal damage.[11] Any of these maneuvers can potentially result in quadraplegia, so neck flexion and extension must be avoided until cervical spine injury can be ruled out. Patients who obstruct despite chin lifting, and those failing to appropriately respond to simple questions, are candidates for intubation. Indications for the intubation of trauma patients are listed in Table 16–4. Advantages of the properly placed and secured cuffed endotracheal tube in the traumatized patient appear in Table 16–5. Selection of the intubation method depends on the type of injury, urgency, and the skills of the anesthesiologist.

Orotracheal intubation is appropriate when the patient is cyanotic or has arrested; presents with na-

TABLE 16-5. ADVANTAGES OF ENDOTRACHAEL TUBE PLACEMENT

Aspiration protection
Means for hyperventilation
Means for continuous positive pressure ventilation
Protection against upper airway obstruction
Route for drug administration

somaxillary trauma or basal skull fracture; or whenever it is deemed the easiest access to a controlled airway. This can be accomplished with (preferred whenever possible) or without topicalization and intravenous drugs, maintaining cricoid pressure just prior to and during laryngoscopy. If cervical spine instability is suspected, it is imperative that the patient's head be secured in a fixed position, avoiding hyperextension or hyperflexion and with minimal cricoid pressure.

Awake nasotracheal intubation in the traumatized patient is appropriate when the patient is cooperative or somnolent; breathing spontaneously; after mandibular trauma where the larynx, trachea, and tongue are intact; or possibly after cervical spine injury. Preparation of the nasal mucosa bilaterally using cocaine or phenylephrine is important to reduce bleeding. Blind nasal intubation, although simple, is associated with a first attempt success rate of only 30%, requiring from four to twelve attempts in 40% of cases.[12] Risk of further airway trauma, especially hemorrhage and maxillary sinusitis, from acute insertion or prolonged intubation, must be considered when electing to intubate nasally. It is contraindicated if basal skull fracture is suspected, as cephalad insertion into the brain is possible.

Useful adjuncts to facilitate oral or nasal tracheal intubation include pharmacologic means and mechanical aids. Sedatives and neuromuscular blocking drugs need to be used judiciously as virtually all traumatized patients are considered to have a full stomach. Sedation and muscle relaxation can be used when the airway is considered to be anatomically easy. Muscle relaxants should be avoided in patients with obviously difficult airways. Instead, sedated awake oral or nasal intubation using mechanical aids (lighted stylet, fiberoptic endoscopy) to achieve airway control is recommended as first choice, together with pulse oximetry monitoring whenever possible. Cricothyroid retrograde intubation methods have been highly successful in adults and children, in patients awake or under general anesthesia when a fiberoptic endoscope is not readily available.[13] Needle cricothyroidotomy has been used successfully during emergent conditions, for resuscitation and during routine surgery for the ventilation/oxygenation of the trauma patient.[14]

Surgical means for airway control include cricothyroidotomy and tracheostomy. Under emergent conditions the cricothyroidotomy is preferred for rapid access for oxygenation and ventilation as it is associated with less bleeding. When time permits and prolonged neck ventilatory assistance is indicated, a tracheostomy under controlled conditions is placed between the second and third tracheal rings, necessitating incision of the thyroid gland with the potential for bleeding.

Avoidance of Prolonged Shock

Pathophysiology of Shock. Although cardiogenic or septic etiologies for hypotension in the trauma patient are possible, a hemorrhagic cause for shock is almost always found. Decreased intravascular volume reduces tissue perfusion, causing tissue ischemia and hypoxia, evoking the microcirculation to redistribute blood flow to the heart and brain while reducing flow to splanchnic, renal, skeletal muscle, and cutaneous vasculature in response to intense sympathetic nervous system activation. Vasoactive mediators (norepinephrine, epinephrine, angiotensin) further contribute to shock by producing disseminated vasoconstriction, instigating platelet aggregation with thrombus formation, and increasing capillary permeability. During the acute shock phase and throughout prolonged fluid resuscitation, several mechanisms are proposed that lead to cellular hypoxia and anaerobic metabolism. Increased interstitial edema reduces cellular oxygen delivery by increasing the capillary to cellular diffusion distance. Microembolization within capillaries reduces perfusion/tissue ratio and interferes with autoregulation. Reperfusion syndrome resulting in massive tissue edema and endothelial swelling promotes further ischemia with hypoxia. Tissue acidosis disables the sodium–potassium ATPase pump of cellular membranes, leading to increased intracellular water locally while intracellular water deficits occur elsewhere.[15]

Diagnosis and Classification of Shock. Patients in moderate to severe hypovolemic shock manifest one or more of the following clinical signs: hypotension; tachycardia; narrowed pulse pressure; low central venous pressure; oliguria; pallor; cyanosis; cool extremities; diaphoresis; confusion; and restlessness. Degree of blood loss and clinical signs frequently correlate, making them useful for determining degree of shock and guiding treatment. Acute hemorrhagic shock is categorized into four classes according to volume lost and associated signs by the American College of Surgeons (Table 16-6). Patients who are anemic; taking diuretics, narcotics, or phenothiazines; or are in the geriatric group; exhibit signs out of propor-

TABLE 16-6. AMERICAN COLLEGE OF SURGEONS CLASSES OF ACUTE HEMORRHAGE

	Class I	Class II	Class III	Class IV
Blood loss (mL)	≤750	1000–1250	1500–1800	2000–2500
Blood loss (%)[a]	≤15	20–25	30–35	40–50
Pulse rate[b]	72–84	>100	>120	≥140
Blood pressure (mmHg)[c]	118/82	110/80	70–90/50–60	<50–60 systolic
Pulse pressure (mmHg)	36	30	20–30	10–20
Respiratory rate	14–20	20–30	30–40	>35
Urine output (mL/hr)[d]	30–35	25–30	5–15	neglible
CNS–mental status	slightly anxious	mildly anxious	anxious and confused	confused and lethargic
Fluid replacement (use 3:1 rule for fluid resuscitation)	crystalloid	crystalloid	crystalloid + blood	crystalloid + blood

[a]Percent of blood volume in a 70-kg adult.
[b]Assume normal of 72/min.
[c]Assume normal of 120/80.
[d]Assume normal of 40–50 mL/h.

tion to the volume lost. Tachycardia may not be a presenting sign in those patients taking beta-adrenergic or calcium-entry antagonists.[16]

Acute blood loss of 15% of total blood volume (TBV = 75 mL/kg in adults) in most healthy adults will result in minimal hemodynamic changes, courtesy of the intact autonomic nervous system. Fluid replacement for these Class I patients is 3 mL of balanced salt solution for each mL of blood lost to maintain euvolemia (3:1 rule). Acute blood loss of 20 to 25% TBV causes tachycardia (> 100/min), narrowing pulse pressure (30 mm Hg), tachypnea (20 to 30/min), and a reduction in urine output (< 0.5 mL/kg/h). These Class II patients require balanced salt solution 3:1 with blood and/or colloid as needed to maintain hemodynamic stability. In Class III, acute blood loss (30 to 35% reduction of TBV), patients are confused and anxious in addition to exhibiting marked changes in vital signs and urine output. Blood infusion must be started immediately to restore oxygen-carrying capacity and to supplement balanced salt/colloid infusion in reestablishing an effective circulating volume. A Class IV hemorrhage patient (> 40% of TBV) is lethargic and very confused, with extreme changes in vital signs. Blood, colloid, and balanced salt solutions are infused as rapidly as possible utilizing all available intravenous sites.[16]

Hemorrhage Control. After the airway is secured, external sites of hemorrhage should be controlled using compression or digital pressure. Use of hemostats for bleeding control frequently leads to further bleeding and trauma to nerves, tendons, and surrounding tissue.[17] Tourniquets are useful only if applied proximal to a traumatic amputation. Disadvantages of tourniquet use include insufficient pressure to occlude arterial bleeding but sufficient to occlude venous return,

increasing blood loss; interference of collateral blood flow, increasing warm ischemia time; and increases in the amputation rate.[17] Military anti-shock trousers (MAST) are helpful in splinting and bleeding control in cases of pelvic and multiple leg fractures. Blood pressure in the shock victim is supported by an increase in peripheral vascular resistance using this device. MAST deflation must be slow, with the abdominal section first, followed by the legs one at a time, during continuous monitoring of the blood pressure. Deflation is stopped and fluid increased if the blood pressure drops more than 5 mm Hg.

Fluid Resuscitation. Clinical and physiologic endpoints to successful fluid resuscitation include the return towards normal of the heart rate; diastolic blood pressure; urine output; central venous pressure; mental status; peripheral pulses; capillary refill; arterial pH; and base deficit. Both the intravascular and the extravascular spaces must be restored if the patient is to be stabilized. If the response to a reasonable quantity of fluids is slow or negligible, intravenous lines must be checked and the patient reassessed for other sites of bleeding previously overlooked. Blood pressure by cuff or doppler and ECG activity are monitored continuously while blood is drawn for type and crossmatch, arterial blood gas, and toxicology screen as soon as intravenous cannulation is achieved.

Adequate peripheral intravenous access in the hypovolemic patient can be difficult to obtain, or is occasionally lost to malfunction and excessive handling during transport or bicarbonate injection. The upper extremity is preferred, when suitable, to the lower extremity, as the risk of deep-vein thrombosis is less and drugs are more likely to reach the heart and the brain during cardiopulmonary resuscitation.

Although cannulation of the basilic or cephalic veins using large-bore cannulae are often sufficient, saphenous vein cutdown with insertion of intravenous tubing or femoral vein cannulation are used for more rapid infusion. In cases where the abdomen is traumatized, use of a lower extremity intravenous route may lead to pooling of resuscitative fluids in the abdomen. Central venous access is accomplished by internal jugular, external jugular, or subclavian routes, supplying a means for infusion and monitoring fluid replacement.

Preventing end organ dysfunction is a critical step in the reduction of serious morbidity and mortality in the traumatized. Avoidance of prolonged shock and protection of end organs after multiple trauma is effectively accomplished by rapid restoration of the circulating volume. Five factors have been identified that influence the rate of infusion: cannula size; method of fluid delivery; number of simultaneous infusions; fluid type; and fluid temperature. Poiseuille-Hagen stated that resistance to fluid flow in a tube can be expressed as follows:

$$R = \frac{8\,nL}{\pi r^4}$$

where R = resistance, n = viscosity, L = length of vessel, and r = radius.

Because the rate of fluid infusion is proportional to the size of the cannula inserted, 16-gauge or larger cannulae are suggested for rapid volume replacement. When insertion of a large-gauged cannulae is impossible, multiple smaller-gauge, or central lines, must be started. Fluid infusion rates using different methods of administration have been studied (Table 16–7). In decreasing rate order, these are pressure bag, 200 mm Hg; syringe in-line; hand pump in-line; and infusate 1 meter above cannula.[18] Fluid type and fluid temperature will effect the fluid viscosity, which is inversely proportionate to the rate of infusion. Whole blood will infuse at twice the rate of packed cells. Whole blood at room temperature infuses 66% faster than whole blood at 4°C.[19]

Fluid Selection. Fluids available for intravenous infusion include crystalloid, balanced salt solutions, hypertonic salt solutions, colloid solution, blood, and blood components. "Artifical blood" such as perfluorochemicals (fluosol-DA) and stroma-free hemoglobin are still experimental and unavailable for general use. Strictly defined, crystalloid solutions contain nonionizing solutes (eg, dextrose in water), and are therefore dangerous for massive resuscitation as they cause hyponatremia, hyperglycemia, and osmotic diuresis, leading to hypovolemia.[20] Comparison between the constituents of some asanguinous solutions and plasma are summarized in Table 16–8.

Balanced Salt Solutions. Advantages of Ringer's lactate are lowered blood viscosity (slightly hypotonic), improving flow in the microcirculation; metabolism of the L isomer of lactate in the liver to bicarbonate, buffering the metabolic acidosis associated with shock; low cost; and nonallergenicity. Disadvantages include the large volume necessary (short circulatory half-life), because of diffusion into the interstitial space; decreased serum osmolarity, producing intracellular edema; and increased intracranial pressure. Although infusion of large amounts of Ringer's lactate does decrease plasma oncotic pressure, in the absence of a marked elevation of pulmonary artery wedge pressure (PAWP > 25 mm Hg), pulmonary edema does not occur and it is otherwise effective for

TABLE 16–7. FLUID FLOW RATES WITH VARIOUS METHODS OF ADMINISTRATION

Catheter	Gravity (1m)	Pump	Syringe	Pressure Bag (at 200 mm Hg)
In Vitra Flow Rates in mL/min Using Water and Deseret Angiocaths				
0.12-inch IV tubing	180	285	200	665
14G	125	215	180	330
16G	100	180	165	285
18G	60	150	140	200
Whole Blood at Room Temperature				
0.12-inch IV tubing	140	335	125	400
14G	90	200	120	200
16G	65	125	100	180
18G	35	80	100	100

From Dula DJ, Muller HA, Donovan JW: Flow rate variance of commonly used intravenous infusion techniques. J Trauma 1981; 2:480.

TABLE 16–8. COMPARISON OF ASANGUINOUS FLUID CONTENTS TO PLASMA (mEq/L)

	9NS	LR	Normisol	Plasmalyte	Plasma
MOsmol/L	308	272	295	294	285
Cations (mEq)					
Na^+	154	130	140	140	142
K^+	—	4	5	5	4
Ca^{++}	—	3	—	—	5
Mg^{++}	—	—	3	3	2
Anions					
Cl^-	154	109	98	98	102
Lactate	—	28	—	—	—
Acetate	—	—	27	27	—
Gluconate	—	—	23	23	—
HCO_3^-	—	—	—	—	26

resuscitation.[21] Because normal saline is devoid of base buffer, infusion of large volumes dilute body buffers, resulting in hyperchloremic metabolic acidosis.[22] Aside from this, normal saline differs little from Ringer's lactate in its advantages and disadvantages in massive fluid replacement. The use of hyperosmolar salt solutions for massive fluid repletion, although still under investigation, has the following proposed advantages: a smaller volume is needed to restore adequate intravascular volume; renal and coronary capillary vasodilation occurs; blood pressure is rapidly elevated and inotropism improved; intracranial pressure is decreased by lowering intracerebral water content, thus improving cerebral perfusion; and the solutions are inexpensive and nonallergenic. Disadvantages include the risks of hyperosmolarity; hypernatremia; hypokalemia; intracellular dehydration; and acute volume overload.[23]

Colloids. Solutions with a molecular weight greater than 60,000 are considered to be colloids. Because of their size and provided that capillary circulation is intact, their molecules enhance plasma volume, making them potentially useful in hypovolemic shock. Colloid solutions are of two types: protein containing (albumin and plasma protein fraction) and nonprotein containing (dextran and starch). Advantages and disadvantages are listed in Table 16–9. Controversial issues concerning the use of colloid versus balanced salt solutions during hypovolemic shock resuscitation are discussed in Chapter 7.

Blood and Blood Products. Several preparations of blood and blood products can be used during the resuscitation of the severely traumatized patient: whole blood; type O negative low titer; type-specific with or without screening and cross-matching; packed red cells; fresh frozen plasma; platelets; and specific procoagulants. Each differs from the other with respect to contents, infection potential, and proper usage. Risks associated with transfusion of blood and blood products are listed in Table 16–10 and compositional differences appear in Table 16–11.

When irreversable shock is imminent despite colloid/balanced salt solution infusion, un-cross-matched type-specific is used even with a risk of possible transfusion reaction (1/1000 if no previous transfusion history; 1/100 if positive transfusion history). If

TABLE 16–9. COMPARISON OF PROTEIN AND NONPROTEIN-CONTAINING COLLOIDS

	Protein		Nonprotein		
	Albumin	PPF	Dextran		Hetastarch
			70	40	
Allergenicity	+	+	+	+	rare
Blood dyscrasia	—	—	+	+	rare
Cross-matching problem	possible		possible		no
Expense	+ +	+ +	+ +	+ +	+
Volume expansion	+	+	+ +	+ +	24 h
Dose			30 mL/kg		20 mL/kg
Infection	no	no	no	no	no
T-1/2 circulation	short	short	short		+ + +
Molecular size	> 60		70k	40k	
Clearance	short	short			prolonged

+ least; + + moderate; + + + most.

TABLE 16-10. DANGERS OF BLOOD TRANFUSION

Risk	Frequency
Viral hepatitis	Up to 25%, of which 10% will die
Bacteroemia	2%
Incompatibility	Up to 0.7%
Haemolysis	Up to 0.3%
Allergic reactions	Up to 0.2%
Other infections (syphillis, malaria, brucellosis, trypanasomiasis)	0.1%
Citrate toxicity	
Acidity	
Hypothermia	
Hyperkalemia	
Coagulopathy	
Free Hb	
Phagolytic dysfunction	
Increased ammonia	
Hyperbilirubinoemia	
Hyper-phaspharemia	
Total death rate	0.1 to 1.0%

Bristow A, Giesecke AH: Fluid therapy of trauma. Semin Anesth, 1985; 4:128.

type-specific is unavailable, type O Rh negative is used with the following proviso: when more than 50% of the TBV has been replaced, type O Rh negative is continued (despite type-specific availability) or risk high probability of a transfusion reaction. Clinical suggestions for propitious use of blood products are as follows: infusion of whole blood is preferred when available; infuse platelets and fresh frozen plasma only if impaired hemostasis is apparent (no routine infusions); and avoid procoagulants until major surgical hemorrhage is controlled. After massive blood transfusion (more than 10 units of packed red cells), the most common coagulopathy is dilutional thrombocytopenia, and requires platelet infusion. In addition to the immediate demands of administering blood products to the patient, those rendering care must remember to exercise precaution against contracting AIDS or hepatitis when handling fluids (patient or donor) and needles.

TABLE 16-11. Constituents of Blood Products

	Whole Blood	PRBC	FFP	PLTS
Infection	+	+ +	+ + +	+ + +
RBC	Y	Y	N	N
Plasma	Y	Y	Y	Y
Albumin	Y	Y	Y	Y
PLTS	Y(<48h)	N	N	Y
Clotting factors	Y(<1wk)	N	Y	Y

Y = yes; N = no.

+ small risk; + + moderate risk; + + + greatest risk.

Associated Life-Threatening Conditions

Immediately after the airway is secured, clinical signs are sought to ascertain that ventilation and oxygenation are adequate. During fluid resuscitation, trauma victims undergo scrutiny for life-threatening and associated injuries. Pathology considered immediately life-threatening is associated with head, thoracic, airway, and vascular trauma.

Thoracic trauma can be organized into five anatomic areas of involvement: thoracic wall; pleural space; lungs; diaphragm; and the mediastinal organs. Thoracic wall injury of significance includes first rib fracture; flail chest; and open pneumothorax. Cases of severe trauma can cause first rib fracture, leading to damage of underlying structures and requiring careful examination for secondary injury to the aorta and tracheobronchial tree. Blunt anterolateral chest trauma involving three or more segments, where rib fracture occurs on both sides of impaction, results in a flail chest. Paradoxical movement of the chest wall (especially severe with transverse sternal fracture) interferes with normal bellows function, causing increased respiratory effort to overcome inefficient gas exchange. Treatment for a severe flail chest depends on endotracheal intubation to provide positive pressure ventilation for internal stabilization. Penetrating injury to the chest wall (open pneumothorax), larger than the glottic opening, allows rapid equilibration between atmospheric and intrapleural pressures. Immediate therapy includes sterile occlusive dressing and chest tube insertion for reinflation of the lung.

Pleural space pathology of significance, from blunt or penetrating causes, includes tension pneumothorax and hemothorax. Diagnosis of pneumothorax depends on decreased breath sounds, percussion hyperresonance, decreased hemithoracic movement, and tracheal deviation, and is confirmed by chest x-ray. When pleural air accumulates rapidly, increased pressure shifts the mediastinum contralaterally. Cardiovascular collapse is signalled by hypotension, tachycardia, diminished QRS voltage, and jugular venous distension. Rapid conversion to a simple pneumothorax by percutaneous large-bore needle thoracostomy at the ipsilateral second intercostal space midclavicular line is necessary. After a characteristic hiss of air, vital signs should return towards normal and a chest tube should be inserted. Hemothorax may represent significant cardiac and/or large vessel bleeding and is commonly associated with blunt or penetrating injury. Decreased breath sounds and dullness to percussion with shock requires aggressive fluid resuscitation and a chest x-ray in the upright position if possible for diagnosis. Chest drainage of greater than 300 mL/h over three hours, or progressive hypotension during drainage, will require emergency thoracotomy.

Traumatic lung injury with lethal consequences involves massive air leak due to tracheal or bronchial disruption. Massive hemoptysis, airway obstruction, and progressive mediastinal or subcutaneous emphysema accompany these lesions, leading to immediate thoracotomy or fiberoptic bronchoscopy through the endotracheal tube if bleeding is minimal. Double-lumen tube insertion with high-frequency ventilation to the injured lung may be necessary to facilitate surgery. Pulmonary contusion may lead to pulmonary edema with decreased compliance, necessitating positive end-expiratory pressure manipulation to maintain adequate oxygenation and ventilation.

Diaphragmatic injury is possible by blunt or penetrating mechanisms, resulting in acute dyspnea and chest pain. Diagnosis is based on ascultation of bowel sounds in the thorax and presence of bowel and/or a nasogastric tube in the chest on chest x-ray. Immediate surgical repair is indicated to avoid atelectasis and severe infection.

Severe blunt chest trauma resulting in cardiac tamponade is almost uniformly fatal due to myocardial and septal rupture. Penetrating injury to the heart can lead to tamponade resulting in Beck's triad (hypotension, muffled heart sounds, and increased venous pressure with jugular venous distention). A penetrating object (eg, a knife) should remain in place during resuscitation, with removal first attempted under controlled conditions in the operating room. Patients with tamponade can be treated initially by subxyphoid pericardiocentesis but will need immediate thoracotomy. Maintaining peripheral vasoconstriction and a full, fast heart during induction is critical. Rupture just distal to the origin of the left subclavian artery occurs in 80 to 90% of cases involving aortic trauma due to high-speed decelerating injury. These injuries are instantaneously fatal in 90% of cases. Patients with incomplete tears or smaller lesions complain of retrosternal or intrascapular pain and shortness of breath. Signs include acute onset of upper extremity hypertension, harsh systolic murmur, and a widened mediastinum on chest x-ray. Arch aortogram is important to locate the disruption, and leaving the femoral artery cannula in place is helpful for monitoring pressure distal to the tear. The right radial artery is preferred to measure pressure proximal to the lesion. Penetrating injury to the aorta is very lethal and chances of survival are better if the site is intrapericardial (presents as a tamponade).

Airway trauma management depends on several factors: degree of obstruction; level of injury; associated injury; and mechanism of injury. Total or partial obstruction after airway trauma is indeed an emergent situation requiring immediate oropharyngeal intubation, cricothyroidotomy, or tracheostomy. When obstruction is not immediately apparent, continued observation is warranted, as hematoma or edema may narrow the airway suddenly. Blunt mechanisms of injury can distort the airway by fracture and disruption. Penetrating mechanisms can sever vessels and nerves resulting in hemorrhage and a loss of motor control. Trauma to the nose, maxilla, or mandible is generally amenable to oropharyngeal intubation using topical anesthesia with the patient awake. Avoiding techniques that induce sudden obstruction and refraining from passing an endotracheal tube blindly into injured areas is essential. Penetrating suprahyoid injury results in obstruction from the loss of tongue control, and a subhyoid injury leads to obstruction from epiglottic injury. Thyroid cartilage injury is prone to hematoma from bleeding and loss of laryngeal muscle tone if the recurrent larygeal nerve is involved. Injury below the thyroid cartilage can lead to obstruction from damage to the trachea, making fiberoptic intubation necessary if caused by a blunt injury or direct insertion of a small tube through the wound if caused by a penetrating injury. When intrathoracic tracheobronchial injury results (blunt mechanism from high-speed deceleration), fiberoptic bronchoscopy is indicated for insertion of an endotracheal tube beyond the injury. Penetrating injury at this level requires insertion of the endotracheal tube under direct vision through the wound. Associated injuries for cases of blunt trauma to the airway are cervical spine fracture and basal skull fracture; in cases of penetrating trauma, vessel and nerve damage with bleeding are additional causes for concern.[24]

Hemorrhage can be intracavitary or extracavitary. Diagnosis of thoracic intracavitary bleeding is made clinically by the presence of hypotension, decreased breath sounds, and dullness to percussion of the hemithorax. Chest radiography will detect the presence of a hemothorax. Abdominal intracavitary bleeding is ruled out by negative peritoneal lavage or CT scan when appropriate. Mortality from major abdominal vascular trauma is high (30 to 40%) regardless of the cause. Forty percent of these patients arrive at the hospital without a palpable blood pressure. Trauma to abdominal organs leads to significant hemorrhage. Both liver and spleen rupture or subcapsular hematomas can be ruled out by abdominal CT. Extracavitary sources of hemorrhage (laceration or fracture) are frequently responsible for significant volume loss and must be diagnosed early for adequate control.

PREOPERATIVE MANAGEMENT

Patients who come to surgery for multiple trauma are at increased risk for mortality and morbidity on the

TABLE 16-12. MULTIPLE TRAUMA PREOPERATIVE PROTOCOL

Airway secured; oxygenation/ventilation adequate[a]
Fluid resuscitation underway; lines, fluids, medications noted[a]
Blood specimens sent and received by blood bank; blood availability[a]
Vital signs; neurologic assessment; hemodynamic stability[a]
Associated injuries (pneumothorax, spine involvement, etc.)[a]
OR staff notified[a]
Adequate personnel to accompany patient to radiology
Adequate staff and monitoring for transfer to OR[a]
Anesthesia staff ready[a]
Anesthesia equipment ready[a]

[a]Minimum needed for the most urgent cases

basis of the emergency surgery, prior medical history, and associated injuries. A brief history, when possible, using the mnemonic AMPLE[25] is extremely helpful prior to induction:

- A —allergies, airway.
- M—Medications (prescribed or abused).
- P —Past medical, surgical, anesthetic history.
- L —Labs, and last menstrual cycle (if childbearing age).
- E —Eaten (NPO status).

Table 16-12 provides a list of items necessary to facilitate efficient patient transfer and prompt initiation of definitive surgery. Complete physical examination from head to toe is vital, time permitting, to rule out life-threatening and limb-threatening injuries. The Glasgow Coma Scale is used to determine level of consciousness (Table 16–13) and should be repeated periodically.

TABLE 16-13. GLASGOW COMA SCALE

Best verbal response	
None	1
Uncomprehensible sound	2
Inappropriate words	3
Confused	4
Oriented	5
Eyes open	
None	1
To pain	2
To speech	3
Spontaneously	4
Best motor responses	
None	1
Abnormal extensor	2
Abnormal flexion	3
Withdraws	4
Localizes	5
Obeys	6
Total Coma Scale	**15**

Teasdale G, Jennett B: Assessment of coma and impaired consciousness. A practical scale. *Lancet* 1974; 2:81–4.

INTRAOPERATIVE MANAGEMENT

A continuous electrocardiogram, a device for monitoring oxygenation and ventilation, continual blood pressure recording, and continual recording of temperature changes are considered minimal monitoring standards.[26] Surveillance of hemodynamics and volume status is improved by insertion of a Foley catheter, intraarterial catheter, and central venous pressure catheter when appropriate. General anesthesia is indicated whenever the thorax and/or abdomen are involved. Induction of anesthesia must be properly conducted in order to avoid further insult. Preoxygenation, precurarization, and rapid sequence are used when the airway is anatomically normal. Cricoid pressure is maintained from drug injection until the endotracheal tube cuff is inflated and proper placement verified. Aspiration of gastric contents, if not already occurring, is a significant possibility throughout the course of treatment in these full-stomach patients, but especially during intubation and extubation. Nasogastric suction (except with basal skull fracture), anticholinergics, antacids, H_2 receptor antagonists, and metoclopramide are advocated to reduce the volume or acidity of stomach contents but are often impractical. Premedication must be individualized and unless strongly indicated is deleted.

Induction of the hemodynamically unstable patient is accomplished by administering only the smallest doses of ketamine or thiopental, followed by only oxygen and neuromuscular blockade until the mean blood pressure rises near 50 mm Hg. Analgesia, amnesia, and cardiovascular stability are carefully balanced with addition of small doses of benzodiazepine and a volatile agent. Narcotics added in small doses as the patient stabilizes help reduce the concentration of volatile agents. Nitrous oxide should be avoided as it adds to the cardiovascular depressive effects from the volatile agents and diffuses into air-containing cavities. Neuromuscular blockade is best achieved by avoiding agents that release histamine and result in potential hypotension.

POSTOPERATIVE MANAGEMENT AND COMPLICATIONS

Multiple trauma patients typically require several teams of surgeons in series or simultaneously to repair injuries sustained. The consequences are numerous: anesthesia is prolonged; blood loss is increased leading to massive transfusion; and significant hypothermia is common. These and other problems often begin in the operating room and carry over into the recovery period.

On transport to the PACU, multiple infusion tubing and monitoring lines, monitoring hardware, oxygen tanks, and ventilating equipment are moved. Ideally the patient should be in stable condition and after prior communication the PACU personnel should be ready to receive the victim. Patient oxygenation, ventilation, and hemodynamic monitoring are the immediate priorities in the PACU. Vital signs, infusion lines, Foley catheter, nasogastric tube, and other tubes are checked and a report is given. Attention is directed towards present or potential problems as discussed below.

Massive blood loss, requiring transfusion of one or more times the total blood volume, commonly results in coagulopathy of several etiologies. Unless whole blood is administered, the endogenous platelet pool is reduced by infusion of non-platelet-containing blood products, leading to dilutional thrombocytopenia (the most common cause of bleeding diathesis following massive transfusion). Signs of coagulopathy include oozing and generalized bleeding from orifices, mucosa, canula puncture sites, and wounds. Patients with coagulopathy and thrombocytopenia should be transfused 0.1 unit platelet pack/kg, raising the platelet count by 50,000/mm³.[16] Storing platelets at 4°C causes platelet dysfunction and shortens platelet lifespan to less than 48 hours. In vivo, platelets are sequestered from circulation during hypothermia, adding to the problem. Coagulopathy from decreased clotting factors V and VIII is much less common and as little as 30% of the normal levels can lead to effective coagulation. The formation of a good blood clot in a glass tube within 10 minutes indicates a normal clotting time and transfusion of fresh frozen plasma is not necessary. Prothrombin time and partial prothrombin time are not considered useful by some in predicting the need for fresh frozen plasma infusion. Patients who are transfused platelets also receive the clotting factors present in platelet plasma. Infusion of fresh frozen plasma is therefore infrequently indicated.[27]

Binding of serum ionized calcium by citrate can infrequently result in hypocalcemia (hypotension, narrow pulse pressure, elevated capillary wedge and central venous pressures), but only if CPD blood infusion exceeds 2 mL/kg/min. Despite transient reductions in serum ionized calcium, euvolemic patients remain hemodynamically stable because levels return to normal minutes after infusion is terminated.[28] Factors promoting citrate toxicity (by interferring with hepatic metabolism) include liver disease, liver transplantation, or hypothermia. Coagulopathy is not a result of hypocalcemia as previously thought. Although banked blood contains elevated potassium levels, hypokalemia has been reported, but hyperkalemia is possible if the infusion rate is greater than 120 mL/min. Routine or prophylactic calcium administration is not recommended for citrate intoxication but is indicated if peaked T-waves appear when hyperkalemia results from rapid blood infusion. Although banked blood is acidic (from increased lactate, pyruvate, glycolysis, and elevated PA_{CO_2}), it contains ample citrate, frequently producing metabolic alkalosis.[29] Bicarbonate administration must not be given routinely and should be based on arterial (or venous) pH and P_{CO_2}.

Heat production to heat loss ratio is often lowered significantly when managing the unstable multiple trauma patient during surgery. Preventing hypothermia is more expedient than treating it once established. Patients allowed to become hypothermic frequently become management problems in the PACU. Oxygen consumption is elevated 500% during shivering, hemoglobin–oxygen affinity is increased, potassium leaks from red cells, citrate metabolism is impaired, myocardial dysfunction occurs, dysrhythmias can be refractory, and increased systemic vascular resistance impairs cardiovascular function. Patients with ischemic heart disease may require sedation and muscle relaxation to prevent the adverse effects of shivering. Hypothermia prolongs pharmacodynamic drug effects and delays awakening. Warm ambient PACU temperature, blankets, and radiant heat lamps are minimally necessary to make the patient euthermic.

Multiple trauma frequently leads to organ failure from either direct injury or the consequences of shock. The organs most often involved include the lungs and the kidneys. Pulmonary contusion, interstitial edema, and aspiration pneumonitis will increase intrapulmonary shunting and require intensive intraoperative and PACU management. Infusions of blood stored longer than five days contain the fibrin-white blood cell and platelet microaggregates thought to contribute to the development of adult respiratory distress syndrome (ARDS).[30] Micropore (40 μm) filtration of blood transfusion has not significantly decreased the incidence or severity of ARDS as compared to standard (170 μm) filtration.[31] Sepsis and shock (intensity and duration) are therefore more likely to influence the development of ARDS than are microaggregates from tranfusion. Early use of low-level positive end-expired pressure (PEEP) is often helpful in minimizing the onset and severity of ARDS. Periodic blood gas analysis in the PACU is used to guide PEEP and inspired oxygen administration. Fluid administration is guided by urine output, hemodynamics, hematocrit, and if necessary pulmonary artery wedge pressure.

Beside ARDS, prolonged shock is linked to renal failure. Oliguria often begins in the operating room but is also seen in the PACU, and can be managed

(Table 16–14) as suggested by Bristow and Giesecke.[19] Mechanical obstruction of the urinary catheter is usually associated with anuria but this must also first be ruled out in oliguria (less than 0.5 mL/kg/h). The lower limit of renal autoregulation is reached when the systolic blood pressure is below 80 mm Hg. Hypovolemia results in hormonal changes prolonging oliguria: catecholamines reduce renal blood flow; renin and angiotensin reduce renal cortical blood flow; and elevated atrial naturetic peptide and antidiuretic hormone reduce net urine output. Renal hypoperfusion is improved by maximizing preload, cardiac output, and renal blood flow by titrating fluids (crystalloid improves renal cortical ultrafiltration better than colloid), inotropes, and low-dose dopamine (3 to 5 μg/kg/min), respectively. Primary renal tubular damage is suspected in a hemodynamically stable patient with iosostenuria and urinary sodium greater than 40 mmol/L prior to using furosemide. Early treatment of renal failure includes sodium repletion, alkalinization of the urine (pH greater than 6.5), and renal-dose dopamine. Renal failure in the trauma patient is most commonly related to hypovolemic shock, although transfusion reaction, disseminated intravascular coagulation, nephrotoxic drugs, contrast media, dextrans, sepsis, fat embolism, myoglobin, and direct trauma to the kidney are other potential causes. Irreversible renal failure requires hemodialysis to maintain intravascular volume, blood urea nitrogen, creatinine, and electrolytes in balance.

Other issues to be addressed in the PACU include extubation, pain management, delayed return to consciousness, and acute drug withdrawal. Failure of a return to consciousness includes a long differential (Chapter 2). In addition to those modalities of postoperative pain treatment discussed in Chapter 5, patients with chest trauma can have an intrapleural catheter surgically implanted intraoperatively or inserted by the anesthesiologist, prior to awakening or in the PACU. This will reduce postoperative splinting and improve pulmonary function early. Extubation will depend upon the extent and cause of trauma-related injuries; antecedent medical history; duration and profundity of shock; hemodynamic status in addition to the state of consciousness; laboratory reports (electrolytes, hematocrit, acid–base balance); normothermia; and the usual pulmonary parameters. Obviously major injury to the head, airway, thorax, or abdomen will require postoperative ventilatory support, especially after massive transfusion in the hypothermic patient. Anemia should be corrected and nutritional balance must be addressed early by the trauma care team to insure maximum outcome.

Violent traumatic injury is frequently sustained during drug negotiations. When patients abusing drugs or alcohol sustain a multiple trauma injury requiring prolonged surgery, symptoms of acute drug withdrawal may manifest in the PACU. Victims with an abuse history exhibit bizarre behavior during withdrawal and demonstrate signs of catecholamine release requiring sedation, narcotics, and treatment of hypertension, pulmonary edema, tachycardia, or dysrhythmias. Acute intoxication with cocaine ("crack") can result in severe cardiovascular stress culminating with hypertension and intracerebral bleed, myocardial infarction and congestive failure, tachydysrhythmias, or sudden death. Chronic alcoholic patients require treatment for impending delirium tremens and higher concentrations of inhalational agents. Acute alcohol intoxication renders the patient more sensitive to anesthetic agents, predisposing to a delayed recovery period or possible overdosing during anesthesia or in the PACU. Victims on prescriptive med-

TABLE 16–14. SUGGESTED PROTOCOL FOR THE MANAGEMENT OF OLIGURIA IN THE TRAUMA PATIENT

Urine output of < 0.5 mL/kg/h
↓
Ensure urine correctly measured
↓
Ensure catheter not blocked
↙ ↘

Systolic BP < 30 mm Hg	Systolic BP > 100 mm Hg
CVP < 5 mm Hg	CVP > 9 mm Hg
Wedge < 7 mm Hg	Wedge > 10 mm Hg
Cardiac output < 4 L/min	Cardiac output > 5 L/min
Vasoconstricted	Vasodilated
Urine osmolarity > 400 mOsm	Urine osmolarity ≡ Plasma
Urine sodium < 10 mmol/L in absence of low serum sodium	Urine sodium > 40 mmol/L
↓	↓
Δ Hypoperfusion	Δ Primary renal damage or established ATN
↓	↓
Give fluids and/or inotropes as indicated	Treat sodium until serum level greater than 140 mmol/L

Give bicarbonate until base excess greater than 5
↓
5–10 mg furosamide ──→ Dopamine @ 3–5 μg/kg/min
↓
Δ Established renal failure
↓
Restrict intake to (output + 1 L/day)
↓
Restrict potassium and sodium
↓
Give calories to prevent tissue catabolism
↓
Early hemodialysis or ultrafiltration

Adapted from Bristow A, Giesecke AH: Fluid therapy of trauma. *Semin Anesth* 1985; 4:130.

ications must be continued as necessary. The PACU is also that area charged with controlling the interface between the patient and family wishing to visit, law enforcement officials wishing to question, and press members wishing to gather information. For this reason patients should be designated a special area in the PACU where one-on-one (often more) nursing care can be administered without disturbing other patients.

It is clear that proper management of the multiple trauma patient requires an intensive coordinated effort incorporating the skills of numerous medical personnel in succession. The rapidity, efficiency, and accuracy with which each phase is carried out often determines morbidity and mortality. The anesthesiologist is charged with a major role in the initial care of the patient, providing anesthesia under the most emergent circumstances, and initial postoperative care. This requires intimate familiarity with a vast body of information, of which only the highlights have been presented.

REFERENCES

1. Shackford SR, Perel A: Forward. Problems in critical care. *Trauma* 1987;1:525.
2. Dolev E: The management of trauma: Historic perspective. Problems in critical care. *Trauma* 1987;1:527–537.
3. Watt J: Doctors in the wars. *J Roy Soc Med* 1984;77:265–266.
4. Ravdin IS: Foreword. *J Trauma* 1961;1:8.
5. Trunkey DD: Overview of trauma. *Surg Clin North Am* 1982;62:3–11.
6. Bzik KD, Bellamy RF: A note on combat casualty care statistics. *Milit Med* 1984;149:229–233.
7. Boyd DR, Adams CR: Comprehensive regional trauma/emergency medical services (EMS) delivery system: The United States experience. *World J Surg* 1983;7:149–153.
8. Cales RH: Trauma mortality in Orange County: The effect of implementation of a regional trauma system. *Ann Emerg Med* 1984;13:15–20.
9. Trunkey DD: Trauma. *Sci Am* 1983;249:28–31.
10. Baker CC, Oppenheimer L, Stephens B, et al: Epidemiology of trauma deaths. *Am J Surg* 1980;140:144–148.
11. Auerbach PS, Geehr EC: Inadequate oxygenation and ventilation using the esophageal gastric tube airway in the prehospital setting. *JAMA* 1983;250:3067–3069.
12. Davies JAH: Blind nasal intubation with propanidid. *Br J Anaesth* 1972;44:528–531.
13. Dhara SS: Guided blind endotracheal intubation. *Anaesthesia* 1980;35:81–82.
14. Latto IP: Management of difficult intubation, in *Difficulties in Tracheal Intubation*. London, Bailliere Tindall, 1987 pp 99–142.
15. Shires GT, Cunningham JN, Baker CRF: Alterations in cellular fluid during acute hemorrhagic shock in primates. *Ann Surg* 1972;176:288–289.
16. Berman JA: The trauma victim, in Frost EAM (ed): *Preanesthetic Assessment.* Vol 1, Boston, Birkhauser, 1988, pp 10–20.
17. Shackford SR: Initial management of patients with multiple injuries. Problems in critical care. *Trauma* 1987;1:550–559.
18. Dula DJ, Muller HA, Donovan JW: Flow rate variance of commonly used intravenous infusion techniques. *J Trauma* 1981;2:480–482.
19. Bristow A, Giesecke AH: Fluid therapy of trauma. *Semin Anesth* 1985;4:124–133.
20. Roth E, Lax LC, Maloney JV: Changes in extracellular fluid volumes during shock and surgical trauma in animals and man. *Surg Forum* 1967;18:43–49.
21. Metildi LA, Shackford SR, Virgilio RW, et al: Crystalloid versus colloid in fluid resuscitation of patients with severe pulmonary insufficiency. *Surg Gyneccol Obstet* 1984;158:207–213.
22. Oh MS, Carroll HJ: The anion gap. *N Engl J Med* 1977;78:213–215.
23. Shackford SR: Fluid resuscitation of the trauma victim. Problems in critical care. *Trauma* 1987;1:576–587.
24. Bogetz MS, Katz JA: Airway management of the trauma patient. *Semin Anesth* 1985;4:114–123.
25. Advanced Trauma Life Support Course. American College of Surgeons, 1981.
26. American Society of Anesthesiologists 1989 Directory of Members. Standards for Basic Intra-operative Monitoring, p 609.
27. Braunstein AH, Oberman HA: Transfusion of plasma components. *Transfusion* 1984;24:281–286.
28. Denlinger JK, Narhwold ML, Gibbs PS, et al: Hypocalcemia during rapid blood transfusion in anaesthetized man. *Br J Anaesth* 1976;48:995–997.
29. Miller RD, Tong MJ, Robbins TO: Effects of massive transfusion of blood on acid–base balance. *JAMA* 1971;216:1762–1769.
30. Miller RD, Brzica SM: Blood, blood components, colloids and autotransfusion therapy, in Miller RD (ed): *Anesthesia*, ed 2. New York, Churchill Livingstone, 1986, vol 2, pp 1348–1350.
31. Durtschi MB, Haisch CE, Reynolds L, et al: Effect of micropore filtration in pulmonary function after massive transfusion. *Am J Surg* 1979;138:8–10.

17 | The Geriatric Patient

Patricia S. Underwood

Physiologic aging processes, and age-related medical derangements and their associated medications, contribute to the special management concerns for the elderly in the postanesthetic care unit (PACU).

Between ages 30 and 40, a gradual decline in all organ function begins. This chapter reviews some of these important physiologic changes of aging in major organ systems, age-related diseases, and methods for management of commonly encountered complications in this age group.

We classify patients past the age of 75 as elderly. A patient this old can expect to live ten more years.[1] Since 1900, when the life expectancy at birth was 49.2 years, this age has risen gradually. In 1984, the number of persons between the ages of 75 and 84 was eleven times larger, and the 85-plus group 21 times greater, than in 1900. Fifty percent of all people past the age of 75 can expect to have at least one operative procedure prior to their death.[2] At Montefiore Medical Center patients past 75 comprise more than 20% of the PACU population.

In caring for the elderly it is immediately apparent that aging is a uniquely individual process and patients must also be evaluated in terms of their vitality. Most physicians have treated 80 year olds who have the stamina of 60 year olds, and the reverse, 60 year olds with the physiologic age of 80. Ease of postoperative recovery can be closely coordinated with preoperative activity level. For example, patients who are bedridden have a greater risk of a postoperative myocardial infarction.[3]

Postoperative complications occurring in elderly patients in the PACU include not only all those usually associated with the surgical procedure performed but also those that are related to the aging process itself. The incidence of postoperative and life-threatening complications is three times higher in patients 75 years and older as compared to those aged 65 to 74 years.[4] All geriatric patients have less functional organ reserve and thus any untoward events in the perioperative period have more pronounced effects. Good intra- and postoperative management dictate that the body's homeostatic mechanisms remain stable. The elderly may not be able to compensate for any derangements.

CARDIOVASCULAR DERANGEMENTS

Cardiovascular derangements are the predominant cause of morbidity and mortality in the aged in the PACU.[5] Physiologic changes and age-related cardiac disease contribute to a higher incidence of these abnormalities in the elderly than in younger patients undergoing the same surgical procedures.

Myocardial Ischemia or Infarction

Coronary artery disease is the single most common pathologic defect in the elderly, both in pathologic and functional terms.[6] Stephen reported that 26.9% of 2000 patients over the age of 70 had a history of arteriosclerotic cardiovascular disease (ASCVD), 18.5% had had a myocardial infarction, and 6.4% complained of angina preoperatively.[7]

Even though the degree of atheromatous change is highly variable, it can be assumed that it is present to some degree in all the aged. Between the ages of 55 and 64, 50 to 60% of all patients at postmortem examination have a significant narrowing of some coronary vessels.[8] This process is accelerated in patients who also have hypertension and diabetes, who smoke, and who are inactive or obese.[9]

Unfortunately the warning signs of coronary disease may be masked in the aged. This is especially true in patients with diabetes and those emerging from the effects of anesthesia. Complaints of chest pain are rare in this setting. The first indication that cardiac disease exists may be an acute cardiac catastrophy, myocardial ischemia, infarction, or failure. Stresses of surgery and anesthesia, pain, anxiety, perioperative fluid shifts, tachycardia, shivering, hypertension, or hypotension can increase myocardial oxygen demand to levels higher than can be supplied through diseased coronary arteries.

In the following section, the recognition and management of this problem in the elderly PACU patient will be reviewed.

Diagnosis. Myocardial ischemia in the PACU may be minimal with only minor changes, such as temporary T-wave inversion, in cardiovascular parameters, requiring little medical intervention. Conversely, cardiac decompensation may occur precipitously if coronary occlusion occurs. It is important to remember that such a potentially disastrous event can follow simple procedures such as cataract extractions, performed under local anesthesia. Intubation, hypo- or hypertensive episodes, and tachycardia can initiate myocardial ischemia during the operative procedure. Often, providing an adequate plane of anesthesia and stabilizing blood pressure, pulse rate, and low central pressures can correct the problem. If not, pharmacologic intervention, as described below, may be necessary, not only intraoperatively but also in the PACU. It is essential that PACU personnel be informed of any such intraoperative event so they will anticipate a recurrence in the PACU. Unfortunately, although T-wave inversion occurs in the operating room (OR), such changes are not always easily identified on the OR ECG monitor. Moreover, T-wave changes are late signs of ischemia and may not occur until the patient arrives in the PACU. Therefore, all patients in this age group should have a 12-lead ECG in the PACU as soon as possible after arrival in the unit.

Although the clinical picture may be ill-defined, the sudden onset of hypotension, dysrhythmias, and acute pulmonary edema should suggest myocardial ischemia or infarction until proven otherwise in the PACU, and immediate aggressive therapy should be instituted. The ability of the elderly heart to adapt to acute ischemia is reduced by previous myocardial damage and diminished myocardial reserve. Prompt treatment is essential to prevent pump failure and death.

Management

Pain. Opiates are given intravenously if needed for pain and restlessness. The fact cannot be emphasized too greatly that the elderly metabolize drugs more slowly and have a high pain threshhold, tolerate pain well, and require less narcotic because the number of opiate receptors decreases with age. Moreover, restlessness secondary to hypoxia must not be misdiagnosed as secondary to pain. Intravenous opiates, such as morphine in 1-mg increments, should be titrated with allowance made for the patient's circulatory time.

Because morphine is vagotonic and vagal responses are enhanced, an atropine 0.5 to 1.0 mg bolus may be necessary to treat bradycardia, nausea, vomiting, atrioventricular block, or nodal rhythm.[10] Judicious use of atropine is essential to avoid sinus tachycardia and an inordinate increase in myocardial oxygen demand.

Care should be taken to prevent hypoxia, respiratory depression, or hypotension following the morphine administration.[11] Pulse oximetry is indicated.

Coronary Ischemia. Nitroglycerin is the cornerstone of therapy and in the PACU is more appropriately given intravenously. An infusion, 50 mg in 250 D5/w, is titrated at 10- to 100 μg/min. Significant improvement of left ventricular function and decrease in the extent of the myocardial ischemia has been reported with the use of this agent.[12,13]

Hypotension. Hypotension occurs when the pump fails and cardiac output falls. To correct this situation, dobutamine 5 to 15 μg/kg/min is recommended. This inotropic agent increases contractility and lowers the systemic vascular resistance slightly.[14]

An alternate treatment is to use dopamine to improve cardiac output for its inotropic effect, and nitroprusside to decrease afterload. This combination should reduce left ventricular filling pressures, reduce the myocardial work, and increase cardiac output.[15]

Ventilatory Support. Although inhalation of an oxygen-enriched atmosphere may be all that is required, there should be no delay in intubating the trachea and instituting mechanical ventilation in patients at the first sign of respiratory decompensation. An increase in arterial PO_2 has been shown to significantly reduce the magnitude of myocardial ischemia.[11]

Monitoring. Because hypotension from cardiogenic shock secondary to ischemia or infarction is difficult to differentiate from that due to hypovolemia in the postoperative period, pulmonary artery and capillary wedge pressures and cardiac output monitoring are usual in unstable, elderly patients. Arterial cannulation for pressure and arterial blood gas monitoring is indicated. Immediate control of pain, dysrhythmias, and hypoxemia; administration of medication to alleviate coronary spasm; reduction of preload and afterload; and institution of inotropic support; are essential to ensure optimal outcome.

Acute Hypertension

Hypertension during emergence from anesthesia is common even in elderly patients who are well controlled preoperatively. The incidence of hypertension in the elderly patient approaches 60%.[16] Expeditious control is essential to prevent postoperative surgical or intracranial bleeding, increased intracranial pressure, and myocardial infarction or cardiac failure.

Diagnosis. A rapid evaluation of the patient to immediately identify the etiology of the hypertension is mandatory. Common causes include pain, hypercarbia, hypothermia, urinary retention, relative volume overload, and emergence delirium. Therapy, therefore, should include appropriate airway and ventilatory management, warming to normothermic state, drainage of a distended bladder, analgesics for pain, and hypnotics for delirium.

Volume overload as a cause of hypertension may first be observed in the PACU as the vasodilating effects of the anesthetic agents dissipate. This physiologic process is especially evident in the aged, all of whom have a diffuse thickening of all vascular walls, which progresses at an extremely individualistic but relentless rate. Connective tissue content increases in the subendothelial level. Calcification and lipid deposition occur near the internal elastic membrane and in the media. Vessels become increasingly less compliant. As a result small changes in intravascular volume are reflected as major changes in blood pressure.[17,18]

As a corollary, because the degree of compliance decreases radically in the elderly, either vasopressor or vasodilators must be administered with extreme caution because of the risk of exaggerated responses.

Management. Because acute emergence hypertension is usually short-lived, a short-acting agent such as nitroprusside, titrated cautiously intravenously, is appropriate for therapy. Nitroprusside is administered in a concentration of 100 μg/cc (50 mg/500 cc) at a dosage range of 0.5 to 5 μg/kg/min. Theoretically, there is the hazard that coronary steal may occur when nitroprusside is used in the myocardium with compromised blood supply. For that reason nitroglycerine is preferred by some anesthesiologists. If the hypertension is accompanied by a tachycardia greater than 120, a short-acting beta blocker, such as esmolol, may be effective. To administer esmolol, begin with a loading infusion of 500 μg/kg/min for one-half minute followed by 25 μg/kg to 50 μg/kg as needed. Esmolol's ultrashort duration of action and ease of titration make it especially advantageous.[19] A combination of sublingual diltiazem and nitropaste has been suggested for less severe hypertensive episodes. Hydralazine and other longer-acting agents are less appropriate for acute management. Because of diminished baroreceptor sensitivity, elderly patients are less likely to develop a reflex tachycardia but are more apt to suffer acute hypotension with hydralazine. The patient's own antihypertensive medication should be continued up to the time of surgery and reinstituted as soon as possible in the postoperative period.

Discontinuing antihypertensive agents preoperatively can accentuate the postoperative hypertension. Clonodine, in particular, is associated with dangerously high rebound hypertension if a periodic dose is missed as the half-life of this drug is short (about eight hours).

Monitoring. Potent antihypertensive agents should only be given when arterial pressures can be monitored continuously, either by direct intraarterial cannulation or finger plethysmography. Because vessels are constricted, the intravascular volumes may be decreased. Relaxation of vessels results in precipitous changes in pressures.

Cardiac Dysrhythmias

Cardiac irregularities are commonly seen in elderly patients following surgery and may or may not be clinically significant. If all other cardiovascular parameters are within the patient's normal range, then treatment is usually unnecessary.

An explanation for these dysrhythmias is that there is an increase of fibrous, fatty, and collagenous tissue in the aging myocardium, especially around the sinus node (Figs 17–1 and 17–2). Associated with this infiltration there is a progressive decrease in the number of pacer cells. Only 10% of the number of pacer cells present in 30-year-old adults are found at the age of 75.[20] Because of the reduced number of pacer cells, minor to severe conduction defects occur. Sick sinus syndrome requiring cardiac pacing is common. Premature atrial and ventricular contractions, and atrial fibrillation, are also frequently seen. Chronic slow, stable dysrhythmias present preoperatively do not generally require treatment. Moreover, pharmacologic treatment of a stable conduction defect, in the aged, may lead to more serious dysrhythmias.[21,22]

Management

Sinus Bradycardia. A new sudden onset of sinus bradycardia in the PACU may herald an abrupt dysrhythmic death from an acute myocardial infarction, congestive heart failure, or hypoxemia. On the other hand, elderly patients with a chronic sinus bradycardia above 40 beats per minute are often asymptomatic. Such a rate in the PACU may reflect a residual effect of opiate anesthesia, or it may be due to the effects of cardioactive drugs such as digitalis, calcium channel blockers, and beta blockers.

Additionally, vagal responses are exaggerated in the elderly initiating bradycardia postoperatively. Fright, pain, emotional stress, distended bladder, or a precipitous blood loss may all evoke such a response. Bradycardia is a frequent occurrence in elderly patients who have undergone transurethral resections and bladder irrigation. If the cardiac output as indicated by the blood pressure is maintained, the abnormal rhythm is usually benign. If blood pressure falls

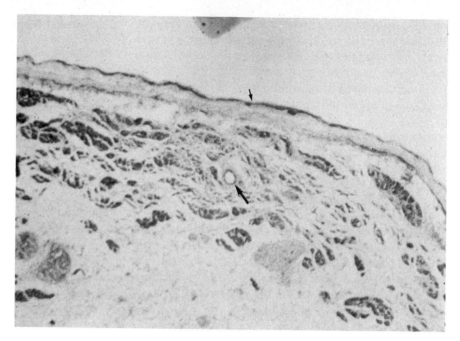

Figure 17-1. Sinus node in elderly patient (40 ×) showing increase of fibrous, fatty, and collagenous tissue in the aging myocardium. Small arrow indicates endocardium, large arrow points to sinus node. (Courtesy of Sumi Mitsudo, Department of Surgical Pathology, Montefiore Medical Center, Bronx, New York.)

or if rate dependent ventricular irregularities occur, treatment with atropine (0.5 to 1 mg IV) usually corrects the problem. If this management is not effective, isoproterenol (0.015 to 0.15 μg/kg/min) infusion may be necessary and should be titrated intravenously. Care must be taken to avoid tachycardia. If the bradycardia persists, cardiac pacing may be required.

Sick Sinus Syndrome. Sick sinus syndrome, although usually associated with other cardiovascular derangements, may appear without warning postoperatively.

Manifestations of this entity include persistant, inappropriate sinus bradycardia; sinus pause or arrest; replacement of normal rhythm with an ectopic pacemaker; paroxysmal atrial fibrillation or atrial standstill with no sinus node activity; paroxysmal supraventricular tachycardia; abnormal sinus node function unrelated to drug therapy; or carotid sinus hyperactivity.[23]

If the patient's symptoms (eg, tachycardia, bracdycardia) cannot be controlled with appropriate medication, cardiac pacing may be required.

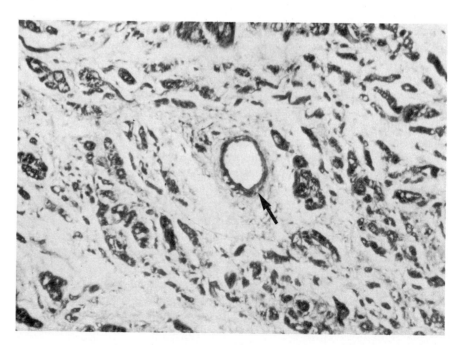

Figure 17-2. Sinus node (100 ×). (Courtesy of Sumi Mitsudo, Department of Surgical Pathology, Montefiore Medical Center, Bronx, New York.)

Supraventricular Tachycardias. The initial goal in the management of tachydysrhythmias is to identify any underlying cause such as hypovolemia, pain, congestive heart failure, myocardial ischemia, or electrolyte or metabolic imbalances. Abnormal rhythms may also be associated with digitalis toxicity and hypokalemia. A prompt attempt then should be made to control the irregularity with verapamil, digitalis (if the serum level is not in a toxic range), or beta blockade, if the cause is cardiac. Electrical cardioversion should be reserved for patients with marked deterioration of hemodynamic status. It is essential to control the tachycardia as quickly as possible to prevent myocardial infarction. Carotid sinus stimulation is not recommended in the elderly because of the hypersensitive sinus node. Sinus arrest or atrioventricular block occurs in the elderly when the node is stimulated.

Ventricular Dysrhythmias. Premature ventricular dysrhythmias are especialy common in the elderly. Usually they are isolated ectopic beats which, along the nonsustained ventricular tachycardia, do not require therapy unless associated with symptoms. However, premature ventricular contractions, supraventricular tachycardias, and rapid atrial fibrillation may herald myocardial ischemia or infarction. If the patient does have advanced unstable or decompensated cardiac disease, aggressive therapy is essential using antidysrhythmics such as lidocaine, pronestyl, or verapamil.[24]

Lidocaine is usually effective acutely in preventing ventricular fibrillation and management of premature ventricular contractions.[25] Lower doses are needed in the elderly, especially those with heart failure (0.5 mg/kg), followed by a second bolus if necessary and then a continuous infusion of 2 mg/min titrated as needed. Because they metabolize local anesthestics slowly, the elderly are prone to develop toxic levels of these agents. Central nervous system (CNS) confusion may be the first indication of drug accumulation. Dosage should be adjusted appropriately on an individual basis. Although lidocaine may be given at the appearance of premature ventricular contractions, prophylactic use is probably unnecessary.[26] In the presence of acute myocardial infarction, cardioversion should be used to reverse the acute onset of rapid atrial fibrillation. Intravenous verapamil, titrated in 2.5 mg doses, is effective in converting supraventricular tachycardia to normal sinus rhythm.

Decreased Cardiac Output and Response to Stress

Cardiovascular reserve has classically been described as falling 1% per year after the age of 30.[27] Recent data from the Baltimore Longitudinal Study indicate that this process may be slowed by regular aerobic exercise.[28] This decrease with age is evidenced by a reduced chronotropic response to exercise and stress. The fact remains that the elderly are less able to increase cardiac output in response to the increased metabolic and oxygen requirements of the perioperative period. Maximum O_2 uptake (MVO_2) with aerobic exercise, as determined by A–VO_2 difference, and heart rate, decreases with aging. This may be in part because of a reduced sensitivity to adrenergic activity.

Also a decrease in ejection fraction and an increase in wall motion abnormalities even in apparently healthy volunteers over age 60 has been reported. These changes, exacerbated with exercise, may be related to unsuspected coronary artery disease.[28]

It is not surprising that the aging heart is at risk of failing in the perioperative period.

PULMONARY DERANGEMENTS

Respiratory Failure

Physiologic changes of aging added to residual respiratory depressant effects of anesthetic agents and the increased metabolic demands of surgical stress make respiratory failure a common, but entirely avoidable, complication in the early postoperative period. Respiratory fragility is a hallmark of the elderly, in whom functional reserve is depleted. Respiratory fatigue develops precipitously in the face of increased metabolic demands and respiratory work load.[29]

In the elderly emphysematous alveolar changes and progressive alveolar duct enlargement increase parenchymal compliance and decrease elastic recoil (Figs. 17–3 and 17–4). As the elastic recoil decreases, the stability of the terminal airways is also reduced, and airway closure occurs at higher lung volumes. When the closing volumes encroach upon tidal volume, gas exchange is affected. With earlier airway closure lung bases are underinflated but still well perfused. Ventilation–perfusion mismatch ensues. This sequence of events explains the fall in arterial PO_2 with aging.

The decreased elastic recoil coupled with the increased chest wall rigidity of the elderly limit maximal expiratory flow rate. The FEV-1 decreased about 30 mL/year in healthy nonsmokers. Ventilatory work increases. Coughing becomes much less effective, secretions are retained, and atelectasis develops more easily.[30]

In the young individual ventilation is controlled by chemoreceptors in the brainstem that respond to hyperpnea and cells in the carotid and aortic bodies sensitive to changes in PO_2. Minute ventilation and oxygen transport is altered as needed. This reflex is

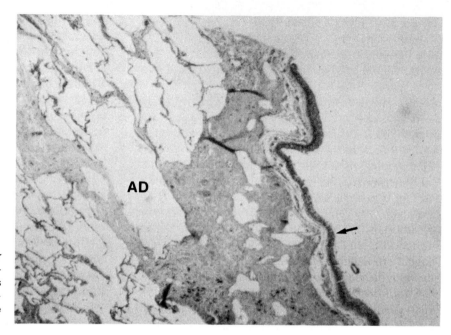

Figure 17–3. Emphysematous alveolar changes and alveolar duct (AD) enlargement in the aging lung. Arrow indicates bronchiole. (Courtesy of Sumi Mitsudo, Department of Surgical Pathology, Montefiore Medical Center, Bronx, New York.)

decreased in the aged who do not respond appropriately to hypercarbia and hypoxemia by increasing ventilation. Pneumonia, postoperative atelectasis, oversedation or residual muscle paralysis, and pulmonary edema do not elicit the tachypnea and tachycardia that normally occur in the young. The only evidence of ventilatory compromise may be restlessness and disorientation.[31] It is imperative that these findings are not misinterpreted and immediately attributed to pain or apprehension. Disastrous hypoxia can occur if more sedation is administered inappropriately.

Properly managed ventilatory depression has little adverse effect. Supplemental oxygen may be all that is required, but in the face of a falling oxygen tension and rising CO_2, immediate intubation and mechanical support are essential and can be life-saving. Reversal of residual effects of muscle relaxants and opiates are an adjunct to therapy of respiratory depression. Arterial blood gas analyses should be performed on any unstable patients in the PACU to rule out aypoxemia. A chest x-ray also aids in establishing this diagnosis. Insertion of a balloon flotation catheter to measure pulmonary pressures may be required to differentiate cardiac from noncardiac pulmonary edema.

RENAL DERANGEMENTS

The patient past 75 has about 50% of the functioning nephrons of the 30 year old. Moreover, at this age renal blood and glomerular filtration rate are mark-

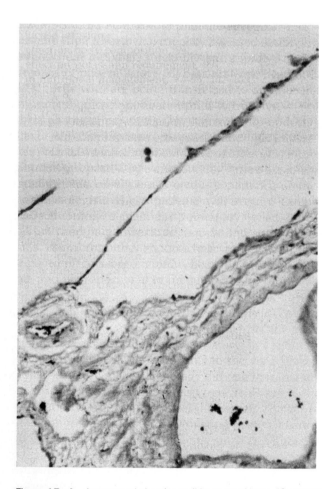

Figure 17–4. Attenuated alveolar wall in an aged lung. (Courtesy of Sumi Mitsudo, Department of Surgical Pathology, Montefiore Medical Center, Bronx, New York.)

edly reduced. Total renal mass, number and surface area of glomeruli, and length and volume of the proximal tubules all decrease with age. There is a parallel decline in tubular function. Intrinsic renal failure is common in the elderly, who are also much more susceptible to nephrotoxic injuries from drugs such as the aminoglycosides, radiographic contrast agents, and prolonged ischemia secondary to hypovolemia and decreased cardiac output.

Oliguria

Oliguria, less than 20 mL/hr of urine, may be a result of prerenal, postrenal, or intrinsic renal failure. Prerenal failure—usually secondary to hypovolemia, cardiac insufficiency, or both—results in decreased renal blood flow and glomerular filtration rate, and is common in the elderly patient postoperatively. Prompt recognition and treatment are especially important, as protracted and uncorrected hypoperfusion may lead to tubular necrosis. Assessment of oliguria is difficult in part due to the fact that normal baroreceptor responses to decreased intravascular volume are depressed in the aged; hypotension occurs late and precipitously; and tachycardia is limited. Normally each nephron may be operating under maximal conditions in this age group to maintain stability in solute and water excretion. When the stress of surgery and anesthesia are added, the senescent kidney may not be able to compensate.

Management. Usually the management of oliguria in the PACU is simple; most patients are hypovolemic. In patients who have had no history of cardiac failure, a fluid challenge or appropriate blood replacement may be all that is required to increase urine output. However, since most of the elderly also have some degree of cardiac insufficiency, central venous or pulmonary artery catheterization may be required to determine appropriate volume replacement and for administration of inotropic agents. Low dosage of dopamine, 3 to 5 μg/kg, will improve the renal blood flow. Diuretics may reestablish urine flow, but should only be used after intravascular volume is optimized. Osmotic diuretics in a well-hydrated elderly patient should be used cautiously. Intravascular volume expansion can cause cardiac insufficiency if given in the presence of intrinsic renal failure. Furosemide and ethacrynic acid deplete renal interstitial electrolytes and interfere with the definitive diagnosis of renal failure. But, because their toxicity is low, some clinicians believe that their use to convert an oliguric to a polyuric renal failure improves outcome.[32]

Polyuria

Urine output in excess of 100 mL per hour suggests the possibility of polyuric renal failure with large quantities of urine in the face of rising BUN and creatinine. Another reason for polyuria in the aged is osmotic diuresis, caused either by hyperglycemia or the presence of some other solute load such as intravenous radiographic contrast agents and diabetes insipidus, is a possibility in the elderly who are prone to CNS vascular derangements. In the presence of polyuria, hypokalemia develops rapidly in the aged patient. Moreover, since many aged patients have received diuretic therapy chronically and already have a low total body potassium, an increase in urinary potassium excretion can cause dangerously low levels of total body and serum potassium.

Conversely, decreased plasma renin activity and aldosterone production in the elderly alter the kidney's ability to conserve sodium. Because potassium excretion in exchange for sodium is decreased, hyperkalemia may develop rapidly. Monitoring serum potassium and appropriate replacement are essential functions in the perioperative management of the elderly patient.[33]

CENTRAL AND AUTOMATIC NERVOUS DERANGEMENTS

As a person ages there is a progressive loss of neural cells, a decline in cerebral perfusion and oxygen consumption, a decreased rate of synthesis, and an increased rate of destruction of neurotransmitters (Figs. 17–5 and 17–6). All these factors enhance the sensitivity of the central nervous system to depression from anesthetic agents. These changes, coupled with a decrease in basal metabolism and elimination of drugs by the aging kidney, can easily explain the CNS derangements seen in the elderly after anesthesia.[34]

Prolonged Awakening and Delirium Following Anesthesia

Prolonged coma that is associated with delerium can be very disturbing for those caring for the aged patient. Fortunately, the usual cause of prolonged awakening is only CNS depression and slow elimination of anesthetic agents.

Hyperreflexia, shivering, and abnormal neurologic signs—not uncommon in young patients—are exaggerated in the elderly.[35] In addition, disorientation is seen in about 10% of the elderly surgical population, and frank delerium in a lesser number.[36] These symptoms usually resolve spontaneously within a matter of hours, but the PACU physician should be vigilant as changes in the pattern of awakening may herald the presence of more serious CNS complications.

Acute brain syndrome in the immediate postoperative period is caused by metabolic abnormalities such as hyperosmolarity, hyponatremia, hypoglycemia, hypothermia, hypoxia, and hypercarbia, and should be easily correctable.[37]

Fortunately castrophic undiagnosed CNS insults are extremely rare, but they do occur. Prolonged hypotension or hypertension, cerebral emboli, or other causes of CNS hypoxia, can prolong awakening indefinitely. Patients with persistent neurological derangements require immediate neurological evaluation including CT scan.

Depressed Laryngeal Reflexes

Age-related CNS depression of protective laryngeal reflexes makes aspiration pneumonitis a constant danger in elderly patients.[38,39] Pneumonia follows only surgical complications and cardiac derangements as a leading cause of death in the elderly. Any patient suspected of having increased gastric contents, recent food ingestion, slow gastric emptying, bowel obstruction, or gastrointestinal bleeding should remain intubated with the balloon cuff inflated until recovery of laryngeal reflexes is certain.

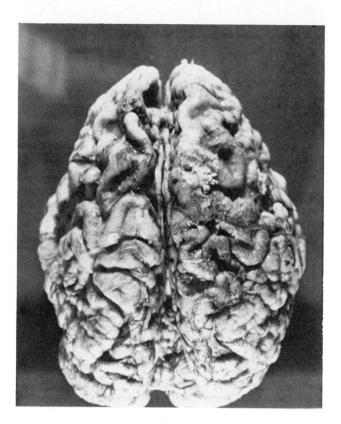

Figure 17–6. Atrophic brain from elderly patient. (Courtesy of Josephina Llena, Department of Neuropathology, Montefiore Medical Center, Bronx, New York.)

Hypothermia

Impaired central thermoregulatory mechanisms, coupled with a decrease in basal metabolism in the elderly, make temperature maintenance a challenge. These patients frequently arrive in the PACU with subnormal temperatures. A compensatory vasoconstriction and shivering, to conserve heat, increase systemic vascular resistance oxygen requirements to a degree that a compromised old heart may decompensate.[40] Heated, humidified air, heating blankets, and heat lamps may help alleviate this problem.

COMMENT

The elderly usually are taking a number of medications for the management of their assorted problems. A survey of 149 patients undergoing vascular surgery found that the patients were receiving a wide variety of cardiac medications.[41] In addition, smaller numbers of patients were taking insulin, oral antidiabetic, mood elevating, thyroid, bronchodilator, and antacid drugs. The interaction of all these is considered in Chapter 3.

Even though the potential for a complicated

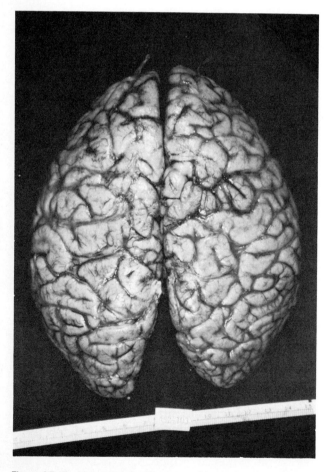

Figure 17–5. Normal brain. (Courtesy of Josephina Llena, Department of Neuropathology, Montefiore Medical Center, Bronx, New York.)

course in the PACU is high, elderly patients tolerate the immediate effects of surgery and anesthesia surprisingly well. In a review of 1176 patients past the age of 75, who were operated upon at our institution from July through December 1987, 92% had a completely uneventful stay in the PACU.[41] Transfer to the surgical intensive care unit (SICU) was required for 5.4%. Of these, 3.8% had undergone open heart surgery; such patients are routinely sent to the SICU. Therefore, only 1.6% of the aged had surgical or medical problems severe enough to require further intensive care. In a previous 5-year study, the overall in-hospital mortality rate in surgical patients past the age of 75 was 9.3%.[41] These statistics suggest that the elderly patient, undergoing uncomplicated elective surgery, should have an uncomplicated postoperative recovery. The PACU staff should be ever alert with this age group, however, because the margin of safety is narrow and the potential for disaster always present.

REFERENCES

1. US Census Bureau: *Current Population Reports,* series P-23, no. 138, Demographics and socioeconomic aspects of aging in the United States. Washington, DC, Government Printing Office, 1984.
2. McLeskey CH: Anesthesia for the geriatric patient *Adv Anesthesia* 1984;2:31–68.
3. Goldman NL, Caldera DL, Nussbaum SR, et al: Multifactorial index of cardiac risk in noncardiac surgical procedures. *N Engl J Med* 1977;207:846–853.
4. Dunn FG: Arteriosclerotic heart disease in the elderly. *Cardiol Clin* 1966;4:253–261.
5. Registrar Generals' Mortality Statistics for Scotland. HMSO, 1974.
6. Medalia L, Sandwhite PD: Disease of the aged: Analysis of pathological observations in 1,251 autopsy protocols in old persons. *JAMA* 1952;149:1433–1437.
7. Stephen CR: Risk factors and outcome in elderly patients: An epidermologic study, in *Geriatric Anesthesia: Principles and Practice.* Boston, Butterworths 1986, 345–362.
8. White NR, Edwards JE, Dry TJ: The relationship of the degree of coronary atherosclerosis with age in men. *Circulation* 1950;1:645–654.
9. Ackerman RF, Dry TJ, Edwards JE: Relationship of various factors to the degree of coronary atherosclerosis in women. *Circulation* 1950;1:1345–1354.
10. Russel RO: Initial management of acute myocardial infarction in the coronary care unit omitting use of streptokinase and angioplasty. *Cardiovasc Perspect* 1988;2:1–2.
11. Madias JE, Madias NE, Hood WB Jr: Precordial ST segment mapping. Effects of oxygen inhalation on ischemic injury in patients with acute myocardial infarction. *Circulation* 1976;53:411–417.
12. Awan NA, Amsterdam EA, Vera Z, et al: Reduction of ischemic injury by sublingual nitroglycerin in patients with acute myocardial infarction. *Circulation* 1976;54:761–765.
13. Flaherty JT, Reid PR, Kelly DT, et al: Introvenous nitroglycerin in acute myocardial infarction. *Circulation* 1975;51:132–139.
14. Keung ECH, Siskind SJ, Sonnenblick EH, et al: Dobutamine therapy in acute myocardial infarction *JAMA* 1981;245:144–146.
15. Richard C, Ricome JF, Rimailho A, et al: Combined hemodynamic effects of dopamine and dobutamine in cardiogenic shock. *Circulation* 1983;67:620–626.
16. Kannel WB, Dawber TR, McGee NL: Perspectives on systolic hypertension: The Framingham study. *Circulation* 1980;61:1179–1182.
17. Milch RA; Matrix properties of the aging arterial wall. *Monogr Surg Sci* 1965;2:261–341.
18. Wellman NE, Edwards JE: Thickness of the media of the thoracic aorta in relation to age. *Arch Pathol* 1950;50:183–188.
19. Leslie J, Kalayjian W, Sirgo M, et al: Intravenous labetalol for treatment of postoperative hypertension. *Anesthesiology* 1987;67:413–416.
20. Lev M: Aging changes in the human sinoatrial node. *J Gerontol* 1954;9:1–9.
21. Lev M, Bharati S: Age related changes in the cardiac conduction system. *Intern Med Specialist* 1981;2:19–27.
22. Dreifes LS: Cardiac arrhythmias in the elderly: Clinical aspects. *Cardiol Clin* 1986;4:273–283.
23. Dreifes LS, Michelson EL, Kaplinsky E: Bradyarrhythmias: Arrhythmias: Clinical significance. *J Am Coll Cardiol* 1983;1:327–338.
24. Fleg JL, Kennedy HL: Cardiac arrhythmias in a healthy elderly population. *Chest* 1982;81:301–307.
25. Lie, KI, Wellens HJ, van Capelles FJ, Durrer D: Lidocaine in the prevention of primary ventricular fibrillation. A double-blind randomized study of 212 consecutive patients. *N Engl J Med* 1974;291:1324–1326.
26. Carruth JE, Silverman ME: Ventricular fibrillation complicating acute myocardial infarction: Reasons against the use of Lidocaine. *American Heart Journal:* 1982;104:545–50.
27. Brandtonbrener M, Lan Boune M, Schock NW: Changes in cardiac output with age. *Circulation* 1955;12:557–566.
28. Port S, Cobb FR, Coleman RE, et al: Effect of age on the response of the left ventricular ejection fraction to exercise. *N Eng J Med* 1980; 303:1133–1136.
29. Edelman NH, Mittman C, Norris AH, et al: Effects of respiratory pattern on age differences in ventilation uniformity. *J Appl Physiol* 1968; 24:49–53.
30. Wright RR: Elastic tissue of normal and emphysematous lungs: A tridimensional histologic study. *Am J Pathol* 1961; 39:355–367.
31. Kronenberg RS, Drage CW: Attenuation of the ventilatory and heart rate responses to hypoxia and hypercapnia with aging in normal men. *J Clin Invest* 1973; 52:1812–1819.
32. Eliahou HE: Mannitol therapy in oliguria of acute onset. *Brit Med J* 1964; 1:807–810.

33. Crane MG, Harris JJ: Effect of aging on renin activity and aldosterone excretion *J Lab Clin Med* 1976; 87:947–951.

34. Greenblatt DJ, Seller EM, Shader RI: Drug disposition in old age. *N Eng J Med* 1982; 306:1031–1088.

35. Rosenberg H, Clofine R, Bialik O: Neurologic changes during awakening from anesthesia. *Anesthesiology* 1981; 54:125–130.

36. Gauthier JL, Hamelberg W: Hip fractures: Influence of anesthesia on patient's hospital course. *Anesth Analg* 1963; 42:609–615.

37. Haugen FP: The failure to regain consciousness after general anesthesia. *Anesthesiology* 1961; 22:657–666.

38. Bedford PD: Adverse cerebral effects of anesthesia on old people. *Lancet* 1955; II:259–263.

39. Potoppidan H, Beecher HK: Progressive loss of protective reflexes in the airway with the advance of age. *JAMA* 1960; 174:2209–2213.

40. Collins KJ, Easton JC, Exton-Smith AN: The aging nervous system: Impairment of thermoregulation. *Adv Med* 1982;18:250–257.

41. Underwood PS: Unpublished data.

HEART AND HEART-LUNG TRANSPLANTATION

Laboratory investigation of heart transplantation began in the early twentieth century; however, the first clinical orthotopic human heart transplantation was performed by Barnard in 1967.[1] The following year, the Stanford clinical heart transplantation program was initiated, and through its research contributed substantially to the refinement of recipient selection criteria, operative technique, organ preservation, and treatment of complications.[2] Indications and contraindications for both heart and heart-lung transplantation are presented in Tables 18–1 to 18–3. The 1-year survival of heart-transplant recipients is approximately 80% and 60% at 5 years in cyclosporine-treated patients at Stanford University (Fig. 18–1).[3,4] At Stanford survival of heart-lung recipients is 74% at 1 year and 59% at 2 years postoperatively.[5] Full discussion of recipient selection, donor management, anesthetic management, and operative procedure is beyond the scope of this chapter.

Heart Transplantation

Physiology of the Denervated Heart. The operative procedure requires removal of all but a small portion of the posterior wall of both the left and right atria. This portion includes the S-A node, which in itself remains innervated by the sympathetic and parasympathetic nervous systems. The resultant heart rate is controlled by the S-A node of the donor heart, which has no direct innervation. Frequently the ECG shows two P-waves; the administration of atropine will only increase the rate of the recipient P-wave. The responses of the denervated heart to direct-acting inotropes (epinephrine, norepinephrine, isoproterenol) and adrenergic antagonists are similar to those in normal patients.[6,7] However, indirect-acting agents (autonomic effects) such as ephedrine, pancuronium, cholinergic antagonists, and anticholinesterases, will have no effect on the denervated heart. No evidence

of reinnervation of the transplanted orthotopic heart has been shown to date. Most heart transplant recipients return to NYHA Class I by 1 year.[8] Normal physiologic mechanisms such as the Frank-Starling effect, conduction and response to alpha and beta adrenergic stimuli, are maintained in the denervated heart. Unlike the normal heart, the denervated heart responds to stresses such as exercise, hypovolemia, or hypotension in two phases: (1) cardiac output increases secondary to increases in preload; and (2) cardiac output, heart rate, and systolic blood pressure increase several minutes later as plasma catecholamines increase. Thus, the early warning signs of hypovolemia may not be evident until severe hypotension occurs.

The effects of the commonly used antidysrhythmics, digoxin and quinidine, deserve mention. Short-term digoxin therapy has no effect on the heart rate of the denervated heart, suggesting an indirect autonomically mediated effect of digoxin. However, chronic use of digoxin will prolong the A-V conduction and slow the heart rate. This last effect suggests a direct effect on the heart.[9] Quinidine slows intraventricular conduction (as in the intact heart) as well as sinus rate and atrioventricular conduction (unlike the effect on intact hearts).[10] The denervated heart has a resting rate of 90 to 120 beats per minute, due to the lack of vagal inhibition. Dysrhythmias are common in the first 6 months, with episodes worsening during rejection of the transplanted heart. The coro-

TABLE 18–1. INDICATIONS FOR HEART TRANSPLANTATION

Diagnosis	Frequency (%)
Cardiomyopathy	48.4
Coronary artery disease	43.0
Valvular disease with cardiomyopathy	5.4
Congenital heart disease	1.5
Other	1.7

Adapted from Wyner J, Finch EL: Heart and heart-lung transplantation, in Gelman S (ed): Anesthesia and Organ Transplantation. Philadelphia, Saunders, 1987, p 116.

TABLE 18–2. INDICATIONS FOR HEART-LUNG TRANSPLANTATION

Diagnosis	Frequency (%)
Primary pulmonary hypertension	44.5
Eisenmenger's syndrome	40.0
Emphysema	2.7
Alpha-1-antitrypsin deficiency	2.7
Other	10.1

Adapted from Reitz BA: Cardiac and cardiopulmonary transplantation, in McGoon DC (ed): Cardiac Surgery, ed 2. Philadelphia, Davis, 1987, p 348.

TABLE 18–3. CONTRAINDICATIONS TO HEART AND HEART-LUNG TRANSPLANTATION

Age over 55 years
Presence of active infectious disease
Systemic illnesses (insulin-dependent diabetes mellitus, renal, hepatic, severe peripheral disease or a malignancy)
Cerebral vascular disease
Recent pulmonary infarction (unresolved)
History of substance abuse or mental instability
Severe pulmonary hypertension (heart transplant only)

Adapted from Reitz BA: Cardiac and cardiopulmonary transplantation, in McGoon DC (ed): Cardiac Surgery, ed 2. Philadelphia, Davis, 1987, p 348.

nary arteries in the denervated heart have a higher resting blood flow due to loss of the normal basal alpha-adrenergic tone, but the response to metabolic demands and to adrenergic agents is maintained. Of concern is the lack of classic chest pain (angina pectoris) to myocardial ischemia and infarction in the denervated heart.

Postoperative Considerations

Infection. The heart transplant recipient is immunosuppressed; therefore, strict reverse isolation is maintained in the intensive care unit. Attempt is made to extubate the patient early if clinically indicated, as well as to remove unnecessary intravenous or urinary catheters. Infection is the leading cause of death in these patients.[11] A wide array of bacterial (55%), viral (22%), fungal (13%), protozoal (6%), and nosocomial (4%) organisms has been described.[12] The early appearance of fever should be taken seriously and not attributed to atelectasis. Early diagnosis and treatment will improve survival. Many institutions include routine, daily clinical evaluation, chest x-ray, and cultures of sputum, urine, and chest tube drainage. In addition, transtracheal aspirates and bron-

chial aspirates may be required. Bacterial, fungal, and protozoal infections are treated with the appropriate drugs. Commonly occurring viral infections such as herpes simplex, herpes zoster, and cytomegalovirus are often treated successfully with acycloguanosine with minimal toxicity. Patients treated with azathioprine for immunosuppression are more prone to infection than the cyclosporine-treated patients. Mediastinitis may occur late (4 to 6 weeks postoperatively), and is relatively asymptomatic (low-grade fever and leukocytosis).[13] Its treatment includes irrigation with 5% povidone-iodine solution and follow-up by serial CT-scans. Of concern is the high incidence (28%) of general surgical complications in heart transplant recipients, with a mortality rate of 10 to 40%.[14-16] These include sigmoid and small bowel perforations, cholecystitis, pancreatitis, and cecal perforation.

Hemodynamic Support. Frequently, isoproterenol infusion (by careful titration) is necessary to maintain a heart rate greater than 90 beats per minute. Postbypass myocardial dysfunction is often treated with dobutamine 2 to 10 $\mu g/kg/min$, especially if residual pulmonary hypertension is present. However, with

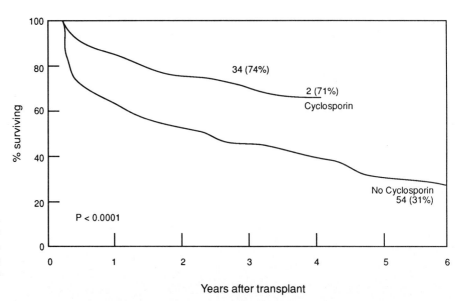

Figure 18–1. Survival of cardiac transplant patients, operations peformed after 1978, comparing those treated with cyclosporine with those not receiving such treatment. (From Kaye et al.,[1] with permission).

good organ preservation and surgical technique there is less of a need for inotropic support postoperatively. Careful attention to temperature normalization is recommended to avoid shivering and increased oxygen consumption in a patient with a denervated heart due to the latter's poor response to stress. Antidysrrhythmic agents other than digoxin and quinidine that may be used are lidocaine for ventricular ectopy (caution for liver toxicity); procainamide for acute control of atrial and ventricular tachydysrhythmias (serum levels must be measured); bretylium for resistant ventricular dysrhythmias; and verapamil for supraventricular dysrhythmias (caution for negative inotropic effects).[17]

Electrolyte imbalance is common in patients on prolonged diuretic therapy. Hypomagnesemia, hypophosphatemia, and hypokalemia should all be corrected with slow intravenous supplements to prevent dysrhythmias and myocardial depression.

Postoperative evaluation of bleeding disorders is the same as following routine open heart surgery. However, it is generally agreed that if chest tube drainage is greater than 200 mL/h, then surgical reexploration is indicated.

Immunosuppression. Immunosuppression begins preoperatively with cyclosporine 12 to 16 mg/kg and azathioprine 4 mg/kg intravenously. Methylprednisolone 500 mg is given intravenously when the patient is weaned off bypass and is followed by three divided doses of methylprednisolone 125 mg IV. Postoperatively, oral prednisone 1.5 mg/kg/day is started and gradually tapered to 0.1 mg/kg/day at the time of discharge. Oral azathioprine 1 to 2.5 mg/kg/day is started and titrated on a long-term basis to maintain a white blood cell count greater than 5000/μL.[18] Cyclosporine is given orally at 9 mg/kg/day, adjusted to achieve whole blood levels of 600 to 800 ng/dL for the first month of therapy, and gradually tapered thereafter to maintain blood levels of 200 to 400 ng/dL. Cyclosporine levels are measured by radioimmunoassay. The introduction of cyclosporine has improved survival by 20 to 25%.[19] Cyclosporine therapy has been associated with nephro-, neuro-, and hepatoxicity.[20-22] Horse antithymocyte globulin 10 mg/kg/day given for seven days has been used at Stanford University. However, currently at the Pittsburgh Presbyterian Hospital rabbit antithymocyte globulin is being used with favorable outcome. A relatively new murine-derived monoclonal antibody (OKT_3) is being investigated.[23] The effect of these globulins may be monitored by examing circulating T-lymphocytes and erythrocyte rosette formation.[12]

Rejection of the transplanted heart usually occurs within the first 3 months and markedly decreases after the sixth month of transplantation. Clinical recognition of rejection may include fever, fatigue, heart failure, dysrhythmias, and voltage decrease on the ECG. Routine myocardial biopsies are performed under fluoroscopy weekly in the first 2 months and then every 3 to 4 months. Histologically, rejection manifests itself with infiltration by mononuclear cells of perivascular structures in the early phase, to be followed by interstitial edema and necrosis in the advanced state.[24] Patients treated with cyclosporine have less rejection episodes, and when rejection occurs, it is easier to treat. Rejection episodes are aggressively treated with methylprednisolone, 1 g bolus per day for three days followed by prednisone 1.5 mg/kg/day. Rabbit antithymocyte globulin is also given. Immunosuppressed patients have a higher propensity to develop malignancies such as lymphomas, skin cancer, colon cancer, and acute myclogenous leukemia.[5,25]

Other complications in the heart transplant patient include advanced occlusive coronary artery disease.[26] It is believed that immunolgical injury to the donor endothelium, with subsequent platelet adhesion and plugging, is the responsible mechanism. Advanced artherosclerosis correlates positively with HLA-A_2 incompatibility, donor age over 35 years, and high triglycerides.[11] As mentioned earlier, no angina symptoms are described; therefore, yearly coronary angiograms are recommended as well as retransplantation if the occlusive disease is severe.[26] Oral dipyridamole prophylaxis is strongly recommended for prevention of platelet aggregation.

Heart-Lung Transplantation

Physiology of the Denervated Heart and Lungs. The transplanted lungs are denervated and lack lymphatic drainage as well as bronchial blood supply. Loss of vagal innervation causes an increase in end-tidal CO_2, loss of the cough reflex below the tracheal anastomosis, loss of ciliary action, and loss of the Hering-Breuer inflation reflex. Consequently, patients without awareness may accumulate dangerous amounts of secretions. Thus patients must be told to actively cough and be suctioned thoroughly. Vagotomy in the heart-lung recipient may prevent bronchospasm in reponse to small airway irritation.[27] However, during acute rejection, bronchospasm can still occur. Due to poor lymphatic drainage, pulmonary edema develops readily with volume loading. Platelet aggregates from transfused blood are not cleaned and may lead to chronic hypoxemia and recurrent infections.[27] Due to the growing concern of lung drainage from oxygen-free radicals, attempts are made to provide the lowest inspired oxygen concentration that can maintain a $PaO_2 > 70$ mm Hg. Pulmonary vascular resistance markedly decreases following transplantation.[17] Left ventricular function is normal. Pulmonary evaluation posttransplantation shows moderate restrictive disease that improves with time.[28] However, late pulmonary complications such as infectious bronchitis, bronchiectasis, and bronchiolitis obliterans may be present.[29] Pulmonary fibrosis secondary to cyclosporine therapy has also been described.

Postoperative Considerations. Many of the principles described earlier for heart transplantation apply to heart-lung recipients. In addition to isoproterenol, a nitroprusside infusion may be required to lower afterload to both the right and left ventricles. Weaning from mechanical ventilation is usually possible within 18 hours. However, if reintubation is required, a sterile tray with all the necessary equipment (laryngoscope, endotracheal tubes, airways, lubricant, topical spray, and tongue blade) should be available. The endotracheal tube cuff should not be overinflated to avoid ischemia of the poorly vascularized anastomosed tracheal mucosa.

Following extubation, emphasis is placed on coughing and clearing of secretions. As with heart transplant recipients, a gradual program of physical therapy is initiated with careful nutritional evaluation. Immunosuppression preoperatively includes oral cyclosporine 18 mg/kg in addition to rabbit antithymocyte globulin. Intraoperatively methylprednisolone 500 mg IV is given and followed by three doses of 125 mg IV for three days. Oral cyclosporine is resumed postoperatively at 10 mg/kg/day adjusted to blood levels. Rabbit antithymocyte globulin is given for three days. In order to avoid steroid interference with healing of the tracheal anastomosis, azathioprine is given orally 1.5 to 2.0 mg/kg/day for 2 weeks and then replaced with prednisone 0.2 mg/kg/day along with cyclosporine maintenance.

Myocardial biopsies are routinely performed, as well as pulmonary function studies and chest radiography. Pulmonary rejection may not occur simultaneously with cardiac rejection,[30] although it also commonly occurs within the first three months. Pulmonary edema immediately following transplantation has been associated with fever and respiratory distress, and will usually respond to steroid therapy.[31] Rejection is treated similarly to heart transplant rejection.

Of equal concern is infection. Vigilance and routine cultures are necessary to diagnose and treat opportunistic infections. The wide array of causative organisms is again similar to those found in heart transplant recipients.

Hepatic dysfunction is common in patients with preoperative right heart failure, pulmonary hypertension, and tricuspid regurgitation.[32] As with heart transplant recipients, those patients may have silent coronary ischemia as well as silent pulmonary insufficiency due to loss of lung stretch reflexes. Renal insufficiency and arterial hypertension are common in cyclosporine-treated patients.

KIDNEY TRANSPLANTATION

Kidney transplantation is the treatment of choice for children and adults with end-stage renal disease (ESRD). The overall success of this procedure is continuing to rise. Several factors contribute to this success over the last few decades. The most significant is the development of excellent transplant centers that emphasize careful donor selection, superb anesthetic and surgical technique, as well as postoperative intensive care. Kidney transplantation offers many patients the opportunity to resume a normal life including successful pregnancies.[26] Common indications for kidney transplantation, as well as survival rates, are shown in Tables 18-4 to 18-6. Some contraindications to kidney transplantation include age over 60 years, active untreatable infection, and disseminated malignancy.

Pathophysiological Findings in Renal Failure

Cardiovascular. Most patients have arterial hypertension, accompanied by left ventricular hypertrophy (LVH). LVH, however, may be caused by chronic volume overload, anemia, and pericarditis. Patients may develop myocardial dysfunction from metabolic acidosis, and elevated serum potassium and magnesium levels. Patients with ESRD have an accelerated mortality rate from ischemic heart disease greater than in normal persons or those with hypertension. Uremic pericarditis is a late sequela of uremia associated with minor symptoms and a clear fluid that responds to dialysis treatment.[33] Dialysis-related pericarditis, however, is associated with pain, fever,

TABLE 18-4. INDICATIONS FOR KIDNEY TRANSPLANTATION IN ADULTS AND CHILDREN

Disease	Frequency (%)
Glomerulonephritis	41
Hypertension	17
Diabetes mellitus	9
Idiopathic	7
Pyelonephritis	6
Polycystic disease	5
Other	15

Modified from Graybar GB, Tarpey M: Kidney transplantation, in Gelman S (ed): Anesthesia and Organ Transplantation. Philadelphia, Saunders, 1987, p 81.

TABLE 18–5. GRAFT SURVIVAL RATES FOLLOWING KIDNEY TRANSPLANTATION

Time	Parent (%)	Donor Sibling (%)	Cadaver (%)
10 years	46	43	24
20 years	29	35	19

Adapted from Lee HM, Mendez-Picon G, Goldman T, et al: The course of long-term survival in kidney transplantation: One center's experience. Transplant Proc 1985; 17:106.

leukocytosis, hemorrhagic fluid, and does not respond to dialysis. Pericardial effusions may be seen as well as conduction abnormalities, especially with electrolyte imbalance.

Pulmonary. Pleural effusions may be seen. Abnormal oxygenation may be explained by arteriovenous malformations, abnormal breathing patterns, or pleural effusions.

Hematologic. The severe anemia observed in ESRD patients may have several causes (Table 18–7). Uremia induces platelet dysfunction responsible for prolonged bleeding times, and coagulopathies.

Metabolic. Metabolic acidosis is common. Hyperparathyroidism, secondary to hypocalcemia and phosphate retention, may lead to calcium deposits in the brain, cornea, heart, nerves, skin, blood cells, and the vasculature. Consequences of this hormonal imbalance are anemia, myocardial dysfunction, dysrhythmias, hyperglycemia, osteomalacia, and osteitis fibrosa cystica.[34] Osteoporosis and osteosclerosis may also be seen. Muscle pain and weakness are common.

Gastrointestinal. Dysfunction of the alimentary tract may occur at any level. Commonly, patients complain of anorexia, nausea, vomiting, bowel habit disturbances, hematemesis, and bowel distension. Delayed gastric emptying is of special importance to anesthesiologists. In addition to platelet dysfunction, a major cause of bleeding in ESRD patients is gastrointestinal hemorrhage.

TABLE 18–6. PATIENT SURVIVAL RATES FOLLOWING KIDNEY TRANSPLANTATION

Time	Parent (%)	Donor Sibling (%)	Cadaver (%)
10 years	63	51	40
20 years	45	38	30

Adapted from Lee HM, Mendez-Picon G, Goldman T, et al: The course of long-term survival in kidney transplantation: One center's experience. Transplant Proc 1985; 17:106.

TABLE 18–7. CAUSES FOR ANEMIA IN PATIENTS WITH ESRD

Decreased erythropoietin production
Bone marrow suppression
Hemolysis
    Oxidizing drugs
    Microangiopathic lesions
    Dialysis
Iron Deficiency
    Blood loss
    Malabsorption
Folate deficiency
Vitamins B_6 and B_{12} deficiency
Secondary hyperparathyroidism
    Inhibition of erythropoiesis
    Rapid RBC turnover
    Myelofibrosis

Adapted from Fried W: Hematological abnormalities in chronic renal failure. Seminar Nephrol 1981; 1:176.

Neuropsychiatric. A peripheral neuropathy is common. Behavioral problems are very common, and in fact suicide accounts for as many as 15% of all deaths following kidney transplantation.[35] Sexual and fertility problems are also common.

Postoperative Considerations

General Measures. Following the completion of surgical repair, the central venous pressure (CVP) should be maintained above 5 and closer to 10 cm H_2O.[36] Urine output is replaced milliliter for milliliter. Systolic blood pressure should be within the 120 to 140 mm Hg range. Hypo- or hypertension may lead to graft damage and should be treated aggressively. Dopamine is the drug of choice for treating hypotension in a euvolemic patient due to its effect of improving urine output. For treating hypertension, one may use clonidine, prazosin, minoxidil, labetalol, captopril, or enalapril. Pure beta-adrenergic blockers may decrease glomerular filtration rate.

Cardiovascular morbidity and mortality is high among post-kidney-transplantation patients. Dysrhythmias occur in 5 to 10% of patients, myocardial infarction in 0.5%, and death from cardiac disease in 1%.[37] A urinary catheter is left for 3 to 5 days for careful evaluation of fluid status. Controversy exists whether or not to extubate patients immediately following kidney transplantation due to high CVP pressures and propensity for developing pulmonary and airway edema. Certainly, if doubt exists, the endotracheal tube should be left in place while the patient is kept well sedated. Careful attention to electrolyte balance is essential. In order to evaluate renal function, daily blood urea nitrogen (BUN) and creatinine levels are monitored. A renal sonogram and renal scan are also performed after transplantation. Diabetic patients require close monitoring of glucose levels.

Rejection. Rejection usually presents with oliguria, graft enlargement and tenderness, fever, leukocytosis, hypertension, weight gain, peripheral edema, and rise in BUN and creatinine levels. Hyperacute (within a few hours of transplantation) rejection is the result of preformed cytotoxic antibodies. The kidney will remain pale and not regain normal turgor. The treatment for hyperacute rejection is immediate nephrectomy. Acute rejection is one that occurs one to three days to a few months after transplantation. Treatment here is with augmenting steroid therapy and administering antithymocyte globulin. Early treatment is essential in preventing permanent damage to the graft. A similar presentation to acute rejection is seen with acute tubular necrosis (ATN). ATN is present in the majority of cadaveric transplants but only in 3% of living related donor grafts. A renal scan often is beneficial in differentiating ATN from acute rejection. In acute rejection the renal scan shows decreasing renal blood flow; however, in ATN the renal flow is actually gradually improving.

Immunosuppression. Several protocols exist. A sample protocol is outlined in Table 18–8. Treatment for rejection, as mentioned earlier, involves steroid "recycling" with antithymocyte globulin administration 15 to 20 mg/kg for ten days or monoclonal OKT$_3$ 5 mg/day for ten days.

Of interest is that very few centers require reverse isolation precautions for kidney transplant recipients. Those centers that do not isolate, however, do limit the volume of family visitations to minimize exposure. There is also some doubt as to whether the cost and anxiety involved with reverse isolation justify its use when compared with the benefit derived.

Infection. As immunosuppressed patients, kidney transplant recipients are prone to a wide array of bacterial and opportunistic infections. Table 18–9 represents a relatively predictable pattern of infections in kidney transplant recipients. Cytomegalovirus (CMV) infection is the most common cause of infection in kidney transplant recipients. In one study, CMV was implicated in 50% of febrile episodes among 433 kidney transplant recipients.[38] CMV infections typically occur within the first 4 months of transplantation. Unlike immunocompetent patients, immunosuppressed patients rarely develop lymphadenopathy or splenomegaly in response to a CMV infection.[39] The clinical presentation of a prolonged febrile episode with or without pneumonitis strongly suggests a CMV infection. Treatment for CMV infection is supportive; while antiviral agents may be tried, they have not yet been shown to be successful in controlling these infections.[40]

Other Complications. Patients receiving cadaveric grafts have a higher overall mortality from infection due to the higher requirements of immunosuppression. As in other immunocompromised patients, the incidence of malignant neoplasms is higher. Gastrointestinal hemorrhage occurs in 10 to 20% of patients and is associated with greater than a 50% mortality. Prophylactic administration of cimetidine has not been shown to be efficacious in lowering the incidence of bleeding.[38] Hypertension posttransplantation may be due to rejection or induced by the native kidneys or due to fluid retention secondary to the Cushing's syndrome these patients develop on chronic steroid therapy.

Hyperparathyroidism and steroid therapy may cause avascular necrosis of the femoral head, requiring total hip replacement.

POSTANESTHETIC CARE OF THE ORTHOTOPIC LIVER TRANSPLANTATION PATIENT

Since the first clinical orthotopic liver transplantation in humans by Starzl and associates in 1963,[41] many advances in surgical technique, organ procurement, anesthetic management, postoperative care, and im-

TABLE 18–8. PERIOPERATIVE IMMUNOSUPPRESSION REGIMEN

| Time Period | Immunosuppressive Agents | |
	Cyclosporine	Steroids
Preoperative	2 mg/kg IV	
Intraoperative		Methylprednisolone 1 gm IV
Postoperative	1–5 days level 800–100 ng/mL	Prednisone 7–10 mg/kg PO *or* methylprednisolone 200 mg/day IV 200 mg/day in 4 divided doses
Long term	Taper to blood level of 500–700 ng/mL therapeutic response	Taper to 5 mg/day by 6 months

TABLE 18–9. PATTERN OF INFECTION IN KIDNEY TRANSPLANT RECIPIENTS

Time	Organisms
0–1 month	Bacterial (wound infections, pneumonias, urinary tract infections)
1–6 months	CMV, fungi, pneumocystis, Listeria, other vital agents
Minimal immunosuppression	Community-acquired (influenza, pneumococci)
Significant immunosuppression	Opportunistic infections

munosuppression have lead to a 1-year survival rate of greater than 80% by 1984.[42] The indications, surgical techniques, and pre- and intraoperative management for liver transplantation have been extensively reported.[43–49] With further advances, the number of medical centers performing liver transplantation will undoubtedly increase, requiring anesthesiologists to be thoroughly familiar with the perioperative management of one of the most challenging procedures.

As most of the experience in liver transplantation has been reported from the Starzl group in Pittsburgh and the Calne group in Cambridge, this section will draw from their results. Proper postoperative management requires knowledge of the preoperative and the intraoperative assessment and management in terms of hepatic, hemodynamic, hematologic, coagulation, pulmonary, metabolic, and biochemical status, as these derangements may continue postoperatively.

The intraoperative course of liver transplantation involves tremendous fluctuations in hemodynamic, hematologic, coagulation, metabolic, and biochemical status (see Figs. 18–2 to 18–8). However, unless unusual medical or surgical complications arise, most of the physiological derangements have stabilized by the end of surgery and admission into the intensive care unit.

General Care

In the intensive care unit, the liver transplantation patients will require monitoring as other critically ill postoperative patients. The invasive hemodynamic monitors, arterial line, and pulmonary artery catheter with continuous mixed venous oxygen saturation capability, are present from the intraoperative period, and full hemodynamic monitoring continues postoperatively. Baseline vital signs, temperature, and hemodynamic profile are immediately obtained and recorded every 15 minutes, as needed, until the patient status is stabilized, and are then recorded every hour. Postoperative ECG and chest x-ray are also obtained.

Intake and output are recorded hourly to guide fluid therapy and maintain urine output. The nasogastric tube is placed to suction and antacid therapy is initiated if the nasogastric drainage tests positive for blood. Surgical, biliary T-tube, and chest tube drainage are recorded and examined for amount as well as color and character. A complete laboratory profile consisting of complete blood count, platelets, electrolytes, glucose, coagulation profile, and liver function tests, is obtained immediately and every six hours until the patient is stable.

Pain is controlled with intravenous opioids (morphine sulfate or fentanyl) in small, carefully titrated doses, as the metabolism of opioids may be altered with transplanted livers.

Cardiovascular Considerations

Due to improved intraoperative monitoring and management (Figs. 18–2 to 18–4) the incidence of postoperative hemodynamic instability, dysrythmias, and requirement for vasoactive therapy has decreased. Postoperative hemodynamic monitoring is a continuation of the intraoperative monitoring, consisting of arterial line, central venous pressure, pulmonary artery pressures with mixed venous oxygen saturation monitoring, and derived hemodynamic parameters. Fluid management and pharmacologic intervention with inotropes, vasopressors, vasodilators, and diuretics are guided by clinical evaluation. As postoperative pulmonary edema may occur at lower pulmonary artery pressures after liver transplantation, adequate urine output is maintained with diuretics,

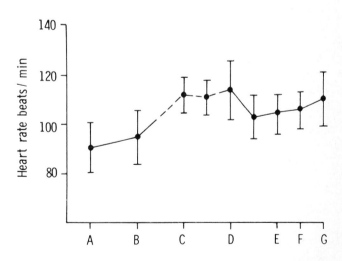

Figure 18–2. Changes in heart rate at the various phases during liver transplantation. Mean ± SEM for nine patients. Phase A, induction; B, dissection; C, anhepatic; D, partial anhepatic; E, gall bladder anastomosis; F, skin closure; G, end of procedure. (From Carmichael FJ, Lindop MJ, Farman JV: Anesthesia for hepatic transplantation: cardiovascular and metabolic alterations and their management. *Anesth Analg* 1985;64:108–116.

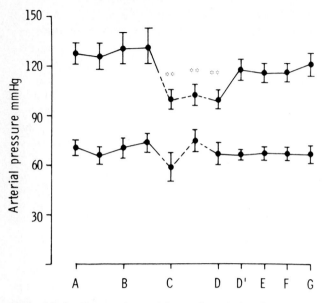

Figure 18–3. Changes in arterial systolic and diastolic pressure during liver transplantation. Mean ± SEM for nine patients. **Differences from preclamping values statistically significant *P* < 0.01. See Fig. 18–2 for details of A–G. From Carmichael FJ, Lindop MJ, Farman JV: Anesthesia for hepatic transplantation: Cardiovascular and metabolic alterations and their management. *Anesth Analg* 1985;64:108–116.

renal dose dopamine (3 to 5 μg/kg/min), and careful fluid replacement therapy. Hypotension is avoided to maintain perfusion to the kidneys and the transplanted liver. Hypertension is common in the early postoperative period and therapy is often required.

Medications with potential for hepatotoxicity, such as alpha methyldopa, should be avoided.

Pulmonary Considerations

Patients arrive into the ICU intubated and require ventilatory support. Frequent blood gas monitoring and daily chest x-ray are mandatory during weaning from ventilatory support, which is usually required for two days postoperatively. Criteria for extubation require patients to be awake and alert to be able to protect their airway against aspiration; to be normothermic; to be hemodynamically stable; and to have satisfactory blood gas values, chest x-ray, and weaning parameters (tidal volume > 5 mL/kg, vital capacity > 10 mL/kg, and negative inspiratory force > − 20 cm H_2O).

Aggressive pulmonary toilet and physiotherapy is initiated to prevent atelectasis. Pleural effusions should be drained by a thoracostomy tube. Daily chest x-ray is obtained to detect pulmonary edema, infiltration, and atelectasis. The occurrence of adult respiratory distress syndrome (ARDS) may herald the onset of fulminant hepatic rejection and failure, or sepsis, and requires aggressive appropriate therapy.

Renal Considerations

Renal dysfunction is common in the postoperative period of liver transplantation. Preoperative renal dysfunction and intraoperative factors—including hemodynamic instability, inferior vena cava clamp-

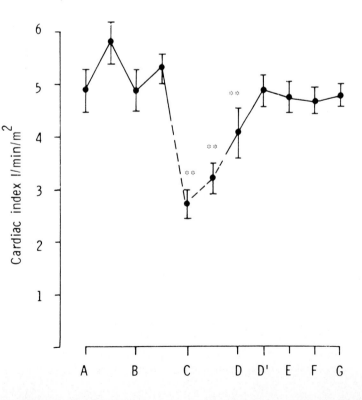

Figure 18–4. Changes in cardiac index during liver transplantation. Mean ± SEM for nine patients. **Differences from preclamping values statistically significant *P* < 0.01, *P* < 0.05. See Fig. 18–2 for details of A–G. From Carmichael FJ, Lindop MJ, Farman JV: Anesthesia for hepatic transplantation: Cardiovascular and metabolic alterations and their management. *Anesth Analg* 1985;64:108–116.)

ing, fluid shifts, hemoglobinuria, and myoglobinuria secondary to massive transfusions—may contribute to postoperative renal dysfunction. Clinical assessment, ventricular filling pressures, and hemodynamic parameters should guide fluid therapy. Urine output should be maintained at greater than 0.5 mL/kg/h by judicious use of fluids, diuretics, and renal-dose dopamine therapy.

With successful liver transplantation, renal dysfunction is corrected even in patients with preoperative renal dysfunction. However, persistent renal dysfunction may be a harbinger of sepsis, liver rejection or failure, or nephrotoxic effects of antibiotic or cyclosporine therapy.

Temperature

Despite intraoperative use of warming blankets, respiratory humidification, and the use of warm intravenous and irrigation fluids, hypothermia is common in the postoperative period due to the long abdominal procedure[50] and the transplantation of cold, preserved donor liver. Towards the end of surgery, there is generally a gradual increase in temperature (Fig. 18–5). As hypothermia may interfere with cardiovascular and coagulation function and shivering increases oxygen consumption, temperature is monitored postoperatively. Warming blankets and adequate ambient temperatures are used to promote the return to normothermia.

Central Nervous System

Preoperative neurologic dysfunction—including hepatic encephalopathy, dysfunction of the transplanted liver, delayed emergence from prolonged an-

esthesia, and impaired metabolism of anesthestics and analgesics—may result in diminished mental status postoperatively. Furthermore, intraoperative emboli, particulate or air, may cause postoperative seizures or coma.[51] Postoperative CNS dysfunction requires a complete neurologic evaluation, search for systemic or metabolic causes, and supportive therapy. Seizures are controlled with phenobarbitol. Reversible cyclosporine CNS toxicity—which may cause confusion, cortical blindness, seizures, or coma—requires reduction in cyclosporine dosage.[52]

Potassium Balance

Potassium levels, which fluctutate greatly intraoperatively, are usually stabilized by the end of the surgery (Fig. 18–6). Postoperative hypokalemia may occur due to preoperative total body depletion, reabsorbtion of potassium into the transplanted liver, and diuretic therapy with inadequate potassium replacement. Hyperkalemia may be present in the postoperative period due to renal failure or inadequate flushing of the hyperkalemic liver preservative solution at the time of liver reperfusion. Persistent hyperkalemia in the postoperative period may be due

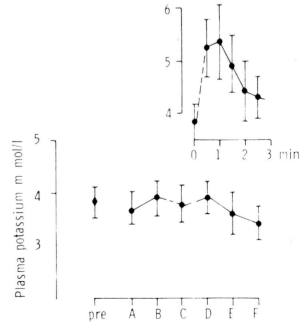

Figure 18–6. Changes in pulmonary arterial plasma potassium concentrations during liver transplantation. Mean ± SEM for nine patients. Inset: plasma potassium samples taken from the pulmonary artery catheter over 30-sec periods after the release of clamps from the portal vein and suprahepatic artery in eight patients. **Differences from preclamping values statistically significant $P < 0.01$, *$P < 0.05$. See Fig. 18–2 for details of A–G. From Carmichael FJ, Lindop MJ, Farman JV: Anesthesia for hepatic transplantation: Cardiovascular and metabolic alterations and their management. *Anesth Analg* 1985;64:113.

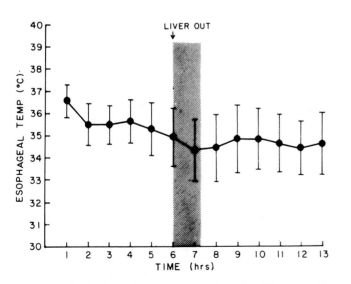

Figure 18–5 Esophageal temperature vs time. $N = 36$, mean and SD are represented. The shaded area represents the anhepatic period. From Borland LM, Roule M, Cooke DR: Anesthesia for pediatric orthotopic liver transplantation. *Anesth Analg* 1985;64:123.

to nonfunction or rejection of the transplanted liver. Routine electrolyte monitoring is required and potassium abnormalities corrected.

Sodium Balance

Sodium level will usually normalize by the end of surgery. Hyponatremia may be due to preoperative inability to excrete free water, vigorous diuretic therapy, or intraoperative iatrogenic causes. Hypernatremia is commonly due to excessive sodium bicarbonate therapy of intraoperative metabolic acidosis.

Calcium Balance

Hypocalcemia, which occurs frequently intraoperatively due to massive transfusions and citrate levels, may continue into the postoperative period. With a functioning liver graft, citrate should be metabolized without affecting calcium levels. Ionized calcium levels should be monitored, and if low, with hemodynamic consequences, calcium chloride should be administered.

Glucose Balance

Usually, with successful liver transplantation, glucose levels are high, even without intraoperative administration of glucose due to the stress of surgery (Fig. 18–7).[48] Hypoglycemia in the postoperative period is a poor prognostic sign. Boluses of D50W and infusion of D10W may be required to maintain glucose level above 100 mg/dL.

Acid–Base Balance

Postoperative metabolic alkalosis, which is common in successful liver transplantation (Fig. 18–8), is due

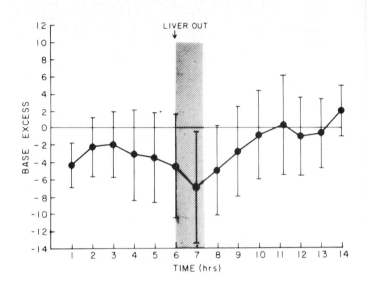

Figure 18–8. Base excess vs time, $N = 42$, mean and SD are represented. The shaded area represents the anhepatic period. From Borland LM, Roule M, Cooke DR: Anesthesia for pediatric orthotopic liver transplantation. *Anesth Analg* 1985;64:123.

to preoperative total body potassium depletion, excessive intraoperative administration of sodium bicarbonate, postoperative metabolism of lactate and citrate, and vigorous diuretic therapy. As metabolic alkalosis may cause lethargy, hypokalemia, and decreased pulmonary ventilation, treatment consisting of potassium chloride replacement, acid solutions, or acetazolamide is required. Refractory metabolic acidosis in the postoperative period may result from nonfunctioning or rejection of the transplanted liver.

Hepatic Function

A successful transplanted liver should show a gradual and steady improvement of liver function with production of bile within 24 hours of graft reperfusion. However, hepatic dysfunction may occur due to primary nonfunction, surgical/technical complications, rejection of the transplanted liver, infections, or a combination of these complications. Primary nonfunction is manifested by coma, fever, coagulopathy, renal failure, metabolic acidosis, cardiogenic shock, and abnormal liver function tests. Pretransplantation ischemia time may be the cause of primary nonfunction. Retransplantation is required.

Technical complications include biliary obstruction and leakage, surgical bleeding, and occlusion or thrombosis of the vascular anastomosis. Fever, malaise, and subsequent sepsis may be the presentation of these complications. The situation requires immediate angiography and reexploration or anticoagulation in cases of portal vein thrombosis. Biliary tree complications of biliary obstruction or leak are investigated by diagnostic modalities, including T-tube

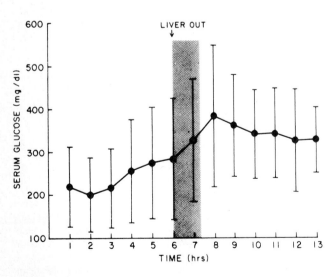

Figure 18–7. Serum glucose vs time, $N = 42$, mean and SD are represented. The shaded area represents the anhepatic period. From Borland LM, Roule M, Cooke DR: Anesthesia for pediatric orthotopic liver transplantation. *Anesth Analg* 1985;64:122.

cholangiogram, percutaneous transhepatic cholangiogram, and computerized tomography.

The signs and symptoms of rejection include fever (usually the first sign), anorexia, depression, abdominal pain with a hard and swollen liver and ascites, and abnormal liver function tests. Differential diagnosis of rejection from sepsis is crucial as the first requires increased immunosuppression, while the second requires decreased immunosuppression.

Although hyperacute liver rejection has not been reported, fever, diminished mental status, hypoglycemia, coagulopathy, production of dilute bile, and abnormal liver function tests in the first 48 hours postoperatively indicate rejection and require retransplantation. Late rejection (> 30 days) is not infrequent and T-tube cholangiogram and computerized tomography reveal decreased attenuation of rejected areas. Immunosuppression is increased and retransplantation may be necessary.

The criteria and considerations for liver retransplantation have been reported.[53] The retransplantation rate is 20% at the University of Pittsburgh, with an overall 1-year survival rate of 49%.[53]

Immunosuppressive Therapy

The introduction of cyclosporin A in 1980 has been by far the most significant reason for increased success of liver transplantation. Presently, cyclosporine and corticosteroids are the mainstay of immunosuppressive therapy. Steroid therapy consists of methylprednisone sodium succinate, administered 1g IV after revascularization of the transplanted liver followed by a six-day postoperative course tapered from methylprednisolone, 50 mg IV q 6 h, to oral maintenance prednisone of 20 mg daily. Acute rejection is treated by a similiar six-day tapered corticosteroid ''pulse'' therapy. Cyclosporin A, an extract of two fungi, has a proposed mechanism of interfering with a monkine interleukin-2, which serves as a growth factor of T-lymphocytes. Cyclosporine is administered 2 mg/kg IV on call to the operating room, followed by 2 mg/kg IV three times a day postoperatively. With return of gastrointestinal function, cyclosporine is given 17.5 mg/kg/day orally in three divided doses.

Cyclosporine trough level monitoring is mandatory to minimize the dose-related cyclosporine toxicities. Optimal trough levels of 800 to 1000 ng/mL should be maintained. Nephrotoxicity, the most common adverse reaction to cyclosporine; lymphoproliferative dysfunction; and CNS toxicity; are reversible with downward adjustments of cyclosporine dosage.

OKT3, T-cell antilymphocyte globulin is used for acute rejections. Bronchospasm, the most important adverse reaction of OKT3 therapy, is treatable with systemic racemic epinephrine. Other adverse reactions include fever, rigors, diarrhea, nausea, vomiting, chest tightness, and exacerbation of pulmonary edema.

Infections

Infections are common complications in liver transplantation as a result of immunosuppression, malnutrition, and prophylactic use of antibiotics. Infectious complications develop in 81% of all liver transplantation patients and fungal infections in 42%.[54]

Fever in the postoperative period is evaluated by physical examination, chest x-ray, gram stain and culture, and sensitivity of sputum, surgical drainage, Foley catheter, and blood. Cultures are obtained for bacteria, virus, and fungus. To diagnose specific infections, diagnostic modalities include ultrasound, computerized tomography, percutaneous transhepatic and T-tube cholangiogram, endoscopic retrograde cholangiopancreatogram, fiberoptic bronchoscopy with lavage, and open lung biopsy.

Strict adherence to aseptic technique by all those in contact with the immunosuppressed patient is essential. Prophylactic mycostatin mouthwash against oral candidiasis and broad-spectrum antibiotic coverage is instituted postoperatively. Judicious reduction in immunosuppression, supportive care including adequate oral or parental nutrition, and specific antibiotic, antiviral, or antifungal agents, are utilized to minimize and treat infectious complications.

Coagulation System

Through the introduction of thromboelastography[55] and heparinless veno-veno bypass, the incidence of postoperative coagulopathy has decreased. Complete coagulation profile, including prothrombin time, partial prothrombin time, platelets, fibrin split products, and fibrinogen levels, is evaluated upon arrival into the intensive care unit. The thromboelastogram may be used to monitor and guide therapy for postoperative bleeding. Epsilon aminocaproic therapy for prevention of hypercoagulable states after successful liver transplantation is controversial.[56,57] Persistent postoperative bleeding is usually due to surgical bleeding, or rejection or nonfunction of the transplanted liver.

Liver transplantation has evolved from an experimental endeavor to an accepted clinical medical therapy in only 25 years. Great advances in many areas—including immunosuppression, hemodynamic monitoring, management of biochemical and metabolic, and coagulation derangements—have contributed to the present-day success of liver transplantation.

With advance and refinement of pre- and intraoperative management, the postoperative course has become much more stable. However, improved and meticulous postoperative management of immunosuppression, infection, coagulation, and metabolic complications will further increase the success and decrease the morbidity of the liver transplantation patient.

POSTANESTHETIC CARE OF THE REPLANTATION PATIENT

Replantation is the surgical restoration of an organ to its original site in the same patient.[58] Replantation of the upper and lower extremities, scalp, ear, lip, penis, and composite grafts have been performed. As microsurgical techniques have improved to allow anastomosis of blood vessels as small as 0.3 mm in diameter, the success of replantation should be judged not in terms of revascularization, but in terms of functional return. The factors that favor or discourage replantation attempts have been reviewed.[59]

This section will review the postoperative care of replantation patients as related to the perioperative factors, such as trauma with resultant blood loss; risk of aspiration pneumonitis during induction of anesthesia; psychological aspects; long surgery and anesthesia and their effects on fluid, electrolyte, acid–base balance, and temperature homeostasis; and metabolism of anesthesic agents. Specific care of the replanted parts will also be addressed.

Psychological Profile

While many amputations are purely accidental or occupation-related, a high percentage of patients who present for replantation surgery have psychological disturbances including psychopathology, substance abuse, or recent stressful events.[60] A complete preoperative psychiatric evaluation may disclose underlying disturbances and will aid in preoperative psychiatric therapy or pharmacologic intervention.[61] Neuroleptic therapy and restraints, if required, should be continued in the immediate postoperative period in the PACU; patients sedated on emergence from anesthesia and the unfamiliar surroundings of the PACU or intensive care unit may further display confusion and agitation and jeopardize the replanted parts. Continuous observation, and psychological and pharmacologic therapy, are necessary to optimize surgical results. Many patients require prolonged psychotherapy and rehabilitation to maximize functional recovery.

Fluid Status

Bleeding from trauma and insidious blood loss during the long surgical procedure may be significant. Frequent serial determination of blood count is required in the perioperative period. Normovolemic hemodi-

lution (hematocrit 25 to 30%) improve rheological properties of blood and improve microcirculation with adequate oxygen delivery unless other coexisting medical considerations are present. Bleeding due to massive transfusions or bleeding diasthesis requires a thorough examination of the coagulation profile and judicious blood component replacement therapy.

Patients with cardiovascular disease or intraoperative hemodynamic instability may require pulmonary artery catheter and full hemodynamic monitoring intra- and postoperatively. Urine output greater than 0.5 mL/kg/h is indicative of adequate intravascular volume status.

Preoperative deficits and/or intraoperative derangements of sodium, potassium, and glucose may be manifested postoperatively and require treatment. Careful evaluation and treatment of acid–base status is imperative, as acidosis on reperfusion has detrimental effects on replanted parts.[62]

Pulmonary Considerations

Careful weaning from ventilatory support is mandatory. The criteria for extubation is similiar as for other critically ill patients, with the following special considerations following prolonged general anesthesia. Patients considered to have a full stomach on induction should also be considered at risk for aspiration upon extubation and should be fully awake and be able to protect their airway. However, awakening may be delayed from prolonged general anesthesia and neuroleptic therapy. Intraoperative maintenance of airway humidity is important in decreasing postoperative pulmonary complications.[63] Neuromuscular agents must be documented to have been fully reversed or metabolized by objective peripheral nerve stimulator criteria.

Temperature

Due to the long procedures, patients may become hypothermic intraoperatively. Maintenance of ambient temperature is the most important factor in prevention of hypothermia.[64] Postoperatively, hypothermia may cause vasoconstriction and increased oxygen consumption due to shivering, both of which are detrimental to survival of replanted parts.

Metabolism of Anesthetics

Prolonged inhalational anesthesia results in significant metabolism and biotransformation of the volatile anesthetics. The result may be manifested by delayed awakening,[65] sedative effects of bromide from halothane metabolism,[66] and renal effects of fluoride from enflurane metabolism.[67]

Postoperative Care of the Replanted Organs

Analgesics are administered to prevent vasoconstriction secondary to pain. To maintain revascularization of the replanted tissue, and to prevent thrombosis, antithrombotic therapy consisting of Rheomacrodex and low-dose aspirin is initiated early in the postoperative period. Heparin may be utilized in cases of thrombosis that will require reexploration. Brachial flexus blocks and continuous epidural anesthesia may also be used to improve blood flow.

Skin temperature is the mainstay of monitoring the viability of the replanted organs.[68] The dorsal aspect of the middle portion of the replanted part is monitored. Successful replants show a rapid and steady increase in skin temperature to above 30°C and remain above 30°C. With arterial complications, the skin temperature will not rise above 30°C and the temperature will decrease to 25 to 27°C, while venous complications will result in skin temperatures in the 28 to 30°C range.

Newer and more sensitive methods of monitoring include transcutaneous oxygen,[69] which has problems of possible burns to the site, and hydrogen ion washout test,[70] which requires implantation of needles in the replanted area. There is evidence that these tests detect changes in microcirculation before skin temperature change or clinical signs and enable earlier salvage surgery before irreversible tissue damage occurs. Pulse oximetry may also be used.

The surgical technology in replantation has advanced to allow revascularization of lost tissue. However, the presence of a nonfunctioning part may have enormous economic, social, and psychological impacts and requires careful preoperative decision making. Once the decision to proceed with surgery has been made, careful and meticulous postoperative care and rehabilitation is necessary for maximal recovery of function.

REFERENCES

1. Barnard CN: A human cardiac transplant: An interim report of a successful operation performed at Groote Schuur Hospital. *S Afr Med J* 1967;41:1257.
2. Baumgartner WA, Reitz BA, Bieber CP, et al: Current expectations in cardiac transplantation. *J Thorac Cardiovasc Surg* 1983;86:639.
3. Reitz BA: Cardiac and cardiopulmonary transplantation, in McGoon DC (ed): *Cardiac Surgery,* ed 2. Philadelphia, Davis, 1987, pp 347–359.
4. Kaye M, Elcombe SA, O'Fallon WM: The international heart transplantation registry—The 1984 report. *J Heart Transplant* 1985;4:290.
5. Weintraub J, Warnke RA: Lymphoma in cardiac transplant recipients: Clinical and histological features and immunological phenotype. *Transplantation* 1982;33:347.
6. Cannom DS, Graham AF, Harrison DC: Electrophysiological studies in the denervated transplanted human heart. *Circ Res* 1973;32:268.
7. Cannom DS, Rider AK, Stinson EB, et al: Electrophysiologic studies in the denervated transplanted human heart: II. Response to norepinephrine, isoproterenol and propranolol. *Am J Cardiol* 1975;36:859.
8. Lough ME, Lindsey AD, Shinn JA, et al: Life satisfaction following heart transplantation. *J Heart Transplant* 1985;4:446.
9. Goodman DJ, Rossen RM, Cannom DS, et al: Effect of digoxin on atrioventricular conduction; studies in patients with and without cardiac autonomic innervation. *Circulation* 1975;51:251.
10. Mason JW, Winkle RA, Rider AK, et al: The electrophysiologic effects of quinidine in the transplanted human heart. *J Clin Invest* 1977;59:481.
11. Wyner J, Finch EL: Heart and heart-lung transplantation, in Gelman S (ed): *Anesthesia and Organ Transplantation.* Philadelphia, Saunders, 1987, pp 111–137.
12. Jamieson SW, Stinson EB: Coronary heart disease, in Conner WE, Briston JD (eds): *Cardiac Transplantation for End-Stage Ischemic Heart Diseases.* Philadelphia, Lippincott. 1985;25:737.
13. Trento A, Dummer GS, Hardesty RL, et al: Mediastinitis following heart transplantation: Incidence, treatment and results. *J Heart Transplant* 1984;3:336–340.
14. Steed DL, Brown B, Reilly JJ, et al: General surgical complications in heart and heart-lung transplantation. *Surgery.* 1985;98:739–745.
15. Leitman IM, Paull DE, Barie PS, et al: Intra-abdominal complications of cardiopulmonary bypass operations. *Surg Gynecol Obstet* 1987;165:251–254.
16. Colon R, Frazier OH, Kahan BD, et al: Complications in cardiac transplant patients requiring general surgery. *Surgery* 1988;103:32–38.
17. Dawkins KD, Jamieson SW, Hunt SA, et al: Long-term results, hemodynamics, and complications after combined heart and lung transplantation. *Circulation* 1985;71:919.
18. Griffith BP, Hardesty RL, Lee A, et al: Management of cyclosporine toxicity by reduced dosage and azathioprine. *J Heart Transplant* 1985;4:410–413.
19. Goldstein JP, Wechsler AS: Heart transplantation. *J Heart Transplant* 1985;20:446–454.
20. Bennet WM, Pulliam JP: Cyclosporine nephrotoxicity. *Ann Intern Med* 1983;99:851–854.
21. Hardesty RL, Griffith BP, Debski RF, et al: Experience with cyclosporine in cardiac transplantation. *Transplant Proc* 1983;15:2553–2558.
22. Klintmalm GBB, Iwatzuki S, Starzl TE: Cyclosporine A hepatotoxicity in 66 renal allograft recipients. *Transplantation* 1981;32:488–489.
23. Gilbert EM, Eiswirth CC, Renlund DG, et al: Use of Orthoclone OKT$_3$ monoclonal antibody in cardiac transplantation: Early experience with rejection prophylaxis and treatment of refractory rejection. *Transplant Proc* 1987;19:45–53.

24. Billingham ME: Diagnosis of cardiac rejection by endomyocardial biopsy. *J Heart Transplant* 1981;1:25.

25. Krikorian JG, Anderson JL, Bieber CP: Malignant neoplasms following cardiac transplantation. *JAMA* 1978; 240:639.

26. Guthaner DF, Schnittger I, Wright A, Wexler L: Diagnostic challenges following cardiac transplantation. *Radiol Clin North AM* 1987;25:367–376.

27. Jamieson SW, Dawkins KD, Burke C, et al: Late results of combined heart-lung transplantation. *Transplant Proc* 1985;17:212.

28. Theodore J, Jamieson SW, Burke C, et al: Physiologic aspects of human heart-lung transplantation: Pulmonary function status of the posttransplanted lung. *Chest* 1984;85:349.

29. Burke CM, Morris AJR, Hawkins CGA, et al: Late airflow obstruction in heart-lung transplantation recipients. *J Heart Transplant* 1985;4:437.

30. Scott WC, Haverich A, Billingham ME, et al: Lethal lung rejection without significant cardiac rejection in primate heart-lung allotransplants. *J Heart Transplant* 1984;4:33.

31. Jamieson SW, Stinson EB, Oyer PE, et al: Heart and lung transplantation for pulmonary hypertension. *Am J Surg* 1984;147:740.

32. Jamieson SW: Recent developments in heart and heart-lung transplantation. *Transplant Proc* 1985;17:99.

33. Lee HM, Mendez-Picon G, Goldman T, et al: The course of long-term survival in kidney transplantation: One center's experience. *Transplant Proc* 1985;17:106.

34. Fried W: Hematological abnormalities in chronic renal failure. *Semin Nephrol* 1981;1:176.

35. Crass MF, Moore PL, Strickland ML, et al: Cardiovascular responses to parathyroid hormone. *Am J Physiol* 1985;249:E187.

36. Washer GF, Schroter GPJ, Starzl TE, et al: Causes of death after kidney transplantation. *JAMA* 1983;250:49.

37. Marshland AT, Bradley JP: Anaesthesia for renal transplantation—5 years experience. *Anaesth Intensive Care* 1983;11:337.

38. Grekas D, Nakos V, Theocharides A, et al: Prophylactic treatment with cimetidine after renal transplantation. *Nephron* 1985;40:213.

39. Peterson PK, Balfour HH, Fryd DS, et al: Fever in renal transplant recipients: Causes, prognostic significance and changing patterns at the University of Minnesota. *Am J Med* 1981;71:345–351.

40. Rubin RH, Tolkoff-Rubin NE: The problem of cytomegalovirus infection in transplantation, in Morris PJ, Tilney NC (eds): *Progress in Transplantation.* Edinburgh, Churchill Livingstone, 1984, vol 1, pp 89–114.

41. Starzl TE, Marchioro TL, von Kaulla K, et al: Homotransplantation of the liver in humans. *Surg Gynecol Obstet* 1963;117:609.

42. Starzl TE, Iwatsuki S, Shaw BW Jr, Gordon RD: Orthotopic liver transplantation in 1984. *Transplant Proc* 1985;17:250.

43. Starzl TE, Putnam CW. *Experiences in Hepatic Transplantation.* Philadelphia, Saunders, 1969, p 553.

44. Calne RY: *Clinical Organ Transplantation.* Oxford, Blackwell, 1971, p 539.

45. Starzel TE: Liver transplantation, in Winter PM, Kang YG (eds): *Hepatic Transplantation: Anesthetic and Perioperative Management.* New York, Praeger, 1986, p 3.

46. Carmichael FJ, Lindop MJ, Farman JV: Anesthesia for hepatic transplantation: Cardiovascular and metabolic alterations and their management. *Anesth Analg* 1985;64:108.

47. Whitten CW: Preanesthetic management: The patient for hepatic transplantation. *Anesth News* Jan 1988:8.

48. Borland LM, Martin DJ: Anesthesia considerations for orthotopic liver transplantation, in Brown BB Jr (ed): *Anesthesia and Transplantation Surgery.* Philadelphia, Davis, 1987, p 157.

49. Winter PM, Kang YG: *Hepatic Transplantation: Anesthetic and Perioperative Management.* New York, Praeger, 1986.

50. Aldrete J, Clapp HW, Starzl TE: Body temperature changes during organ transplantation. *Anesth Analg* 1970;49:384.

51. Starzl TE, Schneck SA, Mazzoni G, et al: Acute neurological complications after liver transplantation with particular reference to intraoperative cerebral air embolus. *Ann Surg* 1978;187:236.

52. De Groen PC, Aksamit AJ, Rakela J, et al: Central nervous system toxicity after liver transplantation: The role of cyclosporin and cholesterol. *N Engl J Med* 1987;317:861.

53. Shaw BW Jr, Gordon RD, Iwatsuki S, Starzl TE: Hepatic Retransplantation. *Transplant Proc* 1985;17:264.

54. Ho M, Wajszuk CP, Hardy A, et al: Infections in kidney, heart, and liver transplantation recipients on cyclosporin. *Transplant Proc* 1983;15:2768.

55. Hertert H: Blutgerinnungstudien mit der Thromboelastographie: einem neuen Untersuchingsverfahren. *Klin Wochenschr* 1948;16:257.

56. Von Kaulla KN, Kaye H, von Kaulla E, et al: Changes in blood coagulation, before and after hepatectomy or transplantation in dogs and man. *Arch Surg* 1966;92:71.

57. Kang YG, Navaglund A, Russel M, et al: Antifibrinolytic therapy during liver transplantation (abstr). *Anesthesiology* 1985;63:A92.

58. Gallico GG, Stirrat CR: Extremity replantation. *Surg Ann* 1983;15:229.

59. Ebert JP: Replantation of severed limbs, in Gelman S (ed): *Anesthesia and Organ Transplantation.* Philadelphia, Saunders, 1987, p 187.

60. Strain JJ, DeMuth GW: Care of the psychotic self-amputee undergoing replantation. *Ann Surg* 1983;197:210.

61. Schweitzer I, Rosenbaum MB: Psychiatric aspects of replantation surgery. *Gen Hosp Psychiatry* 1982;4:271.

62. Dell PC, Seaber AV, Urbaniak JR: The effect of systemic acidosis on perfusion of replanted extremities. *J Hand Surg* 1980;5:433.

63. Chalon J, Patel C, Ali M, et al: Humidity and the anesthetized patient. *Anesthesiology* 1979;50:195.

64. Morris RH: Operating room temperature and the anesthetized, paralyzed patient. *Arch Surg* 1971;102:95–97.

65. Caplan RA, Long MC: Prolonged anesthesia—Management and sequelae of a two-day general anesthetic. *Anesth Analg* 1984;63:353.

66. Mazze RI, Calverly RK, Smith NT: Inorganic fluoride

nephrotoxicity: Prolonged enflurane and halothane anesthesia in volunteers. *Anesthesiology* 1977;46:265.

67. Cousins MJ, Greenstein LR, Hitt BA, Mazze RI: Metabolism and renal effects of enflurane in man. *Anesthesiology* 1976;44:44.

68. Vilkki SK: Postoperative skin temperature dynamics and the nature of vascular complications after replantation. *Scand J Plast Reconstr* 1982;16:151.

69. Smith AR, Sonneveld GJ, Kort WJ, van der Meulen J: Clinical application of transcutaneous oxygen measurements in replantation surgery and free tissue transfer. *J Hand Surg* 1983;8:139.

70. Glogovac SV, Bitz DM, Whiteside LA: Hydrogen washout technique in monitoring vascular status after replantation surgery. *J Hand Surg* 1982;7:601.

19 The Ambulatory Surgery Patient

Rhoda D. Levine

Ambulatory surgery (variously known as *day-surgery, same-day surgery, short-stay surgery, in-and-out surgery, day-case surgery,* and *outpatient surgery*) has gained popularity because it is 40 to 80% less costly than a hospital stay for the same procedure and causes less disruption of the patient's daily life by decreasing separation from home and family. In addition, the risk of nosocomial infection, particularly in the immunocompromised or pediatric[1] patient, is decreased. Hospital beds are made available for "sicker" patients.

Ambulatory surgery presents the anesthesiologist with a unique set of problems. The ambulatory surgery patient must go home with minimum risk of airway compromise, hemorrhage, or severe pain. Which surgical procedures should be done on an outpatient basis? Which patients are appropriate candidates for ambulatory surgery? Which anesthetic techniques and agents are best in this setting? What postoperative complications should be anticipated? What criteria should be used to determine when a patient is ready to go home? The choices will determine the scope of problems that will be encountered in the postanesthetic care unit (PACU).

BACKGROUND

Early "experiments" with anesthesia for ambulatory surgery included Dr James Nicoll's experience in Glasgow, published in 1909,[2] and Dr Ralph Waters' "Down-Town Anesthesia Clinic" in Sioux City, Iowa.[3] More recently, Webb and Graves[4] and Cohen and Dillon[5] reported on their experiences in ambulatory surgery, but third-party payors were unwilling to support these ventures. By 1969, Ford and Reed[6] established the first modern, successful, freestanding ambulatory surgery facility in Phoenix, Arizona.

ORGANIZATION

Ambulatory surgery facilities may be either hospital-based (geographically and financially integrated with a hospital) or freestanding. The unit may share operating rooms and recovery facilities (an integrated unit) or may have facilities of its own in the hospital, near the hospital, or occasionally, some distance away.

Hospital-based units, particularly if they are integrated, are less costly to operate, as staffing, admitting, billing, and physical plant may be shared. Disadvantages include possible problems with operating room scheduling, the "inpatient" orientation of the hospital, and the potential for mixing inpatients and outpatients preoperatively and postoperatively. Hospital "satellites" or separated hospital-based units may utilize the administrative services of the hospital while maintaining control over their own operating rooms and recovery area.

Freestanding units have the advantage of being completely independent, with control over scheduling and staff, and can directly serve communities without hospitals. This may become a disadvantage should a complication requiring postoperative hospitalization occur. Freestanding units *must* have an ongoing arrangement with an inpatient facility to accommodate emergency postoperative admissions.

Regardless of the type of facility, each unit must decide what procedures will be performed and what types of patient will be accepted.

PROCEDURES

Ambulatory surgery procedures were initially short (approximately one hour of anesthesia time) elective operations with minimal blood loss, fluid shifts, postoperative pain, airway compromise, or bowel dysfunction. A list of the most frequently performed ambulatory surgery procedures based on a national survey by the Federated Ambulatory Surgery Association[7] is compared with a similar list published by Bruns[8] in Table 19–1.

Many day surgery units (DSUs) now routinely perform procedures that were initially considered inappropriate (eg, T&A, cone biopsy)—even thyroidectomies[9] and pediatric neurosurgical operations[10] have been performed on selected outpatients in some centers. With careful control and monitoring of anes-

TABLE 19-1. TWO LISTS OF THE MOST FREQUENTLY PERFORMED PROCEDURES

FASA Survey	Bruns Data
Myringotomy	D&C
D&C	Tubal ligation
Laparoscopy (including BTL)	Myringotomy
Arthroscopy	Orthopedics
Tonsillectomy and/or adenoidectomy	Excision skin lesion
	Dental
Excision soft tissue mass	Tonsillectomy and adenoidectomy
Excision skin lesion	
Cystoscopy	Diagnostic laparoscopy
Excision breast mass	Cystoscopy
Bunionectomy	
Inguinal hernias	

Left column adapted from Federal Ambulatory Surgery Association: FASA Special Study I. Alexandria, VA, FASA, 1987. Right column adapted from Bruns K: Postoperative care and review of complications, in Woo SW (ed): Ambulatory Anesthesia Care. International Anesthesiology Clinics. Boston, Little, Brown, 1982, vol 20, p 33.

thetic depth and appropriate drug selection, procedures as long as four to five hours can be successfully performed on an ambulatory basis.[11,12] As most facilities do not operate on a round-the-clock schedule, long procedures should start early in the day.

Lists of ambulatory surgery procedures to be performed on outpatients are generally prepared by government, industry, and third-party payors and are intended as guidelines for reimbursement. The staff and administration of the individual DSU must decide which procedures it will actually perform. Reimbursement should be secondary to appropriate patient care. If it is not safe in your setting, *don't do it.*

PATIENT SELECTION

Proper patient selection is in many ways more important for success of an ambulatory surgery program than the procedures that are performed. Patients must be willing to accept the surgery on an ambulatory basis and must be reliable enough to follow all instructions. It is preferable that a patient live within a short distance of a facility that can provide emergency care should a complication arise in the immediate postoperative period. Patients who live alone or are primary caregivers in their household should arrange for someone to stay with them postoperatively. Some ambulatory surgery facilities have considered "step-down" units near the DSU, where patients may stay up to 23 hours and receive "home-care" type nursing assistance.

Ideally the anesthesiologist should see the patient several days preoperatively to obtain an appropriate history, perform a physical examination, evaluate or request necessary laboratory information, and discuss potential anesthetic risks and management options with the patient. The anesthesiologist thus assumes more of a role as a primary care provider, determines the suitability of a particular patient for the proposed surgical procedure, and evaluates the stability of existing medical problems. If medical consultation is needed to help identify problems or optimize the patient's condition, it may then be obtained in a timely manner. Several approaches are commonly used for preoperative evaluation of ambulatory surgery patients (Table 19-2). Wong[13] reported that 7% of unscreened ambulatory surgery patients had their surgery canceled, more than twice the number of those who underwent preoperative evaluation.

A simple "screening" history described by Wilson and associates (Table 19-3)[14] might serve as a basis for identifying patients at increased anesthetic risk. Patients who were "fit" by these criteria, were usually found to be so after a more extensive and "traditional" evaluation. A similar, directed history has been used for pediatric patients (Table 19-4).[15]

Initially, only healthy patients (ASA I or II) were considered for ambulatory surgery. However, experience has shown that many ASA status III and even status IV patients may be acceptable candidates provided that their medical conditions are stable and well-controlled, because most complications are reported to be related to the type of surgery rather than to the patient's prior medical problems.[16] In addition, some studies[7,17] have shown no relationship between stable preexisting disease and the incidence of postoperative complications. In particular, the patient with asthma, diabetes, or morbid obesity can have successful ambulatory surgery provided that the DSU is prepared to deal with the perioperative problems of these more fragile patients.[18]

Neither elderly patients nor infants were originally accepted for ambulatory surgery. The elderly patient is more likely to have multiple medical problems (especially diabetes, coronary artery disease,

TABLE 19-2. EVALUATION OF THE AMBULATORY SURGERY PATIENT

Who evaluates the patient preoperatively
   Anesthesiologist
   Nurse
   Surgeon
   Nobody
Evaluation "tool"
   Preadmission visit to DSU
   Office visit
   Telephone interview
   Computer "interview"
   Preanesthetic assessment in holding area
   No organized evaluation

TABLE 19–3. DIRECTED MEDICAL HISTORY—ADULT

Do you feel ill?

Have you had any serious illnesses in the past?

Do you get more short of breath or exertion than others of your age?

Do you have a cough?

Do you have a wheeze?

Do you have any (anginal) chest pain?

Do you have ankle swelling?

Have you taken any medications in the past 3 months?

Have you any allergies?

Have you had an anesthetic in the past 2 months?

Have you or your relatives had any problems with anesthesia?

Date of LMP?

Adapted from Wilson ME, Williams NB, Baskett PJF, et al: Assessment of fitness for surgical procedures and the variability of anaesthetists' judgments. Br Med J 1980; 1:510.

and cerebrovascular disease), to be on multiple medications, and have decreased pulmonary reserve. Moreover, the home situation may not be suitable. Lean body mass decreases with increasing age, affecting the pharmacokinetics of many drugs. In addition, sensory input such as hearing or vision may be impaired. As with the PS III and IV patient, the DSU must be attuned to the particular needs of this population.

Most DSUs will accept healthy infants. Babies born prematurely, particularly those who required intubation or oxygen therapy, often have blunted airway reflexes, immature respiratory control, a tendency to easy fatigue of the diaphragm, and poor thermoregulation. More significantly, these babies are at risk for postoperative apnea until approximately 6–12 months after the premature birth.[19] Twelve hours of postoperative monitoring is recommended, making them poor candidates for ambulatory surgery. Other pediatric patients not considered good candidates for ambulatory surgery include those with a significant history of muscular, cardiac, or pulmonary problems, especially sleep apnea.

TABLE 19–4. DIRECTED MEDICAL HISTORY—PEDIATRIC

Breath-holding spells; sleep apnea; snoring

Cardiac, respiratory, or major organ dysfunction

History of prematurity

   Oxygen required? Intubated? Lasting effects?

Muscular problems

Developmental delays

Asthma or frequent colds

Sickle cell disease/trait

Medications

Recent exposure to contagious diseases

Adapted from Epstein BS, Hannallah RS: The pediatric patient, in Wetchler BV (ed): Anesthesia for Ambulatory Surgery. Philadelphia, Lippincott, 1985, p 136.

PREOPERATIVE INSTRUCTIONS

The time of arrival at the DSU should be established preoperatively. Adequate time should be allowed so that the preparation for the operating room is not hurried (usually 60 to 90 minutes). Particular consideration should be given to the elderly patient who may have difficulty ambulating, undressing, and so on. Patients must be instructed and reminded not to eat or drink anything after midnight of the preoperative night. Parents of pediatric patients should receive particular instructions about their NPO status.

Patients are also told to notify the surgeon and/or DSU of any change in physical condition preoperatively (eg respiratory infection) or inability to keep the DSU appointment for any reason. Patients should be instructed to leave valuables at home, as most units do not have facilities for securing them. No makeup, nail polish, or jewelry should be worn. Patients must be aware preoperatively that they will need to be escorted home postoperatively if they receive general anesthesia or any sedative medication. Many units state that surgery will be canceled if an escort is not arranged. If this is a policy of the unit, it must be adhered to. These patients should be cautioned that they should not drive or operate machinery, drink alcohol, or take nonprescribed medications for 24 hours after discharge. Patients should also be advised that they may require admission following surgery. Many DSUs require the patient to sign a witnessed statement that he or she has received, read, and complied with the preoperative instructions.[20]

PREOPERATIVE SEDATION

Preoperative medication has classically been used to provide sedation, anxiolysis, vagolysis, and to ensure amnesia for unpleasant events. These drugs may also smooth induction of anesthesia and provide perioperative analgesia. In addition, preoperative prophylaxis against acid aspiration, nausea, and vomiting may be indicated and desirable. In keeping with the "philosophy" of ambulatory surgery, any medication should cause as little physical, psychomotor, or cognitive impairment as possible.

Egbert and associates[21] noted that not all patients require preoperative sedation or anxiolysis; 35% of surgical patients were not anxious preoperatively. The proportion increased to 65% with an anesthesiologist's preoperative visit alone.

Epstein[20] felt that preoperative medication should not be given because it might prolong recovery. Korttila and Linnoila[22] found that 10 mg diazepam or 75 mg meperidine could impair coordination and reaction time for 5 to 12 hours. Meridy[23] found a prolongation of recovery time only when narcotic premedication was used. However, Clark and Hurtig[24] noted that premedication with 1 mg/kg meperidine and atropine 0.01 mg/kg did not prolong recovery to "street fitness"; and Horrigan and co-workers[25] noted that 100 μg IV of fentanyl improved awakening time, presumably the result of a decrease in anesthetic requirement.

Results of these studies are not necessarily contradictory. "Awakening time" and "recovery time" are not synonymous. Recovery from anesthesia can be divided into several stages. In the ambulatory surgery setting, recovery to "home readiness"—the point at which a patient may be discharged home with a responsible adult—is considered the endpoint. Although many patients don't require preoperative sedation and many DSUs prefer their patients not be premedicated, certain patients may benefit from it. Drugs commonly used for premedication are listed in Table 19–5.

Barbiturates provide sedation and although they are associated with minimal cardiovascular and respiratory side effects, they are antianalgesic (the patient may become disoriented when in pain), have a long duration of action, and no antagonist is available. However, rectally administered barbiturates are often used for induction of anesthesia in young pediatric patients.

The preoperative use of narcotic analgesics is less frequent for ambulatory surgery patients than for inpatients. Most ambulatory surgery procedures are associated with minimal postoperative pain; these drugs may cause respiratory depression; and the need to smooth IV induction and decrease anesthetic requirements is controversial. In addition, narcotics are associated with an increased incidence of nausea and vomiting, which may prolong recovery time.[26,27]

Droperidol is frequently employed as an antiemetic. However, because of its ability to produce dysphoria[28] it is seldom used as a premedicant.

Probably the most commonly used premedication in ambulatory surgery is a benzodiazepine. These drugs produce anxiolysis and anterograde amnesia with minimum cardiovascular and respiratory side effects. Thirty minutes after administration of 5 mg diazepam, 50% of patients were amnesic, while after 10 mg, 90% were amnesic.[29] The disadvantages of diazepam include pain on injection and chemical phlebitis related to its solvent, propylene glycol. The distribution half-life of diazepam is 60 minutes[30] but the elimination half-life is 24 to 48 hours.[31] There is a secondary increase in plasma concentration six to eight hours after IV administration due to intrahepatic recirculation[30]; and its metabolites are biologically active, with an elimination half-life of 51 to 120 hours.[31] White and associates[32] found that 8% of patients experienced ataxia and 16% complained of dizziness one hour after 10 mg of diazepam. One hour after administration of 20 mg, 40% were ataxic and 30% were dizzy. These complaints were of significant magnitude to delay discharge.

Midazolam, a water-soluble benzodiazepine, is felt to be a potentially useful premedicant for ambulatory surgery patients.[32,34] Dixon and associates[35] found that 80% of patients receiving 0.1 mg/kg midazolam were awake two hours after administration, compared to 69% of patients receiving 0.18 mg/kg di-

TABLE 19–5. DRUGS USED FOR PREMEDICATION

Drug	Advantages	Disadvantages
Barbiturates	Sedation/hypnosis Minimum cardiovascular or respiratory depression Minimum nausea/vomiting	No analgesia No antagonist Long duration of action Disorientation, especially with pain
Narcotic analgesics	Analgesia Smoother induction[a] Decreases anesthetic requirement[a] Reversal agent available	Respiratory depression Orthostatic hypotension Rigidity Nausea/vomiting Dysphoria (without pain)
Butyrophenones	Tranquilizer Antiemetic	Dysphoria Prolonged sedation Extrapyramidal symptoms Hypotension
Benzodiazepines	Anxiolysis Anterograde amnesia Minimum nausea/vomiting Minimum cardiovascular or respiratory depression	Variability of patient response No analgesia Sequelae of memory impairment Diazepam—long half-life
Anticholinergics	Vagolytic Antisialogogue	Tachycardia Sore throat Dry mouth

azepam. Of the midazolam patients 50% were amnesic after two hours, while only 18% of the patients receiving diazepam were unable to recall. Such profound amnesia may not be desirable in the ambulatory surgery patient, who must be able to remember postoperative instruction. In addition, some patients are uncomfortable when they are unable to recall.[36,37]

One of the major disadvantages of the benzodiazepines as a class is the lack of a specific antagonist. Neither naloxone[38] nor physostigmine[39] reliably reverse the depressant effects of the benzodiazepines. RO15–1788 (flumazenil) is a specific benzodiazepine antagonist with minimal side effects. Although not yet approved by the FDA for use in the United States (1989), American and European trials have shown this to be a very promising drug.[40,41] Specifically in the realm of ambulatory surgery, flumazenil was shown to improve postoperative recall in patients receiving midazolam.[42]

ASPIRATION IN THE OUTPATIENT

A patient may be considered "at risk" for aspiration if the volume of gastric contents is greater than 25 mL. There is also the risk of Mendelsohn's syndrome if the pH of the gastric aspirate is under 2.5. Patients presenting for ambulatory surgery are among those who are more likely to be "at risk" for aspiration. (Table 19–6). Ong and associates[43] found that 85% of outpatients had gastric volumes greater than 25 mL and 19% had volumes over 75 mL and a pH under 2.0.

Various regimens have been advocated to decrease the risk but none has been universally adopted. Premedication with combinations of meperidine, hydroxyzine, diazepam, and proclorperazine do not decrease the volume of gastric contents nor increase the pH.[44] Glycopyrrolate has proven to be ineffective,[45] particulate antacids cause pulmonary damage if aspirated,[46,47] and sodium citrate increases gastric volume.[48]

Two classes of drugs, the H2 receptor antagonists and the gastroprokinetics, have shown more promise. Cimetidine and ranitidine increase gastric fluid pH. Metoclopramide speeds gastric emptying. A combination of 300 mg cimetidine and 10 mg metoclopramide with 20 mL water orally. Two hours before

surgery[49] decreases gastric volume and increases the pH of gastric fluid. Ranitidine may be preferred to cimetidine because it has fewer drug interactions and side effects.

Nonetheless, there is no evidence that the use of these drugs decreases mortality or prevents the pulmonary consequences of aspiration.[50] Data supporting the efficacy of "antacid" prophylaxis in all ambulatory surgery patients are limited despite the suggestion that it be routinely used, particularly for patients receiving anesthesia by face mask.[51] One of the reasons for this disparity is that the actual number of cases of aspiration reported is extremely small—0.5[52] to 0.003%.[7] However, such treatment continues to be strongly recommended for patients at "high risk" for acid aspiration (Table 19–6).

OPTIONS FOR ANESTHETIC TECHNIQUE

Anesthesia for ambulatory surgery should provide analgesia, amnesia for unpleasant events, muscle relaxation when indicated, protection of the airway, and rapid return of function with no long-lasting side effects. Postoperative nausea, vomiting, drowsiness, and pain are to be avoided.

Local anesthesia is associated with the shortest recovery time but is not a suitable alternative for all patients or all procedures. The addition of sedative and/or anxiolytic drugs (see "Preoperative Sedation" earlier in the chapter may improve patient acceptance, but reduces many of the advantages.

General anesthesia is used for approximately 70% of ambulatory surgery.[7] Ultrashort-acting barbiturates are still preferred as induction agents. However, etomidate[53] and midazolam[54] have been used with success in some centers. Ketamine is usually not indicated for ambulatory surgery because of its central nervous system side effects and prolonged recovery. Propofol is becoming increasingly popular both as an induction agent and for maintenance of anesthesia in the outpatient setting. Pandit and co-workers[55] reported that patients undergoing laparoscopic surgery had shorter recovery times, more rapid discharge, and less nausea and vomiting with propofol than with enflurane. Additional recent investigations[56-59] further support the advantages of propofol.

Among the inhalation anesthetics, enflurane is associated with more rapid recovery than halothane.[60] Korttila and Valanne[61] noted that more than 90 minutes of enflurane anesthesia was associated with significantly longer recovery times than shorter (< 40 minutes) enflurane anesthesia. Recovery, even after more than 90 minutes of isoflurane, corresponded to the shorter enflurane anesthetic, suggesting that isoflurane should be preferred in outpatient

TABLE 19–6. FACTORS PREDISPOSING TO ASPIRATION PNEUMONITIS

Pregnancy	Obesity
Pediatrics	Emergency surgery
Hiatus hernia	Diabetes mellitus
Ambulatory Surgery	Errors in judgment

anesthesia. When appropriately administered, all currently available inhalation agents, including halothane,[62] can be used successfully for outpatient surgery.

Compared to the inhalation anesthetics, wakeup time appears to be more rapid with the narcotic-based techniques[63] but the incidence of postoperative nausea and vomiting is 300% higher,[64,65] often resulting in a similar length of stay in the DSU. Fentanyl and alfentanil are the most widely used of the narcotics[66,67] but agonist/antagonists such as butorphanol[68] and nalbuphine[69] are also popular.

Muscle relaxation may be required for some surgical procedures and/or to facilitate endotracheal intubation. Succinylcholine, because of its rapid onset and short duration of action, should be the ideal muscle relaxant for ambulatory surgery. However, the use of succinylcholine is not without complications. There is always the possibility of producing a Phase II block (especially with infusions of succinylcholine), encountering a patient with abnormal pseudocholinesterase, or triggering an episode of malignant hyperpyrexia in a susceptible patient. Succinylcholine is associated with an increased incidence of cardiac dysrhythmias and is alleged to be responsible for postoperative muscle pain reported by 10 to 72% of ambulatory surgery patients.[70,71] However, neither Sosis and associates[72] nor Zahl and co-workers[73] believe that postoperative musculoskeletal pain is not related to the administration of succinylcholine.

Both atracurium[74] and vecuronium[75] have been used as alternatives to succinylcholine for ambulatory surgery. Although the duration of action of these drugs is relatively short, routine reversal of neuromuscular blockade is recommended.

General anesthesia is frequently associated with pain, nausea, drowsiness, and a feeling of malaise.[70] Regional anesthesia would appear to be a logical alternative. Advantages include minimal postoperative nausea and vomiting,[23] shorter recovery time compared to general anesthesia (with proper selection of technique and drugs), and the possibility of providing prolonged postoperative analgesia at the surgical site. The ability to provide postoperative pain relief reduces the need for narcotic analgesics, permitting earlier discharge from the DSU. Regional anesthesia also provides selected patients with the opportunity to "participate" in the surgical procedure, for example, observing their arthroscopy or laparoscopy on a television screen.

On the other hand, regional blocks are time consuming, both in administration and onset of adequate surgical conditions. Supplementary sedation and anxiolysis may be necessary, and may negate one of the major advantages of regional anesthesia, the short recovery time. In addition, particular blocks have technique-related complications and systemic toxicity may result from "inappropriate" use of local anesthetics.

Field blocks and regional anesthesia of the upper and lower extremities are useful techniques in the outpatient setting. For the arm, the axillary approach to the brachial plexus is often preferred because the interscalene approach may be complicated by a high epidural or total spinal, and the supraclavicular approach carries a small but significant risk of pneumothorax. Blocks of the lower extremity (particularly sciatic-femoral) are not widely used because they tend to limit walking, but ankle or popliteal blocks are excellent for surgery of the foot and toes, and will permit ambulation with crutches, even with residual analgesia. Intravenous regional (Bier block) is a reliable and easily performed technique for both upper and lower extremity surgery. Unfortunately, once the tourniquet is released, analgesia is dissipated.

Central nerve blocks (spinal and epidural) have also become popular for ambulatory surgery.[12] Spinal anesthesia is usually considered easier and faster to perform but is associated with the rise of postlumbar puncture headache. Flaaten and Raeder[76] reported a 37% incidence of headache after spinal anesthesia in ambulatory surgery patients. This rate seems unusually high. The more frequently reported 5 to 10% incidence[77] may still be unacceptable, even with a 25-gauge needle and selection of lower-risk patients (eg, older males). There is no evidence that early ambulation increases the incidence of postdural puncture headache.[78,79]

Lumbar epidural block, although theoretically more difficult and time consuming to perform, minimizes the risk of headache, particularly in younger, female patients. Doses should be considered carefully as these patients tend to require larger volumes of drug.[80] The use of catheter makes this technique more flexible, permitting the continued use of shorter-acting drugs.

Epidural and spinal block are associated with the possibility of postoperative urinary retention,[81] although the incidence is less than that found in the inpatient.[12] For this reason, patients who have received these blocks must demonstrate the ability to void before discharge from the DSU.

Regional block to provide postoperative pain relief, combined with general anesthesia, is becoming a popular technique, particularly in pediatric outpatient surgery. Ilioinguinal, iliohypogastric, and caudal blocks have been used most frequently and most successfully[82,83] for patients undergoing surgery of the inguinal region. Caudal block with 0.25% bupivicaine is also useful for pain relief following circumcision. Vater and Wandles[84] noted that patients receiving a dorsal nerve block of the penis experienced less

TABLE 19-7. LOCAL ANESTHETICS IN AMBULATORY SURGERY

	Spinal Duration (min)	Epidural Duration (min)	Recovery Time (h)
Procaine	30–60	Not useful	2
Chloroprocaine	Not useful	45–60	2
Lidocaine	60–90 abd	Not used	4
	90–120 knee		4
Mepivicaine	60–90	60–90	3
Bupivicaine	Used for local infiltration at surgical site or for pediatric blocks		

Adapted from Mulroy MF: Our pharmacologic armamentarium—Regional anesthesia drugs. Proceedings of the third annual SAMBA meeting, Scottsdale, Arizona, 1988.

nausea and vomiting and earlier voiding, resulting in earlier discharge, then circumcision patients receiving caudal block. Unfortunately, this block may be complicated by hematoma formation at the site of the block resulting in gangrene of the skin of the glans.[85] A penile ring block with 0.25% bupivicaine[86] or the topical application of lidocaine in jelly, spray, or ointment form[87] are also useful techniques for relieving pain after circumcision.

LOCAL ANESTHETICS

One of the major drawbacks to the use of regional anesthesia in outpatient surgery is the time reqired for the block. The use of drugs with a short latency (eg, procaine, chloroprocaine, lidocaine) is preferred. Although drugs with a short duration of action would permit a more rapid discharge from the DSU, long-acting drugs (eg, bupivicaine) provide prolonged postoperative analgesia, and when infiltrated into the surgical site or used in peripheral blocks, can be quite useful. Table 19-7[88] presents some facts about local anesthetics and their usefulness in ambulatory surgery.

RECOVERY FROM ANESTHESIA AND DISCHARGE

Postanesthetic care of the ambulatory surgery patient emphasizes "wellness." Nursing care is directed toward encouraging ambulation and self-care. This is contrasted with the inpatient, who generally experiences more pain and requires more monitoring and more intensive nursing intervention. It is therefore preferable to completely separate the postambulatory surgical patient from the recovering inpatient if at all possible, or separate them as soon as the patient is awake and has stable respiratory and cardiovascular parameters.

However, several studies have documented the potential, especially in children, for hypoxemia fol-

lowing procedures performed on an outpatient basis. Healthy children of all ages are at risk for oxyhemoglobin desaturation during transport or in the PACU if they breathe only room air.[89,90] Also, 43% of children can desaturate to a level of 91% or less. The risk of hypoxemia and need for supplemental oxygen does not correlate to the degree of recovery as measured by a typical scoring system.[91] Children with an upper airway infection may be at particular risk for hypoxemia.[92] Although routine use of additional oxygen will probably prevent problems in most patients, the ready availability and ease of use of the pulse oximeter, documents the effectiveness of oxygen therapy or the need for more therapeutic measures. Thus monitoring by pulse oximetry is highly recommended for all patients in the PACU until normal oxyhemoglobin saturation continues after supplemental oxygen has been discontinued.

Korttila has divided recovery from anesthesia into several stages (Table 19-8)[93] and has listed tools for evaluating patients at each stage.

TABLE 19-8. STAGES OF RECOVERY AND CORRESPONDING ASSESSMENT TESTS

Stage of Recovery	Test of Recovery
Awakening	Open eyes, answer questions
Recovery of airway reflexes	Maintain and guard own airway
Immediate clinical recovery	Sit and stand unaided
Home readiness	Walk on straight line
	Paper/pencil tests (eg, Trieger dot)
	Maddox wing test
	Simple coordination and reaction time
Street fitness	Flicker fusion test
	Psychomotor test batteries
Full recovery (complete psychomotor recovery)	Real driving tests
	Selected psychomotor test batteries
Psychological recovery	Psychological tests

Adapted from Korttila K: How to assess recovery from anesthesia. ASA Annual Refresher Course, 224, 1987, p 1.

Quantification of the earliest phase of recovery should be provided by an objective rather than subjective scoring system. The Aldrete postanesthesia scoring system (Table 19–9)[94] requires that a patient achieve a score of 10 before discharge from the PACU. Steward[95] believes that blood pressure is not related to recovery from anesthesia and that color is often difficult to interpret consistently. He has modified Aldrete's scoring system accordingly (Table 19–10). Documentation of adequate recovery is easily accomplished by the PACU staff by using one of these two scoring systems.

Return of gross motor function (eg, negative Romberg, ability to sit and stand unaided) marks the stage of "immediate clinical recovery," but recovery of additional psychomotor function (fine motor coordination and near normal reaction time to external stimuli) is required before a patient can be discharged home. Pegboard tests,[96,97] tapping tests,[98] and coin retrieval and counting[99] have been described to evaluate home-readiness. None of these has achieved the popularity of paper and pencil tests based on the Bender Gestalt model, in particular, the Trieger dot test.[100] This test requires the patient to connect a series of dots to form a figure. It is simple to administer and score, and provides documentation of performance level on discharge.

TABLE 19–10. SIMPLIFIED POSTANAESTHETIC RECOVERY SCORE

Consciousness	
Awake	2
Responding to stimuli	1
Not responding	0
Airway	
Coughing on command or crying	2
Maintaining good airway	1
Airway requires maintenance	0
Movement	
Moving limbs purposefully	2
Non-purposeful movements	1
Not moving	0
Total	_____

Adapted from Steward DJ: A simplified scoring system for the post-operative recovery room. Can Anesth Soc J 1975; 22:111.

Commonly used discharge criteria are listed in Table 19–11. No time limits are set; however, Fragen and Shranks[101] have suggested that a minimum of two and one half hours elapse before discharge if a patient has received a nondepolarizing neuromuscular blocking agent.

"Street readiness" implies that a patient has recovered more psychomotor function than that which is required to go home with an escort, but not sufficiently to drive. This term is used interchangeably

TABLE 19–9. ALDRETE SCORING SYSTEM

	In	15	30	45	__Hrs	Out
Activity						
Able to move voluntarily or on command						
4 extremities	2	2	2	2	2	2
2 extremities	1	1	1	1	1	1
0 extremities	0	0	0	0	0	0
Respiration						
Able to deep breathe and cough freely	2	2	2	2	2	2
Dyspnea, shallow or limited breathing	1	1	1	1	1	1
Apneic	0	0	0	0	0	0
Circulation						
Preoperative blood pressure _____ mm Hg	2	2	2	2	2	2
BP ± 20 mm of preanesth level	1	1	1	1	1	1
BP ± 20 to 50 mm of preanesth level	0	0	0	0	0	0
BP ± 50 mm or preanesth level						
Consciousness						
Fully awake	2	2	2	2	2	2
Arousable on calling	1	1	1	1	1	1
Not responding	0	0	0	0	0	0
Color						
Normal	2	2	2	2	2	2
Pale, dusky, blotchy, other	1	1	1	1	1	1
Cyanotic	0	0	0	0	0	0
Final Total Score						

Dismissal Criteria: Total score of 10, plus stable vital signs and acceptable surgical site.
A physician's order is required for discharge with a lower score.

Adapted from Aldrete JA, Kroulik D: A post-anesthetic recovery score. Anesth Analg 1970; 49:926.

TABLE 19–11. FREQUENTLY USED CRITERIA FOR DISCHARGE

Awake
Stable vital signs
No respiratory distress
Ambulate without dizziness
Dress self (if appropriate)
Tolerate oral fluids with minimum nausea/vomiting
Surgical wound (stable)—no excessive bleeding
Minimal pain
Escort present
Discharge note by MD
Discharge instructions—verbally and in writing signed by MD, patient, and escort

with "home readiness," although according to Korttila's criteria, additional, more sensitive tests are required to document this level of recovery.

Complete recovery, defined as the point where a patient can perform tasks with a "normal" state of alertness, is best evaluated by testing such skills as simulated driving where the time to brake in response to a simulated accident and the number of performance errors (eg, driving off the road) are measured. Such recovery can take up to 24 hours[93] after general anesthesia or sedation. It is unreasonable for the ambulatory surgery patient to remain in a DSU until this stage of recovery has been achieved. These findings, however, form the basis for the recommendation that patients not drive for 24 hours after receiving anesthesia or sedation.

Recovery from regional block deserves special attention. Total return of motor, sensory, and sympathetic function may conflict with plans to provide postoperative pain relief, particularly in blocks of the upper extremity, those limited to the surgical site, or blocks in pediatric patients. Patients and their escorts must receive instructions on the proper care of limbs that have not recovered sensory function. Patients who have received spinal or peridural block should *never* be discharged until all signs of sympathetic block have dissipated, to eliminate the possibility of postural hypotension after discharge. Return of proprioception in the toes[102] or return of perianal sensation[103] is considered a reliable marker for regression of sympathetic blockade and safe ambulation. Because of the high incidence of urinary retention, most centers also require that patients void after spinal or epidural before discharge.

The most recent JCAHO standards for ambulatory surgery[104] require that procedures for preoperative and postoperative observation of patients be established. A licensed practitioner qualified in resuscitative techniques must be present or immediately available until all patients have been evaluated and discharged. Postoperative instructions, including

how to obtain help in the event of a complication, must be reviewed with the patient or another responsible person and be given in writing to patients who have had general anesthesia or any sedative drugs. Patients who have had any anesthesia except unsupplemented local must be evaluated by a physician (or oral surgeon where appropriate) before discharge. A licensed practitioner with appropriate clinical privileges, and who is familiar with the patient, must be responsible for the decision to discharge that patient. If he or she is not physically present, his or her name must appear (legibly) on the medical record, and *relevant discharge criteria, rigorously applied,* must be used to determine if the patient is ready for discharge. These discharge criteria must be approved by the medical staff of the institution. "All patients who have received anesthesia, except those who have received only unsupplemented local anesthesia, are discharged in the company of a responsible adult."[104]

DSUs are becoming more concerned about the quality and quantity of postoperative care. Some DSUs discourage the use of public transportation home, even with an escort; and many centers require that the individual taking the patient home and providing postoperative care be physically, intellectually, and emotionally able to do so.

If the patient has not arranged for an escort home, the surgery should not be performed. Problems arise, however, when the expected escort does not arrive after the surgery and no substitute can be found. If your unit has stated that patients without an escort must be admitted, then you must adhere to this policy. Our ambulatory surgery unit requires that a patient without an escort who refuses hospital admission must sign that he or she is being discharged against medical advice and is permitted to leave only in a taxicab. A responsible physician must be involved in this decision as well as those that must be made when a patient insists on being discharged before a unit's discharge criteria are met.

Written discharge instructions, signed by the patient and escort, should include specifics about the surgery, pain, and other medications; anticipated anesthetic sequelae; what to do and what not to do; and specifically who (names and phone numbers) to contact in case of complications. Patients who have received spinal anesthesia are encouraged to rest in bed for 24 hours but may sit up to eat. They should be accompanied by an escort when walking to the bathroom and should notify the DSU or indicated person if a headache, stiff neck, or temperature not relieved by acetaminophen develops.[102]

Specific instructions prohibiting the use of alcohol, nonprescribed depressant medications, operating machinery, or driving a car for 24 hours must be given. Korttila has suggested that any patient receiving more than two hours of general anesthesia be cautioned not to drive for at least 48 hours.[105] Patients should be instructed not to make ''important decisions'' until they have completely recovered—usually interpreted as 24 to 48 hours. In 1972, Ogg and co-workers[102] found that despite instructions to the contrary, 31% of outpatients studied went home unescorted, 9% of car owners drove home, and 73% drove within 24 hours. Herbert and associates[107] pointed out that patients must be cautioned that ''aspects of mental ability may remain impaired even after they feel that they have made a full recovery.''

Almost all DSUs contact patients the day after surgery to find out how they are recovering from their surgery and anesthesia. Some facilities give patients a stamped, self-addressed postcard to complete and return.

COMPLICATIONS

Complications associated with ambulatory surgery are listed in Table 19–12 and can be classified as minor or major. Minor complications are events that cause discomfort or inconvenience but do not have any long-lasting sequelae or require hospitalization. Major complications are considered those requiring unanticipated admission to an inpatient facility. Most minor complications are associated with general anesthesia but can also occur after regional block or local anesthesia with or without sedation.

Nausea and vomiting has been described as the most common complication of ambulatory surgery,[8,23] occurring in 11 to 15% of all patients. Factors contributing to nausea and vomiting are listed in Table 19–13.

Pain is well-known to be a major cause of postoperative nausea and vomiting[108]; unfortunately, the narcotic analgesics frequently used to treat postoperative pain may stimulate central receptors that trigger nausea and vomiting.[26,27] There is a balance between pain and the use of narcotic analgesics. One of the ways to decrease postoperative nausea and vomiting is to provide rapid pain relief, preferably without narcotic analgesics. This may be done by encouraging

TABLE 19–12. COMPLICATIONS

Minor	Major
Nausea and vomiting	Hemorrhage
Muscles aches	Infection
Sore throat	Anesthesia catastrophes
Dizziness	Admission
Weakness	
Headache	

TABLE 19–13. ETIOLOGY OF POSTOPERATIVE NAUSEA AND VOMITING

Pain
Narcotic analgesics
Type of surgery
History of motion sickness
Obesity
Sudden movement or position change
Nitrous oxide

the surgeon to infiltrate the wound with a local anesthetic such as bupivicaine.

Pataky and co-workers[109] found that the highest incidence of nausea and vomiting was associated with laparoscopic ovum retrieval. Half of these patients experienced this problem, even in the absence of narcotic analgesics. Other laparoscopic procedures, knee arthroscopies,[109] and strabismus repair[110,111] are also associated with a high incidence of postoperative nausea and vomiting. Of all gynecologic patients 19[112] to 49%[105] experience postoperative nausea and vomiting.

Freeman found that 78% of patients with postoperative nausea and vomiting had a significant history of motion sickness, compared with 33% of patients without postoperative nausea and vomiting.[113] Obesity, hypotension, and sudden position changes have also been associated with nausea and vomiting.[8]

Recently a controversy has arisen over the suggestion that eliminating nitrous oxide from the anesthetic technique decreases the incidence of nausea and vomiting.[65,114,115] Nitrous oxide may cause nausea and vomiting through one of several mechanisms: (1) diffusing into the gastrointestinal tract[116]; (2) increasing pressure in the middle ear[117]; or (3) direct stimulation of central receptors.[118] However, Korttila and associates[119] found no difference in the incidence of nausea and vomiting in patients undergoing laparoscopic surgery with or without nitrous oxide.

Preoperative prophylaxis with 50 mg benzquinamide was not effective in decreasing the incidence of postoperative vomiting after outpatient laparoscopic surgery. However, study patients reported less nausea on the first postoperative day than did the controls.[120] Phenothiazines are associated with central nervous system depression and are not a good choice in the ambulatory surgery setting. Metoclopramide was ineffective in patients having midtrimester pregnancy terminations[121] or laparoscopies.[112]

Droperidol has been shown to be an effective antiemetic in the outpatient setting. Recommended doses range from 0.04 to 0.1 mg/kg for adults and 0.01 to 0.017 mg/kg in children. These doses are reported to decrease postoperative nausea and vomiting without prolonging recovery time[122] or producing extrapyramidal side effects.[123] Larger doses have been tried after strabismus surgery, a procedure associated with an extremely high incidence of postoperative nausea and vomiting. Abramowitz and associates[111] found that 75 μg/kg of droperidol administered after induction of anesthesia reduced the incidence of nausea and vomiting from 85 to 43%. Those patients who received droperidol only after they began to vomit had the longest recovery time (369 minutes). Patients who neither vomited nor received droperidol left the DSU most rapidly (309 minutes). Those receiving prophylactic droperidol who did not vomit had an average recovery time of 339 minutes. Using a similar dose, Lerman and colleagues[110] reduced the incidence of nausea and vomiting to 10% following strabismus surgery.

It is possible that a combination of drugs would be as effective as the higher doses of droperidol without the risks of postoperative somnolence. Doze and co-workers[27] found that 10 to 20 mg metoclopramide administered with 0.5 to 1.0 mg droperidol was a better antiemetic than droperidol alone in adults.

Headache, although more commonly associated with spinal anesthesia, is also frequent after general anesthesia.[124] Sore throat may be the result of breathing dry gases or endotracheal intubation. Muscle aches are believed to be associated with the use of succinylcholine, but as previously noted, this is controversial.

Fahy and Marshall[70] reported that 45% of patients had postoperative "symptoms attributable to the anesthetic." Complaints included drowsiness (30%); headache (13%); malaise (12%); nausea (12%); dizziness (6%); and vomiting (4%). Females were more affected than males, especially those having a first anesthetic. Procedures lasting more than 20 minutes or requiring an endotracheal tube were associated with an increased morbidity.

Importantly, 4% of these patients had symptoms for more than 24 hours postoperatively. In a study of patients after laparoscopy with general anesthesia, Collins and associates[124] reported that 96% of their patients had some complaint at 24 hours and 75% at 48 hours. Some 80% of their patients complained of neck and shoulder pain, 50% had sore throat, and 25% had headache. Only 37% were able to resume their normal activities 24 hours after surgery.

Complications are least frequent in patients receiving regional or local anesthesia only and appear to be most frequent with local anesthesia and supplemental sedation.[7] Patients with cardiovascular disease, particularly if the patient experiences symptoms within three months prior to surgery, were reported to have a higher complication rate than "healthy" patients or even patients with pulmonary disease or diabetes.[125] Approximately two thirds of complications

TABLE 19-14. POSTOPERATIVE ADMISSION FOLLOWING AMBULATORY SURGERY

Surgery (73%)	Anesthesia (20%)	Other (7%)
Extensive surgery	Dizzy	No escort
Misadventure	Nausea and vomiting	Monitoring
Positive pathology	Headache	No home care
Hemorrhage		
Pain		

occurred after discharge and most of these were associated with the surgery (hemorrhage, infection).[7]

Less than 1.5% of all ambulatory surgery patients should require postopertive hospitalization. Reasons for unanticipated postoperative hospitalization of ambulatory surgery patients are presented in Table 19-14.[102,126] Complications of surgery (bleeding, extensive surgery, change of surgical procedure) account for 54 to 63% of postoperative admissions. Anesthesia complications such as nausea and vomiting, airway compromise, intractable pain, sleepiness, and dizziness constitute 12 to 15% of postoperative admissions. The remaining 25 to 30% of admissions are for "other" reasons, including lack of an escort, medical monitoring, and urinary retention, to name a few.

Certain types of surgery are more frequently associated with unanticipated hospital admission. Table 19-15 presents the procedures responsible for the majority of unplanned admissions. Gold and associates[125] noted that patients having laparoscopy were almost four times more likely to be admitted than patients having other procedures.

Postoperative bleeding accounted for 4.2% of admissions reported by Bruns.[8] Tonsillectomy and/or adenoidectomy patients experienced the highest incidence of postoperative bleeding, most occurring after discharge.[16] Those patients who bled during laparoscopy, did so in the operating room or PACU.

Epstein[20] reported an overall admission rate of 0.2% in his facility. However, patients more than 64 years old had a 0.54% admission rate. Physical status III patients were admitted seven times more frequently than PS I or II patients.

TABLE 19-15. PROCEDURES MOST FREQUENTLY REQUIRING POSTOPERATIVE ADMISSION

Laparoscopy
Cystoscopy (plus any additional procedure)
Minilaparotomy
D&C
Arthroscopy
Hernia
Plastic
Dental

SUMMARY

The pressures to perform more and more ambulatory procedures on patients who have complicating medical conditions will very likely continue. This will present the anesthesiologist with a constant challenge in selecting appropriate anesthetic techniques and drugs, evaluating and preparing patients preoperatively, anticipating and preventing perioperative complications, and establishing and maintaining rigorous discharge criteria. The anesthesiologist must take an active role in the postanesthetic care and discharge of ambulatory surgery patients.

REFERENCES

1. Otherson HB, Clatworthy HW: Outpatient herniorrhaphy for infants. *Am J Dis Child* 1968; 116:78–80.
2. Nicoll JH: The surgery of infancy. *Br Med J* 1909; 2:753–757.
3. Waters RM: The down-town anesthesia clinic. *Am J Surg* 39 (suppl):1919; 71–73.
4. Webb E, Graves H: Anesthesia for the ambulatory patient. *Anesth Analg* 1959; 38:359–363.
5. Cohen D, Dillon JB: Anesthesia for outpatient surgery. *JAMA* 196:1966; 1114–1116.
6. Ford JL, Reed WA: The surgicenter—An innovation in the delivery and cost of medical care. *Ariz Med* 1969; 26:801–804.
7. Federated Ambulatory Surgery Association: FASA Special Study I. Alexandria, VA, FASA, 1987.
8. Bruns K: Postoperative care and review of complications, in Woo SW (ed): *Ambulatory Anesthesia Care.* International Anesthesiology Clinics. Boston, Little, Brown, 1982, vol 20, pp 27–34.
9. Steckler RM: Outpatient thyroidectomy: A feasibility study. *Am J Surg* 1986; 152:17–19.
10. Peters KR: Outpatient pediatric neurosurgery. Poster presentation at third annual SAMBA meeting, Scottsdale, Arizona, 1988.
11. Apfelbaum JL, Conahan TJ, Lecky JH: Patient Management in Day Surgery. Anaquest form No. 04-0087, 1986.
12. White PF: Current controversies in outpatient anesthesia. International Anesthesia Research Society Refresher Course, 1986, pp 40–46.
13. Wong HC: Preanesthesia evaluation of ambulatory surgery patients. *ASA Newsletter*, Feb 1987.
14. Wilson ME, Williams NB, Baskett PJF, et al: Assessment of fitness for surgical procedures and the variability of anaesthetists' judgments. *Br Med J* 1980;1:509–512.
15. Epstein BS, Hannallah RS: The pediatric patient, in Wetchler BV (ed): *Anesthesia for Ambulatory Surgery.* Philadelphia, Lippincott, 1985, pp 124–175.
16. Natof HE: Complications associated with ambulatory surgery. *JAMA* 1980; 244:1116–1118.
17. Natof HE: Pre-existing medical problems. Ambulatory surgery. *Illinois Med J* 1984; 166:101–104.
18. Apfelbaum JL: Controversies in ambulatory surgery: The adult patient at risk. Proceedings of the second annual SAMBA meeting, Washington, DC, 1987.
19. Kurth CD, Spitzer AR, Broennle AM, Downes JJ: Postoperative apnea in preterm infants. *Anesthesiology* 1987; 66:483–488.
20. Epstein BS: Outpatient anesthesia. ASA Annual Refresher Course Lectures, 1983, 125, pp 1–6.
21. Egbert LD, Battit GE, Turndorf H, Beecher HK: The value of the preoperative visit by an anesthestist. *JAMA* 1963; 185:553–555.
22. Korttila K, Linnoila M: Psychomotor skills related to driving after intramuscular administration of diazepam and meperidine. *Anesthesiology* 1975; 42:685–691.
23. Meridy HW: Criteria for selection of ambulatory surgical patients and guidelines for anesthetic management: A retrospective study of 1553 cases. *Anesth Analg* 1982; 61:921–926.
24. Clark AJM, Hurtig JB: Premedication with meperidine and atropine does not prolong recovery to street fitness after outpatient surgery. *CAn Anaesth Soc J* 1981; 28:390–393.
25. Horrigan RW, Moyers JR, Johnson BH, et al: Etomidate vs thiopental with and without fentanyl—A comparative study of awakening in man. *Anesthesiology* 1980; 52:362–364.
26. Metter SE, Kitz DS, Young ML, et al: Nausea and vomiting after outpatient laparoscopy: Incidence, impact on recovery room stay and cost (abstract). *Anesth Analg* 1987; 66:S116.
27. Doze VA, Shafer A, White PF: Nausea and vomiting after outpatient anesthesia—Effectiveness of droperidol alone and in combination with metoclopramide (abstract). *Anesth Analg* 1987; 66:S41.
28. Zauder HL: Anesthesia for patients who have terminal renal disease, in Hershey SG (ed): ASA *Refresher Courses in Anesthesiology.* Philadelphia, Lippincott, 1976, vol 4, pp 163–173.
29. Dundee JW, Pandit SK: Anterograde amnesic effects of pethidine, hycosine, and diazepam in adults. *Br J Pharmacol* 1972; 44:140–144.
30. Klotz U, Antonin KH, Bieck P: Pharmacokinetics and plasma binding of diazepam in man, dog, rabbit, guinea pig, and rat. *J Pharmacol Exp Ther* 1976; 199:67–73.
31. Mandelli M, Tognoni G, Garattini S: Clinical pharmacokinetics of diazepam. *Clin Pharmacokinet* 1978; 3:72–91.
32. White PF, Coe V, Shafer A, Sung ML: Comparison of alfentanil with fentanyl for outpatient anesthesia. *Anesthesiology* 1986; 64:99–106.
33. Vinik HR, Reves JG, Wright D: Premedication with intramuscular midazolam—A prospective randomized double-blind controlled study. *Anesth Analg* 1982; 61:933–937.
34. Fragen RJ, Funk DI, Avram MJ et al: Midazolam versus hydroxyzine as intramuscular premedicants. *Can Anaesth Soc J* 1983; 30:136–141.
35. Dixon J, Power SJ, Grundy EM, et al: Sedation for local anesthesia. Comparison of intravenous midazolam and diazepam. *Anaesthesia* 1984; 39:372–376.

36. Conner JT, Katz RL, Bellville JW, et al: Diazepam and lorazepam for intravenous surgical premedication. *J Clin Pharmacol* 1978; 18:285–292.

37. Philip BK: Hazards of amnesia after midazolam in ambulatory surgical patients. *Anesth Analg* 1987; 66:97–98.

38. Christensen KN, Huttel M: Naloxone does not antagonize diazepam-induced sedation. *Anesthesiology* 1979; 34:9–13.

39. Garber G. Ominsky AJ, Orkin FK, Quinn P: Physostigmine-atropine solution fails to reverse diazepam sedation. *Anesth Analg* 1980; 59:58–60.

40. Doenicke A, Suttmann H, Kugler J, et al: Pilot study of a benzodiazepine antagonist. *Br J Anaesth* 1982; 54:1131.

41. Wolff J, Carl P, Clausen TG, Mikkelson BO: RO15-1788 for postoperative recovery. *Anaesthesia* 1986; 41:1001–1006.

42. Sung YF, Reiss N: Flumazenil reduces postoperative amnesia after midazolam anesthesia in ambulatory surgery patients. Abstract presented at third annual SAMBA meeting, Scottsdale, Arizona, 1988.

43. Ong BY, Palahnuik RJ, Cumming M: Gastric volume and pH in outpatients. *Can Anaesth Soc J* 1978; 25:36–39.

44. Manchikanti L, Canella MG, Hohlbein LJ, Colliver JA: Assessment of effect on various modes of premedication on acid aspiration risk factors in outpatient surgery. *Anesth Analg* 1987; 66:81–84.

45. Manchikanti L, Roush JR: Effect of preanesthetic glycopyrrolate and cimetidine on gastric fluid pH and volume in outpatients. *Anesth Analg* 1984; 63:40–46.

46. Kumar N, Pandit SK, Detmer MD: Pulmonary lesions after antacid and cimetidine aspiration. *Anesth Analg* 1980; 59:547–548.

47. Gibbs CP, Hempling RE, Wynne JW: Antacid pulmonary aspiration in the dog. *Anesthesiology* 1979; 51:380–385.

48. Manchikanti L, Grow JB, Colliver JA, et al: Bicitra (sodium citrate) and metoclopramide in outpatient anesthesia for prophylaxis against aspiration pneumonitis. *Anesthesiology* 1985; 63:378–384.

49. Rao TLK, Madhavareddy S, Chinthagada M, El-Etr AA: Metoclopramide and cimetidine to reduce gastric fluid pH and volume. *Anesth Analg* 1984; 63:1014–1016.

50. Stoelting RK: Gastric fluid pH in patients receiving cimetidine. *Anesth Analg* 1978; 57:675–677.

51. Coombs DW: Aspiration pneumonia prophylaxis. *Anesth Analg* 1983; 62:1055–1058.

52. Kallar SK: Survey on risk of aspiration. Presented at third annual SAMBA meeting, Scottsdale, Arizona, 1988.

53. Miller BM, Hendry JGB, Lees NW: Etomidate and methohexitone: A comparative clinical study in outpatient anesthesia. *Anaesthesia* 1978; 33:450–453.

54. Berggren L, Eriksson I: Midazolam for induction of anesthesia in outpatients: A comparison with thiopentone. *Acta Anaesth Scand* 1981; 25:492–496.

55. Pandit S, Kothary SP, Randel GI, Levy L: Recovery after outpatient anesthesia: Propofol versus enflurane (abstract). *Anesthesiology* 1988; 69:A565.

56. Doze VA, Wesphal LM, White PF: Comparison of propofol with methohexital for outpatient anesthesia. *Anesth Analg* 1986; 65:1189–1195.

57. Johnston R, Noseworthy T, Anderson B, et al: Propofol versus thiopental for outpatient anesthesia. *Anesthesiology* 1987; 67:431–433.

58. Sung YF, Freniere S, Tillette T, Powell RW: Comparison of propofol and thiopental anesthesia in outpatient surgery: Speed of recovery (abstract). *Anesthesiology* 1988; 69:A562.

59. Cork RC, Scipione P, Vonesh MJ, et al: Propofol infusion vs thiopental/isoflurane for outpatient anesthesia (abstract). *Anesthesiology* 1988; 69:A563.

60. Davidson SH: A comparative study of halothane and enflurane in pediatric anesthesia. *Acta Anaesth Scand* 1978; 22:58–63.

61. Korttila K, Valanne J: Recovery after outpatient isoflurane and enflurane anesthesia (abstract). *Anesth Analg* 1985, 64:239.

62. Kingston HGG: Halothane and isoflurane anesthesia in pediatric outpatients. *Anesth Analg* 1986; 65:181–184.

63. Azar I, Karambelkar DJ, Lear E: The arousal state and incidence of abnormal neurological signs during recovery from balanced anesthesia, enflurane, and isoflurane (abstract). *Anesthesiology* 1982; 57:A343.

64. Rising S, Dodgson MS, Steen PA: Isoflurane v fentanyl for outpatient laparoscopy. *Acta Anaesth Scand* 1985; 29:251–255.

65. Melnick BM, Johnson LS: Effects of eliminating nitrous oxide in outpatient anesthesia. *Anesthesiology* 1987; 67:982–984.

66. White PF: Use of continuous infusion versus intermittent bolus administration of fentanyl or ketamine during outpatient anesthesia. *Anesthesiology* 1983; 59:294–300.

67. White PF, Coe V, Shafer A, Sung ML: Comparison of alfentanil with fentanyl for outpatient anesthesia. *Anesthesiology* 1986; 64:99–106.

68. Pandit SK, Kothary SP, Pandit UA, Mathai MK: Comparison of butorphanol and fentanyl for outpatient anesthesia. *Can Anaesth Soc J* 1987; 35:130–134.

69. Robinson DM, Kitz DS, Conahan TJ, Lecky JG: Fentanyl vs nalbuphine in the day surgery setting. Abstract presented at the second annual SAMBA meeting, Washington, DC, 1987.

70. Fahy A, Marshall M: Postanesthetic morbidity in outpatients. *Br J Anaes* 1969; 41:433–435.

71. Melnick B, Chalasani J, Lion Uy NT, et al: Decreasing post-succinylcholine myalgia in outpatients. *Can Anaesth Soc J* 1987; 34:238–241.

72. Sosis M, Goldberg M, Marr AT, et al: Succinylcholine does not contribute to postoperative pain after outpatient laparoscopy. Abstract presented at second annual SAMBA meeting, Washington, DC, 1987.

73. Zahl K, Apfelbaum JL, Kitz DS, Conahan TJ: Does vecuronium ''cause'' less muscle pain than succinylcholine? (abstr.) *Anesthesiology* 1986; 65:A114.

74. Pearce AC, Williams JP, Jones RM: The use of atracurium for short surgical procedures in day-case patients (abstract). *Anesthesiology* 1983; 59:A265.

75. Caldwell JE, Braidwood JM, Simpson DS: Vecuro-

nium bromide in anaesthesia for laparoscopic sterilization. *Br J Anaesth* 1985; 57:765–769.

76. Flaaten H, Raeder J: Spinal anesthesia for outpatient surgery. *Anaesthesia* 1985; 40:1108–1111.

77. Burke RK: Spinal anesthesia for laparoscopy: A review of 1,063 cases. *J Reprod Med* 1975; 21:59–62.

78. Carbaat PAT, van Crevel H: Lumbar puncture headache: Controlled study on the preventive effect of 24 hours' bed rest. *Lancet* 1981; 2:1133–1135.

79. Jones RJ: The role of recumbency in the prevention and treatment of post-spinal headache. *Anesth Analg* 1974; 53:788–796.

80. Mulroy M, Bridenbaugh LD: Regional anesthetic techniques for outpatient surgery, in Woo SW (ed): *Ambulatory Anesthesia Care.* International Anesthesiology Clinics. Boston, Little, Brown, 1982, vol 20, pp 71–80.

81. Ryan JA, Adye BA, Jolly PC, Mulroy MF: Outpatient inguinal herniorrhaphy with both regional and local anesthesia. *Am J Surg* 1984; 148:313–316.

82. Hannallah RS, Broadman LM, Belman AB, et al: Control of post-orchidopexy pain in pediatric outpatients: Comparison of two regional techniques. *Anesthesiology* 1987; 66:832–834.

83. Shandling B, Steward DJ: Regional analgesia for postoperative pain in pediatric outpatient surgery. *J Pediatric Surg* 1980; 15:477–480.

84. Vater M, Wandles J: Caudal or dorsal nerve block? A comparison of two local anaesthetic techniques for postoperative analgesia following day case circumcision. *Acta Anaesth Scand* 1985; 29:175–179.

85. Sara CA, Lowry DJ: A complication of circumcision and dorsal nerve block of the penis. *Anaesth Intens Care* 1984; 13:79–85.

86. Elder PT, Belman AB, Hannallah RS, et al: Post-circumcision pain—A prospective evaluation of subcutaneous ring block of the penis. *Reg Anaesth* 1984; 9:48–49.

87. Tree-Trakarn T, Pirayavaraporn S: Postoperative pain relief for circumcision in children: Comparison among morphine, nerve block, and topical analgesia. *Anesthesiology* 1985; 62:519–522.

88. Mulroy MF: Our pharmacologic armamentarium—Regional anesthesia drugs. Proceedings of the third annual SAMBA meeting, Scottsdale, Arizona, 1988.

89. Motoyama EK, Glazener CH: Hypoxemia after general anesthesia in children. *Anesth Analg* 1986; 65:267–272.

90. Kataria BK, Harnik EV, Mitchard R, et al: Postoperative arterial oxygen saturation in the pediatric population during transportation. *Anesth Analg* 1988;67:280–282.

91. Soliman IE, Patel RI, Ehrenpreis MB, et al: Recovery scores do not correlate with postoperative hypoxemia in children. *Anesth Analg* 1988; 67:53–56.

92. DeSoto H, Patel RI, Soliman IE, et al: Changes in oxygen saturation following general anesthesia in children with upper respiratory infection signs and symptoms undergoing otolaryngological procedures. *Anesthesiology* 1988; 68:276–279.

93. Korttila K: Postanesthetic cognitive and psychomotor impairment, in Hindman BJ (ed): *Neurological and Psychological Complications of Surgery and Anesthesia.* International Anesthesiology Clinics. Boston, Little, Brown, 1986; vol 24, pp 59–74.

94. Aldrete JA, Kroulik D: A post-anesthetic recovery score. *Anesth Analg* 1970; 49:924–934.

95. Steward DJ: A simplified scoring system for the postoperative recovery room. *Can Anaesth Soc J* 1975; 22:111–113.

96. Denis R, Letourneau JE, Londorf D: Reliability and validity of psychomotor tests as measures of recovery from isoflurane or enflurane anesthesia in a day-care surgery unit. *Anesth Analg* 1984; 63:653–656.

97. Craig J, Cooper GM, Sear JM: Recovery from day-care anesthesia *Br J Anaesth* 1982; 54:447–450.

98. Azar I, Karambelkar DJ, Lear E: Neurologic state and psychomotor function following anesthesia for ambulatory surgery. *Anesthesiology* 1984; 60:346–349.

99. Sikh SS, Dhulia PN: Recovery from general anesthesia: A simple and comprehensive test for assessment. *Anesth Analg* 1979; 58:324–326.

100. Newman MG, Trieger N, Miller JC: Measuring recovery from anesthesia—A simple test. *Anesth Analg* 1969; 48:136–140.

101. Fragen R, Shanks CA: Neuromuscular recovery after laparoscopy. *Anesth Analg* 1984; 63:51–54.

102. Wetchler BV: Problem solving in the PACU, in Wetchler BV (ed): *Anesthesia for Ambulatory Surgery.* Philadelphia, Lippincott, 1985, pp 275–320.

103. Pflug AE, Aasheim GM, Foster C: Sequence of return of neurological function and criteria for safe ambulation following subarachnoid block. *Canad Anaesth Soc J* 1978; 25:133–139.

104. JCAHO: *Surgical and Anesthesia Services.* Ambulatory Health Care Standards Manual No. 9. JCAHO, Chicago, 1988, pp 31–36.

105. Korttila K: How to assess recovery from anesthesia. ASA Annual Refresher Course, 224, 1987, pp 1–7.

106. Ogg TW, Fischer HBJ, Bethune DW, Collis JM: Day care anaesthesia and memory. *Anaesthesia* 1979; 34:784–789.

107. Herbert M, Healy TEJ, Bourke JB, et al: Profile of recovery after general anesthesia. *Brit Med J* 1983; 286:1539–1542.

108. Anderson R, Crohg K: Pain as a major cause of postoperative nausea. *Can Anaesth Soc J* 1976; 23:366–369.

109. Pataky AO, Kitz DS, Andrews RLO, Leeky JH: Nausea and vomiting following ambulatory surgery: Are all procedures created equal? (abstract.) *Anesth Analg* 1988; 67:S163.

110. Lerman J, Eustis S, Smith D: The effect of pretreatment with droperidol in children undergoing strabismus surgery (abstract). *Anesthesiology* 1985; 63:A473.

111. Abramowitz MD, Oh TH, Epstein BH et al: The antiemetic effect of droperidol following outpatient strabismus surgery in children. *Anesthesiology* 1983; 59:579–583.

112. Williams JJ, Goldberg ME, Larijani GE, et al: A blinded prospective comparison of different methods of reducing nausea and/or vomiting after out-patient surgery. (abstract). *Anesthesiology* 1988; 69:A907.

113. Freeman LA: Ephedrine and hydroxyzine as treat-

ment for postoperative nausea and vomiting—A study of 40 problem patients. Abstract presented at third annual SAMBA meeting, Scottsdale, Arizona, 1988.

114. Alexander GD, Skupski JN, Brown EM: The role of N_2O in postoperative nausea and vomiting. *Anesth Analg* 1984; 63:175.

115. Muir JJ, Warner MA, Buck CF, et al: The role of nitrous oxide in producing postoperative nausea and vomiting (abstract). *Anesthesiology* 1986; 65:A641.

116. Palazzo MGA, Strunin L: Anesthesia and emesis. I: Etiology. *Can Anaesth Soc J* 1984; 31:178–187.

117. Davis I, Moore RJM, Sahiri SK: Nitrous oxide and the middle ear. *Anaesthesia* 1979; 34:147–151.

118. Gillman MA: Nitrous oxide at analgesic concentration—An opiate agonist: Further evidence. *Anesth Analg* 1982; 61:394–395.

119. Korttila K, Havorka J, Erkola O: Nitrous oxide does not decrease the incidence of nausea and vomiting after after isoflurane anesthesia. *Anesth Analg* 1987; 66:761–765.

120. Johnston JF, Silverstein PI, Bollander MA, deSoto H: Effect of prophylactic benzquinamide on perioperative nausea and vomiting in outpatients. Abstract presented at third annual SAMBA meeting, Scottsdale, Arizona, 1988.

121. Cohen SE, Woods QA, Wyner J: Antiemetic efficacy of doperidol and metoclopramide. *Anesthesiology* 1984; 60:67–69.

122. Korttila K, Linnoila M: Skills related to driving after intravenous diazepam, flunitrazepam, or droperidol. *Br J Anaesth* 1974; 46:961–969.

123. Rita L, Goodarzi M, Seleny F: Effect of low dose droperidol on postoperative vomiting in children. *Can Anaesth Soc J* 1981; 28:259–262.

124. Collins RM, Docherty PW, Plantevin OM: Postoperative morbidity following gynaecological outpatient laparoscopy. A reappraisal of the service. *Anaesthesia* 1984; 39:819–822.

125. Gold BS, Kitz DS, Lecky JH, Neuhaus JM: Factors associated with unanticipated hospital admission following ambulatory surgery: A case-control study (abstr.). *Anesthesiology* 1988; 69:A719.

126. Natof HE: Complications, in Wetchler BV (ed): *Anesthesia for Ambulatory Surgery.* Philadelphia, Lippincott, 1985, pp 325–356.

Appendix A | Standards

The American Society of Anesthesiologists adopted "Standards for Postanesthesia Care" during the 1988 ASA annual meeting in San Francisco. The Standards for Postanesthesia Care comprise five individual standards that set forth the minimum levels of postanesthesia care that should be provided to patients who have received general anesthesia, regional anesthesia, or monitored anesthesia care.

STANDARDS FOR POSTANESTHESIA CARE

These Standards apply to postanesthesia care in all locations. These Standards may be exceeded based on the judgment of the responsible anesthesiologist. They are intended to encourage high-quality patient care, but cannot guarantee any specific patient outcome. They are subject to revision from time to time as warranted by the evolution of technology and practice.

Standard 1
All patients who have received general anesthesia, regional anesthesia, or monitored anesthesia care shall receive appropriate postanesthesia management.

1. A postanesthesia care unit (PACU) or an area that provides equivalent postanesthesia care shall be available to receive patients after surgery and anesthesia. All patients who receive anesthesia shall be admitted to the PACU except by specific order of the anesthesiologist responsible for the patient's care.
2. The medical aspects of care in the PACU shall be governed by policies and procedures that have been reviewed and approved by the department of anesthesiology.
3. The design, equipment, and staffing of the PACU shall meet requirements of the facility's accrediting and licensing bodies.
4. The nursing standards of practice shall be consistent with those approved in 1986 by the

American Society of Post Anesthesia Nurses (ASPAN).

Standard II
A patient transported to the PACU shall be accompanied by a member of the anesthesia care team who is knowledgeable about the patient's condition. The patient shall be continually evaluated and treated during transport with monitoring and support appropriate to the patient's condition.

Standard III
Upon arrival in the PACU, the patient shall be reevaluated and a verbal report provided to the responsible PACU nurse by the member of the anesthesia care team who accompanies the patient.

1. The patient's status on arrival in the PACU shall be documented.
2. Information concerning the preoperative condition and the surgical/anesthetic course shall be transmitted to the PACU nurse.
3. The member of the anesthesia care team shall remain in the PACU until the PACU nurse accepts responsibility for the nursing care of the patient.

Standard IV
The patient's condition shall be evaluated continually in the PACU.

1. The patient shall be observed and monitored by methods appropriate to the patient's medical condition. Particular attention should be given to monitoring oxygenation, ventilation, and circulation. While qualitative clinical signs may be adequate, quantitative methods are encouraged.
2. An accurate written report of the PACU period shall be maintained. Use of an appropriate PACU scoring system is encouraged for each patient on admission, at appropriate intervals prior to discharge, and at the time of discharge.
3. General medical supervision and coordination of patient care in the PACU should be the responsibility of the anesthesiologist.

4. There shall be a policy to assure the availability in the facility of a physician capable of managing complications and providing cardiopulmonary resuscitation for patients in the PACU.

Standard V

A physician is responsible for the discharge of the patient from the postanesthesia care unit.

1. When discharge criteria are used, they must be approved by the department of anesthesiology and the medical staff. They may vary depending upon whether the patient is discharged to a hospital room, to the ICU, to a short stay unit, or home.

2. In the absence of the physician responsible for the discharge, the PACU nurse shall determine that the patient meets the discharge criteria. The name of the physician accepting responsibility for discharge shall be noted on the record.

Index

f refers to figures; *t* refers to tables

---

f refers to figures; *t* refers to tables

---

f refers to figures; *t* refers to **tables**

---

f refers to figures; *t* refers to **tables**

f refers to figures; t refers to **tables**

f refers to figures; *t* refers to **tables**